MEDICAL RADIOLOGY

Diagnostic Imaging and Radiation Oncology – Softcover Edition

Springer
Berlin
Heidelberg
New York
Budapest
Hong Kong
London
Milan
Paris
Singapore
Tokyo

A.R. Margulis (Ed.)

Modern Imaging of the Alimentary Tube

With Contributions by

M. Ando · S.M. Ascher · Y. Baba · A.L. Baert · C.I. Bartram · A. Chonan · K.S. Dua
C.S. Easterling · M.P. Federle · G.G. Ghahremani · R.M. Gore · D.H.W. Grönemeyer
S. Kai · S. Kaku · K. Koizumi · J.C. Lappas · D.D.T. Maglinte · A.R. Margulis
M. Maruyama · A. Melzer · M.A. Meyers · F.H. Miller · R.E. Mindelzun · F. Mochizuki
D.J. Nolan · S.H. Ominsky · J. Plassmann · T. Sakai · A. Schmidt · R. Seibel
C. Smith · E.T. Stewart · N. Takemoto · Z.C. Traill · D. Vanbeckevoort · L. Van Hoe
T. Vogl · S.D. Wall · J. Yee

Foreword by
J. E. Youker

Preface by
A.R. Margulis

With 372 Figures in 599 Separate Illustrations

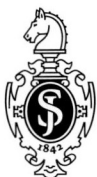

Springer

ALEXANDER R. MARGULIS, MD
Professor of Radiology
University Advancement and Planning
University of California, San Francisco
3333 California Street
Laurel Heights, Suite 16
San Francisco, CA 94143-0292, USA

MEDICAL RADIOLOGY · Diagnostic Imaging and Radiation Oncology

Continuation of
Handbuch der medizinischen Radiologie
Encyclopedia of Medical Radiology

ISSN 0942-5373
ISBN 3-540-66345-2 Springer-Verlag Berlin Heidelberg New York

Library of Congress Cataloging-in-Publication Data applied for

Die Deutsche Bibliothek – CIP-Einheitsaufnahme. Modern imaging of the alimentary tube / A. R. Margulis (ed.). With contribution by M. Ando . . . Foreword by J. E. Youker. Preface by A. R. Margulis. – Berlin; Heidelberg; New York; Barcelona; Hong Kong; London; Milan; Paris; Singapore; Tokyo: Springer 2000. (Medical radiology). ISBN 3-540-66345-2. Modern imaging of the alimentary tube. – 2000

Printed in Germany

The use of general descriptive names, registered names, trademarks, etc. in this publication does not imply, even in the absence of a specific statement, that such names are exempt from the relevant protective laws and regulations and therefore free for general use.

Product liability: The publishers cannot guarantee the accuracy of any information about dosage and application contained in this book. In every individual case the user must check such information by consulting the relevant literature.

Cover design: Joan Greenfield, New York

Typesetting: Best-set Typesetter Ltd., Hong Kong

Printing and binding: Universitätsdruckerei H. Stürtz AG, Würzburg

SPIN: 10741886   21/3135 – 5 4 3 2 1 – Printed on acid-free paper

Foreword

The diagnosis and treatment of diseases of the alimentary tract remains an extremly important part of medical practice. Cross-sectional imaging and interventional radiologic techniques have had a profound impact on the understanding and treatment of these disorders.

This book is edited by Dr Alexander Margulis, who though world renowned as a gastrointestinal radiologist and founder of the Society of Gastrointestinal Radiologists is also recognized as a leader in the development of computerized tomography and magnetic resonance imaging of the abdomen. The volume clearly reflects Dr. Margulis' expertise, broad interests, and renaissance outlook.

Dr. Margulis has assembled an outstanding authorship of experts from around the globe for this volume. The continued importance of contrast examinations of the alimentary tract is emphasized in several chapters describing how contrast studies can be improved, such as the chapter on enteroclysis of the small bowel. Several chapters are devoted to the cross-sectional imaging techniques of ultrasound, CT and MR. Appropriate application of these imaging modalities to each region of the gastrointestinal tract, as well as to specific diseases entities, is explained in detail.

The text goes far beyond a discussion of the common and familiar disorders of the gastrointestinal tract such as ulcer disease, inflammatory disease, and neoplasm. Recently recognized disease processes such as those secondary to immunosuppression are thoroughly covered, and there are chapters on trauma and post-operative changes which will be of great value to the practicing radiologist or gastroenterologist.

The management of alimentary tract disease has been profoundly affected by interventional techniques. Dr. Margulis, in collaboration with the late Dr. J. Burhenne, originated the term "interventional radiology". Dr. Margulis and his authors have clearly and completely elucidated the techniques of interventional radiology, their application to alimentary tract disorders, and the supportive role of imaging in these procedures.

A sound grasp of the physiology and anatomy of the alimentary is necessary to effectively apply imaging studies, and the author have provided landmark chapters in these critical areas.

The purpose of the editor has been to discribe the advances in imaging and therapeutic interventional techniques crucial to caring for patients with diseases of the gastrointestinal tract. This book will be of value not only to radiologists but also to gastroenterologists and surgeons working in this area.

Milwaukee   JAMES E. YOUKER

Preface

Imaging of the alimentary tube has kept pace with the rest of radiology and has greatly benefited from advances in cross-sectional techniques. Endoluminal ultrasonography, helical computed tomography, new fast magnetic resonance imaging sequences (eg., single shot), digital radiography, new contrast media for magnetic resonance imaging, ultrasonography, and computed tomography – all these advances have kept alimentary tract radiology as a vibrant, relevant, and modern subspecialty.

It was not long ago that predictions were made that alimentary tract radiology would disappear to be totally replaced by fiberoptic endoscopy. Not only did this not occur but imaging and endoscopy have established an equilibrium of complementary co-operation, with imaging being dependent on computers starting to make a strong comeback. Multiple new techniques show no sign of abating and keep imaging on the upswing.

This monograph describes and documents many of the advances that are occurring and maintain alimentary tract radiology as a valueable and interesting subspecialty at the turn of the century. The publishers and I are deeply grateful to the participants in this volume for their outstanding contributions. We hope that the readers will agree.

San Francisco   ALEXANDER R. MARGULIS

Contents

Section 4: Surgery Related Advances

1 Overview

A.R. Margulis

1.1 Introduction

Since its inception 100 years ago, gastrointestinal tract radiology has been at the cutting edge of progress in medical imaging, and never has this been more true than during the past 20 years. Like the rest of radiology and indeed all of medical science, it has been the beneficiary of progress in computers, which, while dramatically diminishing in size and price, can now perform almost a trillion functions per second, with the number doubling about every 18 months (Moore's law) (Lenzner 1995). Advances in computers have made computed tomography (CT), magnetic resonance imaging (MRI), digital radiography, digital ultrasonography, and Doppler imaging possible and affordable. The ever-increasing speed of computers has brought many of these modalities to real-time or almost real-time status, increasing their efficiency and their tolerance by gravely ill patients.

1.2 Digital Radiography

Digital radiography has many advantages: It reduces the number of repeat exposures (Fig. 1.1), it in-

A.R. Margulis, MD, DSc (hc), Professor of Radiology, University Advancement and Planning, University of California, San Francisco, 3333 California Street, Laurel Heights, Suite 16, San Francisco, CA 94143-0292, USA

creases flexibility of display by its windowing capabilities, and it makes PACS and teleradiology possible (Huang 1996). With the image intensifiers of the fluoroscopic-radiographic units reaching 16 inches in diameter, direct acquisition of digital images is possible without any intervening steps. This will greatly improve and facilitate plain filming of the abdomen in radiology departments while the portable films will require either digitization or the x-ray sensitive photostimulable plate approach (Thompson 1978).

Digital fluoroscopic imaging provides great flexibility. Magnification for greater detail is possible through reduction of the field of the intensifier down to 9 or even 6 inches. Four to six exposures or video are obtainable, which makes filming of any rapid event routinely demonstrable.

1.3 Barium Studies

The great controversies over the respective advantages of double- versus single-contrast techniques for examination of the alimentary tube are history. It is now well agreed that biphasic examination of the esophagus, stomach, and duodenum is the optimal approach, with the double-contrast images providing the mucosal detail and the single-contrast images supplying information on motility and showing large lesions that can be missed with the double-contrast approach (Montagne et al. 1978; Op Den Orth 1979; Ominsky and Margulis 1981). For the examination of the colon the double-contrast technique should be standard, with the single-contrast examination reserved for patients with suspected obstruction and for debilitated, highly uncooperative, or unconscious patients. If an area of the colon is suspicious for a lesion but the films are not diagnostic, the double-contrast examination can be immediately followed by a single-contrast examination with spot films obtained in the supine and prone positions after the patient has returned from evacuating (Demas

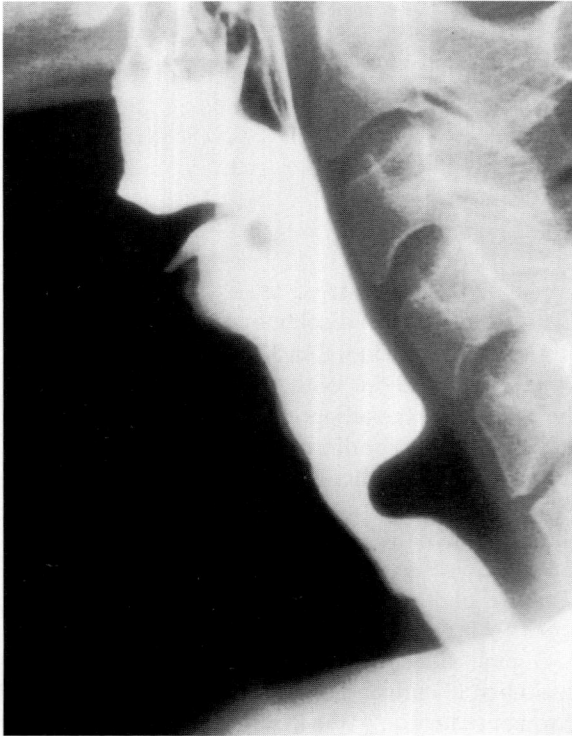

Fig. 1.1. By programming six or more digital exposures per second, superbly detailed views of the pharynx, hypopharynx, and upper esophagus during swallowing are routinely obtainable. This is a lateral view showing hypertrophy of the cricopharyngeal muscle (upper esophageal sphincter), producing symptoms of disturbed swallowing

and MARGULIS 1984). For a high-quality diagnostic examination the patient should never be released before the images have been reviewed and a tentative diagnosis established.

1.4
Enteroclysis

As described in Chap. 7, enteroclysis is the most precise small bowel imaging examination (NOLAN and BARTRAM 1996). It suffers, however, from certain handicaps: the radiation dose is higher than for either the conventional barium small bowel examination or CT, and it does not provide data about small bowel motility or width (Fig. 1.2). These objections hold particularly in systemic sclerosis and nontropical sprue. It is also held that CT, being less invasive and providing more general information, should be the initial examination for confirming, identifying

the cause, and localizing the site of small bowel obstruction (MEGIBOW et al. 1991) (Fig. 1.3).

1.5
Computed Tomography

Helical (spiral) CT has improved the quality of gastrointestinal imaging by reducing motion artifacts from both peristalsis and breathing. The high quality of spiral imaging has made it the screening method of choice for acute abdomen episodes and one of the preferred methods for localizing and guiding the drainage of abscesses as stressed by Groenemeyer. Electron beam tomography, with its great speed and extensive coverage, is also ideal for performing virtual colonoscopy, a procedure in which the computer program eliminates all anatomic structures except for the gas-distended colonic lumen and permits virtual passage through it (HARA et al. 1996).

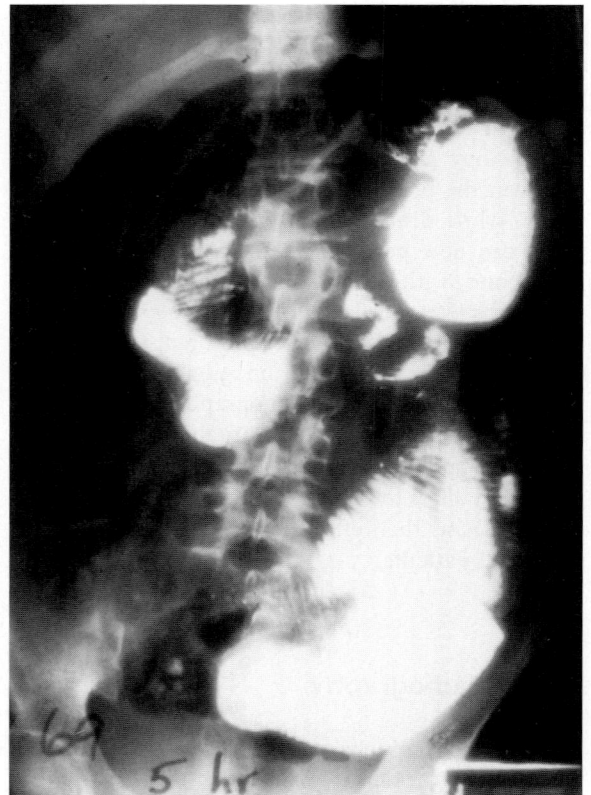

Fig. 1.2. Five-hour delayed conventional small bowel barium study film in a patient with systemic sclerosis (scleroderma). The slow progress of barium and the disturbed motility evidenced as areas of marked bowel dilatation could present diagnostic difficulties for enteroclysis

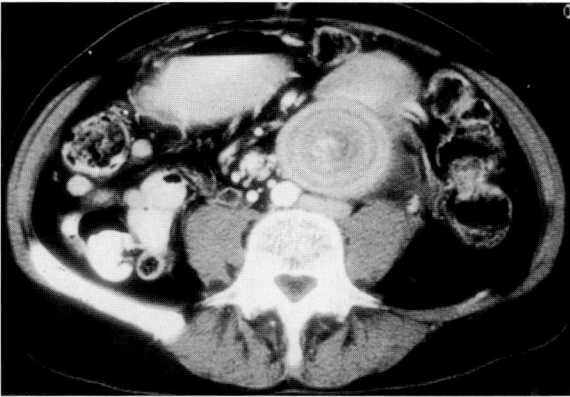

Fig. 1.3. Spiral CT image showing the concentric rings of duodenal intussusception. Enteroclysis could yield equally diagnostic images but more invasively and with a higher radiation dose

Small (even 3-mm) polyps can be seen (Fig. 1.4). If sensitivity and specificity studies now in progress in several centers bear out the early promise, a new, less invasive, easily tolerated and much less costly study may replace diagnostic colonoscopy, making the latter a purely therapeutic procedure.

1.6
Magnetic Resonance Imaging

As described in Chap. 3, MRI has moved from being only useful in a few cases of rectal disease and occasionally in the evaluation of carcinoma of the esophagus to becoming a competitor to CT thanks to the new HASTE (single-shot) sequence, which is so

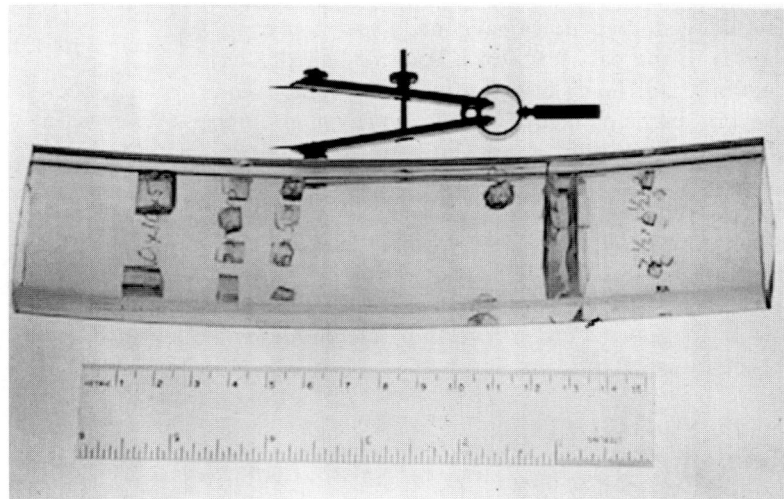

a

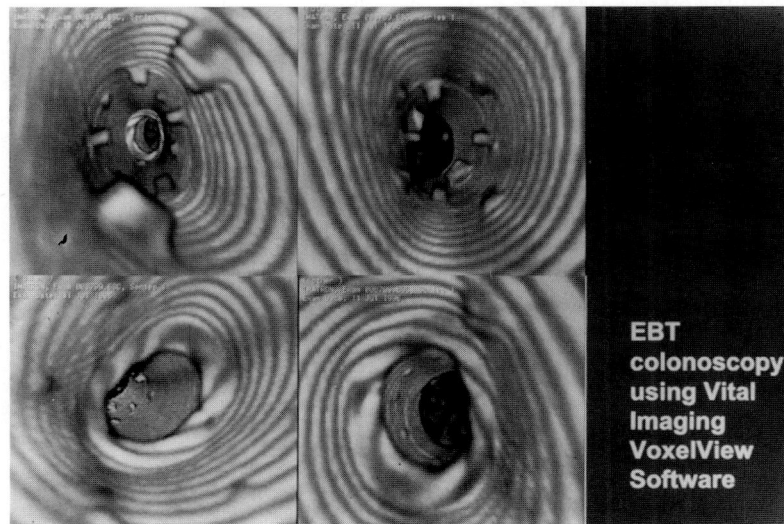

EBT colonoscopy using Vital Imaging VoxelView Software

b

Fig. 1.4. Colon phantom CT virtual colonoscopy performed on an electron beam scanner (Imatron, South San Francisco, Calif.) with implanted plastic "polyps" measuring 3–10 mm (**a**). All of the structures were clearly visible using Vital Imaging VoxelView Software (**b**). (Courtesy of Drs. Juergen Scheidler, Douglas Boyd, and Cameron Ritchie)

fast that it stops motion (KEIFER et al. 1994). As it is T2 weighted, fluid in the bowel images with high signal makes this sequence competitive with CT in the diagnosis of small bowel obstruction (BEALL and REGAN 1996), particularly as MRI also provides coronal and sagittal images.

Although some of the cross-sectional procedures are costlier than plain films and barium or ultrasound studies, performing the costlier procedure at the start of the diagnostic evaluation in order to obtain the precise diagnosis rather than as the last in a long succession of tests is cost saving, not to mention easier on the patient.

1.7
Alimentary Tube Imaging and Genetic Medicine

Human genome studies have made spectacular advances in the past few years. Loci for genetic susceptibility for many diseases, including some colon cancers, are being identified (DE LATTRE et al. 1989; RUSTGI 1994; JAROFF 1991). Until affordable and reliable screening studies are available and treatment by gene replacement becomes a safe reality, imaging attempting to discover demonstrable lesions at an early stage will continue to play an important role. Virtual endoscopy, neural network computer checking of images, and other developing techniques will be the future of imaging.

References

Beall DP, Regan F (1996) Technical note; MRI of bowel obstruction using the HASTE sequence. J Comput Assist Tomogr 20:823–825

De Lattre O, Olschwang S, Law DJ, et al. (1989) Multiple genetic alterations in distal and proximal colorectal cancer. Lancet II:353–356

Demas BE, Margulis AR (1984) Combined use of double-and single-contrast barium enema in the evaluation of suspected colonic disease. Gastrointest Radiol 9:241–245

Gazelle GS, Goldberg MA, Wittenberg J, Halpern EF, Pinkney L, Mueller PR (1994) Efficacy of CT in distinguishing small-bowel obstruction from other causes of small bowel dilatation. AJR 162:43–47

Hara AK, Johnson CD, Reed JE, et al. (1996) Detection of colorectal polyps by computed tomographic colography; feasibility of a novel technique. Gastroenterol Rapid Commun 110:284–290

Huang HK (1996) Picture archiving and communications systems (PACS) in biomedicine. Wiley, New York

Jaroff L (1991) The new genetics. The Grand Round Press, Whittle Direct Books, New York

Keifer B, Grassner J, Haussmann R (1994) Image acquisition single shot turbo spin-echo. J Magn Reson Imaging (Suppl P):86–87

Lenzner R (1995) The reluctant entrepreneur. Forbes 11:162–168

Megibow AJ, Balthazar EJ, Kyunghee CC, Medwid SW, Birnbaum BA, Noz ME (1991) Bowel obstruction: evaluation with CT. Radiology 180:313–318

Montagne JP, Moss AA, Margulis AR (1978) Double-blind study of single and double contrast upper gastrointestinal examinations using endoscopy as a control. AJR 130:1041–1045

Nolan DJ, Bartram CI (1996) Small bowel enteroclysis: pros and cons. Abdom Radiol Abdom Imaging 21:243–246

Ominsky SH, Margulis AR (1981) Radiographic examination of the upper gastrointestinal tract. Radiology 139:11–17

Op Den Ortho (1979) The standard biphasic contrast examination of the stomach and duodenum, Nijhoff, The Hague

Rustgi AK (1994) Hereditary gastrointestinal polyposis and nonpolyposis syndromes. N Engl J Med 331:1694–1702

Thompson TT (1978) A practical approach to modern x-ray equipment. Little, Brown & Co, Boston, MA

Section 1: Techniques

2 Advances in Computed Tomography

D. Vanbeckevoort, A.L. Baert, and L. Van Hoe

CONTENTS

2.1
Advances in Technique

Conventional CT scanners require the gantry to rotate alternately clockwise and anticlockwise to allow for the rewinding of the x-ray tube cables. As a result, a delay of 5–10 s results between the investigation of two slices. The introduction of a slip-ring gantry system in 1987, however, allowed for continuous one-way rotation of the x-ray tube and detector and provided the technologic basis for helical (spiral) CT (Kalender 1994).

2.1.1
Principles of Helical CT

In helical CT, continuous translation of the patient (and examination table) is combined with continuous rotation of the x-ray tube and detector elements. As a result, a spiral or helix of raw data is obtained

during a single breath-hold through the anatomic region of interest (Kalender et al. 1990). In helical CT, slice-by-slice scanning is replaced by volumetric data acquisition (Kalender 1994; Kalender et al. 1990; Heiken et al. 1993).

2.1.2
Technical Considerations for Helical CT

2.1.2.1
Collimation and Table Feed

Before starting a helical CT scan, the radiologist should specify several scanning parameters, including the duration of the scan, the maximal slice thickness, and the table speed.

In most cases, the scan duration should be chosen to achieve sufficient coverage of the patient in the z-axis direction.

As with conventional scanning, choice of collimation settings for helical scanning is based largely on the organ of interest and the diagnostic goal of the scan. Both the collimation and the density of the lesion relative to background tissue determine the smallest lesion that can be detected. Generally, 5- to 8-mm collimation is acceptable for abdominal imaging.

The pitch is defined as the table speed (in mm/s) divided by the collimation (in mm) multiplied by the time needed to complete one 360° rotation of the x-ray tube around the patient (i.e., the "rotation time"). Modern hardware and software, however, allow the table feed to increase up to twice the collimation (pitch = 2:1). This is referred to as extended helical scanning. With extended helical scans, twice the z-axis coverage may be obtained during the same scanning interval. This choice, however, is associated with a penalty in longitudinal resolution due to an increase in effective slice thickness.

D. Vanbeckevoort, MD, Department of Radiology, University Hospitals K.U. Leuven, Herestraat 49, B-3000 Leuven, Belgium
A.L. Baert, MD, Professor, Department of Radiology, University Hospitals K.U. Leuven, Herestraat 49, B-3000 Leuven, Belgium
L. Van Hoe, MD, Department of Radiology, University Hospitals K.U. Leuven, Herestraat 49, B-3000 Leuven, Belgium

2.1.2.2
Image Reconstruction

In helical CT, a single data set is obtained that represents the volume covered in the given number of spiral turns. Direct reconstruction of images from data obtained over any 360° spiral segment would result in nonuniform section thickness and orientation due to patient transport (HEIKEN et al. 1993). To correct the effect of moving the patient continuously during the scan it is necessary to first calculate a planar data set for each image to be reconstructed (KALENDER 1994). Images can be reconstructed at any position within the scanned volume, with arbitrarily fine spacing and in an overlapping fashion if desired. If overlapping images are preferred for high-quality displays, images can be provided by one spiral scan without additional scanning time or increase in x-ray dose.

A variety of interpolation algorithms are available to correct these raw data from volume scans. The simplest approach is a 360° linear interpolation between spiral projection data sets from adjacent turns. However, 360° linear interpolation (also called full-scan with interpolation) diminishes the longitudinal resolution, which can produce volume-averaging artifacts due to broadening of the section-sensitivity profile (HEIKEN et al. 1993). Currently, the most often used approach is a 180° linear interpolation or half-scan with interpolation (KALENDER 1994). This technique offers the advantage of improved slice sensitivity profiles and, thus, provides improved spatial resolution in the longitudinal direction (POLACIN et al. 1992).

2.1.3
Advantages of Helical CT

Compared with standard incremental CT, helical CT has some clear advantages: during helical scanning the patient holds his breath during the entire acquisition of scan data. This reduces misregistration artifacts that occur during conventional incremental scanning of organs subject to respiratory motion (KALENDER et al. 1990; HEIKEN et al. 1993; ZEMAN et al. 1993).

A significant advantage of helical CT is the increased scan speed. Successive periods of data acquisition in conventional CT are separated by the so-called interscan interval. During the latter time interval, the patient is shifted a small distance through the gantry for the next slice to be measured.

In helical CT, the interscan interval is eliminated since patient translation and data acquisition both occur in a continuous way. As a result, the time required to investigate an organ or body part can be significantly reduced. The rapid acquisition of helical CT images also allows for use of lower total contrast doses as compared with dynamic conventional CT (BLUEMKE et al. 1994; SILVERMAN et al. 1995). In addition, using bolus contrast enhancement, scans can be obtained during optimal vascular opacification.

Another advantage of spiral CT is that high-quality multiplanar (2-D) reformations (Fig. 2.1) and three-dimensional (3-D) reconstructions can be produced from a single scan data set, particularly if image data have been acquired with a thin collimation setting and transaxial images have been generated with a high degree of overlap. The rapid acquisition of continuous data in a single breath-hold with heli-

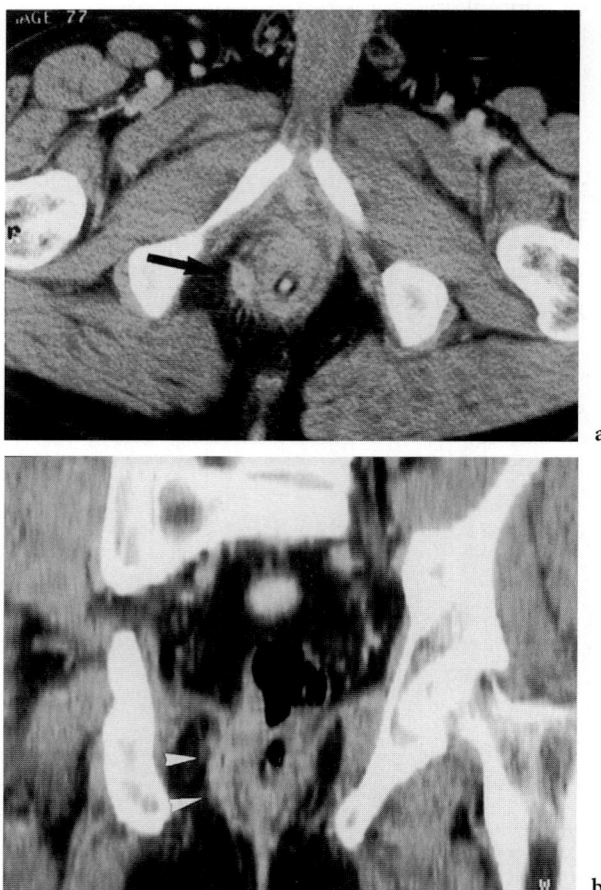

Fig. 2.1. **a** Axial CT scan at the level of the anorectal junction shows a right-sided pararectal inflammatory process (*arrow*). **b** Multiplanar reconstruction in the coronal plane best demonstrates the extension and the relationship of the inflammatory process to the levator muscle (*arrowheads*)

cal CT further eliminates discontinuities in the reconstructions due to motion.

These advantages have improved existing CT applications and have led to new indications, such as CT angiography (RUBIN et al. 1993). By virtue of its ability to collect data with continuous anatomic information within a short period, helical CT is capable of producing detailed three-dimensional displays of blood vessels.

2.2
Clinical Applications

Although gastrointestinal abnormalities are generally detected by conventional barium contrast studies and endoscopy, neither assesses the extramucosal extent of disease. CT, however, permits precise evaluation of both the existence and the degree of extramural involvement. In addition, by imaging both adjacent and distant organs, CT is capable of detecting local disease as well as distant metastases (Moss 1992).

2.2.1
Esophagus

2.2.1.1
Role of CT

Computed tomography is particularly useful in (a) evaluating and staging patients with esophageal carcinoma for planning treatment, (b) assessing tumor response to therapy, (c) determining the presence, location, and severity of esophageal perforations, and (d) evaluating and characterizing the nature of lesions that appear intramural or extrinsic on conventional barium studies.

Currently, there is no clear evidence that CT plays any substantial role in the evaluation of esophagitis and disorders of esophageal motility, such as achalasia and scleroderma. Esophagography and endoscopy remain the initial examinations in these conditions.

2.2.1.2
Techniques of Examination

There is no generally accepted technique for routine CT scanning of the esophagus. Oral administration of 300 ml of a 3% solution of diatrizoate meglumine (Gastrografin) is given 10–15 min before the start of the CT examination to distend the stomach. Just before scanning, with the patient already in the CT gantry and the scout image obtained, an additional swallow of 10 ml Gastrografin mixed with flour is given to identify the esophageal lumen. Some advocate the use of a 3% barium paste to delineate the esophageal lumen and any associated wall thickening (CAYEA and SELTZER 1985; HALVORSEN and THOMPSON 1987). A helical scan is then obtained from the thoracic inlet through the liver following an intravenous injection of 125 ml of 35% iodinated contrast administered as a monophasic injection (2.5 ml/s) via power injector. The table is moved at 7.5 mm/s with a corresponding slice collimation of 5 mm. Overlapping reconstructions are performed at 4-mm increments.

2.2.1.3
Normal Anatomy

The normal intrathoracic esophagus is generally well seen on routine CT scans of the chest and upper abdomen (HALBER et al. 1979). The thickness of the normal esophageal wall as measured by CT in a well-distended esophagus is usually less than 3 mm. Any measurement of more than 5 mm should be considered abnormal regardless of the degree of distension (HALBER et al. 1979; MOSS et al. 1982). Small amounts of air are present in the thoracic esophagus in 40%–60% of the normal population (HALBER et al. 1979; JOST et al. 1978).

The esophagus is surrounded throughout most of its length by periesophageal fat that permits differentiation of the esophagus from adjacent mediastinal structures. The amount of fat depends on body habitus and does not typically surround the esophagus on every CT slice (SAMUELSSON et al. 1984). A visualized fat plane may be focally absent in several anatomic sites, including esophageal contact with the aorta, trachea, left mainstem bronchus, and left atrium (WOLFMAN et al. 1994).

The normal appearance of the gastroesophageal junction is variable. Depending on the degree of gastric distension there may be a normal focal thickening of the gastric wall at the gastroesophageal junction that can mimic a neoplasm (THOMPSON et al. 1982; MARKS et al. 1981).

2.2.1.4
Applications

2.2.1.4.1
MALIGNANT ESOPHAGEAL TUMORS

The most common type of esophageal malignancy is squamous cell carcinoma. Adenocarcinoma is the second most common tumor. The role of CT in evaluating these tumors has been thoroughly studied (HALVORSEN and THOMPSON 1987; HALVORSEN et al. 1986; VILGRAIN et al. 1990).

The CT findings of a primary malignant esophageal tumor may include: (a) an intraluminal mass, (b) focal wall thickening with an eccentric lumen, (c) dilatation of the lumen proximal to an obstructing tumor, (d) loss of periesophageal fat, (e) an esophagobronchial fistula, (f) an irregular or eccentric lumen, and (g) metastatic disease (especially enlargement of mediastinal, retrocrural, left gastric, or celiac lymph nodes, or liver metastasis).

Various CT criteria have been investigated to determine the utility of this modality in predicting invasion of mediastinal structures (Moss et al. 1981b; PICUS et al. 1983). In the normal mediastinum, the esophagus is in direct contact with the posterior wall of the trachea and left mainstem bronchus. Therefore, absence of a fat plane between an esophageal mass and the trachea cannot be used to predict invasion; the demonstration of tracheal displacement or indentation is required (Fig. 2.2) (HALVORSEN and THOMPSON 1987). As in the tracheobronchial tree, the fat plane between the middle third of the esophagus and the aorta is often absent in normal individuals. A small triangle of fat usually is preserved between the esophagus, aorta, and spine in nearly all

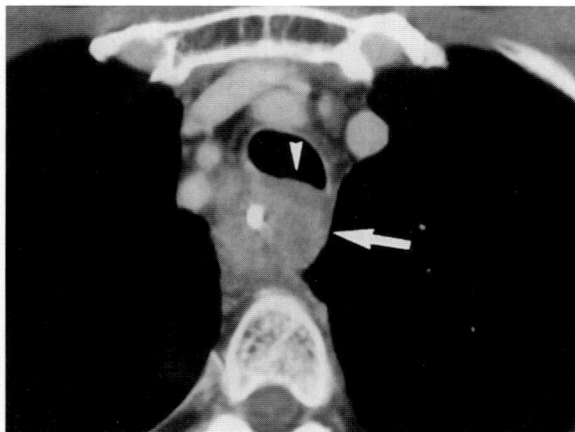

Fig. 2.3. Leiomyoma of the esophagus. CT scan of the lower thorax demonstrates a smooth, well-defined soft tissue mass (*arrows*) arising within the wall of the esophagus and causing deformity of the contrast-filled esophageal lumen

individuals. TAKASHIMA et al. (1991) predicted aortic invasion when esophageal tumor obliterated this fat space. Previously PICUS et al. (1983) described a technique for CT detection of aortic invasion based on the degree of direct contact between the tumor and aorta. If the contact is less than 45°, the aorta is considered normal with no evidence of invasion. When the esophageal contact is greater than 90°, invasion is likely. Contact between 45° and 90° is considered indeterminate.

However, the role of CT in staging esophageal neoplasms has been controversial, with some authorities advocating CT as an effective decision-making tool, whereas others have rejected the ability of CT to stage (HALVORSEN and THOMPSON 1987; VILGRAIN et al. 1990; HALVORSEN and THOMPSON 1984; QUINT et al. 1985). Currently, the fundamental utility of CT relates more to its role in treatment selection (curative or palliative) and follow-up than its ability to place the patient into circumscript staging niches (HALVORSEN and THOMPSON 1989). In many medical centers a multimodal approach including chemotherapy and radiation therapy prior to surgery is used to treat esophageal carcinoma. In these cases CT plays a key role in assessing initial tumor bulk for radiation therapy planning and is also useful in monitoring tumor response to the cytoreductive therapy (WOLFMAN et al. 1994). On the other hand, surgical cure is now frequently attempted by means of transhiatal esophagectomy without thoracotomy. In these circumstances, it is important preoperatively to identify patients with tumor spread to contiguous structures and distant metastases that would preclude an attempt at curative surgery (WOLFMAN et al. 1994).

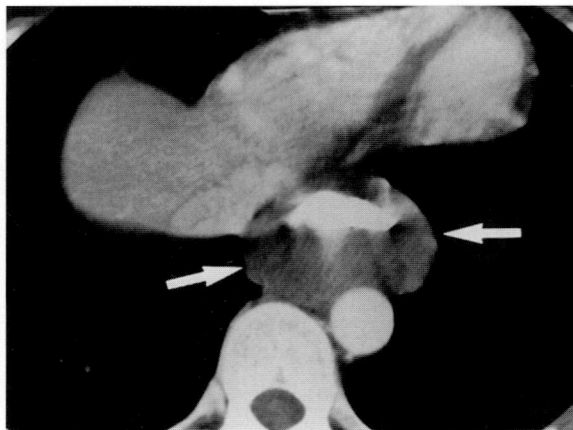

Fig. 2.2. Primary squamous cell carcinoma of proximal esophagus. CT demonstrates marked circumferential but asymmetric esophageal wall thickening (*arrow*), indenting the posterior wall of the trachea inward (*arrowhead*)

2.2.1.4.2
BENIGN ESOPHAGEAL TUMORS

Tumors arising in the wall of the esophagus are usually detected on upper gastrointestinal series. The most common benign lesions are leiomyomas. CT of a leiomyoma typically reveals a well-defined soft tissue mass with soft tissue attenuation and preservation of the surrounding fat (Fig. 2.3) (MEGIBOW et al. 1985). On rare occasions calcification may be definable. Because of the lack of histologic specificity, differentiation from malignant leiomyosarcoma is not always possible.

Esophageal duplication cysts are also easily diagnosed on CT. They appear as well-marginated, low-attenuation (usually near-water-density) spherical masses with preserved surrounding fat planes (KUHLMAN et al. 1985). Sixty percent of esophageal duplication cysts are located in the lower esophagus and are paraesophageal or intramural in location. The differential diagnosis includes abscess, old hematoma, neurofibroma, leiomyoma, and lipoma.

2.2.1.4.3
TRAUMATIC AND IATROGENIC ABNORMALITIES

Esophageal perforation may be iatrogenic in etiology, complicating endoscopy, esophageal dilatation, or attempted intubation (GHAHREMANI 1986). Less frequent sources are ingested foreign bodies, postemetic (Boerhaave syndrome) and postoperative tears, penetrating knife or gunshot wounds, and blunt trauma sustained in whiplash injuries (FLYNN et al. 1989; KIM-DEOBALD and KOZAREK 1992).

In several conditions, CT may provide invaluable information. It can demonstrate some penetrating foreign bodies that are faintly radio-opaque and invisible on conventional radiographs (DOUGLAS and SISTROM 1991). In addition, CT allows the visualization of minute collections of mediastinal air or contrast material due to small tears (ALLEN et al. 1986; BACKER et al. 1990). This information may be helpful in determining which patients require immediate surgical intervention as opposed to those who could be managed conservatively.

2.2.1.4.4
EXTRINSIC LESIONS

Although extrinsic compressions on the esophagus are easily detected by conventional barium studies, differentiation between the various etiologies is frequently problematic. CT, by virtue of its ability to directly image the bowel wall as well as the surrounding mediastinum, may be diagnostic in some cases (PUGATCH et al. 1980; SONES et al. 1982). In the upper mediastinum CT provides an important tool in the diagnosis of vascular abnormalities such as an aneurysmal dilatation of the aorta, a right-sided aortic arch, and an aberrant left or right subclavian artery (SRINIVASAN and SCHOLZ 1980; SCHLESINGER et al. 1984).

Another common cause of extrinsic deviation of the upper thoracic esophagus from the midline is a mediastinal goiter (BASHIST et al. 1983; GLAZER et al. 1982). These lesions are readily identified by CT because of the well-defined borders, the punctate or coarse calcifications, the initial high CT density, and the prolonged enhancement following administration of intravenous contrast material.

Throughout the length of the mediastinum the esophagus may be displaced by enlarged lymph nodes. In patients with advanced pulmonary and mediastinal disease, tuberculosis may rarely involve the esophagus due to direct spread from adjacent lymphadenopathy, most frequently at the level of the carina. In these cases CT demonstrates a heterogeneous, low-density, mediastinal mass with central necrosis adjacent to the esophagus (Fig. 2.4).

2.2.1.4.5
ESOPHAGEAL VARICES

Esophageal varices appear as lobulated or rounded tubular densities in the distal paraesophageal region. Images during an intravenous bolus of contrast material are helpful in distinguishing between varices, which are enhanced, and enlarged lymph nodes or neoplasia (Fig. 2.5).

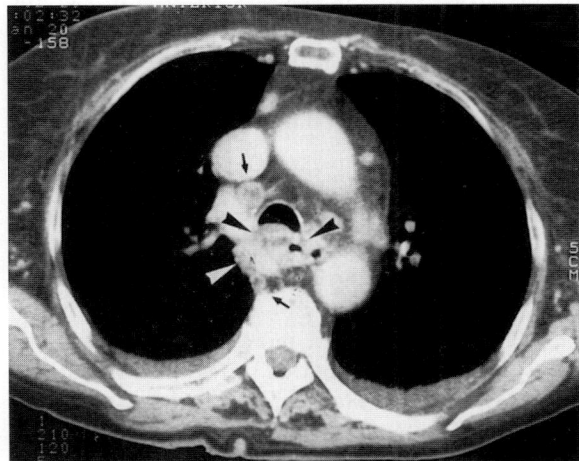

Fig. 2.4. Esophageal tuberculosis. Contrast-enhanced CT scan shows a thickening of the upper esophageal wall with a centrally necrotic mass (*arrowheads*) involving the right lateral wall. There are multiple enlarged mediastinal lymph nodes, some of them showing a hypodense center and peripheral rim enhancement (*arrows*). (From Geusens et al. 1996)

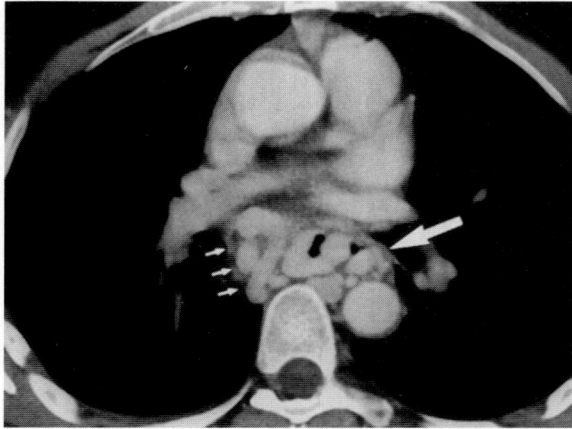

Fig. 2.5. CT scan of esophageal (*large arrow*) and mediastinal (*small arrows*) varices. The enhancement of the esophageal wall is due to enlarged, submucosal, contrast-filled varies

2.2.1.4.6
POSTOPERATIVE ESOPHAGUS

Computed tomography is useful in assessing problems that can arise after esophagectomy. The real strength of CT in this setting is in detecting recurrent tumor in the adjacent mediastinum or upper abdominal lymph nodes, liver, and adrenals.

Computed tomography is the single best way to detect recurrent esophageal carcinoma in the postesophagectomy patient. The study should be performed with oral contrast to adequately distend the interposed stomach. A nondistended stomach may mimic recurrent tumor (GROSS et al. 1985). Gastric distension is especially important near the anastomosis, where an outpouching of the fundus may be confused with a mass (BECKER et al. 1987). Correlating the CT scan with the upper gastrointestinal (UGI) series will clarify the anatomy of the interposition.

The strengths of CT scanning over the UGI series are the ability to identify extraluminal masses in the mediastinum and to detect distant metastases. GROSS et al. (1985) correctly identified seven of nine cases of locally recurrent or residual cancer by CT. Three of these cases were missed by UGI series. The relative usefulness of the UGI series and CT scanning can also be defined with respect to the patient's clinical presentation. In patients presenting with dysphagia, the UGI series may be most helpful in identifying a mucosal lesion or anastomotic stricture. CT is more helpful when symptoms are more general, such as abdominal pain or weight loss (HEIKEN et al. 1984).

2.2.2
Stomach and Duodenum

2.2.2.1
Role of CT

Traditionally, gastroduodenal tumors have been detected by using conventional barium studies and endoscopy. CT, on the other hand, has been used to further evaluate and stage these neoplasms (SCATARIGE and DiSANTIS 1989; KLEINHAUS and MILITIANU 1988). Nowadays, however, CT is being used routinely in patients in whom abdominal malignancy is suspected on the basis of clinical findings. As a result, the initial detection of some of these malignancies is more commonly made by CT, even before conventional barium studies have been performed.

Another new application is the use of CT in planning radiation fields and assessing the response of tumor or metastatic deposits to therapy (NG et al. 1996). Moreover, NAKAJIMA et al. (1994) used CT for the assessment of lymph node volume during chemotherapy in patients with inoperable advanced carcinoma.

In addition, CT remains useful in the differentiation of a primary gastroduodenal process from a process secondarily involving the stomach or duodenal wall. Finally, following partial gastrectomy, CT plays an important role in the evaluation of early postoperative complications and in the detection of tumor recurrence.

2.2.2.2
Techniques of Examination

An optimal CT examination of the gastric and duodenal wall necessitates luminal distension during the period of scanning. Twenty minutes before the CT examination, the stomach is filled with 500 ml of 3% dilute diatrizoate meglumine (Gastrografin) or water. Some prefer the use of water because it is well tolerated and provides an excellent demonstration of mucosa and wall thickness (Fig. 2.6) (BAERT et al. 1989; TSUDA et al. 1995; RICHTER et al. 1996). Because water rapidly passes into the proximal small bowel, an additional 250 ml water should be administered just prior to the beginning of the examination. The use of large volumes of water or diluted contrast media ensures that the stomach and duodenum will be fully distended during the CT scan. The right-side-down decubitus position can be used to better visualize the duodenal loop (HAAGA et al.

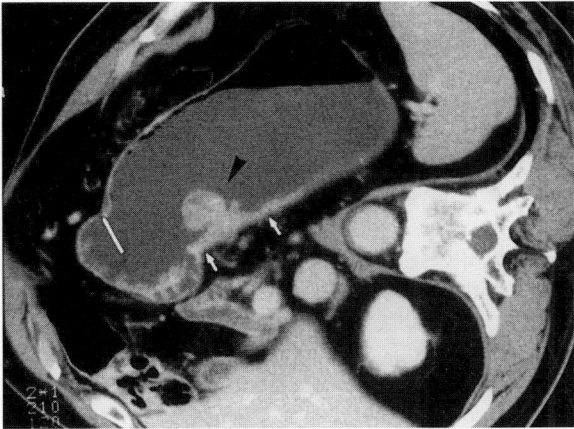

Fig. 2.6. CT in right-side-down position demonstrating an inflammatory pseudopolyp (*arrowhead*) with thickening of the adjacent wall (*small arrows*) using water as an oral contrast agent

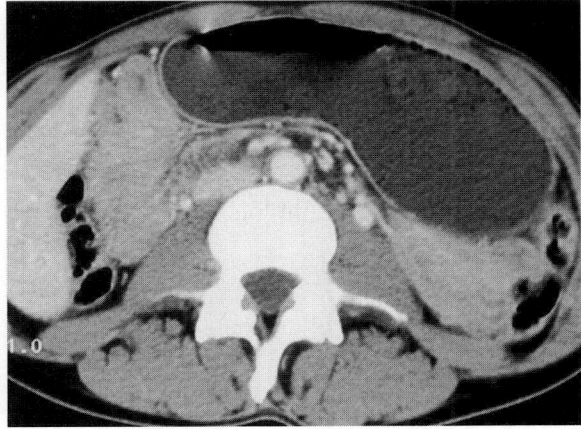

Fig. 2.7. Normal thickness of the gastric wall following intravenous contrast enhancement and optimal distension of the stomach using water as an oral contrast agent

1976). Hypotonic agents (glucagon) are routinely administered and should be employed in all cases of staging neoplasms.

Studying patients after partial gastrectomy requires a modified technique. After oral administration of 300 ml dilute contrast material, 1 mg Glucagon is given intravenously and the patient is slowly turned over his right side to the prone position, then over his left side to a supine posture. This maneuver fills the afferent loop of a Billroth II or Whipple procedure and allows best visualization of the gastrojejunal anastomosis in the majority of cases.

Gas contrast technique is another practical means to achieve expansion of the lumen (THOMPSON et al. 1982). This technique is essential in patients in whom virtual endoscopy is performed.

Helical CT scans are then performed with a collimation of 5 mm, a table speed of 7.5 mm/s, and reconstruction intervals of 4 mm from the xiphoid to the umbilicus with the patient supine. Detection of subtle gastric lesions can be enhanced by repeated scans obtained with the patient prone or in the left or right lateral decubitus positions depending on the location of the lesion. A total of 125 ml of 35% iodinated contrast material is routinely administered intravenously as a monophasic injection (2.5 ml/s) via power injector.

2.2.2.3
Normal Anatomy

The thickness of the gastric wall as measured by CT varies considerably according to the degree of dis-

tension. The normal gastric wall in a well-distended stomach usually ranges from 2 to 5 mm thick (Fig. 2.7), and any measurement greater than 1 cm is considered abnormal (BALFE et al. 1981; MOSS et al. 1980). With proper lumen distension, the normal duodenal wall is thinner than the gastric wall, measuring about 1 mm (MEGIBOW 1986).

2.2.2.4
Applications

2.2.2.4.1
MALIGNANT GASTRODUODENAL TUMORS

Adenocarcinoma. The most frequently demonstrated CT abnormality of gastric carcinoma is focal or diffuse gastric wall thickening with loss of the normal rugal pattern (Fig. 2.8). Other abnormalities frequently seen by CT are irregular outer and inner gastric margins, ulcerated masses, and gastric outlet obstruction.

In order to stage the tumor accurately, the following parameters have to be evaluated: (a) depth of invasion, (b) extension into adjacent organs, (c) regional lymph nodes, and (d) distant metastases. CT, however, is not able to demonstrate the architecture of the gastric wall. Consequently, the invasive depth of cancer limited to the gastric wall cannot be diagnosed.

Direct invasion of gastric tumor into adjacent structures such as the liver, esophagus, spleen, pancreas, and transverse mesocolon and metastatic involvement of the liver, adrenal glands, ovar-

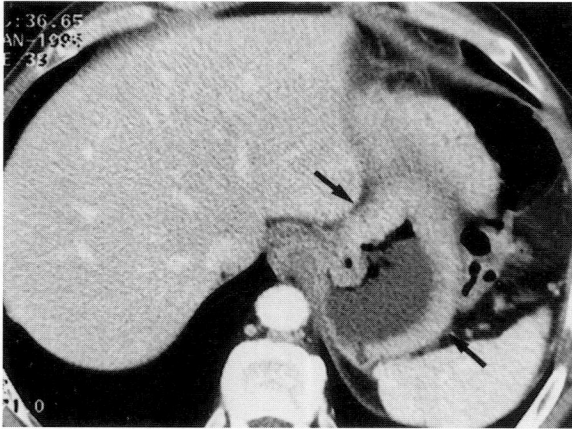

Fig. 2.8. Infiltrating scirrhous carcinoma (linitis plastica) of the stomach. CT scan demonstrates diffuse, moderate thickening of the wall of the gastric fundus (*arrows*)

ies, and peritoneal cavity can be demonstrated on CT.

Initial reports in the late 1970s and early 1980s showed a high accuracy of CT staging of gastric carcinoma in correlation with surgical, laparoscopic, or autopsy findings (BALFE et al. 1981; LEE et al. 1979; Moss et al. 1981a). However, subsequent and more recent studies have proved that the diagnostic accuracy of CT in evaluating tumor invasion to adjacent structures and assessing regional lymph node metastases is not as high as has been reported (SUSSMAN et al. 1988; KOMAKI and TOYOSHIMA 1983; COOK et al. 1986; KLEINHAUS and MILITIANU 1988). In 1988, SUSSMAN et al. concluded in a large series of 75 patients with gastric adenocarcinoma that 31% of patients were understaged and 16% were overstaged when comparing preoperative CT and operative staging. Understaging was due to the inability to detect pancreatic invasion, metastases in normal-sized lymph nodes, and peritoneal carcinomatosis. Direct invasion was predicted if there was a loss of the fat plane between the gastric tumor and an adjacent organ. This sign is unreliable since these patients are often emaciated and will have no fat plane despite a lack of tumor invasion. Surprisingly, pancreatic invasion may be present when the fat plane is intact (SUSSMAN et al. 1988; KLEINHAUS and MILITIANU 1988). Overstaging was due to overdiagnosing adenopathy and invasion of contiguous organs.

Recently, RICHTER et al. (1996) reported that hydro-CT is a reliable screening method for gastric tumors. Staging of gastric carcinomas, however, is not improved.

Based on these results, radiologists must assume a realistic posture when CT is used for staging of gastric tumors. Continued refinement of CT techniques and the recent development of helical CT may improve the ability to stage gastric cancer. However, this has still to be established.

Adenocarcinomas of the duodenum are uncommon, and their features on CT scans have been only occasionally described. FARAH et al. (1987) reported four duodenal adenocarcinomas studied by CT. The most common CT features were thickening of the bowel wall, tumor necrosis, ulceration, and intraluminal defects. More recetly, KAZEROONI et al. (1992) reported a series of 25 duodenal neoplasms, eight of which were adenocarcinomas. CT failed to show pancreatic invasion that was proved pathologically in two of the eight patients. Periduodenal fat invasion was not detected by CT in one patient. CT also failed to detect tumor in normal-sized lymph nodes.

Lymphoma. The stomach is the portion of the gastrointestinal tract most commonly affected by lymphoma (MEGIBOW et al. 1983). In lymphoma, the involvement is predominantly submucosal, so that mucosal imaging by conventional methods may fail to establish the diagnosis. CT, however, well visualizes focal or diffuse wall thickening with distortion of the normal rugal-fold pattern, which is the hallmark of gastric lymphoma (MEGIBOW et al. 1983). The gastric involvement may be isolated, but more commonly is part of a generalized disease process.

Mesenchymatous Tumors. The rare gastric or duodenal leiomyosarcoma has rather distinctive CT features (SCATARIGE et al. 1985). Typically there is a large, sometimes calcified, extraluminal mass (Fig. 2.9). Areas of decreased attenuation within the mass, representing necrosis, are common. There can be direct extension into adjacent organs and metastases to the liver.

2.2.2.4.2
BENIGN GASTRODUODENAL TUMORS

Adenomatous polyps are the most frequent benign neoplastic gastric tumors. They appear on CT scans as a small endoluminal soft tissue mass without thickening of the adjacent gastric wall.

Lipomas are rare. They are submucosal and predominantly occur in the gastric antrum. On CT scan, a lipoma appears as a well-circumscribed mass hav-

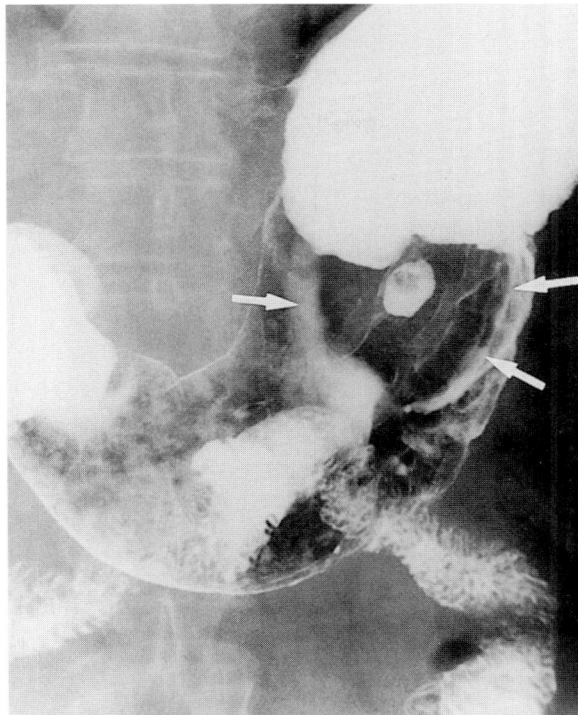

a

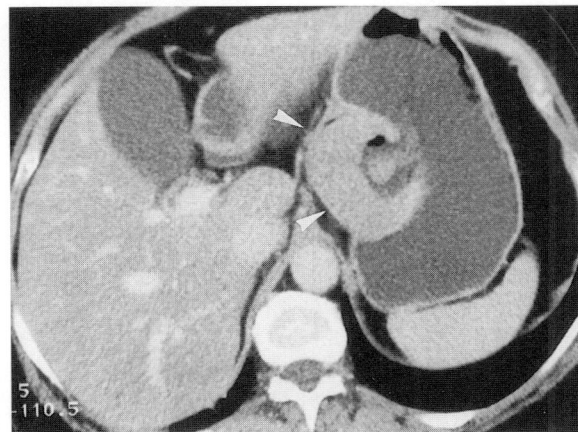

b

Fig. 2.9a,b. Malignant submucosal tumor. **a** Upper gastrointestinal series demonstrates an ulcerated submucosal mass and markedly thickened rugae (*arrows*). **b** CT scan shows an exogastric lesser curvature mass (*arrowheads*) with a deep ulcer. The perigastric fat plane is preserved, indicating absence of perigastric extension

ing a CT attenuation value equivalent to that of fat (Fig. 2.10).

The appearance of a leiomyoma on CT is that of a solid mass of uniform density (Fig. 2.11). The outer border of the leiomyoma is smooth and the fat plane between the tumor and adjacent organs is preserved. Calcifications are frequently identified.

2.2.2.4.3
TRAUMATIC AND IATROGENIC ABNORMALITIES

In the past, gastroduodenal perforations associated with peptic ulcers or necrotic tumors were relatively common, but these have become less frequent due to improved methods for earlier diagnosis and management. However, the incidence of gastroduodenal perforations resulting from iatrogenic and accidental injuries has dramatically increased. Fiberoptic gastroscopy alone accounts for approximately one perforation per one thousand procedures (EIMILLER 1992).

The most common injuries are transmural tears and intramural hematomas. CT findings strongly suggestive of lacerations are extraluminal gas and

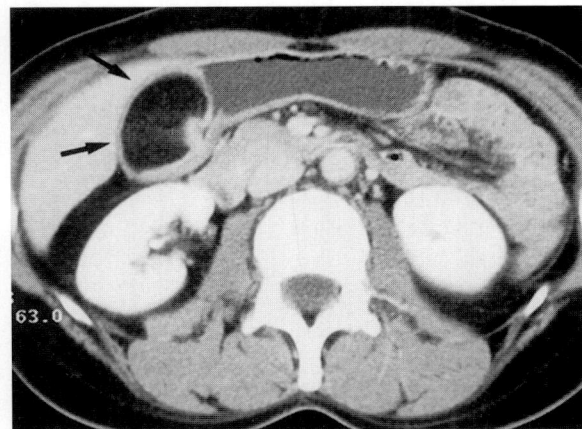

Fig. 2.10. Gastric lipoma. Rounded low-attenuating mass (−74 HU) present in the distal antrum (*arrows*) is consistent with a benign lipoma

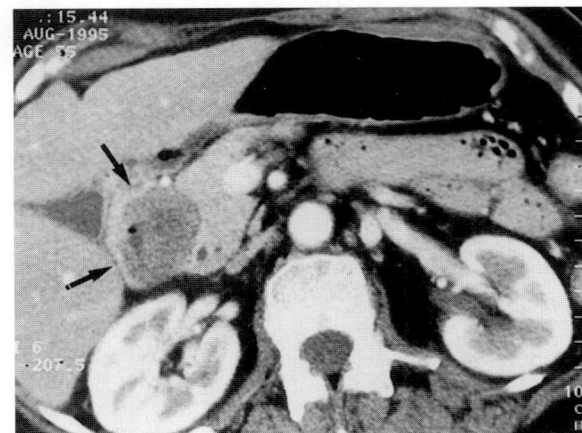

Fig. 2.11. Leiomyoma. CT scan demonstrates a smoothly marginated soft tissue mass (*arrows*) arising from the second portion of the duodenum

extravasation of oral contrast. Depending on the site of perforation, extraluminal gas or contrast may extravasate into the anterior pararenal space or peritoneal cavity. An intramural hematoma results in a focal wall thickening with a measured CT number greater than 30 Hounsfield units (Fig. 2.12).

2.2.2.4.4
EXTRINSIC LESIONS AND SECONDARY INVOLVEMENT

Duodenitis as a secondary manifestation of acute pancreatitis is well depicted by CT, which provides accurate visualization of the pancreatic abnormalities as well as the duodenal inflammation. When a pseudocyst develops and obstructs the descending duodenum, CT allows precise definition of the mass and its relation to the duodenal lumen. Moreover,

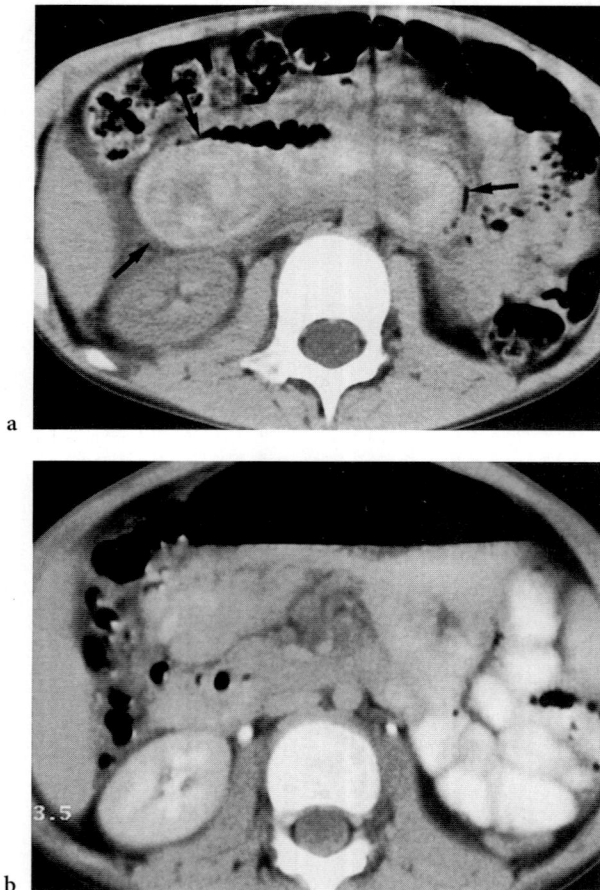

a

b

Fig. 2.13 a,b. Metastatic carcinoma in a patient with a gastrojejunostomy for gastric ulcer. **a** Upper gastrointestinal tract examination demonstrates a tumoral mass (*arrows*) at the medial border of the gastrojejunal anastomosis. **b** CT scan shows an asymmetric circumferential thickening of the wall of the gastric stump near the anastomosis. Endoscopic biopsy revealed a metastatic large cell lung carcinoma

a

b

Fig. 2.12. a Intramural hematoma of the duodenum after gastroduodenoscopy. Note high-density hematoma involving the third part of the duodenum (*arrow*). **b** Follow-up scan 2 months later demonstrates total regression of the lesion

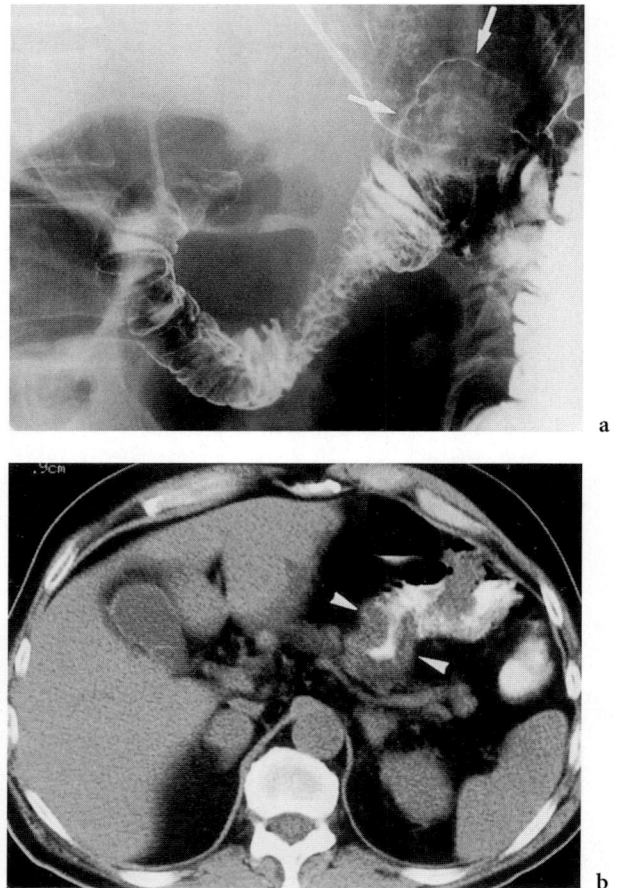

CT can be helpful in demonstrating a safe access route for percutaneous drainage of such pseudocysts.

Metastatic neoplasms to the stomach and duodenum are uncommon (Fig. 2.13). Direct invasion from adjacent structures is the most significant route for spread of malignancy to the duodenum. Although barium studies may reveal mucosal changes in this setting, the ability of CT to depict the extraduodenal as well as the intramural component of the tumor is a major advantage. The most common pattern of spread is involvement of the medial aspect of the C-loop by a contiguous pancreatic carcinoma (SCATARIGE and DiSANTIS 1989). FARAH et al. (1987) reported that in 11 of 14 cases of duodenal

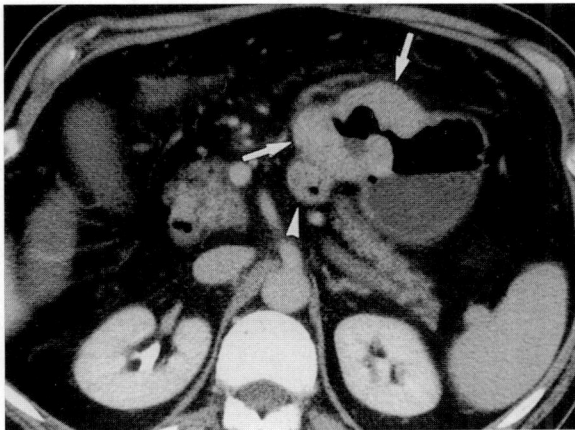

Fig. 2.14. Recurrent cancer following gastric resection (Billroth II) for carcinoma. Tumor encases the wall of the gastrojejunal anastomosis (*arrows*) and invades the adjacent duodenal loop (*arrowhead*)

neoplasms, CT scans revealed that the mass primarily arose from the duodenum.

2.2.2.4.5
CT AFTER GASTRECTOMY

The postoperative stomach may be encountered as an incidental finding on CT examination of the abdomen or the patient may be referred for scanning to evaluate early postoperative complications such as abscesses, intra-abdominal hemorrhages, postoperative pancreatitis, and anastomic leak. In the evaluation of late postoperative complications, CT is useful in demonstrating tumor recurrence as well as metastases to regional lymph nodes or to liver.

Features on CT that suggest tumor recurrence include soft tissue masses in the area of the gastric stump, a thickened wall (Fig. 2.14), afferent loop obstruction, and obliteration of perigastric fat (MULLIN and SHIRKHODA 1985). Therefore in studying these patients, it is important that the anastomosis is well visualized by using sufficient oral contrast or air within the gastric remnant as well as intravenous Glucagon. Metastases in the pancreatic and hepatoduodenal lymph nodes or in the liver are further CT indications of recurrence (MULLIN and SHIRKHODA 1985).

Care must be taken not to confuse tumor recurrence with postoperative fibrosis, hematoma, or unopacified loops of small bowel. A baseline CT examination 2 months after gastrectomy helps to avoid such diagnostic errors (MOSS 1992).

2.2.3
Small Bowel

2.2.3.1
Role of CT

Not being organ-specific, body CT has become a screening modality. In patients with unusual or nonspecific complaints, unexplained bleeding, or clinical suspicion of disease undetected by barium studies or endoscopy, CT may be the first examination to suggest an abnormality of the small bowel wall (HULNICK 1986).

In known neoplastic disorders, CT may provide additional information about tumor extension into the mesentery or adjacent organs and the presence of nodal or hepatic metastases.

In patients with blunt trauma who require further diagnostic evaluation, CT is often the imaging method of choice.

Although barium studies remain the primary method for demonstrating the mucosal extent of Crohn's disease, CT may be valuable in defining the extramural complications of Crohn's disease and in differentiating an abscess from retractile mesenteritis (GOLDBERG 1982; GOLDBERG et al. 1983).

Plain abdominal radiographs and conventional barium studies have been the primary diagnostic methods to evaluate patients with clinically suspected small bowel obstruction. However, when the clinical picture is confusing or plain abdominal radiographs and conventional barium studies are equivocal, further studies are necessary. Recently, CT has been shown to be useful in revealing the site, level, and cause of obstruction and has been increasingly utilized in patients with unusual or unsuspected forms of gastrointestinal obstruction (GAZELLE et al. 1994; FRAGER et al. 1994; MAGLINTE et al. 1993; RUBESIN and HERLINGER 1991).

2.2.3.2
Techniques of Examination

The success of a CT examination of the small bowel depends on the degree to which the small bowel is filled with contrast material. To ensure optimal filling, a cup of 300 ml of 3% dilute diatrizoate meglumine (Gastrografin) is administered every 20 min, beginning 60 min before scanning. Dilute barium suspension has also proved satisfactory (MEGIBOW and BOSNIAK 1980). If an interpretative problem arises in distinguishing unopacified bowel loops from a pathologic mass, administration of more oral contrast material or a change in patient position may be necessary. Rectal contrast is not routinely used.

Intravenous administration of 125 ml of 35% iodinated contrast is always given as a monophasic injection (2.5 ml/s) via power injector. An 80-s delay is used from the initiation of the contrast injection until the onset of scanning. Helical scanning is then performed with 8-mm collimation and a pitch of 1.5. Overlapping reconstructions are obtained at 6-mm increments.

2.2.3.3
Normal Anatomy

On CT, the normal thickness of the small bowel wall varies greatly with the degree of luminal distension. The wall is barely perceptible and no more than 1–2 mm thick in a distended segment and appears thicker (3–4 mm) when the intestine is collapsed or partially distended.

2.2.3.4
Applications

2.2.3.4.1
SMALL BOWEL TUMORS

At CT, small bowel adenocarcinomas are usually seen as a focal area of wall thickening with narrowing of the lumen and prestenotic dilatation. CT may provide unique information about tumor extension and presence of local or distant metastases.

A mesenteric soft tissue mass associated with retraction of surrounding bowel loops with or without hepatic metastases or lymphadenopathy is typically for carcinoid (PICUS et al. 1984).

Lymphoma appears as a focal or diffuse thickening of the bowel wall with the presence of enlarged lymph nodes within the mesenteric loops supplying the involved segment (Fig. 2.15).

Intestinal leiomyosarcomas arise in the submucosa and appear as a large, extraluminal, bulky inhomogeneous and occasionally calcified mass. These tumors have a tendency to spread through the mesentery and/or peritoneal cavity.

Metastatic disease to the small bowel from tumors of the lung, breast, colon, pancreas, kidney, uterus, and skin produce soft tissue nodules adjacent to or impinging on the bowel lumen. Although CT is not

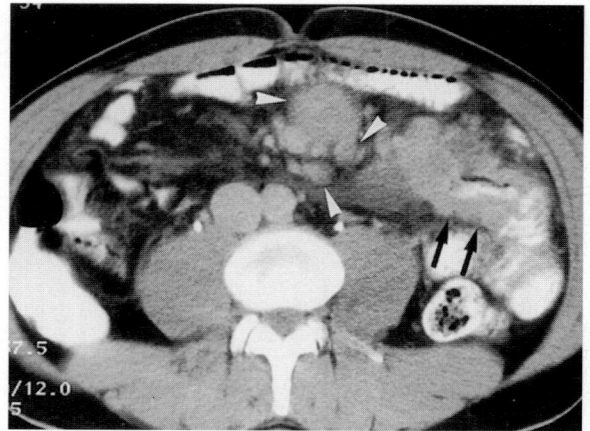

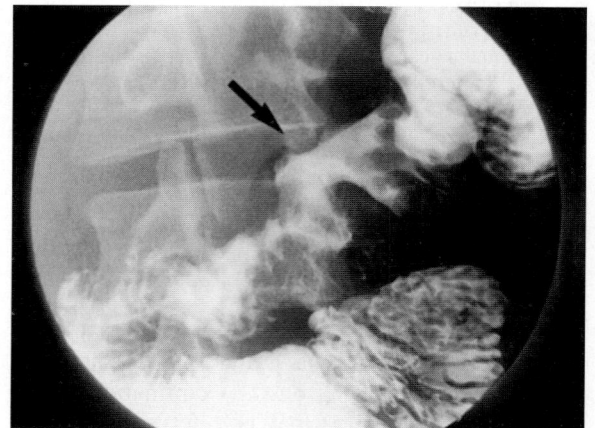

Fig. 2.15a,b. Lymphoma. **a** Marked wall thickening of a proximal jejunal loop (*arrows*) with multiple locoregional adenopathies (*arrowheads*) is seen. **b** Small bowel series demonstrates the presence of a large ulcerated mass (*arrow*) without proximal obstruction.

advocated as a screening method for detecting metastatic disease to the small intestine, it provides unique information about the extent and location of lesions detected or suggested by other diagnostic techniques.

2.2.3.4.2
SMALL BOWEL TRAUMA

The CT signs of small bowel trauma are often subtle and may easily be overlooked. Extravasation of oral contrast and free peritoneal air are the most specific CT findings of bowel injury but CT has a limited sensitivity as these signs may be absent in almost half of the patients (MIRVIS et al. 1992). In addition, pneumoperitoneum is not pathognomonic of perforation and must be interpreted with caution in postsurgical patients and in patients with a

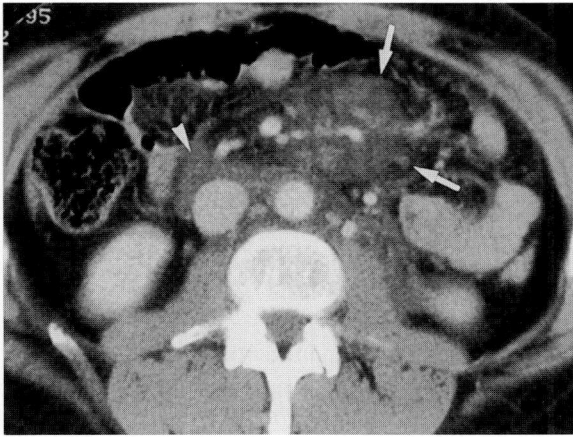

Fig. 2.16. Mesenteric laceration. A small hematoma is noted in the mesentery (*arrows*) and retroperitoneal compartment (*arrowhead*)

degrees of streakiness and poorly defined heterogeneous mesenteric densities (GOLDBERG et al. 1983; CAREY 1980; FISHMAN et al. 1987).

Recently, MEYERS and McGUIRE (1995) reported helical CT imaging features of vascular alterations observed in Crohn's disease. These features include tortuosity, vascular dilatation, and conspicuous prominence and wide spacing of the vasa recta (the "comb" sign) (Fig. 2.19). The identification of these distinct vascular changes may enhance the diagnosis of active, early, or recurrent Crohn's disease.

On CT a Crohn's abscess appears as a circumscribed mass of fluid density with a thick wall that may contain gas (Fig. 2.20). These abscesses repre-

pneumothorax (KANE et al. 1991). Thoracic free air may enter the peritoneal cavity in the absence of bowel perforation.

Fluid or hemorrhage between bowel loops is another key sign of bowel perforation, as hemoperitoneum following solid organ injury usually accumulates in the paracolic gutters and other dependent regions (NGHIEM et al. 1993). Other less specific signs of bowel injury on CT include focal mesenteric hematoma (Fig. 2.16), bowel wall thickening, and hemoperitoneum without apparent solid organ injury (MIRVIS et al. 1992).

Although initial reports stressed the limitations of CT in diagnosis of intestinal injury, CT is nowadays recommended in patients with suspected traumatic and iatrogenic abnormalities who do not require immediate surgery (MARX et al. 1985; MINDELL 1989). In this subset of patients, CT permits the most accurate nonsurgical assessment of the gastrointestinal tract, surrounding organs, and retroperitoneum (MOHAMED et al. 1986).

2.2.3.4.3
INFLAMMATORY DISEASE

The CT features of Crohn's disease are symmetric thickening of the bowel wall to greater than 1 cm, narrowing of the lumen (Fig. 2.17), skipped areas of involvement, and mesenteric abnormalities (SCHNUR and WEINER 1982). Fibrofatty proliferation or "creeping fat" of the mesentery is the most common cause of bowel loop separation and is seen in about 40% of patients (Fig. 2.18). It causes the mesenteric fat to increase in density with various

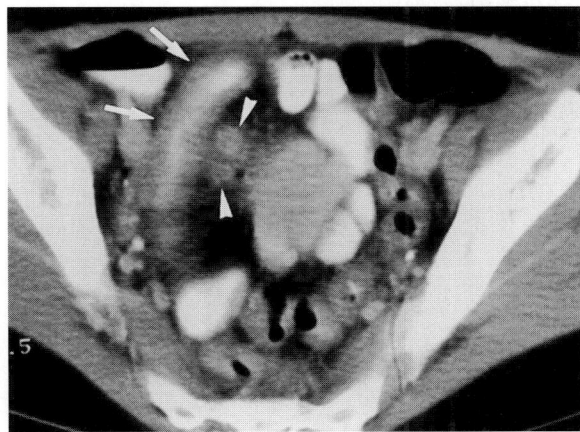

Fig. 2.17. Crohn's disease. CT demonstrates mural thickening of preterminal ileum with narrowing of the lumen (*arrows*) and adenopathies in the surrounding fat (*arrowheads*)

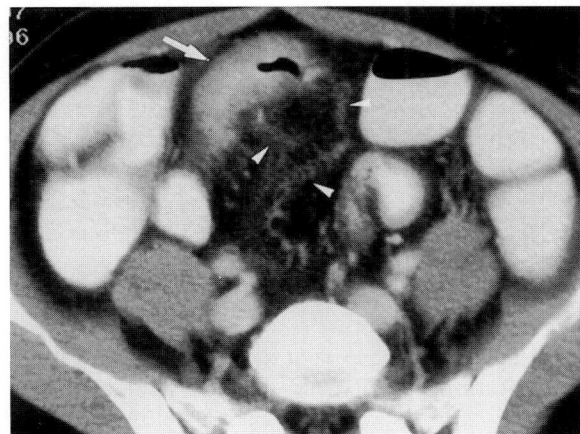

Fig. 2.18. Crohn's disease with mesenteric fibrofatty proliferation. CT scan of the right lower quadrant shows thickening of terminal ileum (*arrow*) and infiltrations in the surrounding mesenteric fat (*arrowheads*)

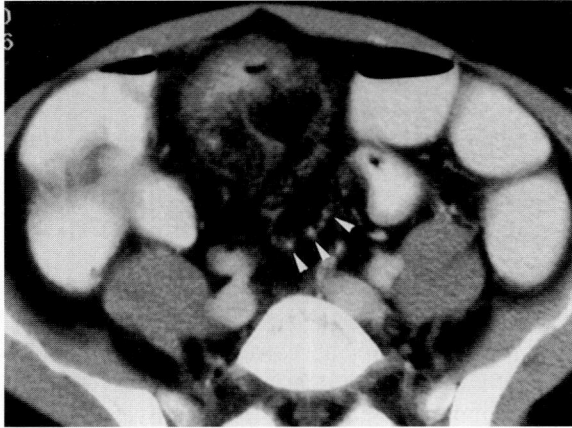

Fig. 2.19. Crohn's disease of distal ileum with hypervascularity. Helical CT demonstrates clearly the dilated vasa recta (*arrowheads*)

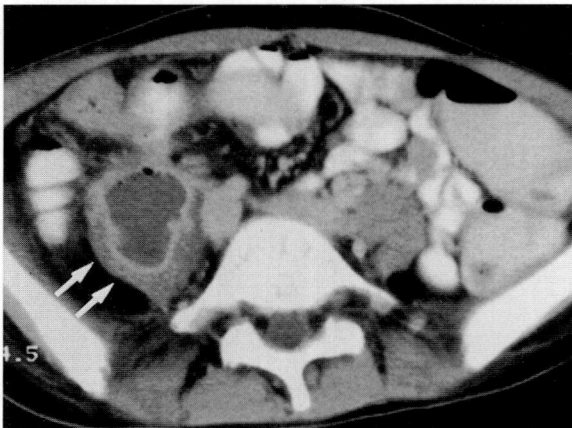

Fig. 2.20. Crohn's abscess. CT scan at the level of the cecum demonstrates a gas-containing abscess in the right psoas muscle (*arrows*)

sent the second most common cause of bowel loop separation observed in Crohn's disease (GORE 1987). Percutaneous drainage has demonstrated mixed results because such abscesses usually have accompanying fistulas (LAMBIASE et al. 1988; CASOLA et al. 1987).

Small regional mesenteric nodes are present in about 20% of patients.

In defining unsuspected local and extraintestinal complications of Crohn's disease, such as enterovesical fistulas, sacral osteomyelitis, venous thrombosis, vascular necrosis of femoral head, and ureteral obstruction, CT may be extremely valuable (GOLDBERG et al. 1983; OREL et al. 1987).

It is clear that CT will continue to play a secondary role in the evaluation of patients with Crohn's dis-

ease and should not be regarded as competing with, but as complementing, barium examinations of the gastrointestinal tract (BALTHAZAR 1991). In patients with acute symptomatology and an abdominal mass, CT is an accurate method for distinguishing among the various causes of the abdominal mass, and, by so doing, avoiding the morbidity and expense of surgical intervention except in patients with frank intraabdominal abscesses (JEFFREY and RALLS 1996). Thickening of the small bowel wall, however, is a nonspecific abnormality that may be seen in other acute and chronic inflammatory bowel conditions imaged by CT. Eosinophilic gastroenteritis appears as a focal wall thickening with edema in the adjacent mesenteric fat (Fig. 2.21). In Whipple's disease, CT shows diffuse intestinal wall thickening, associated with large mesenteric lymph nodes (LI and RENNIE 1981). CT findings in graft-versus-host disease after bone marrow transplantation consist of focal wall thickening, usually of the ileum, with or without target lesions in the bowel caused by submucosal edema or hemorrhage (JONES et al. 1986).

2.2.3.4.4
SMALL BOWEL OBSTRUCTION

The CT diagnosis of small bowel obstruction relies on the demonstration of small bowel dilation (more than 2.5 cm) and identification of a transition zone between dilated and collapsed bowel. The accuracy of CT in diagnosing bowel obstruction ranges from 65% to 95% (MAGLINTE et al. 1993; RUBESIN and HERLINGER 1991; GAZELLE et al. 1994; FRAGER et al. 1994; MEGIBOW 1994).

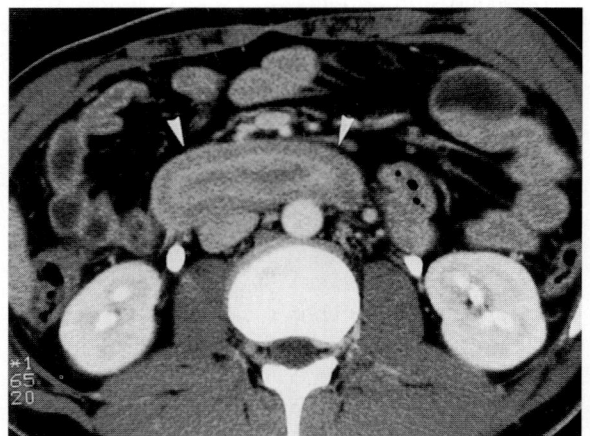

Fig. 2.21. Nonmucosal eosinophilic gastroenteritis. CT after intravenous contrast medium administration shows the three layers of the thickened small bowel wall. The intact mucosal layer is seen as a markedly enhancing inner layer; the thickened submucosal layer is shown as a low attenuation zone (*arrowheads*). (From Van Hoe et al. 1994)

Once the presence of obstruction is identified, the next requirement is to establish the cause. About 50% of intestinal obstructions are caused by adhesions (Fig. 2.22) (BALTHAZAR 1994). Most adhesive bands, however, cannot be seen. Local distortions of the mesenteric fat may be present, but it is extremely difficult to visualize these abnormalities by CT.

Other less common causes of obstruction are intra-abdominal tumors, internal hernias, afferent loop obstruction following Billroth II gastrectomy, gallstone ileus, various types of enteroenteric intussusception, and closed loop obstruction (CUBILLO 1983; GRUMBACH et al. 1986; OSTEEN et al. 1980). Closed loop obstruction is a form of mechanical obstruction in which a loop of bowel is occluded at two points along its course. CT findings are characteristic and include a U-shaped configuration of a distended fluid-filled bowel loop and at the site of obstruction a "beak" or "whirl" sign of the mesenteric vasculature. Because of the localized constriction of the two adjacent segments of bowel, the closed loop may rotate along its long axis, thereby producing a small bowel volvulus. CT signs of intestinal strangulation are a circumferentially thickened loop with high attenuation within the wall or pneumatosis and congestive changes or hemorrhage in the mesentery attached to the closed loop.

Recently, MEGIBOW (1994) reported that in patients who have a history of abdominal malignancy and clinical symptoms suggestive of bowel obstruction, CT is the procedure of choice. In patients who have no history of abdominal surgery and who present with symptoms of bowel obstruction, CT is

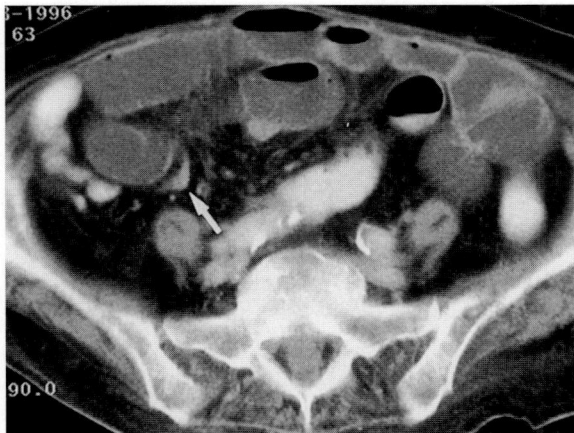

Fig. 2.22. Small bowel obstruction due to adhesions. CT shows markedly distended fluid-filled loops of small bowel with collapsed loop of bowel at the transition zone (*arrow*) in the right lower part of the abdomen

most valuable when there are systemic signs suggestive of infarction, or an associated palpable mass.

2.2.3.4.5
ACUTE ISCHEMIA AND INFARCTION
The CT findings suggestive of acute intestinal ischemia include small bowel dilatation, circumferential wall thickening, and congestive changes in the mesentery. In advanced cases of ischemia in which bowel infarction has already developed, portal or mesenteric venous gas, intramural air (pneumatosis), free intraperitoneal air, and a wall thickening that demonstrates persisting post contrast enhancement may be seen (FEDERLE et al. 1984; PEREZ et al. 1989). In addition to demonstrating findings suggestive of ischemia or infarction of the intestine, CT can sometimes establish the cause of ischemia by showing thrombosis in the superior mesenteric or portal vein, or arterial occlusion (MATOS et al. 1986).

2.2.4
Colon

2.2.4.1
Role of CT

Computed tomography can provide useful information in the preoperative staging and evaluation of patients with known colonic carcinoma (KERNER et al. 1993). In patients who have undergone abdominoperineal resection for rectal carcinoma, CT has become the preferred method for detecting recurrence. In these patients barium enema and endoscopy are of little use.

Barium enema and colonoscopy are still the primary techniques used to detect colon carcinoma. Technologic advances, however, continue rapidly. Recently, helical CT pneumocolon with multiplanar reformatting and three-dimensional reconstruction has become possible. This still evolving technique provides both intra- and extraluminal views, and initial results indicate that it has the potential to replace barium enema (and colonoscopy) for the detection of polypoid colonic lesions (Fig. 2.23) (STEVENSON 1995). AMIN et al. (1996) found that helical CT pneumocolon depicted the morphology of the primary tumor more clearly than barium enema and in one case also detected a 1-cm polyp which was not seen on barium study because the patient was incontinent. Compared to a barium enema, helical CT pneumocolon is quick, with minimal patient discomfort, entails no risk of barium incontinence, and

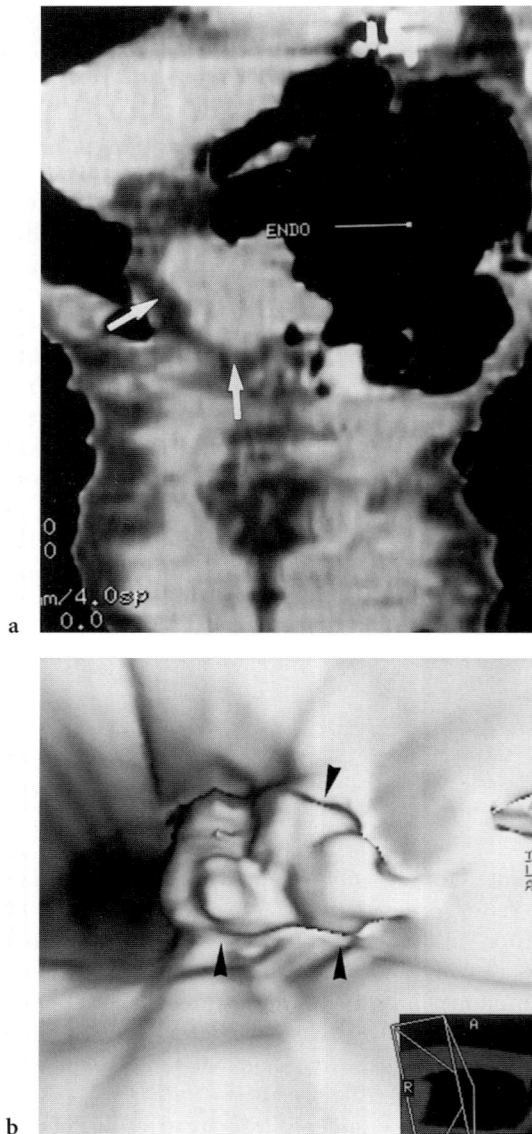

Fig. 2.23. a Coronal reformatting of a nonstenotic adenocarcinoma of the transverse colon (*arrows*). **b** 3-D reconstruction viewed from inside best demonstrates the irregular surface of the polypoid tumoral mass (*arrowheads*)

allows good assessment of local and distant abdominal disease.

Computed tomography can also be useful in detecting and evaluating a variety of diffuse and focal inflammatory conditions of the colon and the appendix. Pericolonic inflammation and abscesses due to diverticulitis or appendicitis can be well seen. In patients with well-localized abscesses, CT-guided percutaneous drainage is performed to help reduce surgical morbidity.

2.2.4.2
Techniques of Examination

Visualization of the intestinal lumen is achieved by the oral administration of 600 ml of 3% dilute diatrizoate meglumine (Gastrografin) to all patients at least 30 min before scanning. In cases of suspected colonic disease an enema of 1000 ml water or dilute Gastrografin is given in order to distend the colon. We prefer the use of water because it provides an excellent CT contrast medium and allows more accurate staging of rectal carcinoma patients (ANGELELLI et al. 1990). Air insufflation per rectum after adequate preparation of the colon is another useful means of distending the colon (CT pneumocolon) (MEGIBOW et al. 1984).

Helical scans with a collimation of 8 mm, a table speed of 12 mm/s, and reconstruction intervals of 6 mm are then performed from the dome of the liver to the anal verge following an intravenous injection of glucagon and contrast material. A total of 125 ml of 35% iodinated contrast material is routinely administered as a monophasic injection (2.5 ml/s) via power injector. Routine scanning is done with the patient supine, but decubitus or prone scans are occasionally performed depending on the location of the lesion.

Currently, helical CT pneumocolon, also known as virtual CT colonoscopy, permits additional three-dimensional reconstruction with a view of the colonic mucosa as seen from inside – similar to the image seen endoscopically (AMIN et al. 1996). Using a mouse, the viewer can then "drive" around the colon to the appendix, turn round, and "drive back," inspecting the other side of the haustral folds.

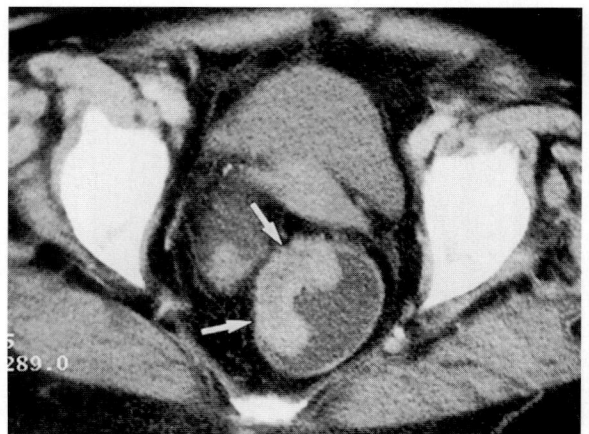

Fig. 2.24. An intraluminal tumor mass (*arrows*) with a central ulcer is present in a patient with a primary adenocarcinoma of the distal rectum

2.2.4.3
Normal Anatomy

On CT, the normal thickness of the wall of the colon is less than 5 mm, provided the lumen is not collapsed. The bowel wall should also have a homogeneous attenuation.

The mesentery and omentum normally contain blood vessels and small lymph nodes less than 3–5 mm in size as well as fat having an attenuation value ranging between −75 and −125 Hounsfield units.

2.2.4.4
Applications

2.2.4.4.1
CT OF COLON CANCER

Preoperative Evaluation. Colon cancer usually involves only a short segment (3–5 cm) and presents on CT as an eccentric focal mass (Fig. 2.24) or as a circumferential asymmetric and irregular thickening of the bowel wall with narrowing of the lumen (Fig. 2.25). Other findings may include extension of tumor into pericolonic fat, lymphadenopathy, invasion of adjacent structures, adrenal or liver metastases, hydronephrosis, ascites, and masses in the abdominal wall, omentum, or mesentery.

Pretherapy staging of a newly diagnosed colorectal cancer involves the determination of depth of spread of tumor in the bowel wall, presence of

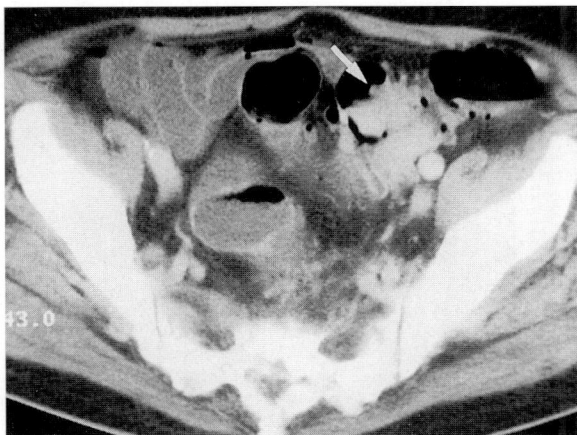

Fig. 2.25. Adenocarcinoma of the sigmoid. CT shows an enhancing tumoral wall thickening in the mid sigmoid and marked luminal narrowing (*arrow*)

lymph node metastases, and presence of remote metastases, particularly in the liver. The early enthusiasm for CT in preoperative staging has not been sustained because of poor accuracy in identification of lymph node metastases and inability to determine local spread. These early studies reported 85%–90% accuracy, which was largely because of the more advanced cases in these series (DIXON et al. 1981). Later, more precise studies in which prospective CT interpretations of all disease stages were correlated with operative findings reported significantly lower accuracy rates (THOMPSON et al. 1986; FREENY et al. 1986). Also disappointing has been the inability of CT to detect intraperitoneal spread of malignant neoplasms. Small nodules implanted on the parietal and visceral peritoneum commonly go undetected on CT.

For primary colon cancer, CT is more accurate in showing extensive invasion of surrounding tissue and distant metastases, such as those in liver and adrenals, than in demonstrating local adenopathy or minimal tumor extension (FREENY et al. 1986)

Postoperative Evaluation. Although the role of preoperative imaging studies for staging is controversial, there is more agreement about the need for postoperative surveillance for recurrence. Recurrence may be local, which is defined as in the suture line, regional to the operative bed or mesentery, or distant (OLSON et al. 1980).

The capacity to detect both local and distant disease currently makes CT the best modality for the detection and staging of recurrent tumors. Because of the high frequency of tumor recurrence in the first 24 months after surgery, a series of follow-up CT scans has been recommended in that interval (CASS et al. 1976). A reasonable timetable includes a baseline study at 2–4 months, then studies every 6 months for 2 years followed by yearly scans (THOMPSON et al. 1986; KELVIN et al. 1983). In addition, a CT scan should be obtained whenever a patient is found to have a rising carcinoembryogenic (CEA) titer.

Almost all recurrences in patients with sphincter-saving resection of a carcinoma and a primary anastomosis develop extraluminally, infiltrating the suture lines. This may be seen as thickening of the colonic wall (Fig. 2.26) or as a mass near the anastomosis (KELVIN and MAGLINTE 1987). Although local recurrence is sometimes identified by a barium enema and not CT, CT often demonstrates the total extent of disease better than the enema (CHEN et al. 1987). Distant tumor nodules may be seen in the liver, peritoneal cavity, adrenal glands,

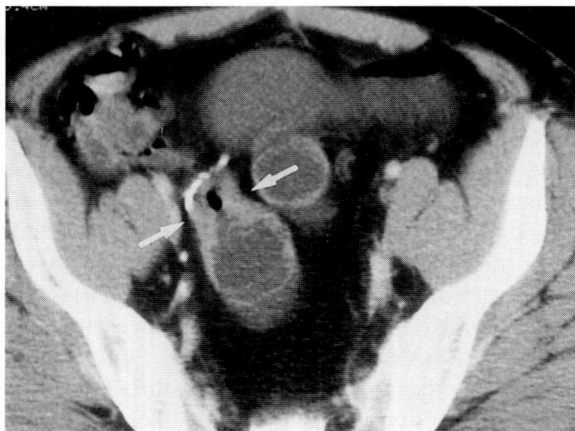

Fig. 2.26. CT scan of the pelvis following previous resection of a sigmoid carcinoma shows recurrence of tumor at the anastomotic site (*arrows*)

lungs, and ovaries (KELVIN and MAGLINTE 1987). Recurrent tumor may also cause enlargement of mesenteric and retroperitoneal lymph nodes (Moss et al. 1981c).

Patients who have undergone an abdominoperitoneal resection of a rectal carcinoma represent a unique situation. Because the rectum is no longer present, endoscopy and barium enema examinations are not possible. In these patients, CT has become the preferred method for detecting recurrence. Recurrent tumor in the pelvis following abdominoperineal resection is most common in the presacral space and appears as a homogeneous, globular soft tissue mass. This appearance is not specific and must be differentiated from postoperative fibrosis (KELVIN et al. 1983; REZNEK et al. 1983). When followed by serial CT scans the benign mass either gets smaller or stays the same size. The borders of the mass become better defined and a fat plane may develop between the mass and the sacrum (KELVIN et al. 1983). Unlike benign lesions, recurrent tumor grows with time and becomes less well defined (KELVIN et al. 1983; REZNEK et al. 1983). CT-directed needle biopsy can prove useful in problem cases (BUTCH et al. 1985).

2.2.4.4.2
CT OF INFLAMMATORY LESIONS

Colitis. In patients with superficial inflammatory colitides only the mucosa is affected and CT findings are either totally absent or minimal and unimpressive. In these cases barium studies remain the most

effective radiographic technique for establishing the diagnosis.

Forms of severe colitis, on the other hand, show a variety of CT abnormalities including concentric thickening of the colonic wall, altered or absent haustral pattern, deep transmural ulcerations, and significant pericolic inflammatory changes. In chronic ulcerative colitis, the muscularis mucosa and submucosa are often involved, and this produces mural thickening and lumen narrowing (Fig. 2.27). The degree of wall thickening and the changes in the pericolonic fat are usually less marked than in Crohn's disease. In patients with Crohn's disease, the colonic wall tends to be even thicker. A "double-halo" appearance has been described (FRAGER et al. 1983). Perirectal abscesses and fistulas may be seen, with displacement of normal structures and inflammation of the pericolonic fat.

The CT abnormalities in other forms of colitis have been documented less frequently. BALTHAZAR et al. (1991) reported that CT was particularly valuable in the initial diagnosis of pseudomembranous colitis affecting debilitated persons on broad-spectrum antibiotic therapy. These patients are often referred for examination because of sepsis and non-specific abdominal complaints with the diagnosis unsuspected at the time of CT scanning. CT shows marked thickening of haustral folds.

Computed tomography may also be helpful in diagnosing typhlitis or necrotizing enteropathy. In these patients, CT shows severe thickening of the cecal wall, with or without intramural gas.

Appendicitis. Throughout the Western world, acute appendicitis is the most common acute abdominal

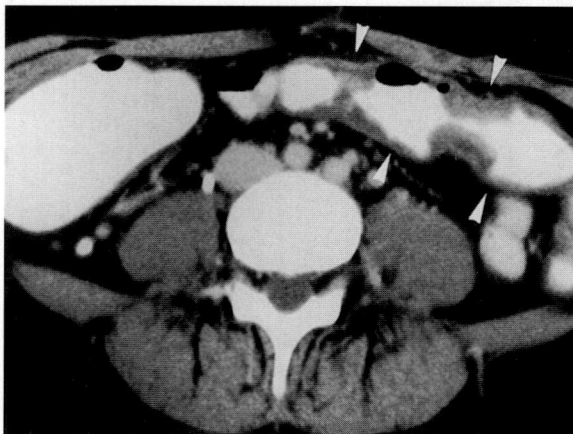

Fig. 2.27. Inhomogeneous mural thickening of transverse colon (*arrowheads*) is seen in this patient with ulcerative colitis

disorder requiring surgery. The diagnosis is usually made on the basis of clinical symptoms and laboratory findings. However, in 20%–30% of patients the clinical findings are atypical, and radiographic examinations are necessary for diagnosis or confirmation (LEWIS et al. 1975). The usefulness and shortcomings of plain abdominal films and barium enema examinations are well established (MEYERS and OLIPHANT 1974; FEDYSHIN et al. 1984). CT, however, has proven to be of considerable value in clinically questionable cases of appendicitis (BALTHAZAR et al. 1986).

The CT findings of appendicitis vary and reflect the stage and severity of the inflammatory process. A specific CT diagnosis of acute appendicitis is based on visualization of a dilated appendix or appendicolith with inflammatory changes in the adjacent fat. In mild cases, the abnormal appendix appears as a slightly distended, fluid-filled, tubular structure that usually measures between 5 and 15 mm in diameter. When severely distended, it may approach 3–4 cm in size (BALTHAZAR et al. 1988). The thickened appendiceal wall may significantly enhance on bolus contrast-enhanced studies (Fig. 2.28). However, a preliminary study by MALONE et al. (1993) suggests that noncontrast CT (without either oral or intravenous contrast) may prove diagnostically useful in patients with acute abdominal pain in the right lower quadrant. If the appendix is not visualized, recognition of an appendicolith in association with pericecal inflammatory changes confirms the diagnosis. Using a high-resolution scanning technique, appendicoliths may be identified in up to 28% of patients with appendicitis (Fig.

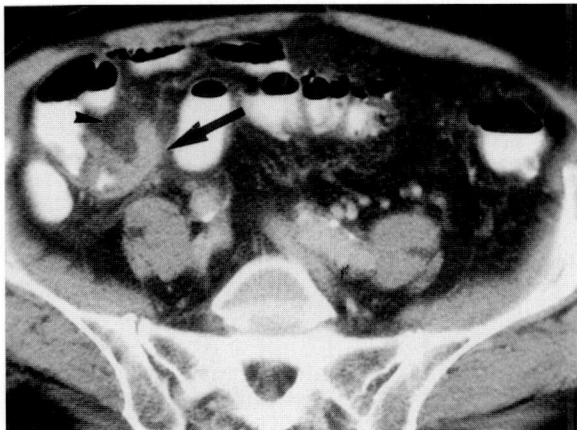

Fig. 2.29. Acute appendicitis. The ring-like calcification (*arrow*) represents an appendicolith

2.29) (BALTHAZAR et al. 1991). If an abnormal appendix or appendicolith is not identified, a definitive CT diagnosis of appendicitis or periappendiceal abscess cannot be made. Other right lower quadrant lesions that may mimic appendicitis on CT include a perforated cecal diverticulum, perforated cecal tumors, and a right-sided thrombosed ovarian vein collateral (VAN HOE et al. 1994). Because the CT findings may be nonspecific in these circumstances, a barium enema should be performed when there is any question regarding the diagnosis, in order to exclude other disease of the cecum or right colon (LEWIS et al. 1975).

The true sensitivity of CT in diagnosing acute appendicitis remains unknown. In a prospective study of 100 patients examined with high-resolution thin-section CT, BALTHAZAR et al. (1991) found a sensitivity of 98%, a specificity of 83%, and an accuracy of 93%. A recently performed prospective, comparative study of high-resolution CT and graded compression sonography revealed that CT had a higher sensitivity (96% vs 76%), accuracy (94% vs 83%), and negative predictive value (95% vs 76%) (BALTHAZAR et al. 1994).

At this time, high-resolution helical CT imaging of the right lower quadrant allows rapid and correct diagnosis of appendicitis in the vast majority of patients and will substantially decrease the number of unnecessary laparotomies performed.

Diverticular Disease. The most common and significant CT abnormality in acute uncomplicated diverticulitis is infiltration of the pericolic fat, seen in 98% of cases (Fig. 2.30) (HULNICK et al. 1984). Other

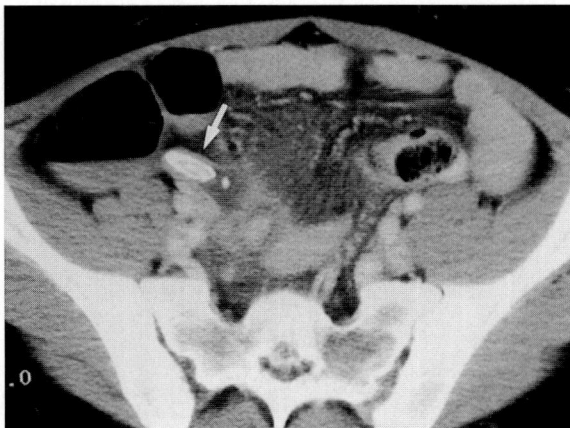

Fig. 2.28. Acute appendicitis with demonstration of an abnormally thickened appendix (*arrow*) and pericecal inflammation (*arrowhead*)

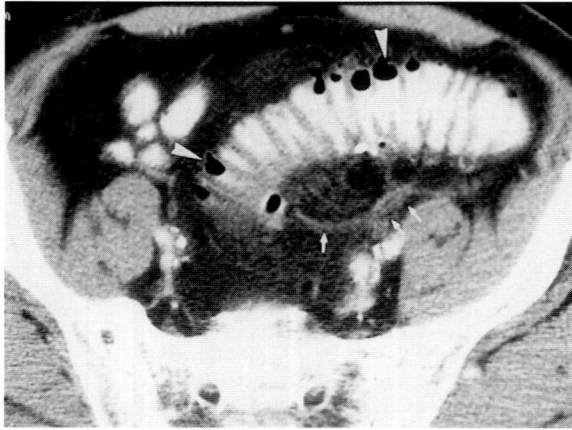

Fig. 2.30. Early sigmoid diverticulitis. Contrast-enhanced CT scan shows small air-filled intramural diverticula (*arrowheads*), streaky densities, and vascular engorgement (*arrows*) within sigmoid mesentery

CT findings of uncomplicated acute diverticulitis include colonic diverticula, mural thickening of the involved segment of colon, edema fluid at the base of the sigmoid mesentery, and engorged mesenteric vasculature (HULNICK et al. 1984; PADIDAR et al. 1994; CHO et al. 1990; BALTHAZAR et al. 1990).

The CT findings of complicated diverticulitis include paracolonic or pelvic abscesses (Fig. 2.31), peritonitis, free perforation, ureteral obstruction, or colovesical fistula (Fig. 2.32) (GOLDMAN et al. 1984). There are two main CT features that suggest the presence of a colovesical fistula: (a) an inflammatory mass encasing the sigmoid colon in close proximity to the bladder, and (b) air within the bladder (GOLDMAN et al. 1984). Although most commonly seen adjacent to the inflamed loop of bowel, diverticular abscesses may be seen into the abdominal wall, groin, or hip joint.

With the use of high-resolution thin-section and helical scanning techniques, the diagnostic sensitivity and specificity of CT are maximized. CHO et al. (1990) reviewed the CT and barium enema findings in 25 patients with sigmoid diverticulitis. CT demonstrated a higher diagnostic sensitivity than barium enema (93% vs 80%) and had a diagnostic specificity of 100%. However, CT findings in diverticulitis are nonspecific and in up to 10% of patients it may not be possible to exclude a perforated carcinoma (PADIDAR et al. 1994). Edema fluid at the root of the sigmoid mesentery and mesenteric vascular engorgement were found to be statistically more common in diverticulitis.

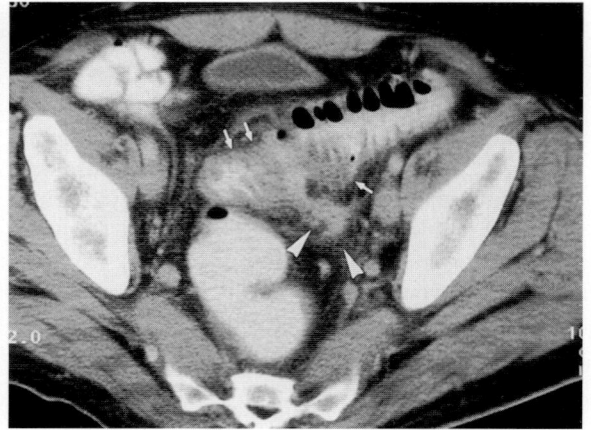

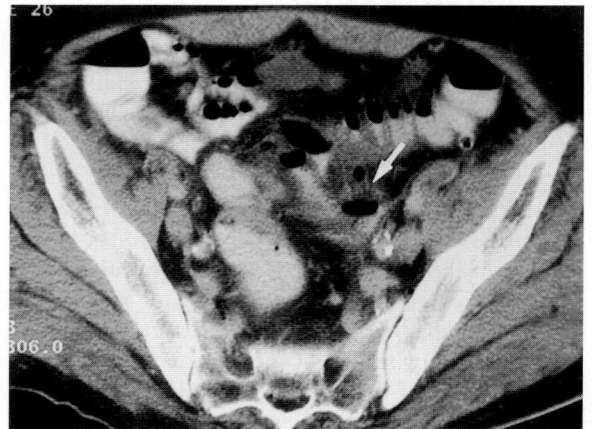

Fig. 2.31a,b. Complicated diverticulitis. **a** CT demonstrates focal wall thickening of the sigmoid colon (*arrows*) and inflammatory changes in the pericolic fat (*arrowheads*). **b** On a higher section, a small gas-containing abscess cavity (*arrow*) is present within sigmoid mesentery

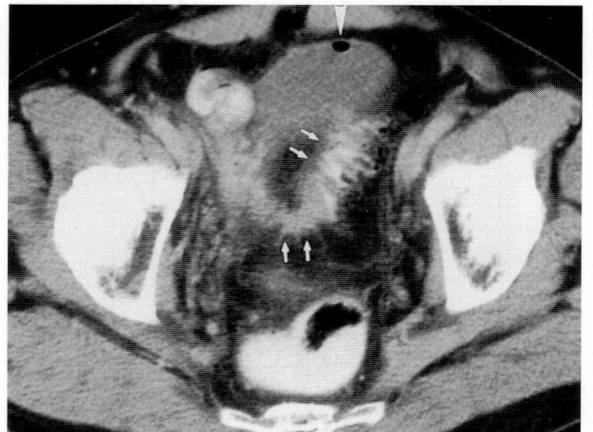

Fig. 2.32. Colovesical fistula. CT shows a thickened sigmoid colon (*arrows*) and a small amount of air in the bladder (*arrowhead*)

Currently CT is the diagnostic modality of choice for evaluating patients with suspected diverticulitis. It is less invasive than contrast enema, is better able to delineate the presence and severity of the pericolic inflammatory process, and has become an essential diagnostic tool for helping the clinician determine whether medical or surgical management is indicated (BIRNBAUM and BALTHAZAR 1994).

References

Allen KS, Siskind BN, Burrell MI (1986) Perforation of distal esophagus with lesser sac extension: CT demonstration. J Comput Assist Tomogr 10:612–614

Amin Z, Boulos PB, Lees WR (1996) Technical report: spiral CT pneumocolon for suspected colonic neoplasms. Clin Radiol 51:56–61

Angelelli G, Macarini L, Lupo L, Caputi-Jambrenghi O, Pannarale O, Memes V (1990) Rectal carcinoma: CT staging with water as contrast medium. Radiology 177:511–514

Backer CL, LoCicero J, Hartz RS, Donaldson JS, Shields T (1990) Computed tomography in patients with esophageal perforation. Chest 98:1078–1080

Baert AL, Roex L, Marchal G, Hermans P, Dewilde D, Wilms G (1989) Computed tomography of the stomach with water as an oral contrast agent: technique and preliminary results. J Comput Assist Tomogr 13:633–636

Balfe DM, Koehler RE, Karstaedt N, Stanley RJ, Sagel SS (1981) Computed tomography of gastric neoplasms. Radiology 140:431–436

Balthazar EJ (1991) CT of the gastrointestinal tract: principles and interpretation AJR 156:23–32

Balthazar EJ (1994) CT of small-bowel obstruction. AJR 162:225–261

Balthazar EJ, Megibow AJ, Hulnick D, Gordon RB, Naidich DP, Beranbaum ER (1986) CT of appendicitis. AJR 147:705–710

Balthazar EJ, Megibow AJ, Gordon RB, Whelan CA, Hulnick D (1988) Computed tomography of the abnormal appendix. J Comput Assist Tomogr 12:595–601

Balthazar EJ, Megibow AJ, Schinella RA, Gordon R (1990) Limitations in the CT diagnosis of acute diverticulitis: comparison of CT, contrast enema, and pathologic findings in 16 patients. AJR 154:281–285

Balthazar EJ, Megibow AJ, Siegel SE, Birnbaum BA (1991) Appendicitis: prospective evaluation with high-resolution CT. Radiology 180:21–24

Balthazar EJ, Birnbaum BA, Yee J, Megibow AJ, Roshkow J, Gray C (1994) Acute appendicitis: CT and US correlation in 100 patients. Radiology 190:31–35

Bashist B, Ellis K, Gold RP (1983) Computed tomography of intrathoracic goiters. AJR 140:455–460

Becker CD, Barbier PA, Terrier F, Porcellini B (1987) Patterns of recurrence of esophageal carcinoma after transhiatal esophagectomy and gastric interposition. AJR 148:273–277

Birnbaum BA, Balthazar EJ (1994) CT of appendicitis and diverticulitis. Radiol Clin North Am 32:885–898

Bluemke DA, Fishman EK, Anderson JH (1994) Dose requirements for a nonionic contrast agent for spiral computed tomography of the liver in rabbits. Invest Radiol 29:195–200

Butch RJ, Wittenberg J, Mueller PR, Simeone JF, Meyer JE, Ferrucci JT (1985) Presacral masses after abdomino-perineal resection for colorectal carcinoma: the need for needle biopsy. AJR 144:309–312

Carey LS (1980) Regional enteritis: the rubbery mesentery. J Can Assoc Radiol 31:269–270

Casola G, vanSonnenberg E, Neff CC, Saba RM, Withers C, Emarine CW (1987) Abscesses in Crohn disease: percutaneous drainage. Radiology 163:19–22

Cass AW, Million RR, Pfaff WW (1976) Patterns of recurrence following surgery alone for adenocarcinoma of the colon and rectum. Cancer 37:2861–2865

Cayea PD, Seltzer SE (1985) A new barium paste for computed tomography of the esophagus. J Comput Assist Tomogr 9:214–216

Chen YM, Ott DJ, Wolfman NT, Gelfand DW, Karsteadt N, Bechtold RE (1987) Recurrent colorectal carcinoma: evaluation with barium enema examination and CT. Radiology 163:307–310

Cho KC, Morehouse HT, Alterman DD, Thornhill BA (1990) Sigmoid diverticulitis: diagnostic role of CT – comparison with barium enema studies. Radiology 176:111–115

Cook AO, Levine BA, Sirinek KR, Gaskill HV (1986) Evaluation of gastric adenocarcinoma. Abdominal computed tomography does not replace celiotomy. Arch Surg 121:603–606

Cubillo E (1983) Obturator hernia diagnosed by computed tomography. AJR 140:735–736

Dixon AK, Fry IK, Morson BC, Nicholls RJ, Mason AV (1981) Pre-operative computed tomography of carcinoma of the rectum. Br J Radiol 54:655–659

Douglas M, Sistrom CL (1991) Chicken bone lodged in the upper esophagus: CT findings. Gastrointest Radiol 16:11–12

Eimiller A (1992) Complication in endoscopy. Endoscopy 24:176–184

Farah MC, Jafri SZ, Schwab RE, Mezwa DG, Francis IR, Noujaim S, Kim C (1987) Duodenal neoplasms: role of CT. Radiology 162:839–843

Federle MP, Chun G, Jeffrey RB, Rayor R (1984) Computed tomographic findings in bowel infarction. AJR 142:91–95

Fedyshin P, Kelvin FM, Rice RP (1984) Nonspecificity of barium enema findings in acute appendicitis. AJR 143:99–102

Fishman EK, Wolf EJ, Jones B, Bayless TM, Siegelman SS (1987) CT evaluation of Crohn's disease: effect on patient management. AJR 148:537–540

Flynn AE, Verrier ED, Way LW, Thomas AN, Pellegrini CA (1989) Esophageal perforation. Arch Surg 124:1211–1215

Frager DH, Goldman M, Beneventano TC (1983) Computed tomography in Crohn disease. J Comput Assist Tomogr 7:819–824

Frager DH, Medwid SW, Baer JW, Mollinelli B, Friedman M (1994) CT of small-bowel obstruction: value in establishing the diagnosis and determining the degree and cause. AJR 162:37–41

Freeny PC, Marks WM, Ryan JA, Bolen JW (1986) Colorectal carcinoma evaluation with CT: preoperative staging and detection of postoperative recurrence. Radiology 158:347–353

Gazelle GS, Goldberg MA, Wittenberg J, Halpern EF, Pinkney L, Mueller PR (1994) Efficacy of CT in distinguishing small-bowel obstruction from other causes of small-bowel dilatation. AJR 162:43–47

Geusens E, Verschakelen JA, Flamaing J, Bogaert J, Ponette E, Decramer M, Baert AL (1996) Esophageal tuberculosis mimicking malignancy. Eur Radiol 6:79–81

Ghahremani GG (1986) Iatrogenic gastrointestinal disorders. In: Taveras JM, Ferruci JT (eds) Radiology: diagnosis – imaging – intervention, vol 4. Lippincott, Philadelphia, pp 1–10

Glazer GM, Axel L, Moss AA (1982) CT diagnosis of mediastinal thyroid. AJR 138:495–498

Goldberg HI (1982) Computed tomographic evaluation of the gastrointestinal tract in diseases other than primary adenocarcinoma. In: Goldberg HI (ed) Interventional radiology and diagnostic imaging modality. University of California Press, San Francisco, pp 236–250

Goldberg HI, Gore RM, Margulis AR, Moss AA Baker EL (1983) Computed tomography in the evaluation of Crohn disease. AJR 140:277–282

Goldman SM, Fishman EK, Gatewood OM, Jones B, Brendler C, Siegelman SS (1984) CT demonstration of colovesical fistulae secondary to diverticulitis. J Comput Assist Tomogr 8:462–468

Gore RM (1987) Cross-sectional imaging of inflammatory bowel disease. Radiol Clin North Am 25:115–131

Gross BH, Agha FP, Glazer GM, Orringer MB (1985) Gastric interposition following transhiatal esophagectomy: CT evaluation. Radiology 155:177–179

Grumbach K, Levine MS, Wexler JA (1986) Gallstone ileus diagnosed by computed tomography. J Comput Assist Tomogr 10:146–148

Haaga JR, Alfidi RJ, Zelch MG, Meany TF, Boller M, Gonzales L, Jelden GL (1976) Computed tomography of the pancreas. Radiology 120:589–595

Halber MD, Daffner RH, Thompson WM (1979) CT of the esophagus. I. Normal appearance. AJR 133:1047–1050

Halvorsen RA Jr, Thompson WM (1984) Computed tomographic evaluation of esophageal carcinoma. Semin Oncol 11:113–126

Halvorsen RA Jr, Thompson WM (1987) Computed tomographic staging of gastrointestinal tract malignancies. I. Esophagus and stomach. Invest Radiol 22:2–16

Halvorsen RA Jr, Thompson WM (1989) CT of esophageal neoplasms. Radiol Clin North Am 27:667–685

Halvorsen RA Jr, Magruder-Habib K, Foster WL Jr, Roberts L Jr, Postlethwait RW, Thompson WM (1986) Esophageal cancer staging by CT: long-term follow-up study. Radiology 161:147–151

Heiken JP, Balfe DM, Roper CL (1984) CT evaluation after esophagogastrectomy. AJR 143:555–560

Heiken JP, Brink JA, Vannier MW (1993) Spiral (helical) CT. Radiology 189:647–656

Hulnick DH (1986) CT of the small intestine. In: Megibow A, Balthazar EJ (eds) CT of the gastrointestinal tract. Mosby, St. Louis, pp 217–278

Hulnick DH, Megibow AJ, Balthazar EJ, Naidich DP, Bosniak MA (1984) Computed tomography in the evaluation of diverticulitis. Radiology 152:491–495

Jeffrey RB, Ralls PW (1996) CT and sonography of the acute abdomen, 2nd edn. Lippincott-Raven, Philadelphia, pp 308–312

Jones B, Fishman EK, Kramer SS, et al. (1986) Computed tomography of gastrointestinal inflammation after bone marrow transplantation. AJR 146:691–695

Jost RG, Sagel SS, Stanley RJ, Levitt RG (1978) Computed tomography of the thorax. Radiology 126:125–136

Kalender WA (1994) Technical foundations of spiral CT. Semin Ultrasound CT MR 15:81–89

Kalender WA, Seissler W, Klotz E, Vock P (1990) Spiral volumetric CT with single-breath-hold technique, continuous transport, and continuous scanner rotation. Radiology 176:181–183

Kane NM, Francis IR, Burney RE, Wheatley MJ, Ellis JH, Korobkin M (1991) Traumatic pneumoperitoneum. Implications of computed tomography diagnosis. Invest Radiol 26:574–578

Kazerooni EA, Quint LE, Francis IR (1992) Duodenal neoplasms: predictive value of CT for determining malignancy and tumor resectability. AJR 159:303–309

Kelvin FM, Maglinte DD (1987) Colorectal carcinoma: a radiologic and clinical review. Radiology 164:1–8

Kelvin FM, Korobkin M, Heaston DK, Grant JP, Akwari O (1983) The pelvis after surgery for rectal carcinoma: serial CT observations with emphasis on non-neoplastic features. AJR 141:959–964

Kerner BA, Oliver GC, Eisenstat TE, Rubin RJ, Salvati EP (1993) Is preoperative computerized tomography useful in assessing patients with colorectal carcinoma? Dis Colon Rectum 36:1050–1053

Kim-Deobald J, Kozarek RA (1992) Esophageal perforation: an 8-year review of a multispecialty clinic's experience. Am J Gastroenterol 87:1112–1119

Kleinhaus U, Militianu D (1988) Computed tomography in the preoperative evaluation of gastric carcinoma. Gastrointest Radiol 13:97–101

Komaki S, Toyoshima S (1983) CT's capability in detecting gastric cancer. Gastrointest Radiol 8:307–313

Kuhlman JE, Fishman EK, Wang KP, Siegelman SS (1985) Esophageal duplication cyst: CT and transesophageal needle aspiration. AJR 145:531–532

Lambiase RE, Cronan JJ, Dorfman GS, Paolella LP, Haas RA (1988) Percutaneous drainage of abscesses in patients with Crohn disease. AJR 150:1043–1045

Lee KR, Levine E, Moffat RE, Bigongiari LR, Hermreck AS (1979) Computed tomographic staging of malignant gastric neoplasms. Radiology 133:151–155

Lewis FR, Holcroft JW, Boey J, Dunphy JE (1975) Appendicitis: a critical review of diagnosis and treatment in 1000 cases. Arch Surg 110:667–684

Li DK, Rennie CS (1981) Abdominal computed tomography in Whipple's disease. J Comput Assist Tomogr 5:249–252

Maglinte DD, Gage SH, Harmon BH, et al. (1993) Obstruction of the small intestine: accuracy and role of CT in diagnosis. Radiology 188:61–64

Malone AJ Jr, Wolf CR, Malmed AS, Melliere BF (1993) Diagnosis of acute appendicitis: value of unenhanced CT. AJR 160:763–766

Marks WM, Callen PW, Moss AA (1981) Gastroesophageal region: source of contusion on CT. AJR 136:359–362

Marx JA, Moore EE, Jorden RC, Eule J Jr (1985) Limitations of computed tomography in the evaluation of acute abdominal trauma: a prospective comparison with diagnostic peritoneal lavage. J Trauma 25:933–937

Matos C, Van Gansbeke D, Zalcman M, Ansay J, Delcour C, Engelholm L, Struyven J (1986) Mesenteric vein thrombosis: early CT and US diagnosis and conservative management. Gastrointest Radiol 11:322–325

Megibow AJ (1986) CT of the duodenum. In: Megibow A, Balthazar EJ (eds) CT of the gastrointestinal tract. Mosby, St. Louis, pp 175–216

Megibow AJ (1994) Bowel obstruction. Evaluation with CT. Radiol Clin North Am 32:861–870

Megibow AJ, Bosniak MA (1980) Dilute barium as a contrast agent for abdominal CT. AJR 134:1273–1274

Megibow AJ, Balthazar EJ, Naidich DP, Bosniak MA (1983) Computed tomography of gastrointestinal lymphoma. AJR 141:541–547

Megibow AJ, Zerhouni EA, Hulnick DH, Beranbaum ER, Balthazar EJ (1984) Air insufflation of the colon as an adjunct to computed tomography of the pelvis. J Comput Assist Tomogr 8:797–800

Megibow AJ, Balthazar EJ, Hulnick DH, Naidich DP, Bosniak MA (1985) CT evaluation of gastrointestinal leiomyomas and leiomyosarcomas. AJR 144:727–731

Meyers MA, McGuire PV (1995) Spiral CT demonstration of hypervascularity in Crohn disease: vascular jejunization of the ileum or the comb sign. Abdom Imaging 20:327–332

Meyers MA, Oliphant M (1974) Ascending retrocecal appendicitis. Radiology 110:295–299

Mindell HJ (1989) On the value of non-contrast CT in blunt abdominal trauma. AJR 152:47

Mirvis SE, Gens DR, Shanmuganathan K (1992) Rupture of the bowel after blunt abdominal trauma: diagnosis with CT. AJR 159:1217–1221

Mohamed G, Reyes HM, Fantus R, Ramilo J, Radhakrishnan J (1986) Computed tomography in the assessment of pediatric abdominal trauma. Arch Surg 121:703–707

Moss AA (1992) Computed tomography of the body, 2nd edn., vol III. Saunders, Philadelphia, pp 643–734

Moss AA, Schnyder P, Candardjis G, Margulis AR (1980) Computed tomography of benign and malignant gastric abnormalities. J Clin Gastroenterol 2:401–409

Moss AA, Schnyder P, Marks W, Margulis AR (1981a) Gastric adenocarcinoma: a commparison of the accuracy and economics of staging by computed tomography and surgery. Gastroenterology 80:45–50

Moss AA, Schnyder P, Thoeni RF, Margulis AR (1981b) Esophageal carcinoma: pretherapy staging by computed tomography. AJR 136:1051–1056

Moss AA, Thoeni RF, Schnyder P, Margulus AR (1981c) Value of computed tomography in the detection and staging of recurrent rectal carcinomas. J Comput Assist Tomogr 5:870–874

Moss AA, Schnyder P, Margulis AR (1982) Computed tomographic evaluation of esophageal and gastric tumors. In: Goldberg HE (ed) Interventional radiology and diagnostic imaging modalities. University of California Press, San Francisco, pp 215–225

Mullin D, Shirkhoda A (1985) Computed tomography after gastrectomy in primary gastric carcinoma. J Comput Assist Tomogr 9:30–33

Nakajima T, Ishihara S, Motohashi H, et al. (1994) Neoadjuvant chemotherapy for inoperable gastric cancer in local and general delivery routes (FLEP therapy). In: Banzet P, Holland JF, Khayat D, et al. (eds) Cancer treatment: an update. Springer, Berlin Heidelberg New York, p 411

Ng VW, Husband JE, Nicolson VM, Minty I, Bamias A (1996) CT evaluation of treatment response in advanced gastric cancer. Clin Radiol 51:215–220

Nghiem HV, Jeffrey RB Jr, Mindelzun RE (1993) CT of blunt trauma to the bowel and mesentery. AJR 160:53–58

Olson RM, Perencevich NP, Malcolm AW, Chaffey JT, Wilson RE (1980) Patterns of recurrence following curative resection of adenocarcinoma of the colon and rectum. Cancer 45:2969–2974

Orel SG, Rubesin SE, Jones B, Fishman EK, Bayless TM, Siegelman SS (1987) Computed tomography vs barium studies in the acutely symptomatic patient with Crohn disease. J Comput Assist Tomogr 11:1009–1016

Osteen R, Guyton S, Steele G Jr, Wilson RE (1980) Malignant intestinal obstruction. Surgery 87:611–615

Padidar AM, Jeffrey RB Jr, Mindelzun RE, Dolph JF (1994) Differentiating sigmoid diverticulitis from carcinoma on CT scans: mesenteric inflammation suggests diverticulitis. AJR 163:81–83

Perez C, Llauger J, Puig J, Palma J (1989) Computed tomographic findings in bowel ischemia. Gastrointest Radiol 14:241–245

Picus D, Balfe DM, Koehler RE, Roper CL, Owen JW (1983) Computed tomography in the staging of esophageal carcinoma. Radiology 146:433–438

Picus D, Glazer HS, Levitt RG, Husband JE (1984) Computed tomography of abdominal carcinoid tumors. AJR 143:581–584

Polacin A, Kalender WA, Marchal G (1992) Evaluation of section sensitivity profiles and image noise in spiral CT. Radiology 185:29–35

Pugatch RD, Faling LJ, Robbins AH, Spira R (1980) CT diagnosis of benign mediastinal abnormalities. AJR 134:685–694

Quint LE, Glazer GM, Orringer MB, Gross BH (1985) Esophageal carcinoma: CT findings. Radiology 155:171–175

Reznek RH, White FE, Young JW, Fry IK, Nicholls RJ (1983) The appearances on computed tomography after abdomino-perineal resection for carcinoma of the rectum: a comparison between the normal appearances and those of recurrence. Br J Radiol 56:237–240

Richter von GM, Düx M, Roeren T, Heuschen U, Kauffmann GW (1996) Gastrointestinale Disgnostik mit Hydrosonographie und Hydro-CT. Fortschr Röntgenstr 164:281–289

Rubesin SE, Herlinger H (1991) CT evaluation of bowel obstruction: a landmark article: implications for the future. Radiology 180:307–308

Rubin GD, Dake MD, Napel SA, McDonnell CH, Jeffrey RB Jr (1993) Three-dimensional spiral CT angiography of the abdomen: initial clinical experience. Radiology 186:147–152

Samuelsson L, Hambraeus GM, Mercke CE, Tylen U (1984) CT staging of oesophageal carcinoma. Acta Radiol Diagn (Stockh) 25:7–11

Scatarige JC, DiSantis DJ (1989) CT of the stomach and duodenum. Radiol Clin North Am 27:687–706

Scatarige JC, Fishman EK, Jones B, Cameron JL, Sanders RC, Siegelman SS (1985) Gastric leiomyosarcoma: CT observations. J Comput Assist Tomogr 9:320–327

Schlesinger AE, Leiter BE, Connors SK (1984) Computed tomography diagnosis of right aortic arch with an aberrant left innominate artery. J Comput Assist Tomogr 8:81–87

Schnur MJ, Weiner SN (1982) The string sign on computerized tomography. Gastrointest Radiol 7:43–46

Silverman PM, Cooper C, Trock B, Garra BS, Davros WJ, Zeman RK (1995) The optimal temporal window for CT of the liver using a time-density anaysis: implications for helical (spiral) CT. J Comput Assist Tomogr 19:73–79

Sones PJ Jr, Torres WE, Colvin RS, Meier WL, Sprawls P, Roger JV Jr (1982) Effectiveness of CT in evaluating intrathoracic masses. AJR 139:469–475

Srinivasan MK, Scholz FJ (1980) Hemiazygos vein as a cause of posterior indentation of the esophagus: a case report. Gastrointest Radiol 5:13–15

Stevenson G (1995) Radiology in the detection and prevention of colorectal cancer. Eur J Cancer 31A:1121–1126

Sussman DK, Halvorsen RA Jr, Illescas FF, et al. (1988) Gastric adenocarcinoma: CT versus surgical staging. Radiology 167:335–340

Takashima S, Takeuchi N, Shiozaki H, et al. (1991) Carcinoma of the esophagus: CT vs MR imaging in determining resectability. AJR 156:297–302

Thompson WM, Halvorsen RA, Williford ME (1982) Computed tomography of the gastroesophageal junction. Radiographics 2:179–194

Thompson WM, Halvorsen RA, Foster WL Jr, Roberts L, Gibbons R (1986) Preoperative and postoperative CT staging of rectosigmoid carcinoma. AJR 146:703–710

Tsuda K, Hori S, Murakami T, Nakamura H, Tomoda K, Nakanishi K, Shiozaki H (1995) Intramural invasion of gastric cancer: evaluation by CT with water-filling method. J Comput Assist Tomogr 19:941–947

Van Hoe L, Baert AL, Marchal G, Spitz B, Penninckx F (1994) Thrombosed ovarian vein collateral mimicking acute appendicitis on CT. J Comput Assist Tomogr 18:643–646

Vilgrain V, Mompoint D, Palazzo L, et al. (1990) Staging of esophageal carcinoma: comparison of results with endoscopic sonography and CT. AJR 155:277–281

Wolfman NT, Scharling ES, Chen MY (1994) Esophageal squamous carcinoma. Radiol Clin North Am 32:1183–1201

Zeman RK, Fox SH, Silverman PM, et al. (1993) Helical (spiral) CT of the abdomen. AJR 160:719–725

3 Magnetic Resonance Imaging of the Alimentary Tube

S.M. Ascher

CONTENTS

3.1
Introduction

Magnetic resonance imaging (MRI) of the alimentary tube became feasible as techniques to (a) arrest bowel motion, (b) remove competing high signal intensity of adjacent fat, (c) increase the dynamic range of intra-abdominal signal intensities, and (d) decrease susceptibility artifacts became widespread. Specifically, fat suppression, breath-hold gradient echo, single-shot echo train T2-weighted sequences, and intravenous gadolinium chelates have all contributed to this endeavor (SEMELKA et al. 1991). Controversy still exists, however, over which oral contrast agent, if any, is necessary for performing diagnostic studies.

This chapter will review current MRI techniques and highlight the MRI findings in congenital, inflammatory, benign, and malignant gastrointestinal processes. A brief discussion of oral agents will be presented at the end.

S.M. ASCHER, MD, Associate Professor of Radiology, Director, Body MRI, Department of Radiology, Georgetown University Medical Center, 3800 Reservoir Road, NW, Washington DC 20007-2197, USA

3.2
Magnetic Resonance Imaging Technique

3.2.1
General Guidelines

To insure reproducible, high-quality gastrointestinal MRI examinations, bowel motion secondary to respiration and/or peristalsis must be, at the very least, limited and preferably eliminated. Many centers have adopted the routine administration of intramuscular glucagon prior to imaging. While this is effective, up to one-third of patients may experience one or more side-effects, including nausea, diaphoresis, and hypotension (CHERNISH and MAGLINTE 1990). Moreover, in a significant number of patients glucagon is contraindicated (e.g., those with diabetes mellitus). As an alternative, fasting patients for at least 4–6h prior to imaging achieves consistent bowel hypotonicity and is well tolerated.

While many regions of the alimentary tube are amenable to imaging with the system's body coil, the widely available phased-array torso surface coil results in improved spatial resolution when employing smaller fields of view and/or increased matrix size (SMITH et al. 1992; HAYES et al. 1992). However, because of the coil's near field sensitivity profile, high signal intensity fat and motion-related phase ghosting may obscure thorough evaluation of certain bowel segments (MCCAULEY et al. 1992). Techniques to moderate this effect include: (a) placement of nonselective saturation pulses over the subcutaneous fat, (b) employment of fat suppression sequences, (c) use of breath-hold sequences, (d) swapping phase and frequency directions, and/or (e) postprocessing the data with a filter to homogenize the signal intensities (OUTWATER and MITCHELL 1994; TEMPANY and FIELDING 1996).

Our preferred imaging protocol includes: (a) precontrast T1-weighted fat-suppressed spin echo (SE) or breath-hold fat-suppressed T1-weighted spoiled gradient echo (SGE), (b) immediate postgadolinium chelate T1-weighted SGE (preferably fat suppressed), (c) 2-min postcontrast T1-weighted fat-suppressed SE or SGE, and (d) T2-weighted (preferably fat-suppressed) SE in select cases. Breath-hold imaging is employed whenever possible as it eliminates respiratory artifact. The long imaging times associated with conventional and even fast T2-weighted SE sequences limit their routine use when evaluating the alimentary tube; however, the advent of half Fourier single-shot turbo spin echo (HASTE) makes high-quality T2-weighted imaging of the bowel possible. The advantages of this sequence include: (a) minimal susceptibility artifact (ideal for gas-filled bowel and in the presence of metal clips), (b) minimal chemical shift artifact, and (c) short acquisition time (1 s/slice, which overcomes the need for sus-

pended respiration). Clinical applications of HASTE are currently under investigation and appear promising (SEMELKA et al. 1996a,b) (Fig. 3.1). Non-breath-hold T2-weighted fast SE sequences are reserved for evaluating the rectum and pelvic organs, and the liver for metastatic disease.

Intravenous gadolinium chelates (Gd) (0.1 mmol/kg) are useful in the evaluation of bowel disease. Images are acquired immediately and at 2 min after contrast administration. This facilitates identification of abnormalities of both capillary blood flow and interstitial accumulation, respectively. Fat suppression increases the conspicuity of abnormal bowel enhancement by removing the competing high signal intensity fat adjacent to the involved bowel segment.

3.2.2
Special Considerations for Specific Bowel Segments

3.2.2.1
Esophagus (Fig. 3.2)

Cardiac pulsations in the phase encode direction degrade esophageal image quality. A saturation band across the heart and/or cardiac gating helps limit this. Cardiac gated gadolinium-enhanced fat-suppressed images demonstrate the esophageal wall well, allowing assessment of esophageal disease including spread to the mediastinum.

3.2.2.2
Stomach (Fig. 3.2)

Gadolinium-enhanced fat-suppressed imaging of the stomach highlights both normal anatomy and gastric disease processes (SEMELKA et al. 1991; HAMED et al. 1992). Distending the stomach with water or another oral agent improves assessment. Since gastric mucosa enhances more than other bowel mucosa, its presence in a Meckel's diverticulum or duplication cyst is well demonstrated. Gastric morphology is highlighted on T2-weighted HASTE images.

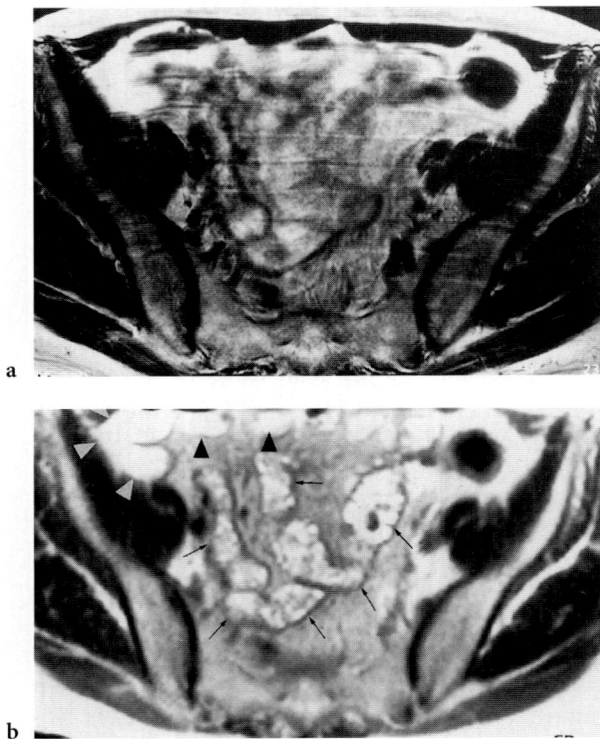

Fig. 3.1. Axial high-resolution T2-weighted fast SE (**a**) and T2-weighted HASTE (**b**) images in the same patient at a comparable location. The longer acquisition times of fast SE sequences are susceptible to respiratory and peristaltic motion. This in turn leads to ghosting and blurring (**a**). In contrast, motion-independent HASTE provides reproducible high-quality T2-weighted images of the alimentary tube. The fluid-filled small (*arrows*, **b**) and large bowel (*arrowheads*, **b**) are well seen

3.2.2.3
Small Bowel (Fig. 3.2)

Successful imaging of the small intestine requires routine fasting or use of an antiperistaltic agent;

pathologic processes will only be reliably seen when the small bowel is immobilized. The combined use of fat suppression and intravenous gadolinium is sensitive for the detection of bowel wall inflammatory or neoplastic disorders (SEMELKA et al. 1991; SHOENUT et al. 1994, 1993a). T2-weighted HASTE appears promising in the evaluation of small bowel pathology, especially neoplasms (SEMELKA et al. 1996b).

3.2.2.4
Large Bowel (Fig. 3.2)

Techniques for imaging the colon parallel those for imaging the small bowel. Gadolinium-enhanced fat suppression is the mainstay of diagnosis. The rectal wall layers are clearly delineated on this sequence. The rectum, with its relatively fixed position, is also amenable to the longer acquisition times of T2-weighted fast SE sequences. T2-weighted images can provide useful information concerning: (a) intrinsic bowel pathology, (b) the relationship between the colonic process and adjacent pelvic viscera and sacrum, and (c) the appearance of recurrent carcinoma versus radiation fibrosis in the post- and perioperative state. Endorectal surface coils optimize spatial and contrast resolution and have had success in demonstrating the rectal wall layers, the anal sphincter complex, and tumors (CHAN et al. 1991; SCHNALL et al. 1994; HUSSAIN et al. 1995). Some investigators favor instilling rectal contrast when using the endorectal coil to improve detection of mucosal abnormalities.

3.3
Disease Processes

3.3.1
Congenital Abnormalities

3.3.1.1
Malrotation

Malrotation is the failure of normal intestinal rotation and fixation. Since the duodenojejunal and cecocolic segments rotate independently, a spectrum of malrotation exists. If the normal process is arrested, nonrotation or incomplete rotation results, whereas if the process proceeds aberrantly, reversed rotation or anomalous fixation/fusion of the mesenteries results. Nonrotation is the most common of

the malrotation abnormalities. It is recognized on tomographic images by noting that the third and fourth portions of the duodenum do not cross the aorta anteriorly.

3.3.1.2
Meckel's Diverticulum

Meckel's diverticulum, a persistent omphalomesenteric duct remnant, is the most common anomaly of the alimentary tube, with a prevalence of about 2% in the general population. It occurs along the antimesenteric border of the ileum, within 1 m of the ileocecal valve. Twenty percent of patients may be symptomatic and experience obstruction secondary to intussusception and/or inflammation. If the diverticulum contains gastric mucosa, ulceration and bleeding may result. Small bowel enema (enteroclysis) and technetium-99 m pertechnetate scintigraphy are the most sensitive imaging examinations to detect Meckel's diverticulum. Contrast-enhanced MRI, like scintigraphy, may detect the presence of a diverticulum if it is lined by gastric mucosa. Specifically, the gastric mucosa of the diverticulum will enhance more than that of the adjacent large or small bowel on the capillary phase of imaging (CHEW and ZAMBUTO 1992) (Fig. 3.3).

3.3.1.3
Duplication Cysts

Mucosal lined gastrointestinal duplication cysts occur throughout the alimentary tube. They reside in or adjacent to a wall of bowel. Their mucosal lining may not be the same as that of the involved segment. Duplication cysts usually present in infancy or childhood with mass effect, infection, peptic ulcer, or pancreatitis. The latter two occur if the cyst contains gastric mucosa or pancreatic tissue, respectively. MRI has been used to demonstrate duplication cysts, especially if barium study or ultrasonography is inconclusive. The cyst's contents are often proteinaceous and are higher in signal than simple fluid on T1-weighted images. The cyst wall may have variable signal intensity (MACPHERSON 1993). Following intravenous gadolinium chelate, the cyst wall enhances while the fluid-filled lumen remains signal void. A gastric mucosa-lined cyst will enhance more than other types of duplication cysts and can suggest the correct diagnosis.

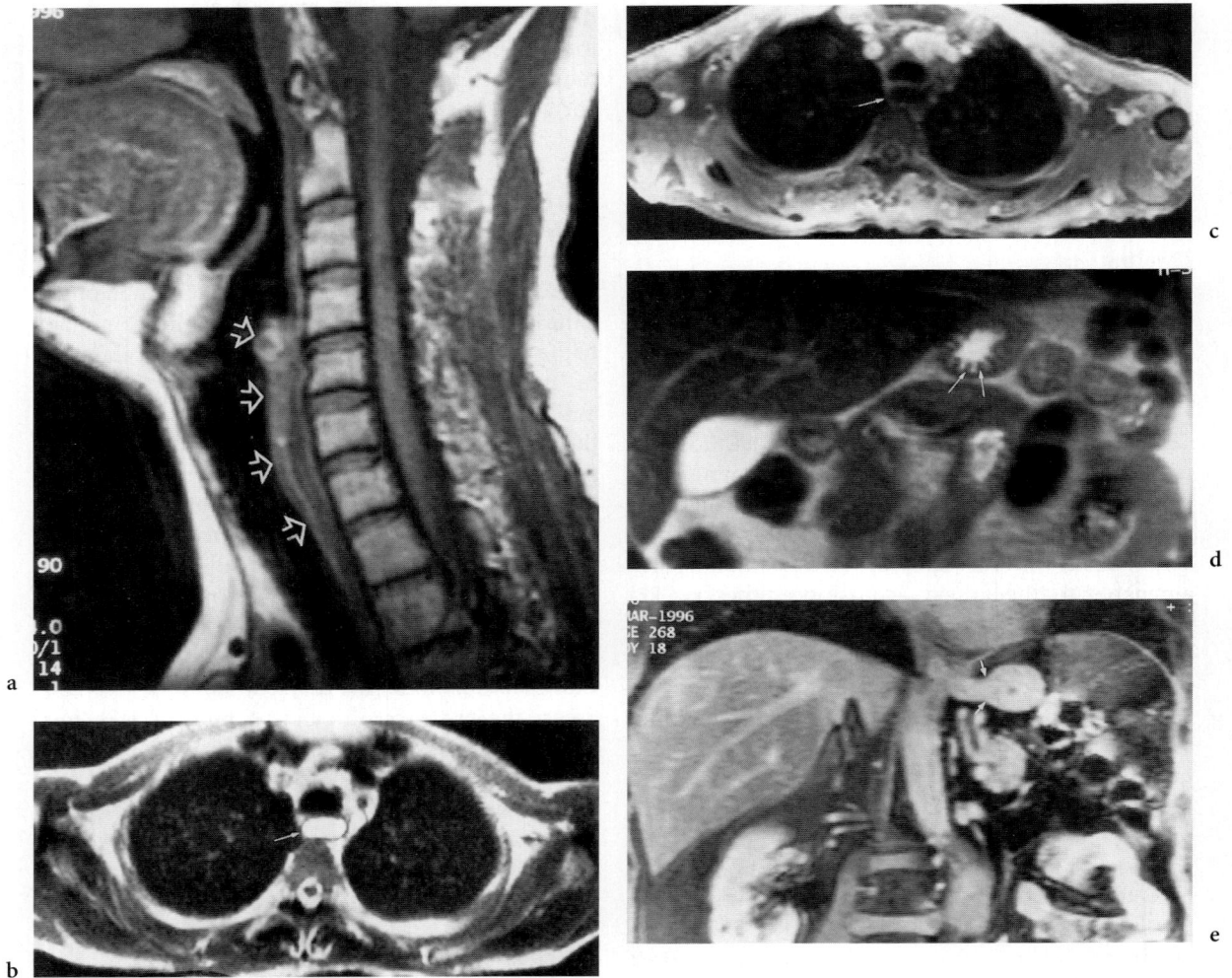

Fig. 3.2a–k. Normal anatomy. **a** Sagittal gadolinium-enhanced T1-weighted SGE, **b** axial T2-weighted HASTE, and **c** transverse gadolinium-enhanced T1-weighted fat-suppressed SGE images of the normal esophagus. The normal esophagus is usually collapsed (*open arrows*, **a**); however, it may be distended by air or fluid, especially if there is a distal obstruction. The T2-weighted HASTE image illustrates the fluid-filled thin-walled esophagus (*solid arrow*, **b**) in a patient with an obstructing carcinoma at the gastroesophageal junction. Following contrast there is normal mural enhancement (*solid arrow*, **c**). **d** Coronal T2-weighted HASTE of the collapsed stomach shows normal rugae (*arrows*). **e** Coronal and **f** axial gadolinium-enhanced T1-weighted fat-suppressed SGE of the stomach. The enhancing gastroesophageal junction (*arrows*, **e**) is well seen. Note that the gastric mucosa enhances more than other bowel segments (*arrow*, **f**). Gastric distension is mandatory to assess the stomach wall; in this case a negative oral agent was ingested (**f**). **g–j** Axial (**g,h**) and sagittal (**i**) T2-weighted HASTE and coronal gadolinium-enhanced T1-weighted fat-suppressed SFE (**j**) of the small (*arrows*, **g–j**) and large (*arrowheads*, **g–j**) bowel. T2-weighted HASTE images excel at demonstrating air- and fluid-filled structures and allow superior visualization of the bowel wall including the valvulae conniventes and haustra. Portions of the duodenum, ileum and jejunum are highlighted. Note how well the terminal ileum (*arrows*, **h**) and cecum (*arrowheads*, **h**) are demonstrated. Following contrast, the walls of the alimentary tube enhance, including the stomach (*curved arrow*, **j**), duodenum (*arrows*, **j**) duodenal diverticulum (*open arrow*, **j**), and right colon (*arrowheads*, **j**). Incidental note is made of an abdominal aortic aneurysm (*aaa*, **j**). **k** Axial gadolinium-enhanced T1-weighted fat-suppressed SGE image of the normal rectum. The combination of intravenous contrast and fat suppression increase the conspicuity of the different rectal wall layers (from outer to inner): low signal intensity muscularis propria (*short arrows*, **k**), high signal intensity submucosa, low signal intensity muscularis mucosae and lamina propria (*long arrow*, **k**), and high signal intensity mucosa

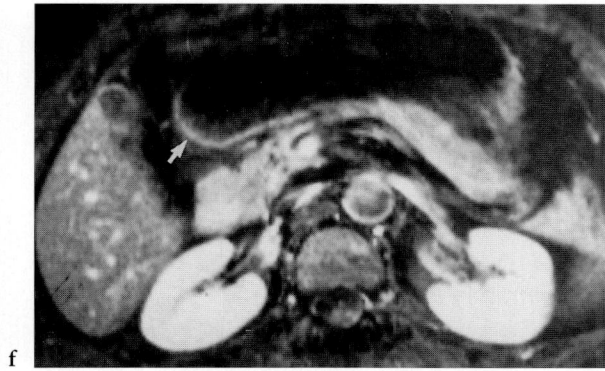

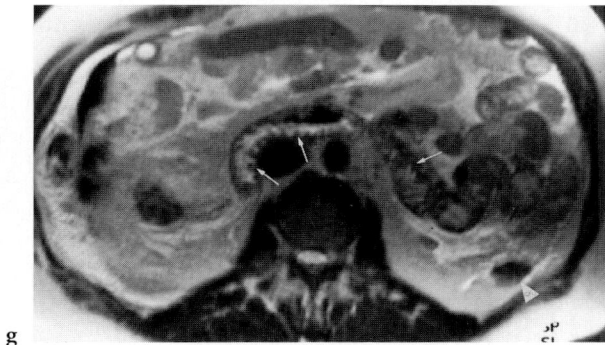

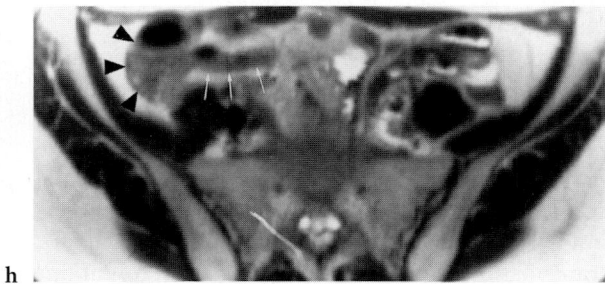

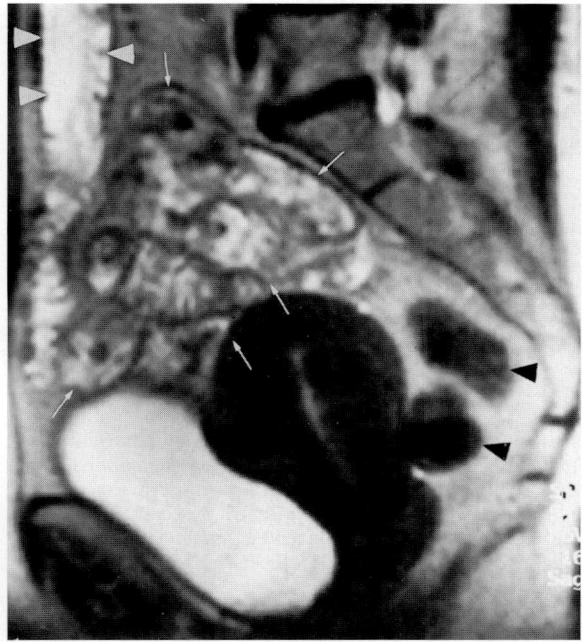

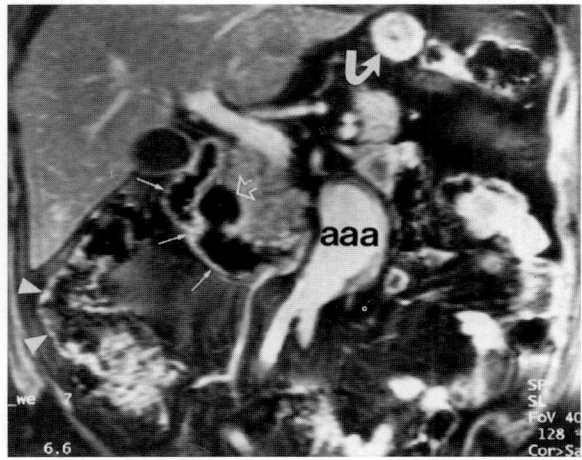

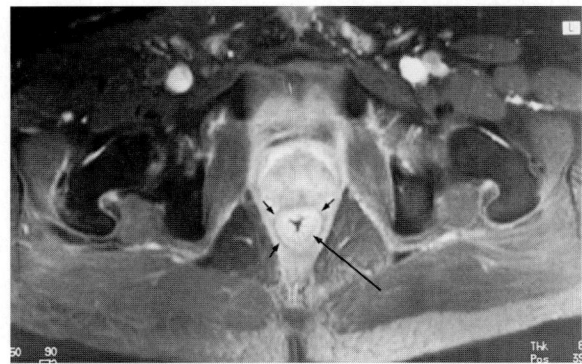

Fig. 3.2a–k. *Continued*

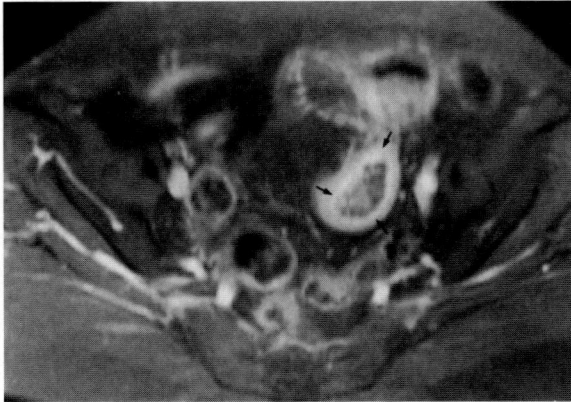

Fig. 3.3. Meckel's diverticulum. Axial gadolinium-enhanced T1-weighted fat-suppressed SE image shows a blinded ended loop originating from the ileum. The marked mucosal enhancement (*arrows*) suggests a gastric-lined structure. Both the location and the enhancement characteristics aid the diagnosis of a gastric-lined Meckel's diverticulum. (From Shoenut et al. 1993d).

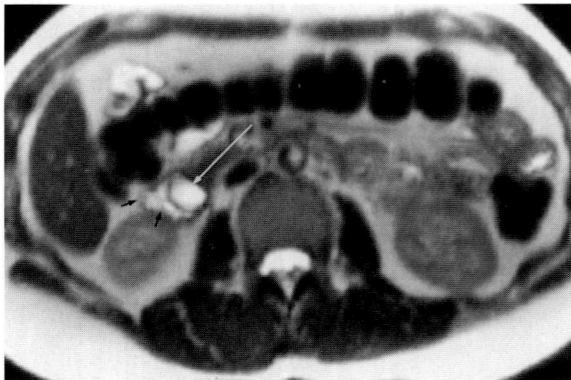

Fig. 3.4. Choledochocele. Axial T2-weighted HASTE shows a fluid-filled cystic structure (*long arrow*) protruding into the duodenum (*short arrows*); this structure proved to be a choledochocele

3.3.1.4
Choledochocele

Choledochocele is a congenital anomaly characterized by cystic dilation of the distal common bile duct near the papilla. It may be associated with abdominal pain, bleeding, jaundice, and pancreatitis. The diverticulum can contain calculi. On diagnostic examinations a choledochocele may mimic papillary edema or carcinoma. When large enough, a choledochocele can protrude into the duodenum and even occlude it. MR cholangiopancreatography (MRCP) and T2-weighted HASTE images facilitate the correct diag-

nosis: a smooth-walled cyst that resides in the duodenum and communicates with the biliary tree (Fig. 3.4).

3.3.2
Inflammation

3.3.2.1
Inflammatory Bowel Disease

Ulcerative colitis and Crohn's disease are the two most common forms of inflammatory bowel disease (IBD) (SHOENUT et al. 1994). Traditionally, patients have been studied with barium examinations, CT, and/or endoscopy; however, MRI is emerging as an imaging alternative. Investigators have found that MRI correlates well with clinical evaluation, endoscopy, and histologic findings (SHOENUT et al. 1993a, 1994; KETTRITZ et al. 1995). These investigators conclude that MRI is promising for diagnosing the type of IBD, for evaluating its severity, and for monitoring response to treatment.

3.3.2.1.1
CROHN'S DISEASE

Crohn's disease is a nonspecific inflammatory process. While any portion of the gastrointestinal tract may be involved, the small bowel is the site of predilection. Crohn's disease occurs in families and has an increased incidence in peoples of Jewish descent. The etiology of Crohn's disease is unknown, but it is probably multifactorial, with genetic factors, transmissible infectious agents, and autoimmune phenomena all being implicated (SPIRO 1993). Patients with Crohn's disease usually present in young adulthood, though onset after age 50 is not unusual. Nonbloody diarrhea, abdominal pain, fever, and weight loss are the most common symptoms.

The distribution of Crohn's disease includes isolated terminal ileum involvement in 30% of patients, synchronous ileal and cecal involvement in 40%, and isolated colon involvement in 20%. When disease is restricted to the colon, differentiation from ulcerative colitis may be difficult (GOLDBERG et al. 1979). Patients with Crohn's disease are at increased risk for developing colon carcinoma.

Crohn's disease is a transmural process characterized by noncaseating granulomas and prominent lymphoid tissue. There is also an associated nonspecific cellular infiltrate. Grossly, aphthous ulcers are one of the earliest manifestations of the disease.

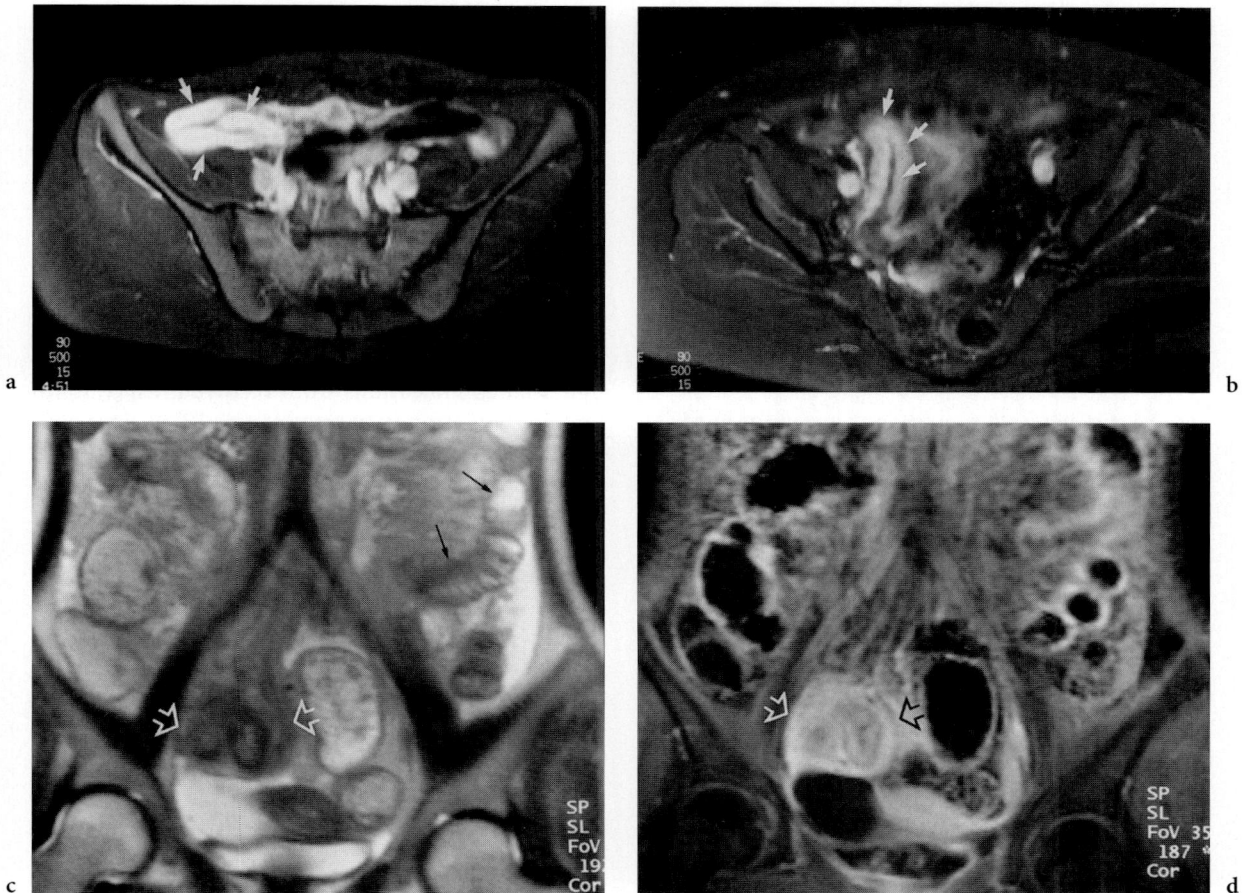

Fig. 3.5a–d. Crohn's disease. **a,b** Gadolinium-enhanced T1-weighted fat-suppressed SGE images characterize the usual findings in two patients with Crohn's disease: bowel wall thickening with transmural enhancement of the involved ileum (*arrows*). **c** Coronal T2-weighted HASTE and **d** gadolinium-enhanced T1-weighted fat-suppressed SGE images in another patient with Crohn's disease. The develop-ment of breathing-independent T2-weighted HASTE allows routine high-quality T2-weighted sequences of the bowel to be obtained. Two adjacent distal ileal loops are thickened (*open arrows*, **c**) compared with disease-free proximal segments (*arrows*, **c**). Similarly, the inflamed and thick-walled ileum demonstrates marked transmural enhancement (*open arrows*, **d**), the hallmark of Crohn's disease

With time the ulcers coalesce to form a system of deep fissures that track transmurally and extend beyond the bowel into adjacent tissues. The bowel wall becomes thickened from fibrosis and edema. Excess mesenteric fat envelops the diseased segments of bowel. Disease is segmental in distribution and skip regions are common. Complications of Crohn's disease include: strictures, sinus tracts, fistulae, abscesses, and inflammatory lymph nodes. Medical therapy is the mainstay of treatment. Surgery is reserved for complications refractive to conservative management; postoperative recurrence is common.

Crohn's disease and its complications are well imaged by MRI. The transmural involvement, skip lesions, and mesenteric inflammatory changes are amenable to gadolinium-enhanced fat-suppressed techniques. Full-thickness bowel wall involvement is circumferential but asymmetric. The most common appearance of Crohn's disease on MR images is a thickened terminal ileum, asymmetric cecal involvement, and transmural enhancement following intravenous contrast (SHOENUT et al. 1993a) (Fig. 3.5). Rectal sparing, sinus tracts, fistulae, abscesses, and strictures are ancillary findings. Inflammatory stranding secondary to dilated vasa rectae and sinus tracts, a profusion of lymph nodes, and abundant fat characterize the mesenteric findings. The MRI features of Crohn's colitis are similar to its small bowel findings. Transmural involvement helps distinguish

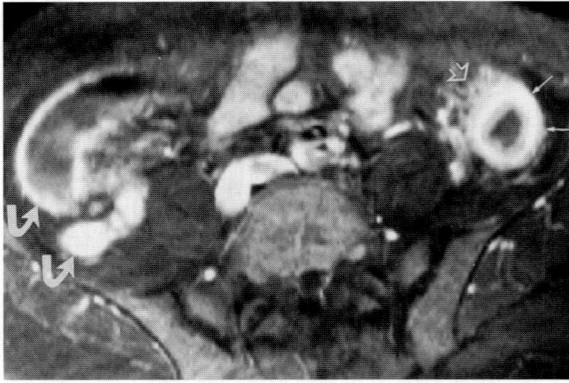

Fig. 3.6. Crohn's colitis. Axial gadolinium-enhanced T1-weighted fat-suppressed SGE in a patient with Crohn's colitis. The findings of Crohn's colitis parallel the small bowel features: bowel wall thickening and full-thickness enhancement (*arrows*). There is also synchronous terminal ileum and cecal involvement (*curved arrows*). Note the inflammatory stranding and prominent vasa rectae that accompany the bowel findings in patients (*open arrow*). (From Shoenut et al. 1993a)

Crohn's colitis from ulcerative colitis; there is no submucosal sparing (Fig. 3.6) (SHOENUT et al. 1993a, 1994). Crohn's disease spares the rectum, which is easily assessed on sagittal images.

There is good correlation between MRI findings and Crohn's disease activity (SHOENUT et al. 1993a, 1994; KETTRITZ et al. 1995). The MRI criteria for mild, moderate, and severe disease have been described by SHOENUT et al. (1994). Severity of disease is based on bowel wall thickness, percent contrast enhancement, and length of involved segment (Fig. 3.7). MRI determinations are made on gadolinium-enhanced T1-weighted fat-suppressed images using the nondependent surface. Mild disease corresponds to wall thickening <5 mm, length of affected bowel wall segment <5 cm, and percent contrast enhancement <50%. To make the diagnosis, bowel wall thickening must be at least 4 mm and one of the other two criteria must be satisfied. Moderate disease produces wall thickening up to 1.0 cm, contrast enhancement between 50 and 100%, and variable length of bowel affected. Severe disease correlates with wall thickening >1.0 cm, contrast enhancement >100%, and length of affected segment >5 cm (typically >10 cm). An MRI product [percentage mural contrast enhancement × wall thickness × length of diseased bowel (MRP)] has been developed to quantify disease activity (KETTRITZ et al. 1995). When compared with

clinical indices [Crohn's Disease Activity Index (CDAI) and modified Index of the International Organization for the Study of Inflammatory Bowel Disease (IOIBD)], linear correlation was found between the MRP and the clinical disease activity indices ($R = 0.633$, $P = 0.0012$ and $R = 0.274$, $P = 0.0373$ for IOIBD and CDAI, respectively). These findings suggests MRI may be the best imaging modality for evaluating the severity of Crohn's disease as barium radiographic findings have limited correlation with clinical symptoms or response. Moreover, MRI is not subject to the potential complications from recurrent exposure to ionizing radiation (GOLDBERG et al. 1979). This consideration is particularly important in the evaluation of patients who are pregnant or of reproductive age (SHOENUT et al. 1993b).

The MRI findings of Crohn's disease complications (e.g., fistula and abscess), save for "pouchitis," are covered separately. "Pouchitis" refers to inflammation of the continent ileal reservoirs constructed in patients who have undergone total colectomy for debilitating IBD (DEUTSCH et al. 1991). The MRI findings in "pouchitis" are nonspecific: a thickened enhancing ileal reservoir wall with stranding in the "peripouch" fat.

3.3.2.1.2

ULCERATIVE COLITIS

Ulcerative colitis is an inflammatory mucosal disease affecting the large bowel. It commonly affects young people and those of Jewish descent. Caucasians and females are affected preferentially and a positive family history is reported in up to 25% of cases (SPIRO 1993). As with Crohn's disease, the etiology of ulcerative colitis is not well understood, but infectious, genetic, psychosomatic, and immunologic factors have all been implicated. Rectal bleeding and intermittent diarrhea are common symptoms. Patients with ulcerative colitis may develop toxic megacolon, a condition characterized by debilitating bloody diarrhea, fever, leukocytosis, and abdominal pain in combination with large bowel dilation. Colon carcinoma is a complication of long-standing chronic ulcerative colitis.

Ulcerative colitis begins in the rectum and spreads in a contiguous fashion proximally. With time, the entire colon may be involved. The small bowel may be affected as well. Backwash ileitis, a sequela of pancolonic disease, may be present in up to one-third of cases. Colonic contents reflux into the ileum via a patulous ileocecal

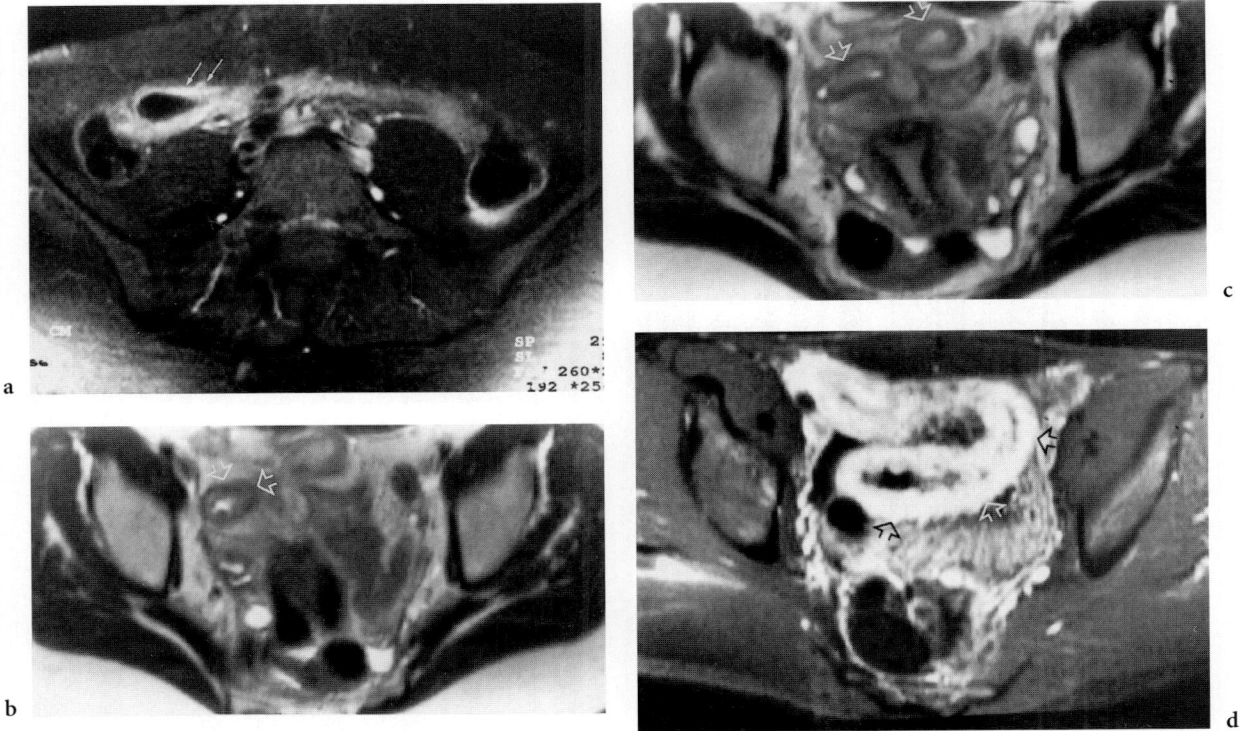

Fig. 3.7a–d. Crohn's disease severity. Axial T1-weighted gadolinium-enhanced fat-suppressed SGE (**a,d**) and T2-weighted HASTE (**b,c**) in patients with differing severities of Crohn's disease. Mild disease is characterized by short segment (<5 mm) involvement that enhances modestly (<50%) (*arrows*, **a**). Moderate disease produces wall thicken-ing up to 5 cm (*open arrows*, **b,c**), enhancement up to 100% (not shown), and variable length of affected bowel, whereas severe disease shows marked wall thickening (>1 cm) and enhancement (>100%) and involves longer bowel segments (>5 cm) (*open arrows*, **d**)

valve and incite small bowel irritation (SPIRO 1993).

Ulcerative colitis is a mucosal process character-ized by microabscesses of the crypts of Lieberkühn. These microabscesses coalesce to form mucosal ul-cers. With long-standing disease, the bowel wall be-comes thick and the colon shortens. There is an associated loss of haustral markings and the colon has a "lead pipe" appearance.

The MRI features of ulcerative colitis reflect the underlying pathology (Fig. 3.8). On gadolinium-enhanced T1-weighted fat-suppressed images there is marked mucosal enhancement with low signal in-tensity sparing of the submucosa (SEMELKA et al. 1991; SHOENUT et al. 1993a, 1994). The vasa rectae are prominent. Long-standing subacute disease leads to submucosal edema and lymphangiectasia which accentuates the low signal intensity of the sub-mucosa on contrast-enhanced images. In contrast to the submucosal sparing that typifies acute exacerba-tions and chronic indolent ulcerative colitis, toxic megacolon is a transmural process with full-thickness enhancement on MRI.

3.3.2.2
Fistula

Fistulae are communicating tracts between viscera or between one of the viscera and the skin and are a common denominator for disease processes that compromise tissue integrity: inflammation (includ-ing IBD), infection, neoplasia, radiation therapy, and ischemia. MRI effectively detects fistulae when surface coils, off-axis imaging planes, and high-resolution T2-weighted and gadolinium-enhanced T1-weighted fat-suppressed sequences are used in concert. Several investigators have described the MRI features of abdominopelvic fistulae (OUTWATER and SCHEIBLER 1993; SEMELKA et al.

a

b

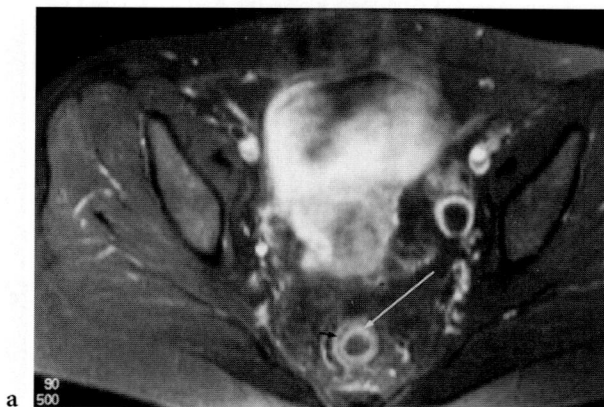

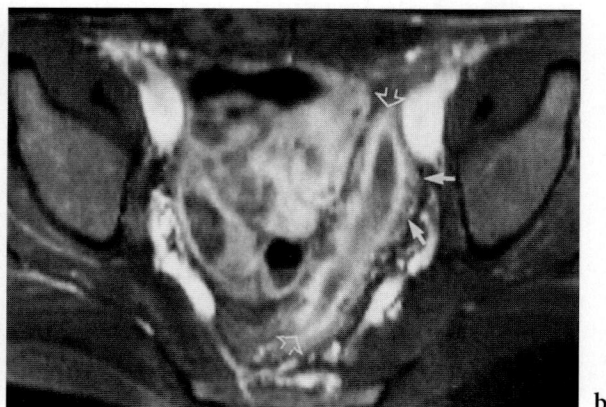

Fig. 3.8a,b. Ulcerative colitis. **a** Axial gadolinium-enhanced T1-weighted fat-suppressed SE image in a patient with ulcerative colitis demonstrates characteristic mucosal enhancement (*long arrow*) with submucosal sparing (*short arrow*). This feature, coupled with differences in distribution, helps distinguish ulcerative colitis from Crohn's disease. **b** Axial gadolinium-enhanced T1-weighted fat-suppressed SE image in a patient with long-standing disease. In chronic cases, the involved segment becomes ahaustral and shortened (*open arrows*, **b**). Associated submucosal edema and lymphangiectasia accentuate submucosal sparing (*solid arrows*, **b**)

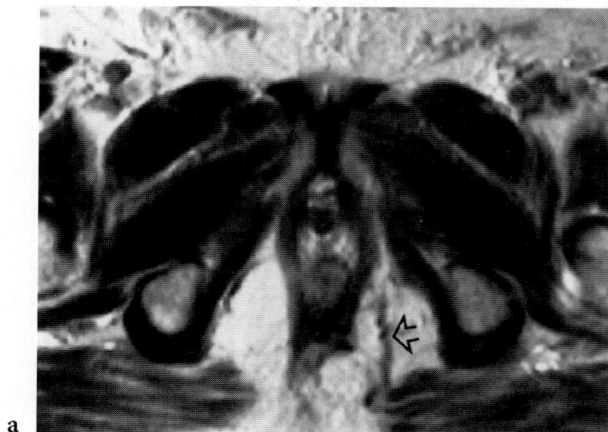

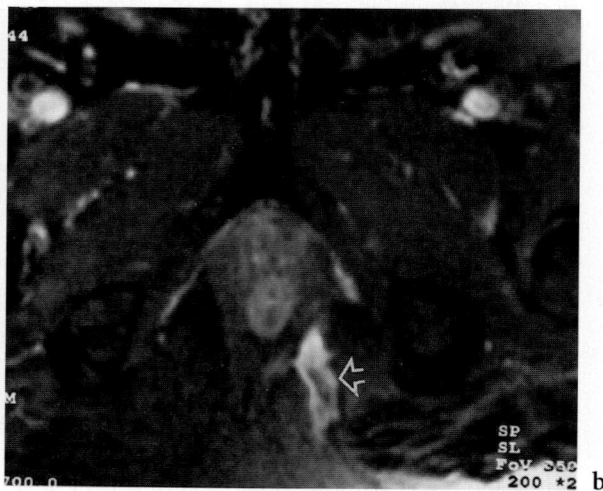

a

b

Fig. 3.9a,b. Fistula. Axial T1-weighted SE (**a**) and gadolinium-enhanced T1-weighted fat-suppressed SE (**b**) in a patient with an enterocutaneous fistula, a complication of surgery. A serpiginous low signal intensity tract (*open arrow*, **a**) enhances after contrast (*open arrow*, **b**). Contiguous images (not shown) showed the fistula connecting the rectum and perineum. Fistulae are most conspicuous on contrast-enhanced fat-suppressed MRI technique. (From Ascher et al. 1996)

1997). Fluid-filled fistulae have high signal intensity on both conventional and fast SE T2-weighted sequences, whereas gas-filled fistulae are signal void. Following intravenous gadolinium chelate, the walls of the fistulae enhance and can be distinguished from the surrounding low signal fat on fat-suppressed T1-weighted images (Fig. 3.9). Focal discontinuity of the involved organ at the site of tract penetration establishes the diagnosis. In another study limited to patients with suspected perianal fistula, dynamic contrast-enhanced MRI was found to be a highly accurate, rapid, noninvasive technique that provided anatomic and pathologic data to guide surgical management (SPENCER et al. 1996).

3.3.2.3
Abscess

Abscesses are complications of gastrointestinal or biliary surgery, diverticulitis, appendicitis, or IBD.

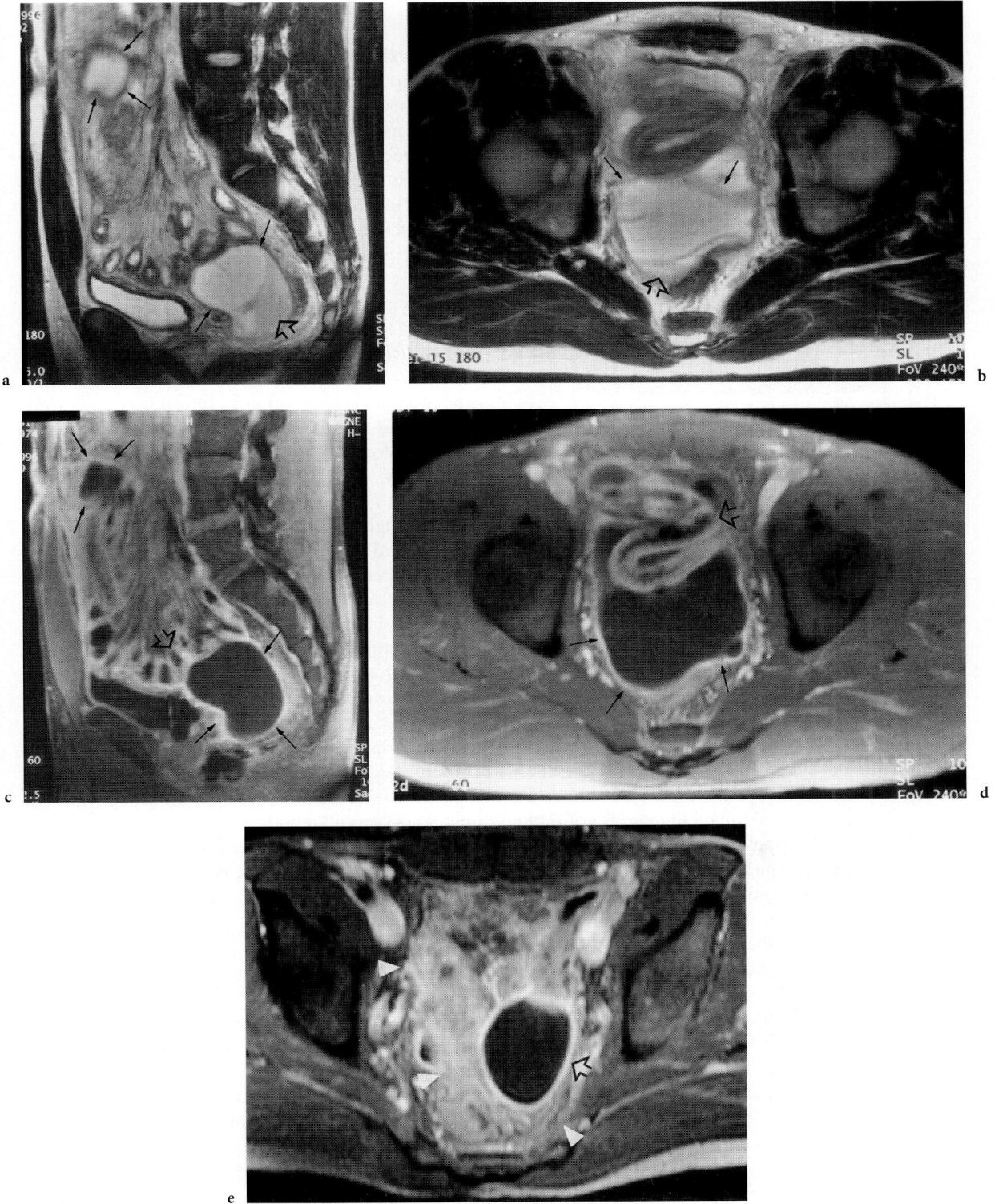

Fig. 3.10a–e. Abscess. Sagittal (**a**) and axial (**b**) T2-weighted HASTE and sagittal (**c**) and axial (**d**) gadolinium-enhanced T1-weighted fat-suppressed SGE images in a patient with multiple bowel-related abscesses. The fluid-filled abscess cavities are well seen on the T2-weighted HASTE images (*solid arrows*, **a,b**). Note that the inferior abscess is complex, with a lower signal intensity component in the dependent portion (*open arrow*, **a,b**). Following contrast administration, the walls of the abscesses (*arrows*, **c,d**) and adjacent bowel (*open arrow*, **c,d**) enhance. **e** Gadolinium-enhanced T1-weighted fat-suppressed SGE image in another patient demonstrates an abscess where the wall enhances (*open arrow*) more than surrounding bowel. Note the inflammatory enhancement in the surrounding fat (*arrowheads*)

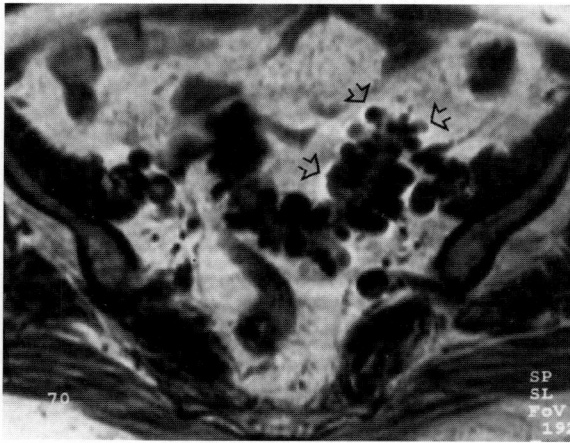

Fig. 3.11. Diverticula. Axial T1-weighted SGE image shows diverticula in the sigmoid colon. Note the susceptibility artifact of the air-filled diverticula, which is accentuated on gradient echo images (*open arrows*)

Computed tomography (CT) and ultrasonography are the first-line imaging modalities in the search for abscesses. They offer both diagnostic and therapeutic capabilities. The emergence of interventional MRI may increase MRI's role in abscess evaluation. Specifically, open MRI systems, automated table motion, MRI-compatible needles and drainage equipment, and rapid single-shot imaging are all commercially available, making abscess diagnosis and percutaneous drainage feasible. On gadolinium-enhanced T1-weighted fat-suppressed images, a fluid collection with an enhancing rim is consistent with the diagnosis of abscess (Fig. 3.10). Signal void gas within the fluid collection helps confirm the diagnosis. The role of an oral or rectal contrast agent to differentiate an abscess from a loop of bowel is, at present, not established. In general, however, abscesses can be distinguished from bowel if T2-weighted HASTE and gadolinium-enhanced fat-suppressed techniques are used. In patients with diminished renal function or iodine contrast allergy suspected of having an abscess, MRI should be performed if ultrasonography is nondiagnostic.

3.3.2.4
Diverticulitis

Diverticula occur throughout the large bowel, though inflamed diverticula tend to occur in the descending and sigmoid colon (Fig. 3.11). CT is comparable and in some cases superior to barium enema

in the evaluation of diverticulitis (Cho et al. 1990). Intravenous gadolinium-enhanced T1-weighted fat-suppressed MRI highlights bowel wall thickening and pericolonic abscesses. Similarly, fistulae and sinus tracts are well visualized on gadolinium-enhanced MRI. On noncontrast T1-weighted SGE images, low signal intensity inflammatory strands stand out in relief amidst the high signal intensity of the pericolonic fat.

3.3.2.5
Appendicitis

Appendicitis is most often a clinical diagnosis without the aid of any imaging modality. However, in cases where the diagnosis is uncertain, ultrasonography and CT are commonly performed (Balthazar et al. 1991; Jeffrey et al. 1988). MRI, with its high contrast resolution for inflammatory disease and lack of ionizing radiation, is an appealing alternative. On gadolinium-enhanced T1-weighted fat-suppressed images the inflamed appendix shows marked enhancement. If present, a calcified appendicolith images as a discrete signal void. Inflammatory stranding in the surrounding fat is best shown on unenhanced T1-weighted SGE images as low signal intensity strands against a background of high signal intensity fat. If appendicitis is complicated by a periappendiceal abscess, the abscess wall will also enhance after contrast, while the abscess cavity will remain a signal void. T2-weighted HASTE may similarly show a high signal intensity fluid-filled collection with associated signal void air (Fig. 3.12).

3.3.2.6
Radiation Enteritis

Radiation therapy in excess of 45 Gy can cause an obliterative endarteritis of the small vessels in the intestinal wall and mesentery. This in turn leads to radiation enteritis: ischemia, an inflammatory infiltrate, and mucosal and submucosal edema. Radiation enteritis has both early and late sequelae. The early complications include: ulceration, necrosis, bleeding, perforation and abscess, and fistula formation. Later, strictures and bowel fixation and angulation are caused by progressive fibrosis and may lead to small bowel obstruction. Gadolinium-enhanced MRI is able to image both the diffuse early ischemic and inflammatory changes of radiation therapy, as well as the more focal late fibrotic

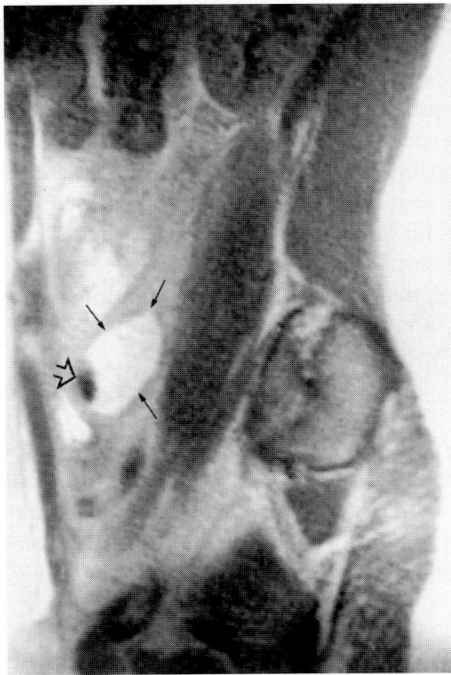

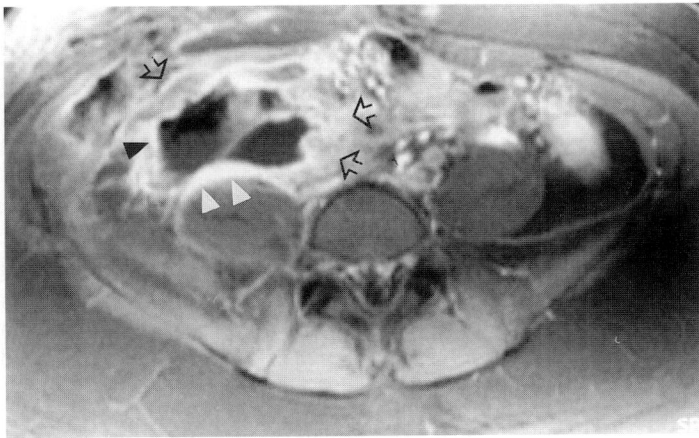

Fig. 3.12a,b Appendicitis. Sagittal T2-weighted HASTE **a** and gadolinium-enhanced T1-weighted fat-suppressed SGE (**b**) images shows a fluid collection (*solid arrows*, **a**) in the right lower quadrant with signal void, air (*open arrow*, **a**), in the nondependent portion, consistent with a periappendiceal abscess. Following contrast the walls of the abscess enhance (*arrowheads*, **b**), as do the inflammatory changes in the surrounding fat (*open arrows*, **b**)

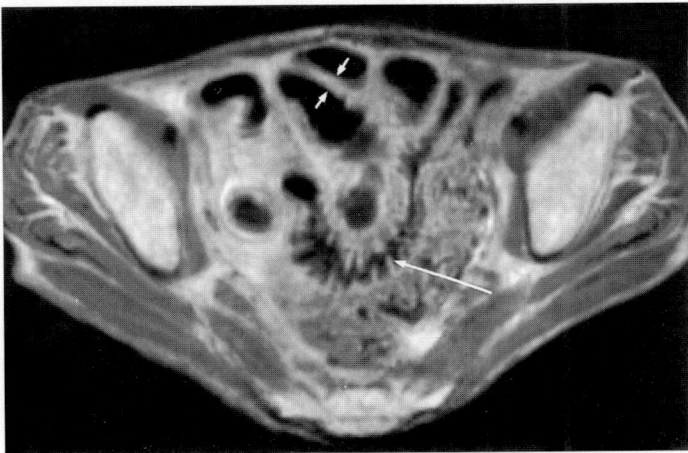

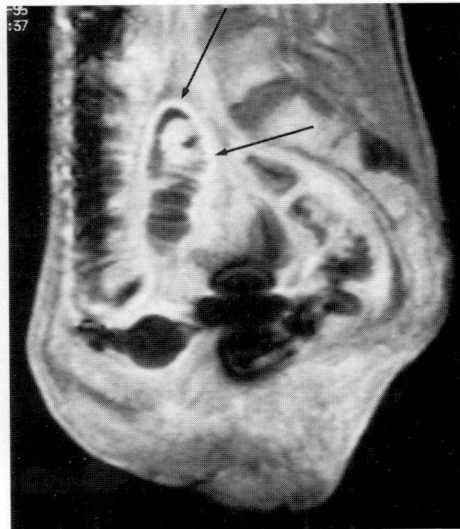

Fig. 3.13a,b. Early radiation enteritis. Axial (**a**) and sagittal (**b**) gadolinium-enhanced T1-weighted SGE in a patient following recent radiation therapy. Ischemia, inflammatory infiltrate, and edema lead to bowel wall thickening (*short arrows*, **a**) and mucosal enhancement (*long arrows*, **a,b**). An associated ileus is also noted, as is stranding in the small bowel mesentery

sequelae. In the former, the bowel is thickened and the mucosa and associated inflammatory stranding markedly enhances [Fig. 3.13]; in the latter, fibrosis can lead to minimally enhancing narrowed segments of bowel with varying degrees of proximal dilation (ASCHER and SEMELKA 1996).

3.3.2.7
Immunocompromised Patient

3.3.2.7.1
OPPORTUNISTIC INFECTIONS
Viral, fungal, mycobacterial, or protozoan gastrointestinal opportunistic infections are common in the immunocompromised patient. When longstanding, they can lead to chronic wasting. While patients may come to MRI for evaluation of fever or suspected abscess, synchronous enteric infections are often present. The MRI findings tend to be nonspecific: focal bowel wall thickening, increased secretions, and mesenteric edema. However, certain features may suggest a specific etiology. For example, cytomegalovirus infection may cause bowel wall thickening secondary to submucosal hemorrhage whereas dilated fluid-filled loops of bowel are characteristic of *Cryptosporidium* infection (JEFFREY et al. 1992) (Fig. 3.14). In patients with chronic wasting and hypoproteinemia, generalized bowel wall thickening, edema, and ascites may be seen.

Patients with human immune virus (HIV) infection and/or acquired immunodeficiency syndrome (AIDS) may also develop opportunistic infections resulting in proctitis and perirectal abscesses. These infections lead to rectal wall thickening with inflammatory stranding in the perirectal space. In extreme cases, frank abscesses are seen. Contrast-enhanced T1-weighted fat-suppressed imaging highlights rectal wall thickening and abscess formation. Soft tissue infiltration, with low signal intensity stranding in the perirectal space, is best shown on unenhanced T1-weighted images.

3.3.2.7.2
GRAFT VERSUS HOST DISEASE
Graft versus host disease is a complication that can occur after heterotopic bone marrow transplantation. Its MRI manifestations include diffuse bowel wall thickening and mucosal enhancement (Fig. 3.15).

3.3.3
Mass Lesions: Benign

3.3.3.1
Leiomyoma

Leiomyomas are the most common benign neoplasms of the proximal gastrointestinal tract. They

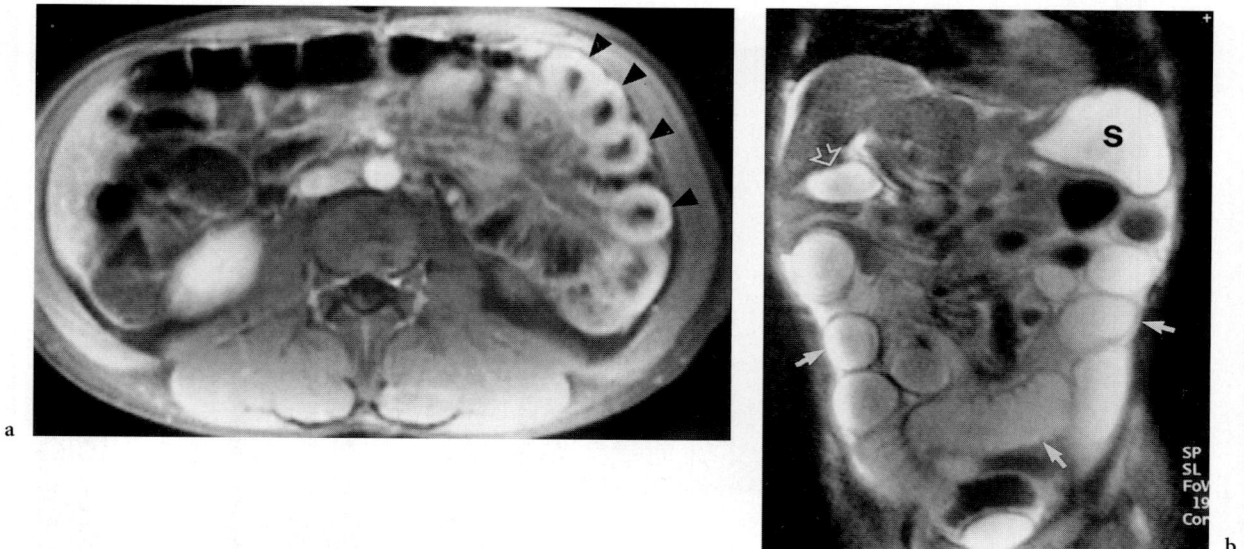

Fig. 3.14a,b. Immunocompromised enteritis. Axial gadolinium-enhanced T1-weighted fat-suppressed SGE (a) and coronal T2-HASTE (b) images in two patients with AIDS. Patients with HIV may have a nonspecific enteritis with bowel wall thickening, increased secretions, and mesenteric edema (*arrowheads*, a). These changes are highlighted on contrast-enhanced fat-suppressed technique. Alternatively, dilated fluid-filled loops of bowel are characteristic of *Cryptosporidium* infection (*arrows*, b). (On b: S, stomach; *open arrow*, gallbladder)

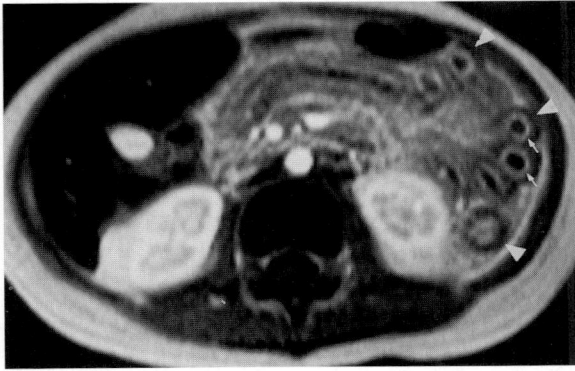

Fig. 3.15. Graft versus host disease. Axial gadolinium-enhanced T1-weighted SGE image in a patient on immunosuppressive therapy following bone marrow transplant. These patients are at risk for graft versus host disease, which images as diffuse bowel wall thickening (*arrowheads*) and mucosal enhancement (*arrows*)

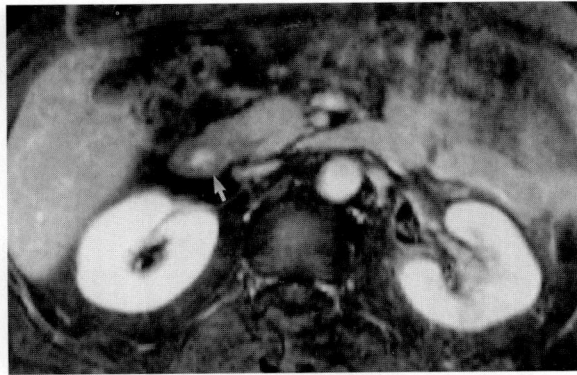

Fig. 3.16. Leiomyoma. Axial gadolinium-enhanced T1-weighted fat-suppressed SE image in a patient with a submucosal mass seen on a conventional upper gastrointestinal series. The corresponding MR image shows a small enhancing lesion (*arrow*) in the submucosa of the duodenum; this is nonspecific. Pathologic correlation revealed a benign leiomyoma

are composed of smooth muscle and tend to be solitary lesions when present in the stomach and small bowel, but are often multiple when present in the esophagus. Leiomyomas originate in the subserosa or submucosa, but can also extend intraluminally. When these tumors enlarge they have a propensity for central necrosis and ulceration leading to gastrointestinal bleeding (EISENBERG 1983a). Leiomyomas image as submucosal or polypoid masses that enhance after gadolinium chelate administration (Fig. 3.16). If complicated by necrosis, signal void areas are noted within them.

3.3.3.2
Lipoma

Lipomas are submucosal neoplasms that occur throughout the alimentary tube. They cluster about the ileocecal valve, either in the distal small bowel or the ascending colon. MRI exploits their fatty composition to establish the diagnosis. Lipomas have high signal intensity on T1-weighted images and will show a characteristic loss of signal on chemically selective excitation fat-spoiled images (Fig. 3.17). Lack of central necrosis, heterogeneous enhancing stroma, and blood products suggest benignancy (YOUNATHAN et al. 1991).

3.3.3.3
Other Mesenchymal Tumors

Fibromas, neuromas, and hemangiomas are uncommon benign alimentary tube neoplasms and present as nonspecific mass lesions on MRI.

3.3.3.4
Polyps

Polyps occur throughout the gastrointestinal tract. They may be hyperplastic, hamartomatous, or adenomatous. And while they can be isolated findings, they are also associated with polyposis syndromes. Adenomatous polyps are the most worrisome of the three histologic types and are at risk for carcinomatous transformation. Malignant potential is related to polyp size. Up to 46% of polyps larger than 2 cm harbor adenocarcinoma (EISENBERG 1983b).

3.3.3.4.1
LARGE BOWEL POLYPS

Colonic adenomas are the most common *large bowel* neoplasm and are classified according to their glandular pattern: tubular, tubulovillous, or villous. While all have malignant potential, villous adenomas, found most often in the rectosigmoid or the cecum, pose the highest risk for cancerous transformation. Patients with Gardner's syndrome and familial polyposis have multiple large bowel adenomatous polyps. Because all of these patients

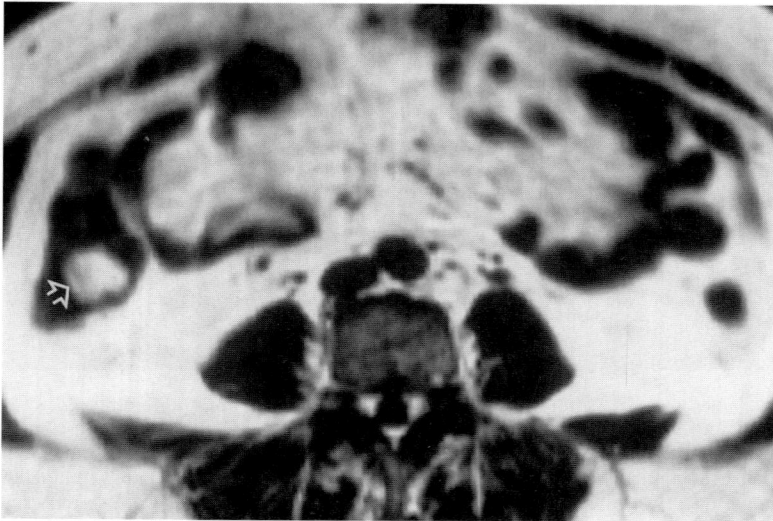

a

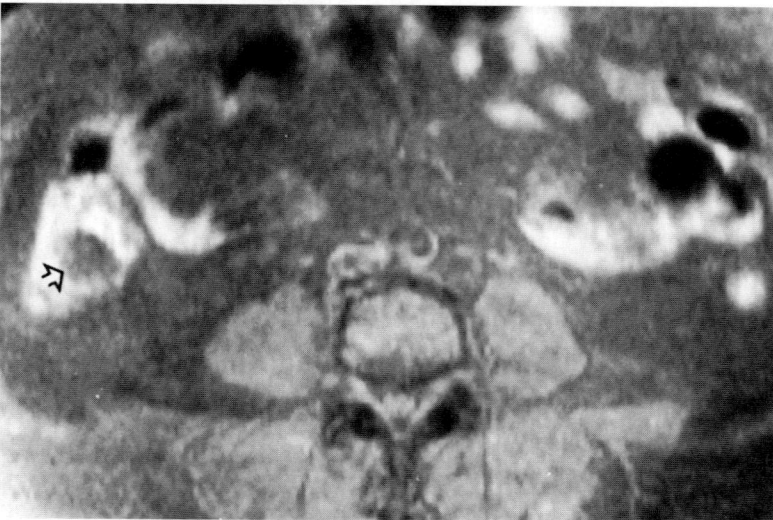

b

Fig. 3.17a,b. Lipoma. Axial T1-weighted (**a**) and fat-suppressed (**b**) SE images. A high signal intensity lesion (*open arrow*, **a**) in the colon fades with fat suppression (*open arrow*, **b**), diagnostic of a lipoma. (From Shoenut et al. 1993b)

will eventually develop colorectal carcinoma, colectomy is recommended at the time of initial presentation. Multiple hamartomas of the large bowel are usually seen in patients with Peutz-Jeghers syndrome and juvenile polyposis.

3.3.3.4.2
MRI APPEARANCE

On gadolinium-enhanced T1-weighted fat-suppressed SGE images, most polyps appear as enhancing masses that arise from the wall of the alimentary tube and protrude into the bowel lumen (ASCHER and SEMELKA 1996) (Fig. 3.18). If enhancing interstices are present, the diagnosis of a villous adenoma should be entertained. Similarly, if an intraluminal mass transgresses the bowel wall, malignant degeneration is almost certain.

3.3.4
Mass Lesions: Malignant

3.3.4.1
Adenocarcinoma

3.3.4.1.1
ESOPHAGUS

Esophageal adenocarcinoma accounts for 5% of esophageal malignancies. They may arise de novo in Barrett esophagus, or they may arise in the stomach and traverse the gastroesophageal junction to in-

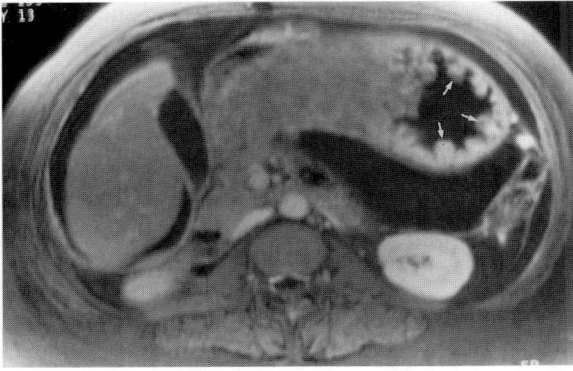

Fig. 3.18. Gastric polyps. Axial gadolinium-enhanced T1-weighted fat-suppressed SGE image in a patient with Gardner's syndrome. Multiple enhancing gastric polyps protrude into the lumen (*arrows*). In the absence of obvious invasion through the stomach wall, MRI cannot distinguish between benign and malignant polyps. MRI, like conventional barium studies, relies on size to suggest a coexisting malignancy; up to 46% of adenomatous polyps greater than 2 cm harbor adenocarcinoma

volve the distal esophagus. Moderate success has been reported for staging esophageal carcinoma with MRI. Accuracies between 75% and 100% have been reported for identifying pericardial, aortic, and tracheobronchial invasion on conventional unenhanced SE technique (HALVORSEN et al. 1987; QUINT et al. 1985; TRENIKER et al. 1994; HALVORSEN and THOMPSON 1991). Identifying invasion into mediastinal fat remains problematic; however, intravenous gadolinium chelate administration improves delineation of tumor extent (TEMPLETON et al. 1994). Currently the best MRI approach for the evaluation of esophageal malignancy is with cardiac gated gadolinium-enhanced T1-weighted fat-suppressed SE (Fig. 3.19). Oral contrast agents have not been routinely used, though some advocate a specially formulated gadolinium dimeglumine barium paste for evaluating esophageal disease (PAVONE et al. 1992). For detection of lymphadenopathy, MRI, like CT, relies on size criteria. Signal intensity alone on noncontrast T1-, T2-, or gadolinium-enhanced T1-weighted images cannot differentiate between normal, reactive, or tumor-replaced lymph nodes. A comprehensive staging MRI for patients with esophageal carcinoma should include an abdominal survey to assess for the presence of hepatic metastases.

3.3.4.1.2

STOMACH

Gastric adenocarcinoma has been linked to dietary, geographic, certain medical conditions including:

pernicious anemia, atrophic gastritis, adenomatous polyps, dietary nitrates, and individuals who are native Japanese. The morphology of stomach cancer is variable. The scirrhous type, linitis plastica, spreads superficially throughout the stomach and results in a nondistensible aperistaltic viscus.

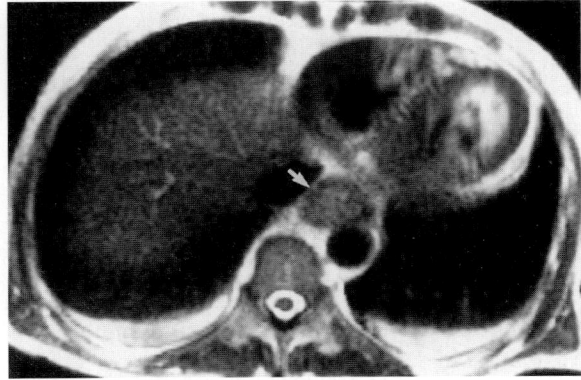

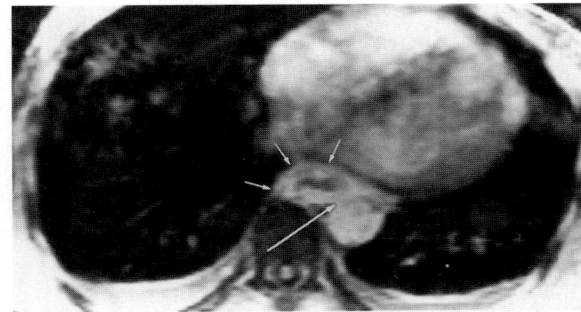

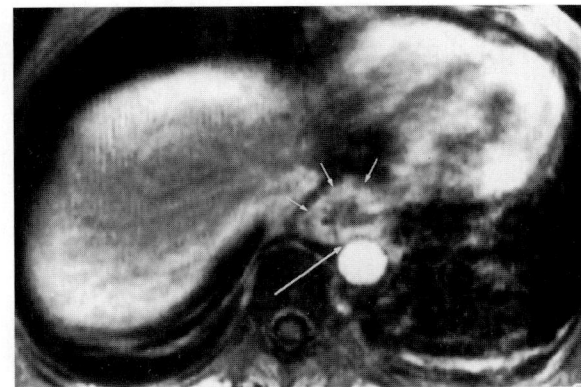

Fig. 3.19a–c. Esophageal adenocarcinoma. Axial T2-weighted HASTE (**a**) and axial gadolinium-enhanced T1-weighted fat-suppressed SGE (**b,c**) images demonstrate a distended soft-tissue filled esophagus (*arrow*, **a**) in a patient with a history of Barrett esophagus. Following contrast, the circumferential tumor enhances (*short arrows*, **b,c**). Note that the fat plane separating the posterolateral esophagus from the aorta is obliterated proximally (*long arrow*, **b**), but preserved distally (*long arrow*, **c**). At surgery, the tumor was adherent to portions of the aorta

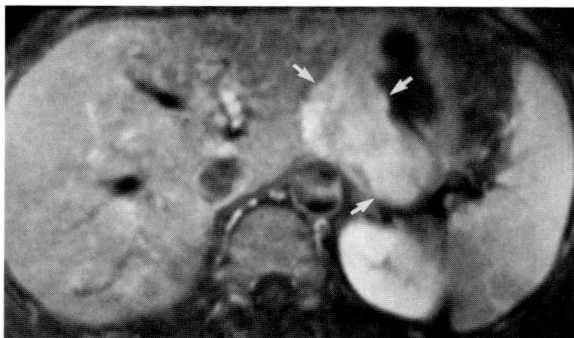

Fig. 3.20. Gastric adenocarcinoma. Axial T1-weighted fat-suppressed SE image in a patient with carcinoma of the stomach. An enhancing tumor infiltrates the lesser curve, causing mural thickening (*arrows*). (From SHOENUT et al. 1993d)

Magnetic resonance imaging is well suited for imaging the primary tumor, assessing depth of invasion, and evaluating intraperitoneal disease (SEMELKA et al. 1993; MATUSHITA et al. 1994). Adequate gastric distension is essential for surveying the gastric wall. Although many tumors are higher in signal than background stomach on T2-weighted images, some gastric cancers, especially those of the scirrhous type, are low in signal intensity compared with stomach wall (WINKLER et al. 1987). This reflects the desmoplastic hypovascular nature of scirrhous carcinoma. The use of intravenous gadolinium chelate increases lesion conspicuity (Fig. 3.20). On gadolinium-enhanced out-of-phase SGE images, irregularity or loss of the low signal intensity band that normally surrounds the stomach implies extraserosal disease. This finding has a 97% sensitivity, a 79% specificity, and an overall accuracy of 92% for determining the presence or absence of extraserosal imaging (MATUSHITA et al. 1994). Gadolinium-enhanced T1-weighted fat-suppressed SGE imaging is useful for identifying both the primary tumor and contiguous and/or intraperitoneal spread of disease. Peritoneal implants and regional lymph nodes enhance and can be easily differentiated from the adjacent low signal intensity fat (SEMELKA et al. 1993). Hepatic metastases are well shown on T2-weighted fat-suppressed and dynamic T1-weighted SGE techniques (SEMELKA et al. 1992). Detection of lymphadenopathy is size dependent and comparable to CT.

3.3.4.1.3
SMALL BOWEL

Small bowel adenocarcinoma accounts for only 1% of gastrointestinal malignancies. Most, 45%, are duodenal and occur in the ampulla region, where they can lead to obstructive jaundice (TRENKER et al. 1994). Regardless of location, small bowel cancer may cause bowel obstruction and/or chronic blood loss. Alternatively, patients may be asymptomatic and present late in the disease with metastases. Lymph node involvement is common. MRI is not the primary modality to diagnose patients with suspected small bowel carcinoma; however, gadolinium-enhanced T1-weighted fat-suppressed imaging can assess tumor bulk and local disease extension. MRI can also be used to evaluate for hepatic metastases.

3.3.4.1.4
LARGE BOWEL

Colonic adenocarcinoma is the most common alimentary tube malignancy. Patients at increased risk for developing adenocarcinoma of the colon include those with familial polyposis, Gardner's syndrome, ulcerative colitis, Crohn's colitis, and previous ureterosigmoidostomies. Advanced age is also a risk factor. Cancers predominate in the rectosigmoid colon, but right-sided lesions are increasing in frequency (KEE et al. 1992). Tumors may be circumferential ("apple core"), polypoid, or plaque-like. Symptoms reflect tumor location and morphology, but some combination of change in bowel habits, bleeding, pain, and weight loss is usually reported.

Initial reports using MRI for assessing colon cancer found that conventional SE compared favorably with CT in terms of overall staging accuracy, which was approximately 80% (BUTCH et al. 1986; THOENI 1991). MRI had the added advantage of multiplanar acquisition, which facilitated identification of local tumor extent. Another group reported good correlation between gadolinium-enhanced T1-weighted fat-suppressed techniques and surgical findings for tumor size, bowel wall involvement, peritumoral extension, and lymph node detection (SHOENUT et al. 1993c). On MRI, cancers are enhancing masses that disrupt the normal bowel layers (Fig. 3.21). Because the spatial resolution of body coil is limited, surface coils are usually used when evaluating depth of bowel wall invasion and local spread of disease (Fig. 3.22).

Commercially available surface coils including the body phased array, Helmholtz, and endorectal coils boost signal-to-noise and improve spatial resolution. A study comparing a prototype body phased array coil and a conventional body coil for pelvic imaging found overall image quality and anatomic

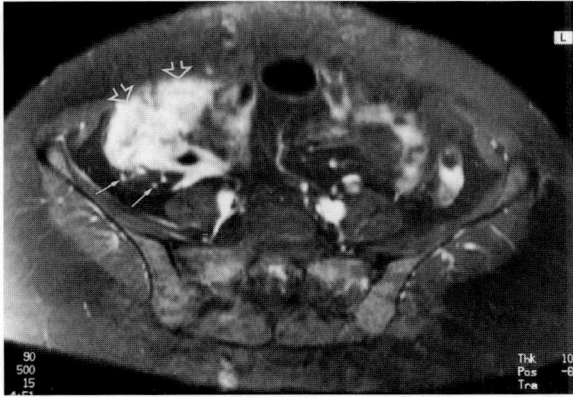

Fig. 3.21. Cecal carcinoma. Axial gadolinium-enhanced T1-weighted fat-suppressed SE image in a patient with colon cancer. A large cecal carcinoma extends to the peritoneum (*open arrows*). Note the enhancing multiple perilesional lymph nodes (*solid arrows*). (From Shoenut et al. 1993d)

detail to be superior with the phased array coil (SMITH et al. 1992). The Helmholtz surface coil has been proven to reliably differentiate rectal tumors confined to the bowel wall from those infiltrating the perirectal fat (DELANGE et al. 1990). Of all the surface coils marketed, the endorectal coil provides the highest signal-to-noise and spatial resolution of the rectum. This reflects the close proximity of the coil to the rectum. Using an endorectal coil permits differentiation of the anatomic layers of the rectal wall on fat-suppressed T2-weighted images (SCHNALL et al. 1994). Moreover, several investigators have shown endorectal coil imaging to perform well at staging local extent of rectal cancer (CHAN et al. 1991; SCHNALL et al. 1994).

Rectosigmoid cancer recurrence rates vary between 8% and 50% depending on the stage of the primary tumor at presentation (DELANGE et al. 1989). Tumors recur locally and curative surgery is feasible in the majority of patients. MRI is well suited for detecting recurrent rectal carcinoma; the relatively fixed anatomic position of the rectum is amenable to imaging directly in the sagittal plane. Employing T1-, T2-, and postcontrast T1-weighted sequences, accuracies of 93.3% have been reported for the detection of recurrent rectosigmoid tumor (BALZARINI et al. 1990). Other investigators have shown that MRI outperforms conventional CT and is more specific than transrectal ultrasonography (TRUS) for identifying recurrent disease (DELANGE et al 1989; GOMBERG et al. 1986; KRESTIN et al. 1988;

PEMA et al. 1994). Specifically, MRI detected recurrent rectal carcinoma in 83.2% of patients, while TRUS detected recurrence in only 41.6% (WAIZER et al. 1991).

Recurrent tumor is usually low in signal intensity on T1-weighted images, gets brighter in signal intensity on T2-weighted images, and enhances significantly after intravenous gadolinium chelate (Fig. 3.23). In contradistinction, post-treatment fibrosis in patients who have undergone surgery more than 1 year previously remains low in signal intensity on both T1- and T2- weighted images and enhances minimally following contrast administration (BUTCH et al. 1986; THOENI 1991; DELANGE et al. 1989; ITO et al. 1992) (Fig. 3.24). Overlap in signal behavior between recurrent tumor and fibrosis exists. Specifically, granulation tissue and inflammation may parallel the signal intensity of recurrent tumor, especially if the patient is within 1 year of treatment. Furthermore, although the signal intensity of fibrosis on T2-weighted images decreases after approximately 1 year, granulation tissue has increased signal intensity on postgadolinium images for a more prolonged period of time – up to 3 years – particularly when using fat-suppressed T1-weighted images. And finally, recurrent tumor may mimic radiation fibrosis when desmoplastic features predominate: recurrence is low in signal on T2-weighted images and enhances minimally after gadolinium chelate administration.

A technical caveat to be aware of concerns the use of T2-weighted fast SE sequences and phased array surface coil imaging. This combination renders intra-abdominal and pelvic fat higher in signal intensity compared with conventional SE and body coil imaging; therefore, recurrent tumor may not be as conspicuously higher in signal intensity than fat. The morphology of the tissue in the resection bed aids diagnosis. Fibrosis is generally plate-like while recurrence appears more nodular. As with all image interpretation, patient symptomatology and laboratory studies must be taken into consideration when formulating a diagnostic impression. A rise in CEA levels and recent onset of presacral pain are harbingers of recurrence.

3.3.4.2
Leiomyosarcoma

Leiomyosarcomas are hypervascular neoplasms. They are often large and exophytic with a propensity for central necrosis. These features may help

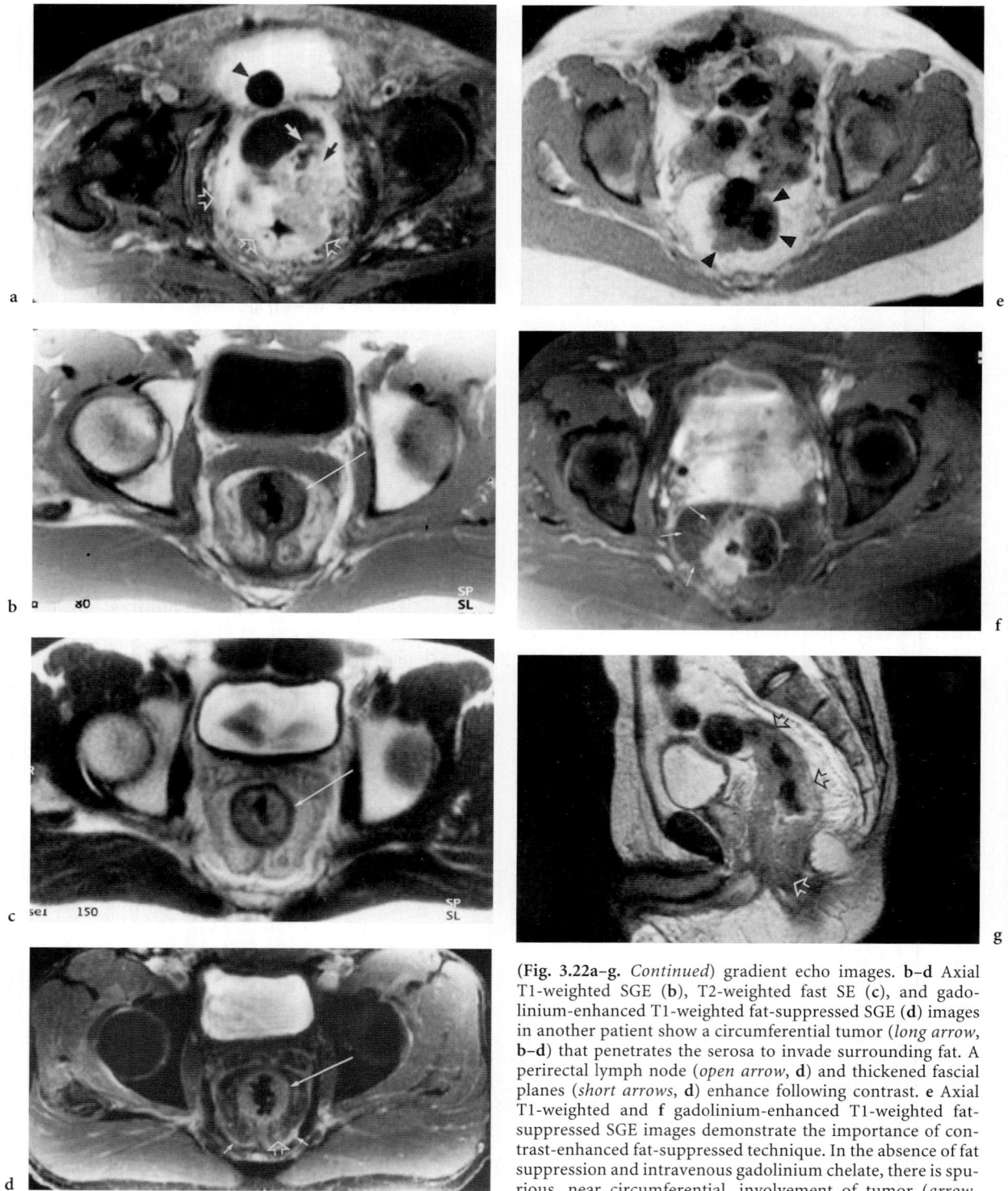

Fig. 3.22a–g. Rectal adenocarcinoma. a Axial gadolinium-enhanced T1-weighted fat-suppressed SGE in a patient with extensive rectal cancer. The tumor produces rectal wall thickening (*open arrows*) that invades adjacent bowel (*solid arrows*) and extends into the perirectal fat. Susceptibility artifact in air-containing bowel "blooms" (*arrowhead*) on

(Fig. 3.22a–g. *Continued*) gradient echo images. b–d Axial T1-weighted SGE (b), T2-weighted fast SE (c), and gadolinium-enhanced T1-weighted fat-suppressed SGE (d) images in another patient show a circumferential tumor (*long arrow*, b–d) that penetrates the serosa to invade surrounding fat. A perirectal lymph node (*open arrow*, d) and thickened fascial planes (*short arrows*, d) enhance following contrast. e Axial T1-weighted and f gadolinium-enhanced T1-weighted fat-suppressed SGE images demonstrate the importance of contrast-enhanced fat-suppressed technique. In the absence of fat suppression and intravenous gadolinium chelate, there is spurious, near circumferential, involvement of tumor (*arrowheads*, e); however, the true extent of tumor is highlighted with the addition of fat suppression and gadolinium chelate. Linear enhancing peri-rectal invasion is also well seen (*arrows*, f). g Sagittal T2-weighted fast SE image underscoring the utility of the sagittal imaging plane for delineating the craniocaudad extent of rectal tumors (*open arrows*). The relatively fixed position of the rectum renders it amenable to the longer acquisition times associated with fast SE imaging

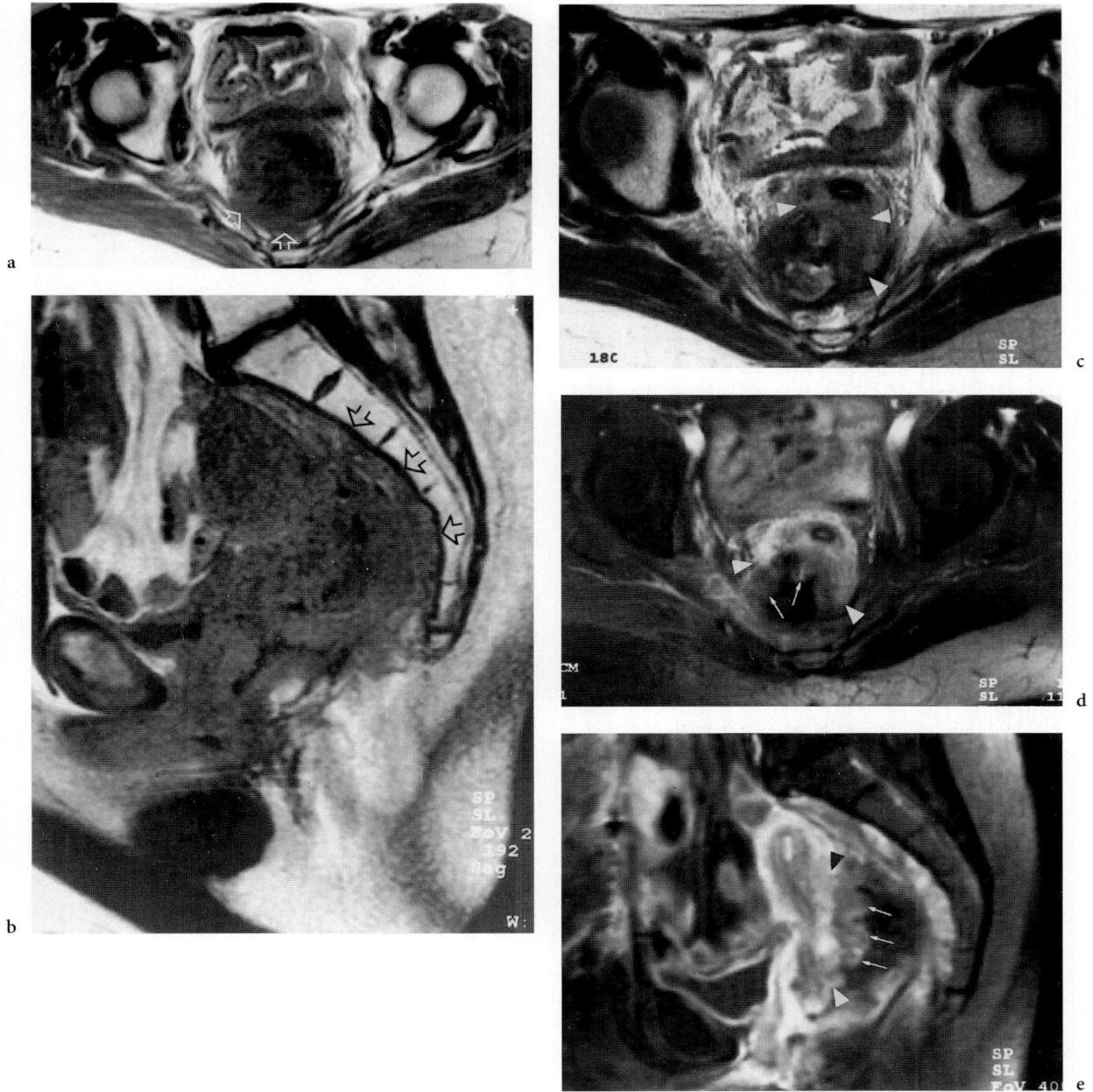

Fig. 3.23a–e. Recurrent rectal adenocarcinoma. Axial (**a**) and sagittal (**b**) T1-weighted SGE, axial T2-weighted fast SE (**c**), and axial (**d**) and sagittal (**e**) gadolinium-enhanced T1-weighted fat-suppressed SGE images in a patient with a history of rectal carcinoma and within 12 months following radiation therapy. A large mass is noted in the pelvis which obliterates the presacral space (*open arrows*, **a,b**). On the T2-weighted fast SE sequence the rectal mass is contiguous with the uterus (*arrowheads*, **c**). Following contrast, the lobulated recurrent tumor enhances (*arrows*, **d,e**) and invades the posterior myometrium (*arrowheads*, **d,e**). The marked enhancement of the bladder wall and fat-replaced sacral marrow is consistent with radiation therapy changes. Note that recurrent tumor need not be very high in signal intensity (**c**); preservation of high signal intensity fat on T2-weighted fast SE sequences obtained with the phased array surface coil decreases the conspicuity between recurrent tumor and surrounding fat

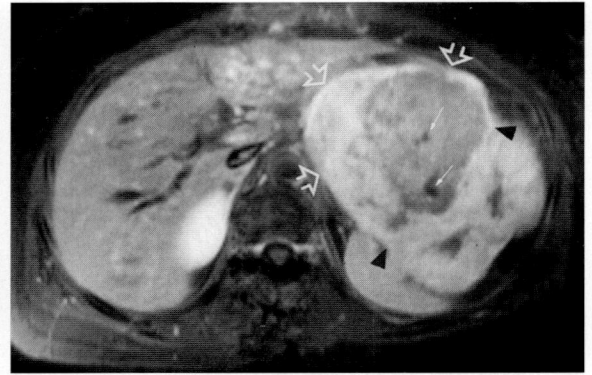

Fig. 3.25. Gastric leiomyosarcoma. Axial gadolinium-enhanced T1-weighted fat-suppressed SE image in a patient with a large tumor (*open arrows*) originating from the lesser curve of the stomach (*arrowheads*). The exophytic nature of the tumor, coupled with areas of necrosis, seen as signal voids (*solid arrows*), is typical of leiomyosarcomas. (From Shoenut et al. 1993d)

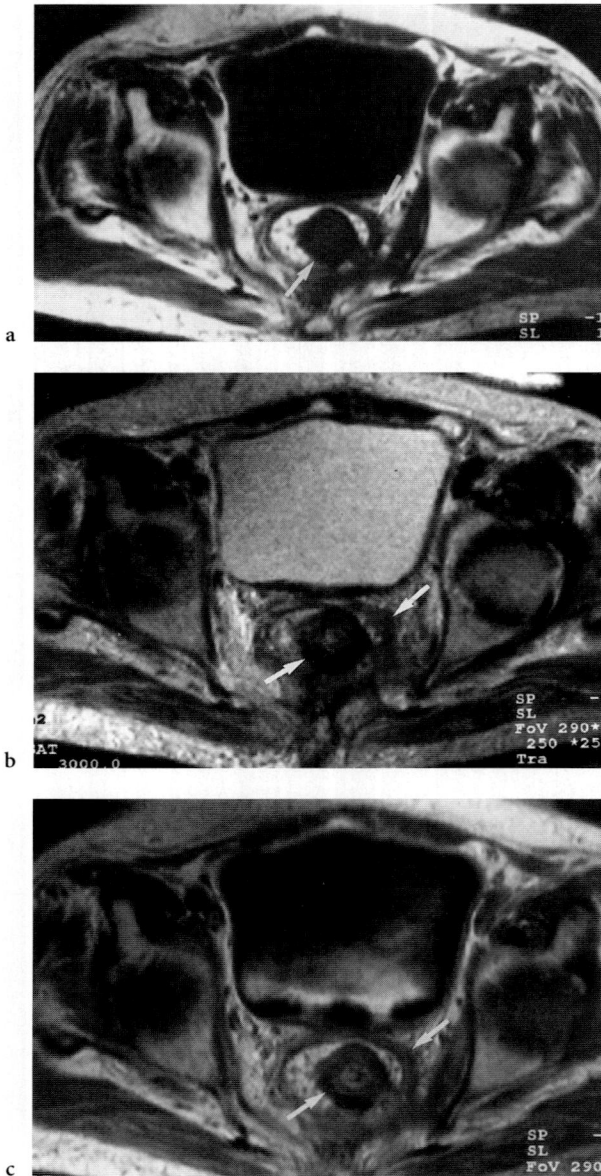

Fig. 3.24a–c. Late post-radiation therapy changes. T1-weighted (a), T2-weighted (b), and gadolinium-enhanced T1-weighted (c) SE images. Rectal wall and perirectal musculature thickening are low in signal intensity on the unenhanced images (*arrows*, a and b) and do not enhance significantly after intravenous contrast (*arrows*, c). There is also tethering of the rectal wall to the perirectal musculature. This constellation of imaging findings is characteristic of the post-radiation therapy changes that occur at least 1 year following treatment. (From Ascher et al. 1996)

differentiate them from adenocarcinoma and lymphoma.

The most common location for leiomyosarcoma is the stomach, followed by the ileum. Tumor spreads contiguously to adjacent viscera or hematogenously. Lymph node involvement is rare.

Leiomyosarcomas are conspicuous on gadolinium-enhanced T1-weighted SGE images because of their increased vascularity. On early postcontrast images they show marked enhancement, while on the delayed interstitial phase images the tumors retain contrast. Fat suppression potentiates the visibility of tumors. The central areas of necrosis do not enhance on postgadolinium images (Fig. 3.25). Due to the frequent occurrence of liver metastases, a dedicated liver survey is mandatory. This is best accomplished with dynamic contrast-enhanced T1-weighted SGE imaging. The hypervascular metastases exhibit early ring enhancement or uniform enhancement and equilibrate rapidly with background liver.

3.3.4.3
Kaposi's Sarcoma

Approximately one-half of patients with AIDS-related Kaposi's sarcoma will have alimentary tube lesions at autopsy; regardless, most patients are asymptomatic. Rarely, gastrointestinal Kaposi's sarcoma may cause obstruction, intussusception, or hemorrhage. If gastrointestinal lesions accompanied by retroperitoneal adenopathy, splenic and hepatic lesions, and infiltration of the psoas or abdominal wall are detected in a patient with AIDS, the diagno-

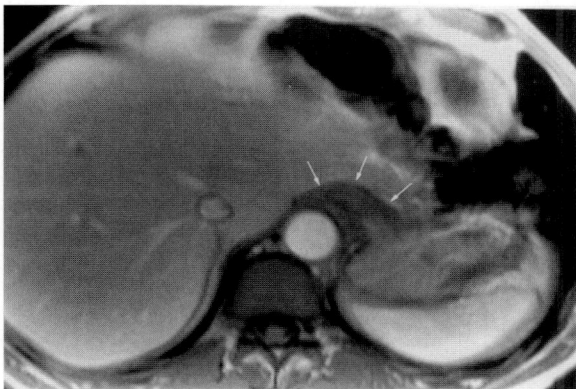

Fig. 3.26. Squamous cell carcinoma of the esophagus. Axial gadolinium-enhanced T1-weighted SGE image 45 s after contrast demonstrates asymmetric circumferential involvement of the distal esophagus (*arrows*)

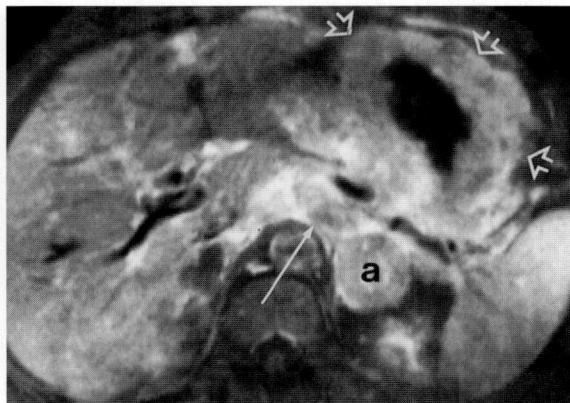

Fig. 3.27. Gastric lymphoma. Axial gadolinium-enhanced T1-weighted fat-suppressed SE image in a patient with non-Hodgkin's lymphoma. Although the entire stomach wall is involved with tumor (*arrowheads*), it remains distensible. Preservation of distensibility is typical of non-Hodgkin's lymphoma involving the bowel and helps distinguish it from a scirrhous adenocarcinoma. Note that the retroperitoneal involvement includes lymph nodes (*solid arrow*) and the adrenal gland (*a*). (From Shoenut et al. 1993d)

sis of Kaposi's sarcoma should be raised (JEFFREY 1992).

3.3.4.4
Squamous Cell Carcinoma

Squamous cell carcinoma accounts for the majority of esophageal (95%) and anal malignancies. In both locations, the imaging characteristics resemble adenocarcinoma. Orthogonal imaging planes and gadolinium-enhanced T1-weighted fat-suppressed images allow evaluation of the primary tumor and local extent of disease (Fig. 3.26).

3.3.4.5
Lymphoma

3.3.4.5.1
STOMACH
Primary gastric lymphoma is rare; rather Hodgkin's and non-Hodgkin's lymphomas are more likely to involve the stomach. Specifically, the stomach is the most common site of extranodal disease, especially in non-Hodgkin's lymphoma. Lymphomatous infiltration is characterized by marked gastric wall thickening. An important diagnostic feature in non-Hodgkin's lymphoma is preservation of gastric distensibility (Fig. 3.27), whereas Hodgkin's lymphoma, like scirrhous adenocarcinoma, incites a desmo-

plastic reaction and a nondistensible aperistaltic viscus results. Synchronous lymphadenopathy is common.

3.3.4.5.2
SMALL BOWEL
Primary small bowel lymphoma, usually poorly differentiated lymphocytic and diffuse histiocytic lymphomas, originates from lymphoid tissue that predominates in the terminal ileum (AL-MONDHIRY 1986). Several morphologic types or patterns have been described: polypoid, infiltrating, or endoexenteric. When endoexenteric, the large extraluminal component may ulcerate and fistulize. In 20% of cases, multiple lesions are present and more than one pattern of disease may coexist. Distensibility of the bowel is preserved and obstruction is rare. The different morphologic patterns enhance on T1-weighted fat-suppressed imaging following intravenous gadolinium chelate administration. This technique also highlights associated lymphadenopathy and fistulae if present.

Secondary extranodal small bowel lymphoma is present in up to half of patients with primary Hodgkin's or non-Hodgkin's lymphoma. Moderately enhancing thickened loops of bowel are seen on contrast-enhanced MRI. Small bowel thickening in the presence of mesenteric and retroperitoneal lymphadenopathy and splenic lesions should raise the diagnosis of lymphoma.

3.3.4.5.3
LARGE BOWEL

Primary large bowel lymphoma is rare. There is a known association with HIV infection or chronic ulcerative colitis (BARTOLO et al. 1982; DRAGOSICS et al. 1985). Non-Hodgkin's lymphoma is the most common histology. Large bowel lymphoma is usually a manifestation of widespread disease and occurs between the fifth and seventh decades. Single or multiple enhancing bowel masses, or diffuse nodularity with wall thickening, typify the MRI findings on gadolinium-enhanced images. As elsewhere in the alimentary tube, coexistent bulky lymphadenopathy and splenic involvement help establish the diagnosis.

3.3.4.6
Carcinoid

Carcinoid tumors are neuroendocrine in origin and are the most common primary small bowel tumor. The majority occur in the distal ileum. The primary tumor is often small and not readily imaged. However, the associated desmoplastic reaction and bulky lymphadenopathy are amenable to imaging. Specifically, on unenhanced T1-weighted and T2-weighted HASTE images, low-intermediate signal intensity strands radiating from the root of mesentery characterize the desmoplastic response (Fig. 3.28), while a profusion and/or enlargement of lymph nodes suggests lymphadenopathy (SEMELKA et al. 1996b). When large enough, the primary tumors produce asymmetric bowel wall thickening which enhances following intravenous gadolinium chelate administration. Carcinoids metastasize to the liver and lung. When present in the liver they cause "carcinoid syndrome." Immediately following contrast administration, these hypervascular metastases demonstrate rim or uniform enhancement.

Carcinoid tumors also occur in the colon with the rectum being the site most frequently affected. Rectal carcinoids are usually malignant. In contrast, carcinoid tumors that occur in the appendix are almost always benign.

3.3.4.7
Metastases

3.3.4.7.1
ESOPHAGUS

Metastases to the esophagus are infrequent. In patients with breast or lung cancer, esophageal in-

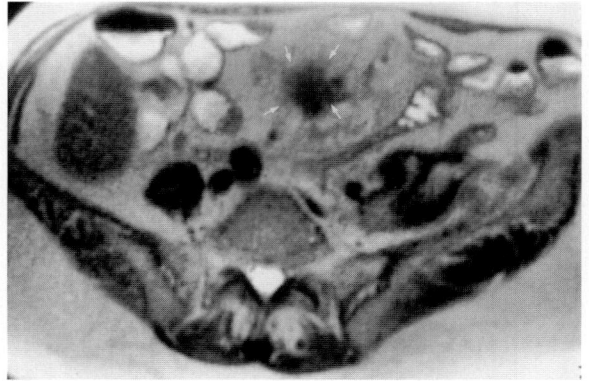

Fig. 3.28. Carcinoid. Axial T2-weighted HASTE image demonstrates a mesenteric mass in a patient with a small bowel carcinoid (*arrows*). The low signal intensity of the mass, coupled with its stellate morphology, is consistent with the desmoplastic reaction known to occur with carcinoid tumor. While the primary tumor is often small and infrequently imaged, the mesenteric and hepatic involvement are amenable to MRI

volvement is via hematogenous and/or lymphatic spread, while in patients with gastric cancer, direct extension is often the cause of esophageal metastases. The MRI findings are nonspecific: an enhancing mass on contrast-enhanced T1-weighted images. Fat suppression increases the conspicuity of the metastases.

3.3.4.7.2
STOMACH

Metastatic disease to the stomach results from direct extension and/or hematogenous or lymphatic spread. For example, a colon carcinoma arising from the transverse colon can spread along the gastrocolic ligament to invade the stomach. Similarly, pancreatic carcinoma that arises from the body of the gland can invade the posterior wall of the gastric body and antrum. In contrast, hematogenous gastric metastases are frequently associated with breast carcinoma. The desmoplastic reaction incited by breast carcinoma metastases may result in an appearance indistinguishable from primary scirrhous adenocarcinoma of the stomach. Finally, lymphatic spread of tumor to the stomach may be secondary to esophageal carcinoma. Save for cases of contiguous spread where the primary tumor can be imaged directly invading the stomach, the MRI findings of gastric metastases are nonspecific, i.e., enhancing masses within the stomach.

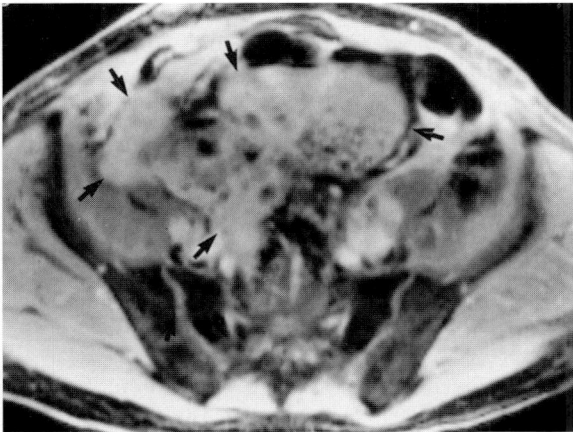

Fig. 3.29. Metastases to the small bowel. Axial T1-weighted fat-suppressed SGE image in a patient with pancreatic adenocarcinoma metastatic to the small bowel. Enhancing tumor coats and envelops the ileum (*arrows*)

3.3.4.7.3
SMALL BOWEL

Metastases to the small bowel are common, though often asymptomatic. They may occur via direct extension, peritoneal/serosal seeding, or, less commonly, hematogenous dissemination. Small intestine metastases from pancreatic carcinoma are the result of contiguous spread along the mesentery, whereas metastases from ovarian or gastric cancer involve the small bowel by peritoneal/serosal seeding. Gadolinium-enhanced T1-weighted fat-suppressed imaging is well suited to defining serosal-based metastases and in some instances is superior to CT (SEMELKA et al. 1993) (Fig. 3.29). Even small enhancing nodules may be seen against the low signal intensity mesenteric fat that surrounds the small intestine. Saline peritoneography, whereby saline is instilled into the peritoneum and imaged with a fast T2-weighted sequence, has met with some success in identifying small peritoneal and serosal metastases (MAGRE et al. 1996). Hematogenous metastases to the small bowel occur in association with breast cancer, lung cancer, or malignant melanoma and lodge on the antimesenteric border. When sufficiently large they may act as the lead point for intussusception.

3.3.4.7.4
LARGE BOWEL

Metastases to the large bowel are usually the sequelae of direct spread. Ovarian cancer is infamous for invading sigmoid colon and the metastases

are well shown on contrast-enhanced fat-suppressed T1-weighted images.

3.4
Intraluminal Contrast Agents

3.4.1
General Considerations

The theoretical benefits of intraluminal contrast agents include reliable marking of bowel from adjacent structures and better definition of bowel wall processes. The ideal oral contrast agent has the following characteristics: (a) patient acceptability in terms of palatability and side-effects, (b) uniform opacification of bowel regardless of concentration

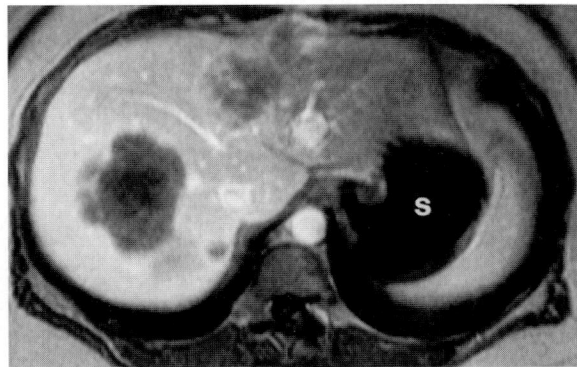

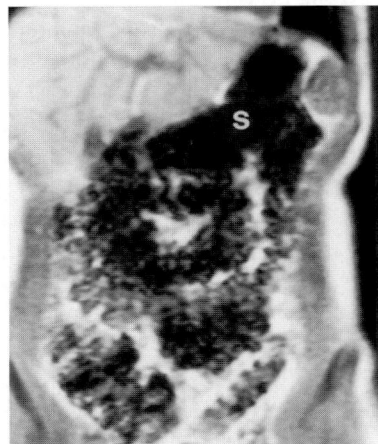

Fig. 3.30a,b. Negative oral contrast agents. **a** Axial gadolinium-enhanced T1-weighted fat-suppressed SGE image in a patient with cervix cancer metastatic to liver. The stomach lumen (*s*) is distended by negative contrast following ingestion of PFOB. **b** Coronal T1-weighted SGE image in a patient after OMP administration. The stomach (*s*) and portions of bowel containing the oral agent possess signal void lumens

and sequence parameters, (c) lack of absorption and complete excretion, (d) no induced motion or susceptibility artifacts, (e) improvement in diagnostic accuracy, (f) high margin of safety, and (g) low cost. For all agents there is a trade-off between these features (TAMMO et al. 1994).

Oral contrast agents fall into two major categories: positive and negative agents. Positive agents shorten T1 relaxation to increase intraluminal signal intensity, while negative agents shorten T2 relaxation or rely on the absence of mobile protons to decrease intraluminal signal intensity. Biphasic agents are high in signal intensity on T1- and low in signal intensity on T2-weighted images.

3.4.2
Positive Contrast Agents

Gadopentetate dimeglumine (Magnevist Enteral, Schering AG, Berlin, Germany) is an oral positive contrast agent. Its method of action is similar to its intravenous counterpart: paramagnetic shortening of T1 and T2 relaxation with the T1 effects predominating. To decrease dilutional effects as it progresses through the gastrointestinal tract, the gadopentetate dimeglumine is mixed with mannitol. It has also been mixed with barium paste for use in the esophagus. Intraluminal gadopentetate dimeglumine is well tolerated, effectively marks the bowel, and can demonstrate bowel wall thickening (KAMINSKY et al. 1991). Currently enteral gadopentetate dimeglumine is not commercially available in the United States.

Oral manganese particles are positive intraluminal contrast agents that work by shortening T1 and T2 relaxation. They occur naturally in green tea and blueberries (SATOH et al. 1993). Manganese chloride (LumenHance, Bristol-Myers Squibb, Princeton, N.J., USA) is an oral manganese agent that, when combined with a polymer, possesses biphasic properties. This agent performs well with fast imaging techniques (BERNADINO et al. 1993).

Ferric ammonium citrate (FAC) is a ferric oral agent that is a positive contrast agent when combined with other edible substances. It is the principal ingredient in the over-the-counter product Geritol (Beecham, Bristol, Tenn., USA). Initial reports found that Geritol was an effective oral contrast agent for marking the proximal small bowel, but its utility was limited by induced peristalsis and the associated degradation in image quality (WESBEY et al. 1985; LI

et al. 1989). FAC combined with sodium bicarbonate, food-grade substances, and water [oral magnetic resonance (OMR), Oncomembrane, Seattle, Wash., USA] is another positive agent that routinely delineates bowel, but gastrointestinal side-effects have been reported in approximately one-fifth of patients at the recommended dose (PATTEN et al. 1993).

3.4.3
Negative Contrast Agents (Fig. 3.30)

Perfluoroctylbromide (PFOB) (perflubon, Imagent GI, Alliance Pharmaceutical, San Diego, Calif., USA) is a negative contrast agent without mobile protons. Because of the associated peristalsis and rapid transit time through the alimentary tube, routine administration of glucagon is advocated when using PFOB (BROWN et al. 1991). Patient tolerance of PFOB is high, though some may complain of an oily taste and/or rectal incontinence for the first 3h after ingestion.

Superparamagnetic particles are negative contrast agents that rely on T2* shortening effects to decrease intraluminal signal intensity. Oral magnetic particles (OMP, Nycomed, Oslo, Norway) are a superparamagnetic ferrite crystal suspension. Patients tolerate ingesting OMP, but susceptibility effects may degrade image quality on gradient echo sequences (BOUDGHENE et al. 1993; OKSENDAL et al. 1991). AMI-121 (Lumirem, Roissy, France) is another superparamagnetic particle that performs well at marking bowel and is well tolerated (ROS et al. 1991; TORRES et al. 1990).

Over-the-counter clay containing substances (e.g., Kaopectate, kaolin-pectate, Upjohn, Kalamazoo, Mich., USA) are negative agents with diamagnetic shortening of both T1 and T2 relaxation times in aqueous solutions. Widespread use is limited as patients find them unpalatable.

Barium sulfate suppresses signal intensity via decreased mobile protons at high concentrations and diffusion of water molecules through susceptibility gradients near the suspended particles (LANGMO et al. 1992). It may be administered safely orally and/or rectally. In an attempt to improve both its palatability and its negative agent properties, barium sulfate has been combined with other negative contrast agents (LIEBIG et al. 1993).

Gas is a negative intraluminal contrast agent that has been used in evaluation of both the proximal and the distal gastrointestinal tract. Susceptibility artifacts predominate at high field strength and preclude its routine use (WEINREB et al. 1984; ZERHOUNI et al. 1986; CHOU et al. 1993).

3.4.4
Other Contrast Agents

Many over-the-counter foods (e.g., milk, green tea, oil, blueberries) have been studied as potential oral agents. They tend to be high in signal intensity on both T1- and T2-weighted sequences, a result of their lipid components/paramagnetic trace elements and fluid state, respectively. These agents perform well in the proximal gastrointestinal tract, but dilutional effects predominate distally and limit their usefulness as a bowel contrast agent (BISSET 1989; BALZARINI et al. 1992).

3.5
Conclusion

The role of MRI for investigating alimentary tube disorders is increasing. Advances in fast scanning and fat suppression techniques coupled with intravenous contrast agents have contributed to MRI's emergence. Current indications for MRI of the gastrointestinal tract include: diagnosing the type and extent of IBD, detecting fistulae, staging rectal malignancy, and differentiating tumor recurrence from postradiation fibrosis.

References

Al-Mondhiry H (1986) Primary lymphomas of the intestine: east-west contrast. Am J Hematol 22:89–105

Ascher SM, Semelka RC (1996) MRI of the gastrointestinal tract. In: Higgins CB, Hricak H, Helms CA (eds) Magnetic resonance imaging of the body. Lippincott-Raven Press, Philadelphia, pp 101–124

Ascher SM, Semelka RC, Brown JJ (1996) Pancreas, spleen, bowel, and peritoneum. In: Hayes CE, Dietz MJ, King BF, et al. Pelvic imaging with phased array coils: quantitative assessment of signal-to-noise ratio improvement. J Magn Reson Imaging 2:231–326

Balthazar E, Megibow AJ, Siegal SE, Birnbaum BA (1991) Appendicitis: prospective evaluation with high-resolution CT. Radiology 180:21–24

Balzarini L, Ceglia E, D'Ippolito G, et al. (1990) Local recurrence of rectosigmoid cancer: what about the choice of MRI for diagnosis? Gastrointest Radiol 15:338–342

Balzarini L, Aime S, Barbero L, Ceglia E, et al. (1992) Magnetic resonance imaging of the gastrointestinal tract: investigation of baby milk as a low cost contrast medium. Eur J Radiol 15:171–174

Bartolo D, Goepel JR, Parsons MA (1982) Rectal malignant lymphoma in chronic ulcerative colitis. Gut 23:164–168

Bernardino ME, Weinreb JC, Mitchell DG (1993) Fast MR imaging of the bowel with a manganese chloride T1/T2 contrast agent (abstract). Radiology 189(P):203

Bisset GS, III (1989) Evaluation of potential practical oral contrast agents for pediatric magnetic resonance imaging: preliminary observations. Pediatr Radiol 20:61–66

Boudghene FP, Bach-Ganso T, Grange JD, et al. (1993) Contribution of oral magnetic particles in MR imaging of the abdomen with spin-echo and gradient-echo sequences. J Magn Reson Imaging 3:107–112

Brown JJ, Duncan JR, Heiken JP, et al. (1991) Perfluoroctylbromide as a gastrointestinal contrast agent for MR imaging: use with and without glucagon. Radiology 181:455–460

Butch RJ, Stark DD, Wittenberg J, et al. (1986) Staging rectal cancer by MRI and CT. AJR 146:1155–1160

Chan TW, Kressel HY, Milestone B, et al. (1991) Rectal carcinoma: staging at MR imaging with endorectal surface coil. Radiology 181:461–467

Chernish SM, Maglinte DDT (1990) Glucagon: common untoward reactions – review and recommendations. Radiology 177:145–146

Chew FS, Zambuto DA (1992) Meckel's diverticulum. AJR 159:982

Cho KC, Morehouse HT, Alterman DD, Thornhill BA (1990) Sigmoid diverticulitis: diagnostic role of CT – comparison with barium enema studies. Radiology 170:111–115

Chou C, Liu G, Chen L, Jaw T (1993) Retrograde air insufflation in MRI: a technical note. Abdom Imaging 18:211–214

de Lange EE, Fechner RE, Wanebo HJ (1989) Suspected recurrent rectosigmoid carcinoma after abdominoperineal resection: MR imaging and histopathologic correlation. Radiology 170:323–328

de Lange EE, Gechner RE, Edge SB, Spaulding CA (1990) Preoperative staging of rectal carcinoma with MR imaging: surgical and histopathologic correlation. Radiology 176:623–628

Deutsch AA, McLeod RS, Cullen J, Cohen Z (1991) Results of the pelvic-pouch procedure in patients with Crohn's disease. Dis Colon Rectum 34:475–477

Dragosics B, Bauer P, Radaasziewicz T (1985) Primary gastrointestinal non-Hodgkin's lymphomas. Cancer 55:1060–1073

Eisenberg RL (1983a) Solitary filling defects in the jejunum and ileum. In: Eisenberg RL (ed) Gastrointestinal radiology. Lippincott Philadelphia, pp 492–504

Eisenberg RL (1983b) Single filling defects in the colon. In: Eisenberg RL (ed) Gastrointestinal radiology. Lippincott, Philadelphia, pp 681–710

Goldberg HI, Caruthers B Jr, Nelson JA, Singleton JW (1979) Radiographic findings of the national cooperative Crohn's disease study. Gastroenterology 77:925

Gomberg JS, Friedman AC, Radecki PD, Grumbach K, Caroline DF (1986) MRI differentiation of recurrent colorectal carcinoma from postoperative fibrosis. Gastrointest Radiol 11:361–363

Halvorsen RA, Thompson WM (1991) Primary neoplasms of the hollow organs of the gastrointestinal tract. Cancer 67:188–189

Halvorsen RA, Herfkins RJ, Wolfe WG (1987) Comparison of magnetic resonance to computed tomography for staging esophageal carcinoma. Miami Beach, American Roentgen Ray Society Proceedings 133

Hamed MM, Hamm B, Ibrahim ME, Taupitz M, Mahfouz AE (1992) Dynamic MR imaging of the abdomen with gadopentetate dimeglumine: normal enhancement pattern of liver, spleen, stomach, and pancreas. AJR 158:303–307

Hayes CE, Dietz MJ, King BF, et al. (1992) Pelvic imaging with phased array coils: quantitative assessment of signal-to-noise ratio improvement. J Magn Reson Imaging 2:231–326

Hussain SM, Stoker J, Lameris JS (1995) Anal sphincter complex: endoanal MR imaging of normal anatomy. Radiology 197:671–677

Ito K, Kato T, Tadokoro M (1992) Recurrent rectal cancer and scar: differentiation with PET and MR imaging. Radiology 182:549–552

Jeffrey RB (1992) Abdominal imaging in the immunocompromised patient. Radiol Clin North Am 30:579–596

Jeffrey RB, Laing FC, Townsend RR (1988) Acute appendicitis: sonographic criteria based on 250 cases. Radiology 167:327–329

Kaminsky S, Laniado M, Gogoll M, et al. (1991) Gadopentetate dimeglumine as a bowel contrast agent: safety and efficacy. Radiology 178:503–508

Kee F, Wilson RH, Gilliland R, Sloan JM, Rowlands BJ, Moorehead RJ (1992) Changing site distribution of colorectal cancer. BMJ 305:158

Kettritz U, Isaacs K, Warshauer DM, Semelka RC (1995) Crohn's disease: pilot study comparing MRI of the abdomen with clinical evaluation. J Clin Gastroenterol 21:249–253

Krestin GP, Steibrich W, Friedman G (1988) Recurrent rectal cancer: diagnosis with MR versus CT. Radiology 168:307–311

Langmo L, Ros PR, Torres GM, Erquiaga E (1992) Comparison of MR imaging after barium administration with CT in pelvic disease. J Magn Reson Imaging 2:89–91

Li KCP, Tart RP, Storm B, Rolfes R, Ang P, Ros PR (1989) MRI contrast agents: comparative study of five potential agents in humans. Proceedings of the Annual Meeting of the Society of Magnetic Resonance in Medicine, p 791

Liebig T, Stoupis C, Ros PR, Ballinger JR, Briggs RW (1993) A potentially artifact-free oral contrast agent for gastrointestinal MRI. Magn Reson Med 30:646–649

Macpherson RI (1993) Gastrointestinal tract duplications: clinical, pathologic, etiologic and radiologic considerations. Radiographics 13:1063–1080

Magre GR, Terk M, Colletti P, et al. (1996) Saline MR peritoneography. AJR 167:749–751

Martin RG (1986) Malignant tumors of the small intestine. Surg Clin North Am 66:779–785

Matushita M, Oi H, Murakami T, et al. (1994) Extraserosal invasion in advanced gastric cancer: evaluation with MR imaging. Radiology 192:87–91

McCauley TR, McCarthy S, Lange R (1992) Pelvic phased array coil: image quality assessment for spin-echo imaging. Magn Reson Imaging 10:513–522

Oksendal AN, Jacobsen TF, Gundersen HG, Rinck PA, Rummeny E (1991) Superparamagnetic particles as an oral contrast agent in abdominal magnetic resonance imaging. Invest Radiol 26:S67–S70

Outwater EK, Mitchell DG (1994) Magnetic resonance imaging techniques in the pelvis. MRI Clin North Am 2:161–188

Outwater EK, Scheibler ML (1993) Pelvic fistulas: findings on MR images. AJR 160:327–330

Patten RM, Lo SK, Phillips JJ (1993) Positive bowel contrast agent for MR imaging of the abdomen: phase 2 and 3 clinical trials. Radiology 189:277–283

Pavone P, Cardone GP, Cisterno S, Di Girolamo M (1992) Gadopentetate dimeglumine-barium paste for opacification of the esophageal lumen on MR images. AJR 159:762–764

Pema PJ, Bennett WF, Bova JG, Warman P (1994) CT vs MRI in diagnosis of recurrent rectosigmoid carcinoma. J Comput Assist Tomogr 18:256–261

Quint LE, Glazer GM, Orringer MGB (1985) Esophageal imaging by MR and CT: study of normal anatomy and neoplasms. Radiology 156:727–731

Ros PR, Green AM, Bernadino ME, Harms SE, Unger P, Hahn PF (1991) Safety and efficacy of superparamagnetic iron oxide: summary of multicenter phase II/III clinical trials (abstract). Radiology 181:93

Satoh S, Munechika H, Ri K, Hishida T, Nagasawa O (1993) Green tea as a positive enhancement agent for MR imaging of the gastrointestinal tract (abstract). Radiology 189:133

Schnall MD, Furth EE, Rosato EF (1994) Rectal tumor stage: correlation of endorectal MR imaging and pathologic findings. Radiology 190:709–714

Semelka RC, Shoenut JP, Silverman R, Kroeker MA, Yaffe CS, Mickflikier AB (1991) Bowel disease: prospective comparison of CT and 1.5T pre- and postcontrast MR imaging with T1-weighted fat-suppressed and breath-hold FLASH sequences. J Magn Reson Imaging 1:625–632

Semelka RC, Shoenut JP, Kroeker MA, et al. (1992) Focal liver disease: comparison of dynamic contrast-enhanced CT and T2-weighted fat-suppressed, FLASH, and dynamic gadolinium-enhanced MR imaging at 1.5T. Radiology 184:687–694

Semelka RC, Lawrence PH, Shoenut JP, et al. (1993) Primary malignant ovarian disease: prospective comparison of contrast enhanced CT and pre- and post intravenous Gd-DTPA enhanced fat-suppressed and breath hold MRI with histological correlation. J Magn Reson Imaging 3:99–106

Semelka RC, Kelekis NL, Thomasson D (1996a) HASTE MR imaging: description of technique and preliminary results in the abdomen. J Magn Reson Imaging 6:698–699

Semelka RC, John G, Kelekis NL, Burdeny DA, Ascher SM (1996b) Small bowel neoplastic disease: demonstration by MRI. J Magn Reson Imaging 6:855–860

Semelka RC, Hricak H, Kim B, et al. (1997) Pelvic fistulas: appearances on MR images. Abdom Imaging 22:91–95

Shoenut JP, Semelka RC, Silverman R, Yaffe CS, Mickflikier AB (1993a) Magnetic resonance imaging in inflammatory bowel disease. J Clin Gastroenterol 17:73–78

Shoenut JP, Semelka RC, Silverman R, Yaffe CS, Mickflikier AB (1993b) MRI in the diagnosis of Crohn's disease in two pregnant women. J Clin Gastroenterol 17:244–247

Shoenut JP, Semelka RC, Silverman R, Yaffe CS, Mickflikier AB (1993c) Magnetic resonance imaging evaluation of the local extent of colorectal mass lesions. J Clin Gastroenterol 17:248–253

Shoenut JP, Semelka RC, Silverman R, et al. (1993d) The gastrointestinal tract. In: Semelka RC, Shoenut JP (eds) MRI of the abdomen with CT correlation. Raven Press, New York, pp 119–143

Shoenut JP, Semelka RC, Magro CM, Silverman R, Yaffe CS, Mickflikier AB (1994) Comparison of magnetic resonance imaging and endoscopy in distinguishing the type and severity of inflammatory bowel diseases. J Clin Gastroenterol 19:31–35

Smith RC, Reinhold C, McCauley TR, et al. (1992) Multicoil high-resolution fast spin echo MR imaging of the female pelvis. Radiology 184:671–675

Spencer JA, Ward J, Beckingham IJ, et al. (1996) Dynamic contrast-enhanced MR imaging of perianal fistulas. AJR 167:735–741

Spiro HM (1993) Inflammatory bowel disease. In: Spiro HM (ed) Clinical gastroenterology. McGraw-Hill, New York, pp 631–760

Tammo HPR, Davis MA, Ros PR (1994) Intraluminal contrast agents for MR imaging of the abdomen and pelvis. J Magn Reson Imaging 4:291–300

Tempany CM, Fielding JR (1996) Female pelvis. In: Edelman RR, Hesselink JR, Zlatkin MB (eds) Clinical magnetic resonance imaging. Saunders, Philadelphia, pp 1432–1465

Templeton PA, Kui M, White CS, Krasna MJ (1994) Use of gadolinium-enhanced MR imaging to evaluate for airway invasion in patients with esophageal carcinoma. Radiology 193:311

Thoeni RF (1991) Colorectal cancer: cross-sectional imaging for staging of primary tumor and detection of local recurrence. AJR 156:909–915

Torres GM, Ros PR, Burton SS, Barreda R, Erquiaga E (1990) Retroperitoneal MR imaging before and after oral administration of superparamagnetic iron oxide contrast material (abstract). Radiology 177:358

Trenker SW, Halvorsen RA, Thompson WM (1994) Neoplasms of the upper gastrointestinal tract. Radiol Clin North Am 32:15–24

Waizer A, Powsner E, Russo I, et al. (1991) Prospective comparative study of magnetic resonance imaging versus transrectal ultrasound for preoperative staging and follow-up of rectal cancer. Dis Colon Rectum 34:1068–1072

Weinreb JC, Maravilla KR, Redman HC, Nunnally R (1984) Improved MR imaging of the upper abdomen with glucagon and gas. J Comput Assist Tomogr 8:835–838

Wesbey GE, Brasch RC, Goldberg HI, Engelstad BL (1985) Dilute oral iron solutions as gastrointestinal contrast agents for magnetic resonance imaging: initial clinical experience. Magn Reson Imaging 3:57–64

Winkler ML, Hricak H, Higgins CB (1987) MR imaging of diffusely infiltrating gastric carcinoma. J Comput Assist Tomogr 11:337–339

Younathan CM, Ros PR, Burton SS (1991) MR imaging of colonic lipoma. J Comput Assist Tomogr 15:492–494

Zerhouni EA, Brennecke CM, Fishman EK, Zimmer R, Soulen RL (1986) Development of gaseous contrast agents for MRI of the abdomen and pelvis (abstr). In: Proceedings of the 34th annual meeting of the Association of University Radiologists. Association of University Radiologists, Reston

4 Endosonography

A. CHONAN, F. MOCHIZUKI, and M. ANDO

CONTENTS

4.1 Introduction

Diagnostic imaging of the alimentary tube has mainly been achieved by roentgenography and endoscopy. However, it is difficult to obtain intramural or extramural information using these modalities. On the other hand, endosonography visualizes the alimentary tube wall with its different layers which are subsequently correlated with histologic layers. Therefore, the effectiveness of endosonography has been widely accepted in various alimentary tube diseases, including submucosal tumors or cancers. In this chapter we shall present the endosonographic findings of representative diseases of the alimentary tube.

A. CHONAN, MD, Department of Gastroenterology, JR Sendai Hospital, 1-3-1 Itsutsubashi Aoba-ku, Sendai 980, Japan
F. MOCHIZUKI, MD, Department of Gastroenterology, JR Sendai Hospital, 1-3-1 Itsutsubashi Aoba-ku, Sendai 980, Japan
M. ANDO, MD, Department of Gastroenterology, JR Sendai Hospital, 1-3-1 Itsutsubashi Aoba-ku, Sendai 980, Japan

4.2 Endosonographic Instruments

Two types of instrument are employed in endosonography. One type, employed in conventional endosonography, is an ultrasound probe mounted on the tip of the endoscope (Fig. 4.1a,b) (STROHM et al. 1980; DIMAGNO et al. 1980). This type uses comparatively low-frequency ultrasonic waves and is appropriate for large, deep lesions. The other is an endoscopic ultrasound probe which is passed through a forceps channel (Fig. 4.1c,d) (SILVERSTEIN et al. 1989; KIMMEY et al. 1990; RÖSCH and CLASSEN 1990). It uses comparatively high-frequency ultrasonic waves to ensure high resolution, and it is therefore appropriate for small, shallow lesions. The specifications of these instruments are shown in Table 4.1.

Concerning the delineation method, endosonography is divided into two subtypes, namely the radial scanning type and the linear scanning type. The radial scanning type is convenient for delineating endosonographic imaging because it possesses a visual ultrasonic field of 360° whereas the linear scanning type has a visual ultrasonic field of only 60°. Therefore, the radial scanning type is widely used in Japan except when assessment of vertical extension is necessary (e.g., in esophageal cancer).

Regarding the technique employed, after insertion of the scope, endosonographic examination is fundamentally performed with the alimentary tube filled with water. However, lesions that cannot be coated with water should be investigated with a water-filled balloon.

4.3 Normal Wall Structure of the Alimentary Tube

In the normal wall of the alimentary tube, a five-layered structure is visualized by endosonography (AIBE et al. 1986; KIMMEY et al. 1989). Figure 4.2a

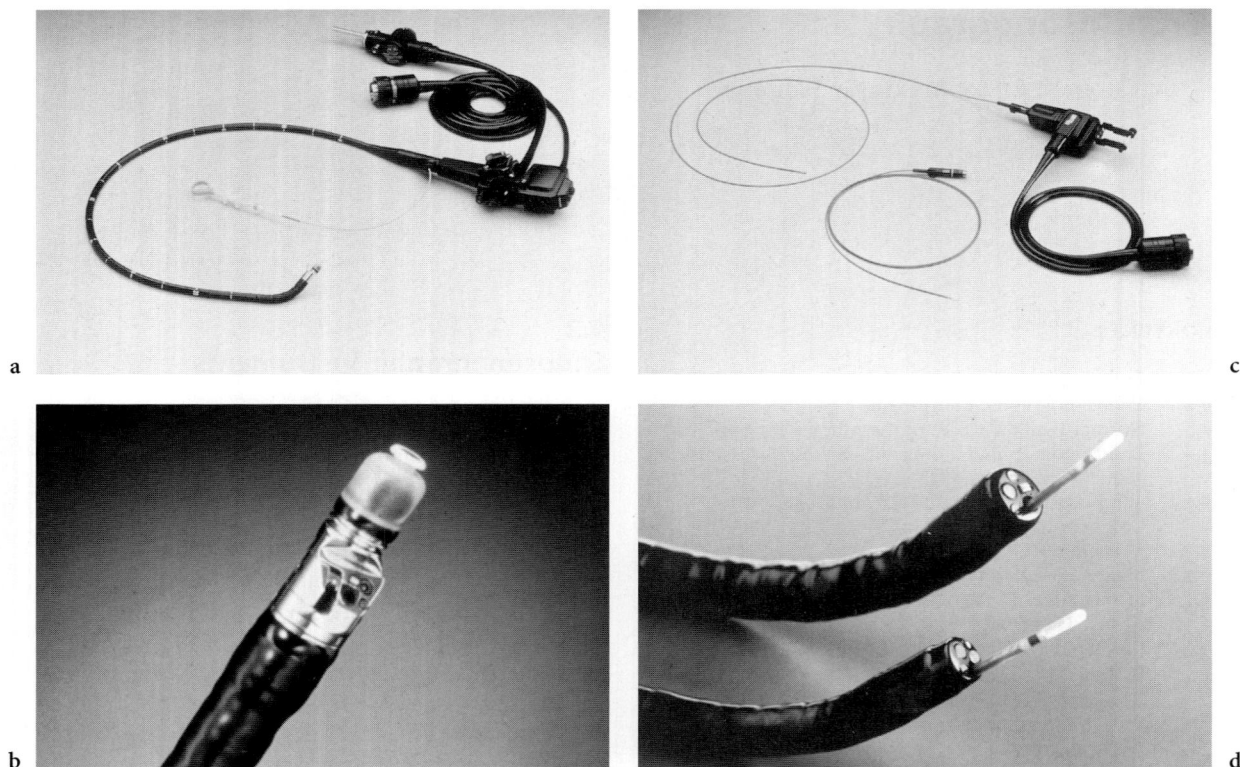

Fig. 4.1. a Conventional endosonographic instrument (0lympus GF-UM200). **b** Ultrasound probe mounted at the tip of the endoscope. **c** Endoscopic ultrsound probe (0lympus UM-2R/3R). **d** The ultrasound probe is passed through the forceps channel of the scope

Table 4.1. Specifications of endosonographic instruments (Olympus and Fujinon) for the alimentary tube

	Conventional type			Endoscopic ultrasound probe	
	GF-UM200[a]/UM20 (Olympus)	GF-UMQ200[a] (Olympus)	CF-UM200[a]/UM20 (Olympus)	UM-2R/3R (Olympus)	SP701PL (Fujinon)
Endoscope	Forward-oblique viewing gastroscope	Forward-oblique viewing gastroscope	Forward viewing colonoscope		
Working length (mm)	1055	1055	1325	2050	1700/1900/2200
Diameter (mm)					
Distal end (outer diameter)	14.2	13.2	17.4	2.5	2.0/2.6
Biopsy channel (inner diameter)	2.2/2.0	2.2	2.8		
Echoprobe	Mechanical radial scanning (360°)	Mechanical radial scanning (360°)	Mechanical radial scanning (300°)	Mechanical radial scanning (360°)	Radial (360°) and linear (switchable)
Frequency (MHz)	7.5 and 12 (switchable)	7.5 and 20 (switchable)	7.5 or 12	12 (UM2R)/20 (UM3R)	12 or 15 or 20
Focusing point (mm)	30 (7.5 MHz) 25 (12 MHz)	30 (7.5 MHz) 22 (20 MHz)	30 (7.5 MHz) 25 (12 MHz)		

[a] Video endoscope.

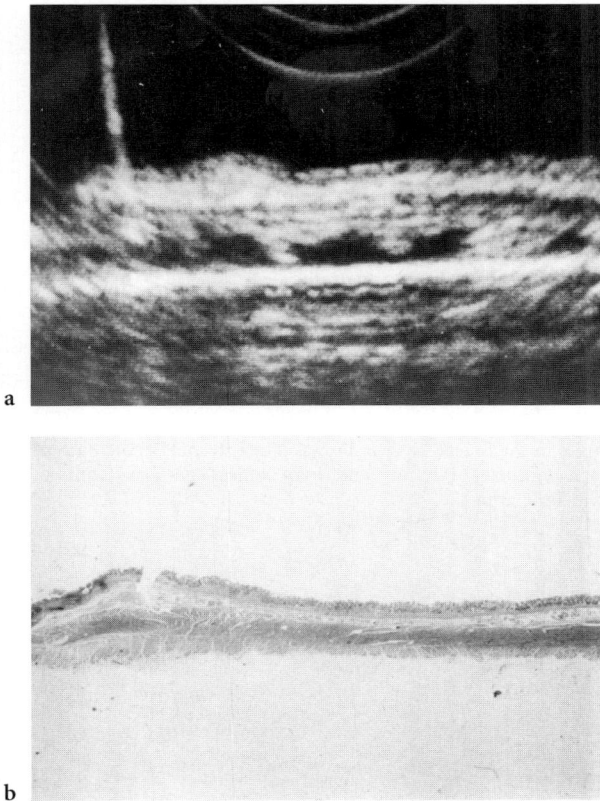

Fig. 4.2. a Appearance of the normal gastric wall of the resected specimen on endosonography (10 MHz). A pin echo is shown at the left end. b Histologic appearance of the same specimen. There is a pin hole at the left end

shows a sonogram of the normal gastric wall of a resected specimen. A pin echo can be seen at the left end. Figure 4.2b presents a cross-sectional view of the wall shown in Fig. 4.2a; a pin hole is visible at the left end. Figure 4.3 shows a schematic drawing of the normal wall structure of the alimentary tube. The first (hyperechoic) layer corresponds to the border of the echo and the mucosa, and the second (hypoechoic) layer constitutes the mucosa and

muscularis mucosae. The third (hyperechoic) layer is the submucosa, and the fourth (hypoechoic) layer is the muscularis propria. The fifth and last (hyperechoic) layer includes the subserosa, the serosa, and the border of the echo. A hyperechoic thin layer is frequently seen in the fourth layer; thus, in these cases, a seven-layered structure is visualized by endosonography. The echo source of this hyperechoic thin layer in the fourth layer is considered to be the border of the two muscle layers and/or the connective tissue between them.

4.4
Endosonographic Findings of Various Diseases of the Alimentary Tube

4.4.1
Submucosal Tumors and Extramural Compression

Both submucosal tumors and extramural compression are covered with normal mucosa. Therefore, it is difficult to differentiate them by roentgenography or endoscopy. Rather, endosonography is the most efficacious imaging modality for their differentiation (YASUDA et al. 1989; HASHIMOTO et al. 1989; CALETTI et al. 1989).

4.4.1.1
Myogenic Tumors

Both leiomyoma and leiomyosarcoma are hard tumors. Tumors derived from the muscularis propria are visible in the fourth layer on endosonographic imaging, while tumors derived from the muscularis mucosae are seen in the second layer. Leiomyoma is frequently demonstrated by endosonography as an intraluminal or intramural homogeneous hypoechoic mass, less than 4 cm in size, with a clear,

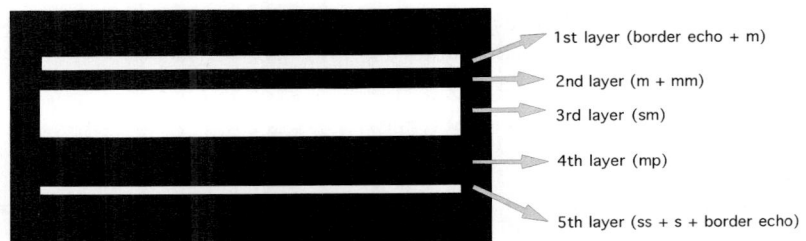

Fig. 4.3. Schematic drawing of the normal wall structure of the alimentary tube as visualized by endosonography. *m*, Mucosa; *mm*, muscularis mucosae; *sm*, submucosa; *mp*, muscularis propia; *ss*, subserosa; *s*, serosa

1st layer (border echo + m)
2nd layer (m + mm)
3rd layer (sm)
4th layer (mp)
5th layer (ss + s + border echo)

m: mucosa, mm: muscularis mucosae, sm: submucosa
mp: muscularis propria, ss: subserosa, s: serosa

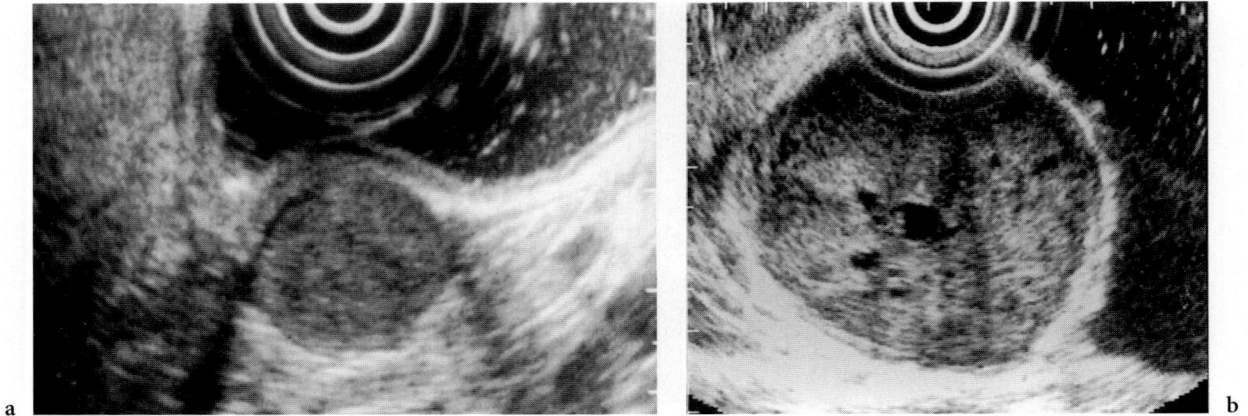

a

b

Fig. 4.4. a Sonogram of gastric leiomyoma (7.5 MHz). A homogeneous hypoechoic mass in the fourth layer with a clear, smooth margin is shown. **b** Sonogram of gastric leiomyosarcoma (7.5 MHz). A heterogeneous hypoechoic mass in the fourth layer is shown. The internal echoic pattern is a mixture of hypo- and hyperechoic patterns with an anechoic area

smooth margin. Figure 4.4a shows a leiomyoma of the stomach, which on endosonography was visualized as a homogeneous hypoechoic mass in the fourth layer (muscularis propia) with a clear, smooth margin. On the other hand, leiomyosarcoma is frequently visualized by endosonography as an extraluminal mass. 4 cm or more in size, with a clear, nodular margin. Sometimes an ulcer is present at the top of the tumor. However, the most characteristic feature of leiomyosarcomas is that their internal echoic pattern is a mixture of hypo- and hyperechoic patterns, often associated with anechoic areas, as in the case of the leiomyosarcoma of the stomach in the fourth layer shown in Fig. 4.4b.

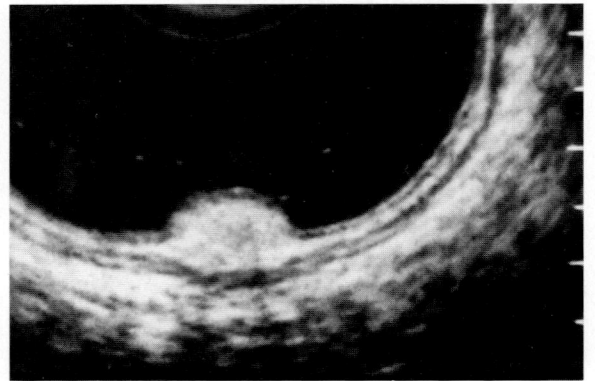

Fig. 4.5. Sonogram of a lipoma of the colon (7.5 MHz). An intraluminal homogeneous hyperechoic mass is delineated in the third layer

4.4.1.2
Lipomas

A lipoma is a soft submucosal tumor delineated in the third layer (submucosa) on endosonographic imaging. Lipomas are frequently revealed by endosonography as intraluminal homogeneous hyperechoic masses with clear, smooth margins. Figure 4.5 shows a lipoma of the colon: a homogeneous hyperechoic mass is visible in the third layer.

and/or submucosa) on endosonographic imaging. They are frequently visualized by endosonography as anechoic lesions with clear, smooth margins. A lymphangioma is demonstrated by endosonography as an anechoic mass extending through the second and third layers, divided by septa. Figure 4.6 shows a gastric cyst as seen on endosonography: an anechoic mass is visible in the third layer.

4.4.1.3
Cystic Lesions

Cystic lesions are very soft submucosal tumors delineated in the second and/or third layer (mucosa

4.4.1.4
Aberrant Pancreas

Aberrant pancreas is an elastic submucosal tumor delineated in the third layer (submucosa) on

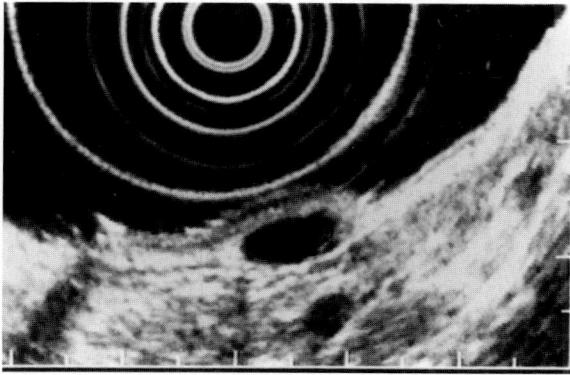

Fig. 4.6. Sonogram of a gastric cyst (12 MHz). An anechoic lesion is visible in the third layer

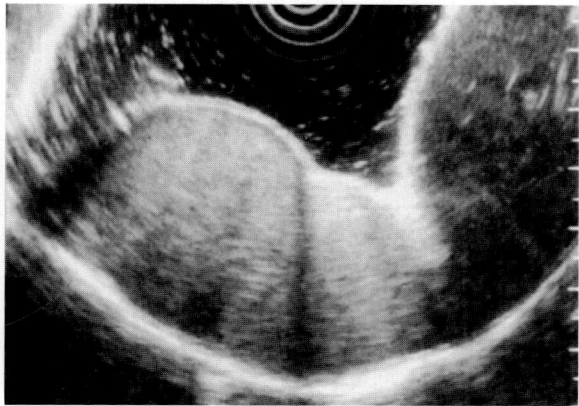

Fig. 4.7. Sonogram of extragastric compression due to a hepatic hemangioma (7.5 MHz). The lesion is shown outside the normal five-layered structure of the stomach

endosonographic imaging. An aberrant pancreas is frequently visualized by endosonography as a spindle-shaped heterogeneous hypoechoic mass with an unclear, irregular margin. A duct-like anechoic area is often present in the mass, and the fourth layer is thickened.

4.4.1.5
Extramural Compression

Extramural compression by neighboring tissue is imaged as a mass outside of the five-layered structure of the wall of the alimentary tube. Therefore, it is easy to differentiate between submucosal tumor and extramural compression endosonographically. Figure 4.7 shows extragastric compression due to a liver hemangioma. The five-layered structure of the wall is intact.

4.4.2
Cancers

Endosonography is efficacious for diagnosing the depth of cancerous invasion (MURATA et al. 1987; RIFKIN et al. 1989; OHASHI et al. 1989; SHIMIZU et al. 1990; TIO et al. 1990; LIGHTDALE 1992; ROUBEIN et al. 1990; KATSURA et al. 1992; RÖSCH et al. 1992; DITTLER and SIEWERT 1993; GRIMM et al. 1993; YANAI et al. 1993; CHO et al. 1993; CHONAN 1993; CHONAN et al. 1995; SMITH et al. 1993; MARUTA et al. 1994). A schematic illustration of the depth of cancerous invasion of the alimentary tube as estimated by endosonography is shown in Fig. 4.8.

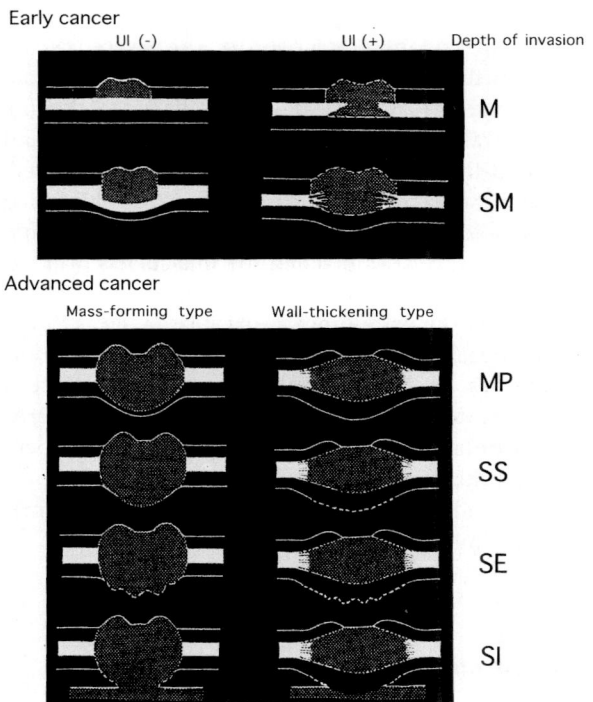

Fig. 4.8. Schematic illustration of the depth of cancerous invasion of the alimentary tube, as estimated by endosonography. Ul (−), Absence of ulcers or ulcer scars; Ul (+), presence of ulcers or ulcer scars; M, mucosa; SM, submucosa; MP, muscularis propria; SS, subserasa; SE, serosa; SI, invasion of adjacent structures

4.4.2.1
Early Cancers

In early cancer without ulcers or ulcer scars, absence of alterations of the third (submucosa), fourth (muscularis propria), and fifth (subserosa–serosa) layers on endosonography is interpreted as showing that the cancer is limited to the mucosa. Involvement of the third layer is interpreted as submucosal invasion. In early cancer associated with ulcers or ulcer scars, the tumor echo is usually associated with a fan-shaped hypoechoic shadow and tapering interruption of the third layer. Absence of thickening of the wall is interpreted as showing that the cancer is limited to the mucosa, while thickening of the wall is interpreted as submucosal invasion.

4.4.2.2
Advanced Cancers

Advanced cancers are divided into two types based on endosonographic findings. In the mass-forming type, cancer is detected as a mass with a clear margin and concomitant destruction of the layered structure. In the wall-thickening type, the layered structure remains relatively intact and marked thickening of the wall is noted. In both the mass-forming and the wall-thickening type, destruction of the first, second, and third layers, as well as irregular narrowing of the fourth layer, is taken as a definite indication that the cancer has invaded the muscularis propria. Complete destruction of the five-layered structure with a smooth extraluminal surface is taken as a definite indication that the cancer has extended to the subserosa. Irregularity of the extraluminal surface in addition to complete destruction of the layered structure is taken to mean that the cancer has penetrated the serosa. An obscure border between the cancer and the neighboring tissue is defined as malignant invasion of adjacent structures.

4.4.2.3
Preoperative Endosonographic Staging

Endosonographic T and N staging has been carried out according to the TNM system (Sobin et al. 1988). Due to the limited penetration depth, assessment of cancer metastasis to distant organs (M stage) is beyond the scope of endosonography. The criteria of T and N staging are as follows: T1 tumor, tumor invading the mucosa or submucosa; T2 tumor, tumor invading the muscularis propria (esophageal or rectal cancer) or subserosa (gastric or colon cancer); T3 tumor, tumor invading the adventitia (esophageal or rectal cancer) or serosa (gastric or colon cancer); T4 tumor, tumor invading adjacent structures; N0, no

lymph node metastasis; N1 – regional lymph node metastasis.

Many studies have compared preoperative T and N staging by endosonography with postoperative histologic staging (Murata et al. 1987; Rifkin et al. 1989; Tio et al. 1990; Lightdale 1992; Roubein et al. 1990; Katsura et al. 1992; Rösch et al. 1992; Dittler and Siewert 1993; Grimm et al. 1993; Cho et al. 1993; Chonan 1993; Chonan et al. 1995; Smith et al. 1993). The overall accuracy of T and N staging is 82%–89% and 66%–89% for esophageal cancer, 71%–90% and 63%–83% for gastric cancer, and 83% and 50%–69% for colorectal cancer, respectively.

4.4.2.4
Case Studies

Figure 4.9a shows a sonogram of a type 0-IIa submucosal cancer of the colon, obtained with an endoscopic ultrasound probe. Though no change of the fourth or fifth layer is visible, the destruction of

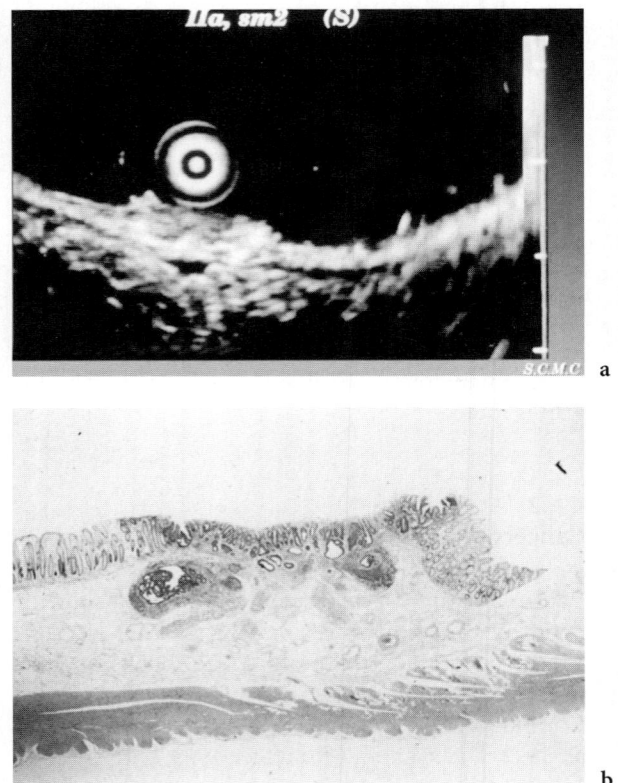

Fig. 4.9. a Sonogram of submucosal cancer of the colon, obtained with an endoscopic ultrasound probe (20 MHz). Destruction of the third layer by the tumor is shown, with no alteration of the fourth or fifth layer. **b** Histologic appearance in the same case. The cancer is seen to invade the middle level of the submucosal layer

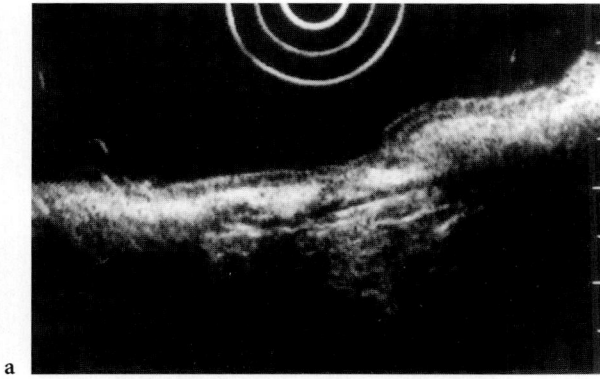

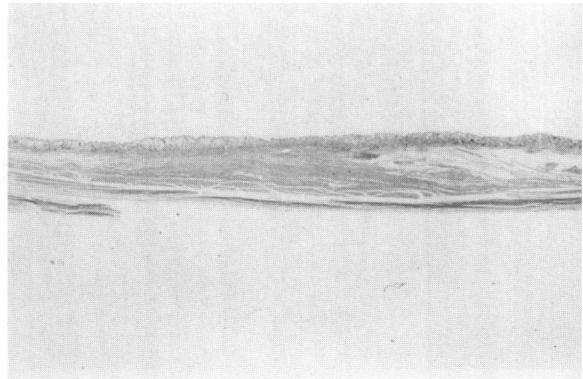

Fig. 4.10. a Ultrasonogram of a type 0–IIc gastric cancer associated with an ulcer scar (7.5 MHz). There is complete destruction of the third layer, but a fan-shaped hypoechoic shadow is present and there is tapering interruption of the third layer. The lack of thickening of the wall was taken to indicate that the cancer was limited to the mucosa. **b** Cross-section of the same case. The cancer is limited to the mucosa. Fibrosis due to the ulcer scar can be seen in the submucosal layer

Fig. 4.11. a Roentgenogram of a type 2 advanced esophageal cancer. **b** Sonogram of the same case (7.5 MHz), showing irregularity of the extramural surface in addition to complete destruction of the layered structure. However, the border between the cancer and the aorta is clear, indicating that the depth of cancer invasion is serosal

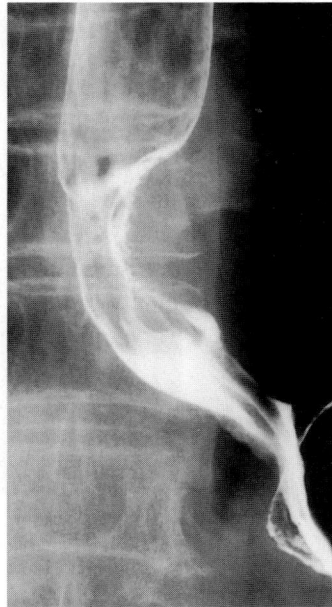

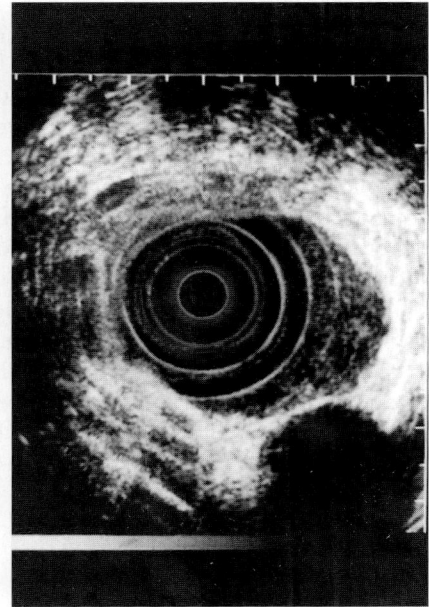

the third layer is obvious. Figure 4.9b is a cross-section of the same case. Cancer has massively invaded the submucosal layer.

Figure 4.10a shows the endosonographic appearance of a type 0–IIc early gastric cancer associated with an ulcer scar. The third layer has been completely destroyed. However, a fan-shaped hypoechoic shadow and tapering interruption of the third layer are visualized, and the absence of thickening of the wall is interpreted as showing that the cancer is limited to the mucosa. Figure 4.10b shows a cross-section of the same case. Fibrosis due to an ulcer scar is visible in the submucosal layer.

Figure 4.11a shows a roentgenogram and Fig. 4.11b an endosonogram of type 2 esophageal cancer. Irregularity of the extraluminal surface in addition to complete destruction of the layered structure is demonstrated by endosonography. However, the border between the cancer and the aorta is clear. The depth of cancer invasion was determined as serosal.

Figure 4.12 shows an endosonogram of type 4 gastric cancer (scirrhous). The layered structure remains relatively intact and marked thickening of the wall is noted. Therefore, on the basis of endosonography this case was diagnosed as wall-thickening type gastric cancer due to scirrhous invasion.

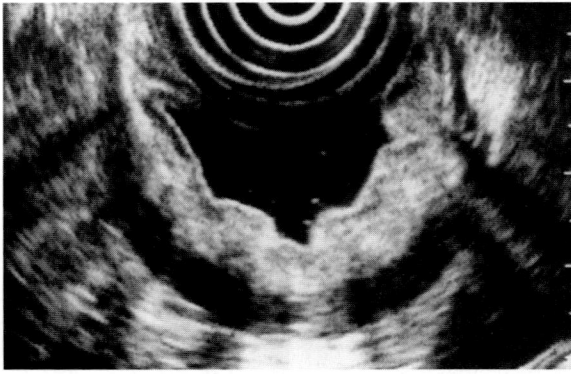

Fig. 4.12. Sonogram of a type 4 gastric cancer (7.5 MHz). The layered structure remains relatively intact and marked thickening of the wall is noted.

4.4.3
Malignant Lymphomas

Malignant lymphomas are commonly demonstrated by endosonography as very hypoechoic masses with a homogeneous echoic pattern (Fig. 4.13a) (TIO et al. 1986; BOLONDI et al. 1987; SUEKANE et al. 1993). Some of them appear as an aggregation of multiple hypoechoic nodules (Fig. 4.13b); histologically, these correspond to follicular lymphomas whose lymph follicles are large on cross-sections (Fig. 4.13c). The appearance of other malignant lymphomas on endosonography is very similar to that of peptic ulcers or ulcer scars, and it is therefore difficult to diagnose them correctly on the basis of this modality.

4.4.4
Esophagogastric Varices

Endosonographic examination assists in treatment selection by providing information on intramural vessels (varices), extramural vessels, and perforated vessels (CALETTI et al. 1990; NAKAMURA et al. 1992). After the treatment of esophagogastric varices, endosonography is effective in assessing the remaining vessels or recurrence of the varices.

4.4.5
Gastric Ulcers

The depth, size, and echoic pattern of gastric ulcers can be objectively estimated by end-osonography (NIWA et al. 1991). Therefore, endosonography is useful for detecting ulcers which are hard to heal or recurrent ulcers, and also for assessing the healing process of gastric ulcers. The healing process of a gastric ulcer at the lesser curvature of the lower body is demonstrated in Fig. 4.14. Figure 4.14a shows the endosonographic findings in respect of an active stage ulcer. A

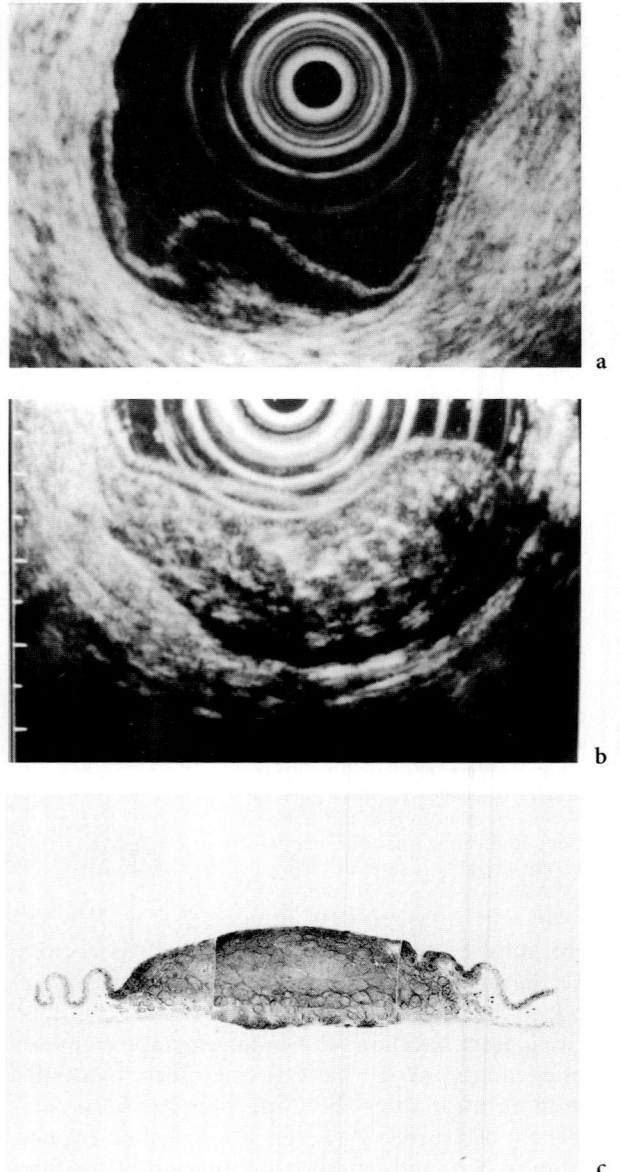

a

b

c

Fig. 4.13. a Sonogram of a gastric malignant lymphoma (7.5 MHz), showing a homogeneous very hypoechoic mass. **b** Sonogram of another gastric malignant lymphoma (7.5 MHz). An aggregation of multiple hypoechoic nodules is demonstrated. **c** Cross-section of the same case as in **b**. Large lymphoid follicles are shown from the submucosa to the serosa

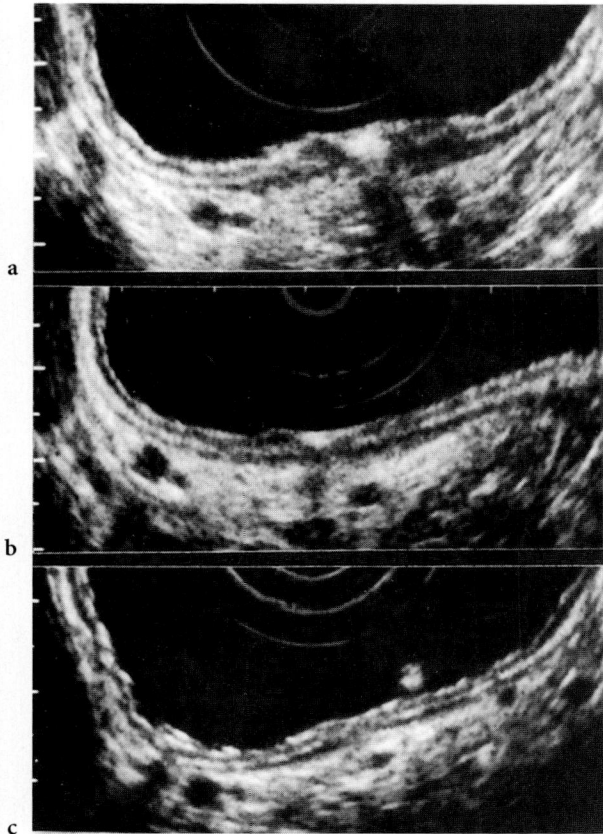

Fig. 4.14. a Sonogram of a Ul IV gastric ulcer in the active stage (12 MHz). A hyperechoic layer due to white coating is present at the bottom of the ulcer. The gastric wall has thickened, and the five-layered structure has been completely destroyed and replaced by a hypoechoic ulcer echo. b Sonogram of the same case in the healing stage (12 MHz), showing contraction of the hypoechoic ulcer echo and disappearance of the wall thickening. c Sonogram of the same case in the scarring stage (12 MHz). The hyperechoic area due to white coating and the hypoechoic ulcer echo have both disappeared

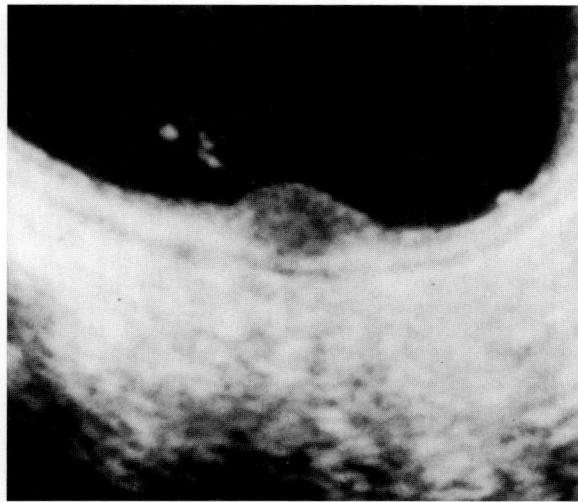

Fig. 4.15. Sonogram of a carcinoid tumor of the rectum (7.5 MHz). Destruction of the third layer is shown

4.4.6
Carcinoid Tumors

Carcinoid tumors are very hard and slightly yellowish masses covered with normal mucosa, similar to submucosal tumors. They are sometimes associated with a central depression at the top of the tumor. Carcinoid tumors are visualized by endosonography as homogeneous and relatively hypoechoic masses in the third layer, with a smooth, clear margin (SHIMIZU et al. 1990; YOSHIKANE et al. 1993). Occasionally, the internal echoic pattern is heterogeneous or relatively hyperechoic, depending on its histologic structure. Figure 4.15 shows the endosonographic appearance of a carcinoid tumor of the rectum. A relatively hypoechoic homogeneous mass is visible in the third layer.

hyperechoic area due to white coating is shown at the bottom of the ulcer, the gastric wall is thickened, and the five-layered structure has been completely destroyed and replaced by a hypoechoic ulcer echo. This ulcer is diagnosed as Ul IV. Figure 4.14b is the sonogram of the same case in the healing stage. The hypoechoic ulcer echo has contracted and the wall thickening has disappeared. A sonogram of the same case in the scarring stage is shown in Fig. 4.14c. The hyperechoic area due to white coating and the hypoechoic ulcer echo have disappeared. The lesion is covered with a normal appearing first layer. These findings suggest that the quality of ulcer healing is very good.

References

Aibe T, Fuji T, Okita K, et al. (1986) A fundamental study of normal layer structure of the gastrointestinal wall visualized by endoscopic ultrasonography. Scand J Gastroenterol 21 (Suppl 123):6–15

Bolondi L, Casanova P, Caletti G, et al. (1987) Primary gastric lymphoma versus gastric carcinoma: endoscopic US evaluation. Radiology 165:821–826

Caletti G, Zani L, Bolondi L, et al. (1989) Endoscopic ultrasonography in the diagnosis of gastric submucosal tumor. Gastrointest Endosc 35:413–418

Caletti G, Brocchi E, Baraldini M, et al. (1990) Assessment of portal hypertension by endoscopic ultrasonography. Gastrointest Endosc 36:S21–S27

Cho E, Nakajima M, Yasuda K, et al. (1993) Endoscopic ultrasonography in the diagnosis of colorectal cancer invasion. Gastrointest Endosc 39:521–527

Chonan A (1993) Clinical evaluation of endoscopic ultrasonography (EUS) in the diagnosis of depressed type early gastric cancers. Gastroenterol Endosc 35:1269–1281 (in Japanese with English abstr.)

Chonan A, Fujita N, Mochizuki F, et al. (1995) Diagnosis of the depth of advanced gastric cancer invasion by endoscopic ultrasonography: effectiveness of the balloon-compression method. Dig Endosc 7:220–225

DiMagno EP, Buxton JL, Regan PT, et al. (1980) Ultrasonic endoscope. Lancet I:629–631

Dittler HJ, Siewert JR (1993) Role of endoscopic ultrasonography in gastric carcinoma. Endoscopy 25:162–166

Grimm H, Binmoeller KF, Hamper K, et al. (1993) Endosonography for preoperative locoregional staging of esophageal and gastric cancer. Endoscopy 25:224–230

Hashimoto H, Mitsunaga A, Suzuki S, et al. (1989) Evaluation of endoscopic ultrasonography for gastric tumors and presentation of three-dimensional display of endoscopic ultrasonography. Surg Endosc 3:173–181

Katsura Y, Yamada K, Ishizawa T, et al. (1992) Endorectal ultrasonography for the assessment of wall invasion and lymph node metastasis in rectal cancer. Dis Colon Rectum 35:362–368

Kimmey MB, Martin RW, Haggitt RC, et al. (1989) Histologic correlates of gastrointestinal ultrasound images. Gastroenterology 96:433–441

Kimmey MB, Martin RW, Silverstein FE (1990) Endoscopic ultrasound probes. Gastrointest Endosc 36:S40–S46

Lightdale CJ (1992) Endoscopic ultrasonography in the diagnosis, staging and follow-up of esophageal and gastric cancer. Endoscopy 24(Suppl 1):297–303

Maruta S, Tsukamoto Y, Niwa Y, et al. (1994) Evaluation of upper gastrointestinal tumors with a new endoscopic ultrasound probe. Gastrointest Endosc 40:603–608

Murata Y, Muroi M, Yoshida M, et al. (1987) Endoscopic ultrasonography in the diagnosis of esophageal carcinoma. Surg Endosc 1:11–16

Nakamura H, Inoue H, Kawano T, et al. (1992) Selection of the treatment for esophagogastric varices. Surg Endosc 6:228–234

Niwa Y, Nakazawa S, Tsukamoto Y, et al. (1991) A new method for evaluating gastric ulcer healing by endoscopic ultrasonography. Scand J Gastroenterol 26:457–464

Ohashi S, Nakazawa S, Yoshino J (1989) Endoscopic ultrasonography in the assessment of invasive gastric cancer. Scand J Gastroenterol 24:1039–1048

Rifkin MD, Ehrlich SM, Marks G (1989) Staging of rectal carcinoma: prospective comparison of endorectal US and CT. Radiology 170:319–322

Rösch T, Classen M (1990) A new ultrasonic probe for endosonographic imaging of the upper GI tract. Endoscopy 22:41–46

Rösch T, Lorenz R, Zenker K, et al. (1992) Local staging and assessment of resectability in carcinoma of the esophagus, stomach, and duodenum by endoscopic ultrasonography. Gastrointest Endosc 38:460–467

Roubein LD, David C, DuBrow R, et al. (1990) Endoscopic ultrasonography in staging rectal cancer. Am J Gastroenterology 85:1391–1394

Shimizu S, Tada M, Kawai K (1990) Use of endoscopic ultrasonography for the diagnosis of colorectal tumors. Endoscopy 22:31–34

Silverstein FE, Martin RW, Kimmey MB, et al. (1989) Experimental evaluation of an endoscopic ultrasound probe: in vitro and in vivo canine studies. Gastroenterology 96:1058–1062

Smith JW, Brennan MF, Botet JF, et al. (1993) Preoperative endoscopic ultrasound can predict the risk of recurrence after operation for gastric carcinoma. J Clin Oncol 11:2380–2385

Sobin LH, Hermanek P, Hutter RVP (1988) TNM classification of malignant tumors: a comparison between the new (1987) and the old editions. Cancer 61:2310–2314

Strohm WD, Phillip J, Hagenmüller F, et al. (1980) Ultrasonic tomography by means of an ultrasonic fiberendoscope. Endoscopy 12:241–244

Suekane H, Iida M, Yao T, et al. (1993) Endoscopic ultrasonography in primary gastric lymphoma: correlation with endoscopic and histologic findings. Gastrointest Endosc 39:139–145

Tio TL, Den Hartog Jager FCA, Tytgat GNJ (1986) Endoscopic ultrasonography of non-Hodgkin lymphoma of the stomach. Gastroenterology 91:401–408

Tio TL, Coene PPLO, Luiken GJHM, et al. (1990) Endosonography in the clinical staging of esophagogastric carcinoma. Gastrointest Endosc 36:S2–S10

Yanai H, Fujimura H, Suzumi M, et al. (1993) Delineation of the gastric muscularis mucosae and assessment of depth of invasion of early gastric cancer using a 20-megahertz endoscopic ultrasound probe. Gastrointest Endosc 39:505–512

Yasuda K, Nakajima M, Yoshida S, et al. (1989) The diagnosis of submucosal tumors of the stomach by endoscopic ultrasonography. Gastrointest Endosc 35:10–15

Yoshikane H, Tsukamoto Y, Niwa Y, et al. (1993) Carcinoid tumor of the gastrointestinal tract: evaluation with endoscopic ultrasonography. Gastrointest Endosc 39:375–383

Section 2: Anatomic Areas

5 Esophagus

K.S. Dua, C.S. Easterling, and E.T. Stewart

CONTENTS

5.1
Introduction

Increasingly, the spectrum of esophageal disorders spans the expertise of a number of subspecialties interested in gastrointestinal pathology, but especially diagnostic radiologists and gastroenterolo-

K.S. Dua, MD, Assistant Professor of Medicine, Medical College of Wisconsin, Division of Gastroenterology & Hepatology, Director, GI Diagnostic Laboratory, VAMC, Froedtert Memorial Lutheran Hospital, 9200 West Wisconsin Avenue, Milwaukee, WI 53226-3596, USA
C.S. Easterling, MS/CCC, Clinical Supervisor, Speech Pathology, Curative Rehabilitation Services, Froedtert Memorial Lutheran Hospital, 9200 West Wisconsin Avenue, Milwaukee, WI 53226-3596, USA
E.T. Stewart, MD, FACR, Professor of Radiology, Medical College of Wisconsin, Chief, GI Radiology, Froedtert Memorial Lutheran Hospital, 9200 West Wisconsin Avenue, Milwaukee, WI 53226-3596, USA

gists. Speech pathologists are now playing an increasingly active role in evaluating patients with dysphagia and assisting with recommendations of oral intake and management of patients with pharyngoesophageal dysphagia.

The contents of this chapter will be primarily directed at a review of some of the advances in the diagnosis and management of pharyngoesophageal disorders. Due to the increasing interest in the evaluation of pharyngeal and esophageal motor disorders, a review of pharyngoesophageal function will be followed by a description of the increasingly employed modified barium swallow by speech pathologists as well as a review of esophageal motility disorders. The recent introduction of expandable metallic stents is a major advancement in the treatment of malignant obstruction of the esophagus and the current application will be reviewed.

5.2
Importance of Understanding Dysphagia

Swallowing is a complex but orderly integration of neuromuscular events for transporting liquids and solids from the mouth to the stomach. For convenience, swallowing may be divided into oropharyngeal and esophageal components; however, in practice, both must be evaluated. Swallowing occurs when the individual is awake and also during eating, up to 1000 times a day. Difficulties are quickly apparent to patients and are broadly referred to as "dysphagia."

5.3
Oral, Pharyngeal, and Esophageal Mechanics

In the mouth and pharynx, there are three important considerations when swallowing is being considered:

5.3.1
Bony and Cartilaginous Structures

Bony and cartilaginous structures include the mandible, palate, base of the skull, hyoid bone, thyroid cartilage, and cervical spine as well as their supporting membranes. These structures form the skeleton that supports the muscular components that participate in mastication and swallowing.

5.3.2
Neural Control

Neural control is modulated by paired mid brain swallowing centers which receive afferent input from the 5th, 7th, 9th, and 10th cranial nerves. Efferent fibers leave the mid brain via the 5th, 7th, 9th, 10th, and 12th cranial nerves. There are two postulated theories to describe control of swallowing. One suggests that the swallowing sequence is preprogrammed and events occur in a predetermined sequence when a swallow is initiated. The second theory suggests that there is sequential propagation of mechanical events which responds to stimuli during bolus movement. A combination of the two is very likely (DODDS et al. 1990a).

Neural control of esophageal function is from the medullary swallowing center via the 9th and 10th cranial nerves.

5.3.3
Muscle Groups

There are 31 pairs of striated muscles encompassing the tongue, palate, muscles of mastication, and pharynx. The constrictors of the pharynx are supported by the pharyngobasilar fascia, which is attached to the base of the skull. Supra- and infrahyoid muscles contribute to the characteristic upward excursion of the hyoid and larynx during swallowing. It is the coordinated action of these muscles that moves the bolus sequentially from the mouth into the pharynx and esophagus.

The cricopharyngeal muscle, which is a defined muscle attached to the cricoid cartilage, is also known as the upper esophageal sphincter (UES) and defines the beginning of the esophagus. The muscularis propria of the esophagus is composed of an inner circular and an outer longitudinal muscle layer, muscle layers which are continuous with the gastric muscularis propria. Circular and longitudinal muscle in the proximal one-half of the esophagus is striated but becomes smooth muscle in the distal one-third of the esophagus. The esophagus ends at the lower end of the lower esophageal sphincter (LES), which is not a defined muscle. The esophagogastric junction corresponds to the "Z" line or squamocolumnar junction seen endoscopically or on dissection. Radiologically the esophagogastric junction is often seen during peristalsis as a thin nondistensible mucosal ring, also known as the "B-ring." The B-ring is only seen when the esophagus is distended by the barium bolus.

It is the constrictors of the pharynx and the circular muscle contractions in the esophagus which impart the characteristic stripping wave that is observed during pharyngoesophageal peristalsis. Observations of peristalsis are directed at the "inverted-V" of the tail of the bolus as it is propelled distally.

The contribution of contraction of longitudinally oriented muscle is dramatically seen during laryngeal elevation as swallowing occurs. Although there is also significant shortening of the esophagus during peristalsis, this is more difficult to observe unless some marker is present such as diverticulum, esophageal web, or ring.

The UES and LES are contracted at rest. When swallowing is initiated, both relax. The UES remains relaxed for about 0.5 s. The LES remains relaxed much longer (6–8 s), until the bolus enters the stomach.

Pharyngeal peristalsis is very rapid, in the range of 10–25 cm/s, whereas the velocity slows to 2–4 cm/s in the esophageal body and even slower as the bolus approaches the LES.

5.4
Qualitative Similarity Between Fluoroscopy and Manometry

Longitudinal excursions complicate the recording of pressures, especially in the pharynx. However, it is now possible to obtain high-fidelity pressure tracings of pharyngoesophageal motility using strain gauge and/or sleeve devices during manometric recordings. When fluoroscopic observations of esophageal motility are compared to simultaneous manometric pressure events, there is striking qualitative similarity between the two modalities (Fig. 5.1). For this reason, the qualitative assessment of esophageal motility is very accurately performed during fluoroscopy (STEWART and DODDS 1994).

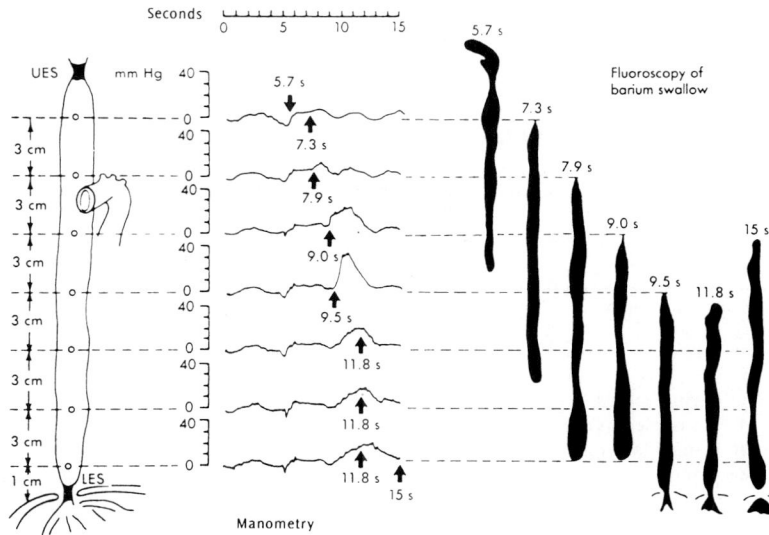

Fig. 5.1. Breaking of the peristaltic wave in the mid esophagus of a recumbent subject. In this patient with a nonspecific abnormality of esophageal motor function, a 5-ml barium swallow was recorded by concurrent videoradiography and intraluminal esophageal manometry. Seven manometric recordings sites, spaced at 3-cm intervals, were distributed along the length of the esophagus. *Vertical arrows* on each manometric tracing indicate the time during swallow sequence that corresponds to video images on right. In the proximal half of the esophagus, normal propagating peristaltic pressure wave strips the swallowed barium bolus toward the stomach. A precise relationship exists between peristaltic pressure wave and video images in that the upstroke onset of peristaltic pressure corresponds to a passage of the tail of the barium bolus. In the middle of the esophagus, the peristaltic wave fails, and only a low-amplitude simultaneous pressure wave is seen in the distal esophagus. Because of the failure of the peristaltic contraction wave, the transport of the barium bolus arrests in the distal half of the esophagus (9.5-s image), and then the barium washes back toward the proximal esophagus (15-s image). (From STEWART and DODDS 1994)

However, because fluoroscopy provides no information about pressure events, manometry may be required to confirm abnormal pressures in the pharynx as well as the esophagus and its sphincters (UES and LES).

5.5
Phases of Swallowing

It is convenient to describe swallowing in four phases: preparatory, oral, pharyngeal, and esophageal (DODDS et al. 1990a).

The introduction of liquid or solid bolus material is handled during the preparatory phase by masticating solid components into a more convenient semiliquid bolus material. Solid material is mixed with saliva, which is produced at a rate of approximately 0.5 ml/min. Satisfactory tongue motions are required to process the bolus during the preparatory phase. During the oral phase of swallowing, the bolus is moved posteriorly into the pharynx by tongue motion. This is accompanied by elevation of the soft palate and occlusion of the nasopharynx, which prevents nasopharyngeal regurgitation. The pharyngeal phase of swallowing is accompanied by closure of the vestibule of the larynx and vocal cords during transport of the bolus as well as relaxation of the cricopharyngeal muscle (upper esophageal sphincter). Also, during the pharyngeal phase of swallowing, there is significant elevation and forward motion of the hyoid and larynx, which may contribute to movement of the epiglottis as it is pushed posteriorly over the airway.

Figure 5.2 diagrammatically describes the events occurring during the oropharyngeal phases of swallowing. The entire swallowing sequence is rapid, in the vicinity of 1.0 s (DODDS et al. 1990a). As the bolus flows through the pharynx, it elongates. Generally, fluoroscopic observations of oropharyngeal swallowing events are satisfactory. However, rapid sequence filming in the lateral as well as frontal projection may be required to record normal and abnormal events and morphology (Figs. 5.3, 5.4). Two to six frames per second is the most commonly employed rate and new digital fluoroscopy equipment provides high-quality images. Video (VHS) recording at 30 frames/s is used

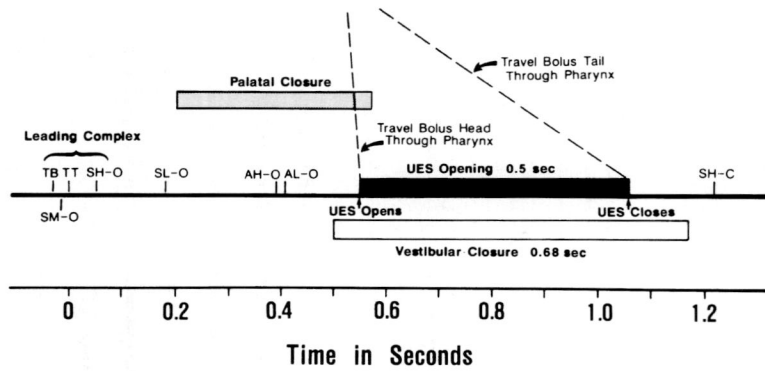

Fig. 5.2. Time line of 50 ml barium bolus swallow in normal subjects. Reference time of zero is used as onset of propulsive tongue tip (*TT*) movement at maxillary incisors. This movement begins to propel bolus toward the pharynx. Other notations include tongue base movement (*TB*), onset on superior hyoid movement (*SH-O*), onset of submental electrical activity (*SM-O*), onset of superior laryngeal movement (*SL-O*), onset of anterior hyoid movement (*AH-O*), onset of anterior laryngeal movement (*AL-O*), and completion of superior hyoid movement (*SH-C*). Palatal closure occurs as barium bolus flows from the mouth into the oropharynx. *Broken lines* indicate flow of bolus head and tail, respectively, through the pharynx. Upper esophageal sphincter (*UES*) opening occurs when the bolus head reaches the UES; UES closes when the bolus tail reaches the sphincter. In this example, closure of laryngeal vestibule straddles the interval that the bolus is in the pharynx. The entire swallowing sequence lasted about 1.2 s. (From DODDS et al. 1990)

Table 5.1. Causes of abnormal oral or pharyngeal swallowing (from DODDS et al. 1990b)

Neurologic disease
   Cerebrovascular
   Posttraumatic
   Degenerative (e.g., Alzheimer)
   Parkinsonism
   Amyotrophic lateral sclerosis/motor neuron disease
   CNS neoplasm
   Bulbar poliomyelitis
   Pseudobulbar palsy
   Friedreich spastic ataxia
   Familial dysautonomia
   Postoperative CNS tumor
Muscle disease
   Muscular dystrophy
   Oculopharyngeal dystrophy
   Myotonic dystrophy
   Dermatomyositis
   Myasthenia gravis
Radiation injury
Gastroesophageal reflux disease?
Pharmacologic agents (e.g., atropine, thorazine)
Malignancy
   Tongue
   Pharynx
   Larynx
Postoperative
   Tongue
   Pharynx
   Larynx

Table 5.2. Abnormalities in the preparatory and oral phases of swallowing (from DODDS et al. 1990b)

Radiologic findings	Types of impairment
Preparatory phase	
Cannot hold barium in mouth anteriorly	Reduced lip closure
Cannot form bolus	Reduced range or coordination of tongue movement
Cannot hold bolus posteriorly (premature spill)	Reduced tongue shaping
Cannot chew	Reduced tongue lateralization
Oral phase	
Hesitancy initiating swallow	Impaired cognitive function, neural function, or oral sensation
Tongue moves forward at onset of swallow	Forward tongue thrust
Stasis in sulci	Reduced labial or buccal tension
Stasis in floor mouth	Reduced tongue shaping
Stasis in mid tongue depression	Tongue scarring
Abnormal lingual peristalsis	Impaired tongue motion
Poor tongue-to-palate contact	Reduced tongue elevation
Repetitive tongue rolling	Parkinson disease
Premature spill of bolus	Reduced tongue or palatal control
Piecemeal deglutition	Abnormal neural control
Slow oral transit movement	Impaired tongue

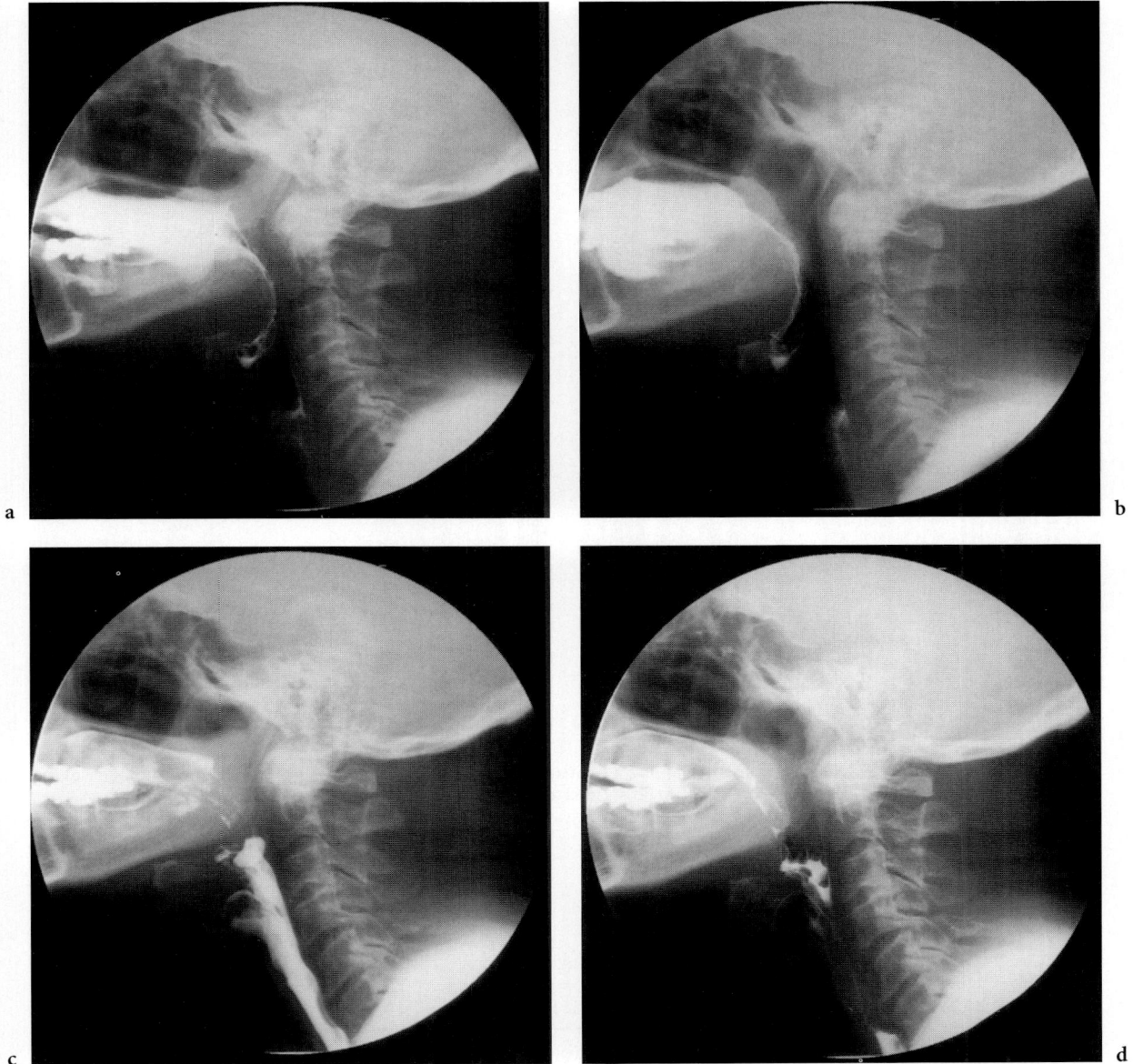

Fig. 5.3a–d. These four lateral images obtained during a normal swallow are representative of oral and pharyngeal swallowing events. During normal swallowing, the bolus is pushed into the oropharynx by the tongue. The soft palate elevates, occluding the nasopharynx and preventing nasopharyngeal regurgitation. The airway is protected by glottic and vestibular closure and the epiglottis inverts. The cricopharyngeal muscle (UES) relaxes and is pushed open by the passing bolus. Significant hyoid motion, upward and anteriorly, takes place.

for research and especially for the modified barium swallow. This avoids excessive radiation exposure to the patient and personnel in the fluoroscopy room.

The etiology of abnormal oral and pharyngeal swallowing is varied (Table 5.1) (DODDS et al. 1990b). One of the most common etiologies in a hospital population is cerebrovascular disease resulting in neuromuscular deficit. In most hospitals and cancer centers, oropharyngeal malignancy or laryngeal malignancy is associated with significant dysphagia and oftentimes results in difficulty swallowing. The postoperative oropharynx is commonly associated with severe difficulties in swallowing. The magnitude of difficulty is directly proportional to the amount of surgery performed, i.e., glossectomy, mandibul-

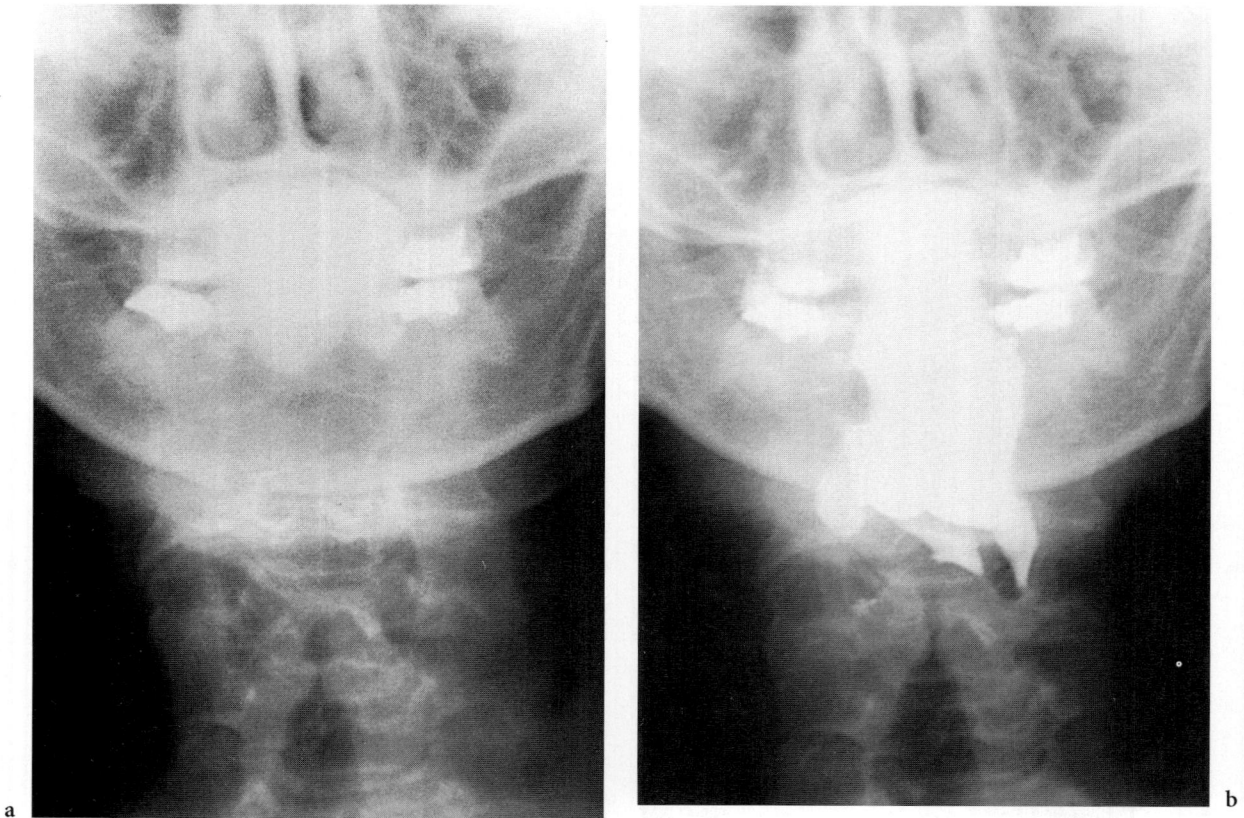

Fig. 5.4a–d. These four images are representative of oral and pharygeal morphology during a normal swallow. Symmetry of the lateral pharyngeal walls is to be expected. The piriform sinuses are effaced and do not re-form until the bolus passes

Table 5.3. Abnormalities in the pharyngeal phase of swallowing (from Dodds et al. 1990b)

Radiologic findings	Generic impairment
Absent or decreased hyoid movement	Feeble contraction, suprahyoid muscle
Absent or decreased laryngeal movement	Abnormal contraction, thyrohyoid
Poor palatal movement	Impaired function of velopharyngeal closure mechanism
Delayed or absent pharyngeal phase	Impaired sensation; damage to neural programming in the brainstem
Increased unilateral residual valleculae and/or piriform sinus	Unilateral impairment of pharyngeal peristalsis
Abnormal movement, epiglottis	Impaired function of thyrohyoids, cervical spur, mass
Laryngeal penetration/aspiration	Early: premature oral spill; during: impaired laryngeal closure; late: pharyngeal residue
Abnormal opening of upper esophageal sphincter (UES)	Impaired UES relaxation; decreased UES compliance; feeble hyoid movement; feeble pharyngeal transport

ectomy, hemilaryngectomy, supraglottic laryngectomy, or total laryngectomy.

Abnormalities in the preparatory and oral phases of swallowing result in radiologic findings which can sometimes be predicted if the impairment is known (Table 5.2) (Dodds et al. 1990b). It is usual to see the result of several types of impairment. Therefore, the radiologic finding is a "summation" of pathology. For example, following surgery there may be neural, muscular, and skeletal alterations producing over-

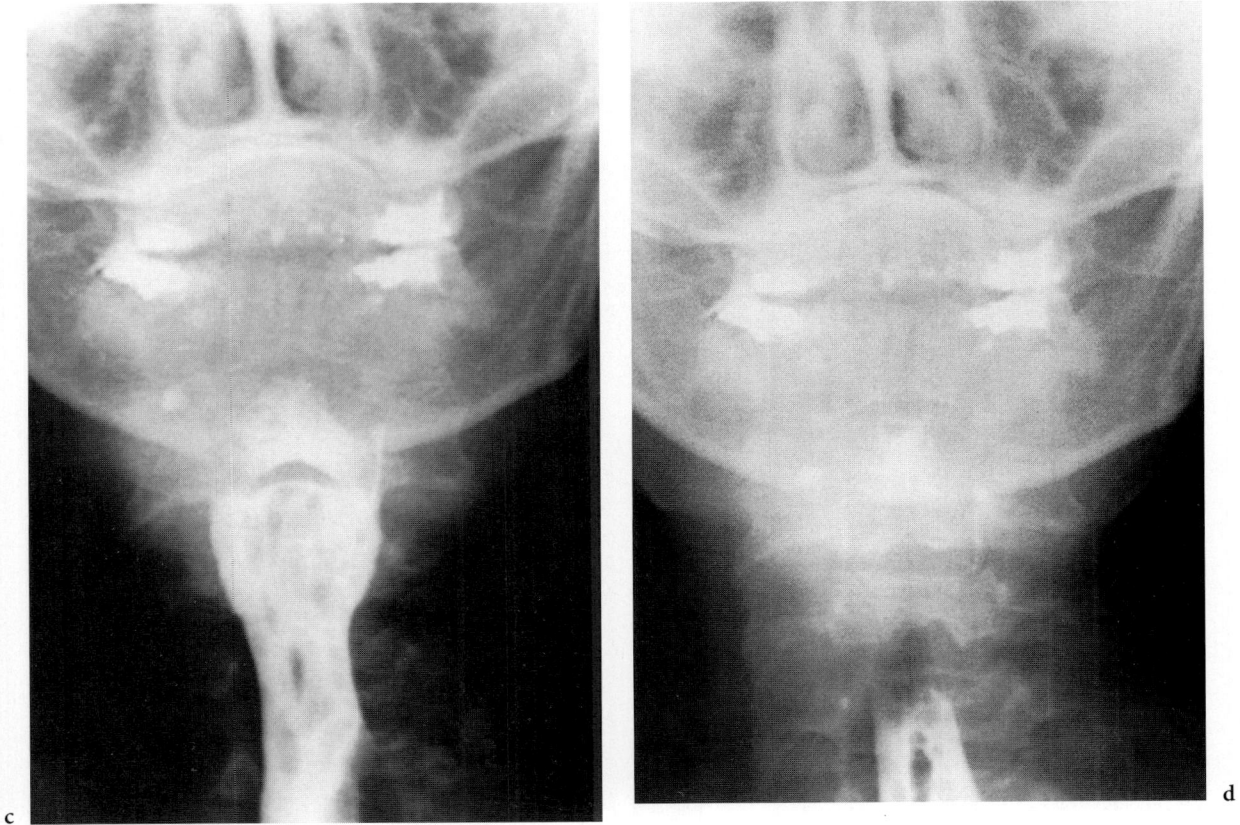

c

d

Fig. 5.4a–d. *Continued*

lapping impairment to oral processing of the bolus. Abnormalities in the pharyngeal phase of swallowing are generally documented (Table 5.3) (DODDS et al. 1990b).

Viewing in the lateral projection is the preferred and most informative projection when evaluating the pharynx. Penetration and/or aspiration is seen best since the airway is easily separated from the pharynx. Penetration is defined as the portion of a bolus entering the vestibule of the airway. Aspiration is bolus material below the true vocal cords.

5.6
Esophageal Peristalsis

Peristaltic activity in the esophagus is defined as follows: *Primary peristalsis* is initiated by the act of swallowing and represents uninterrupted aboral progression of the peristaltic sequence beginning in the pharynx and progressing to the esophagogastric junction (Fig. 5.5). *Secondary peristalsis* is similar to primary peristalsis except in its mode of initiation. Secondary peristalsis is generally initiated by esophageal distention, either by injection of a bolus or possibly gastroesophageal reflux. Since it is identical in every way to primary peristalsis other than its mode of initiation, secondary peristalsis can be used to evaluate esophageal motility. Either primary or secondary peristalsis can be incomplete and there may be escape of material from the peristaltic event or the peristaltic event may break entirely. *Aperistalsis* is the absence of any peristaltic event. An interesting phenomenon often seen superimposed on normal and abnormal events is what has been termed *tertiary contractions* (Fig. 5.6)

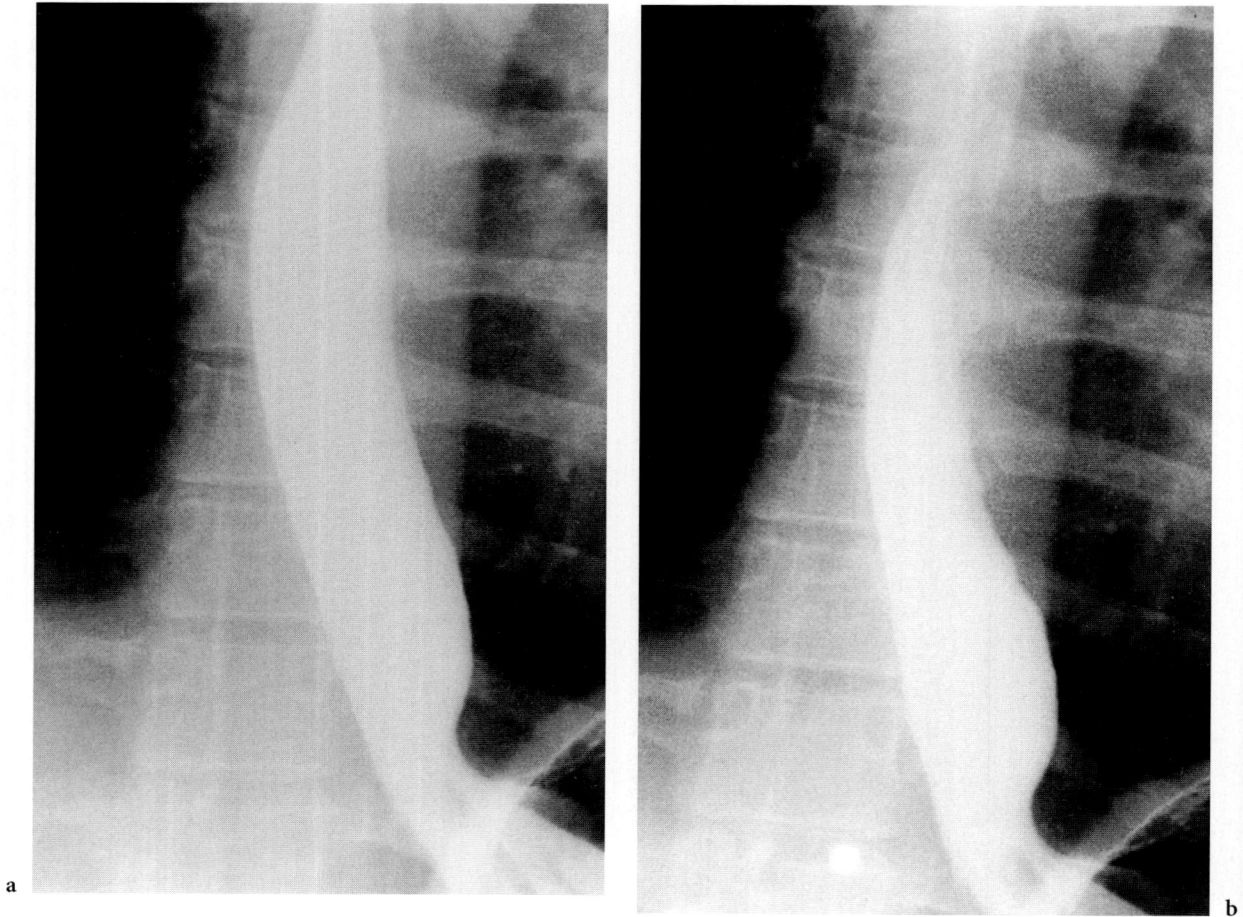

a

b

Fig. 5.5a–f. Normal esophageal peristalsis is seen as a progressive uninterrupted progression of a stripping wave through the entire length of the esophagus. The tail or "inverted-V" is the important region of interest. This appearance is imparted to the barium column by the contraction of circular muscle in the wall of the esophagus. This normal primary peristaltic sequence was initiated by a 10-ml swallow of barium

These *nonperistaltic contractions* may or may not be lumen obliterating. Although they may be superimposed on otherwise normal peristaltic activity, they are often associated with significant motor disturbances (STEWART and DODDS 1994).

5.7
Technical Considerations

Although the oral and pharyngeal phases of swallowing are generally evaluated in the erect position, there is a common misconception that esophageal peristaltic events can be evaluated properly with the patient in the erect position. Because of the influence of gravity, esophageal clearance in the erect position may be complete in the absence of normal esophageal motility. The esophagus is best examined with the patient in the recumbent position, which nullifies the effect of gravity. In the recumbent position, the esophagus must actively contract in order to empty and it is this position that is preferred for evaluation of esophageal motility. Single swallows uninterrupted by repetitive swallowing are required to evaluate peristalsis; this is because repetitive swallowing inhibits peristaltic events, producing abnormalities such as breaking of the peristaltic wave which are difficult to assess. A number of swallows may be required to document motility disturbances since significant motility disorders have reproducible abnormalities. Occasional mild motility disturbances are seen in asymptomatic normal

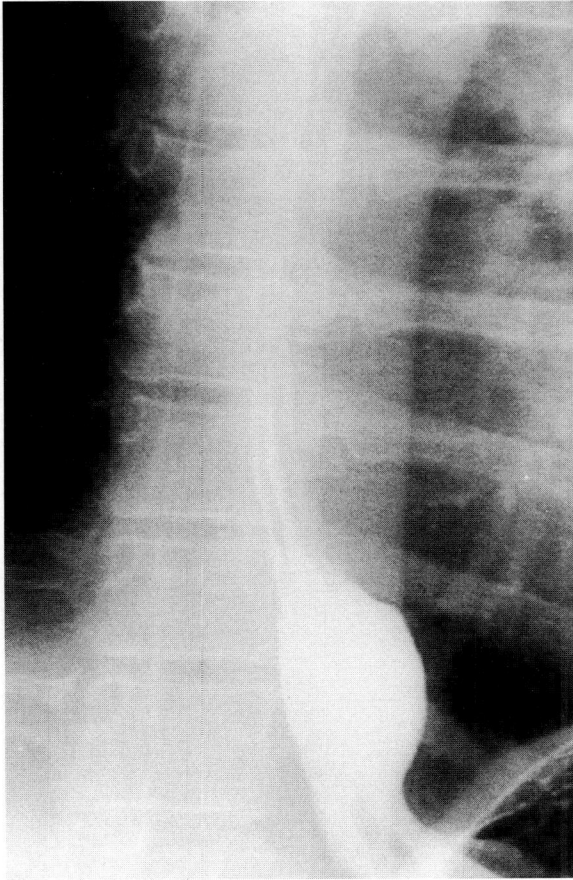

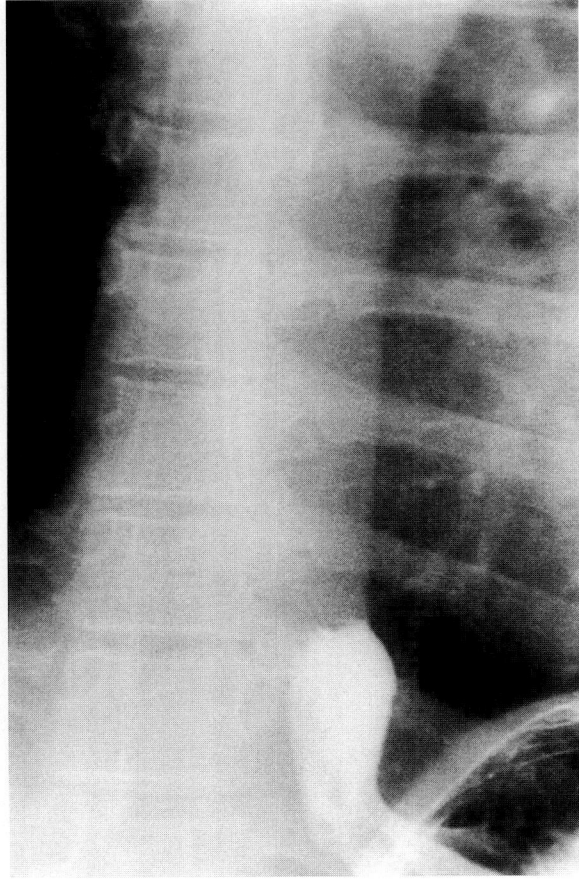

c

d

Fig. 5.5a–f. *Continued*

individuals. For this reason, careful observation of a number of swallows is a requisite for adequate fluoroscopic observation of peristaltic events and determination of a significant abnormal motility pattern.

5.8 Classification of Esophageal Motility Disturbances

It is convenient to classify esophageal motor disturbances as primary or secondary (Table 5.4) (STEWART and DODDS 1994). Primary motor disorders are defined as those that are not related to underlying disease. These are quite limited in number

and relatively uncommon. Secondary motility disorders are more numerous and much more often encountered. These esophageal motor disturbances, related to underlying disease, are termed secondary motility disorders. The frequency with which these abnormalities are encountered varies from institution to institution. The large list of diseases that may be associated with abnormal esophageal peristalsis is shown in Table 5.4 and illustrates how protean these findings may be. It should be remembered that some motility disturbances encountered cannot be easily classified and, oftentimes, etiology is not apparent. Also, motility disturbances without significant symptoms are encountered from time to time and should not initiate expensive and time-consuming further evaluation.

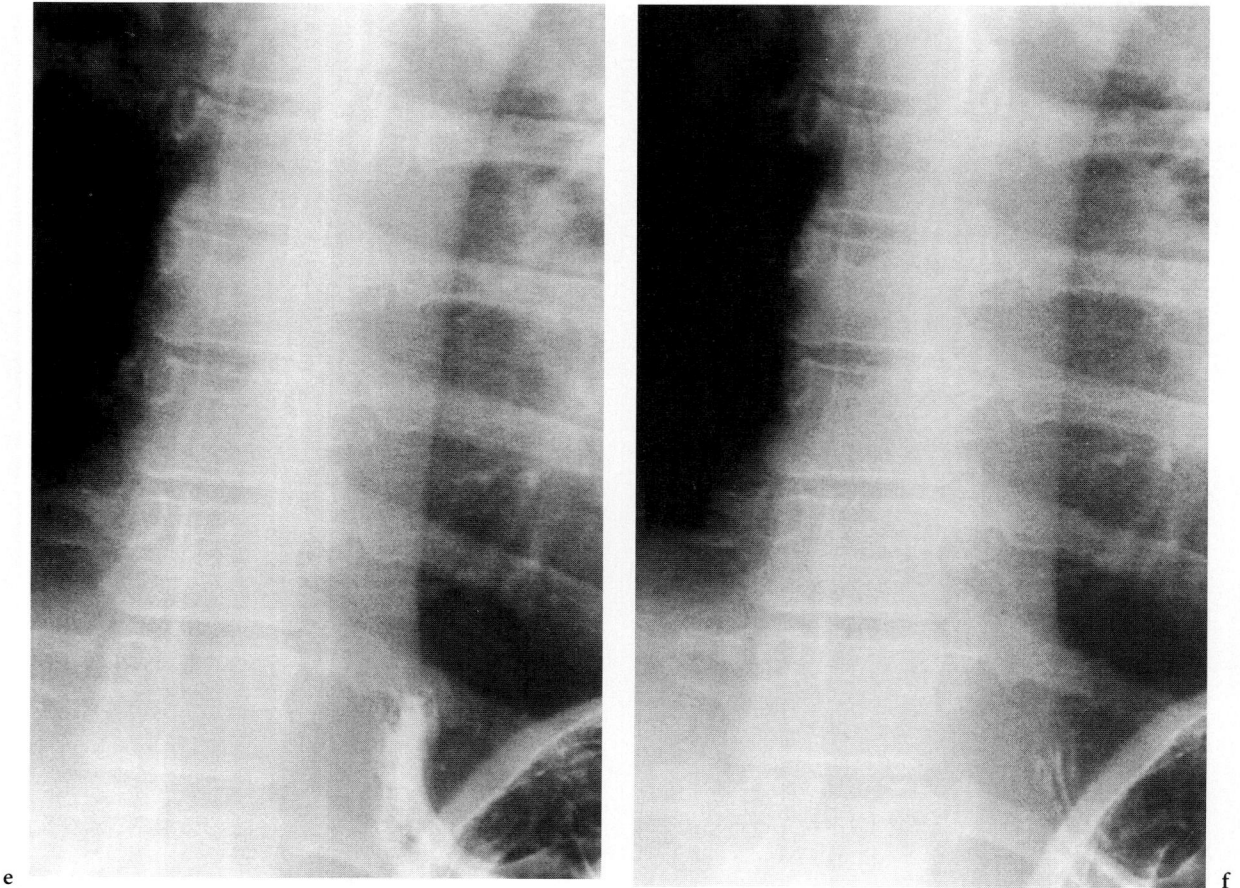

e

f

Fig. 5.5a–f. *Continued*

5.9
Modified Barium Swallow

The modified barium swallow (MBS) is now commonly employed by speech pathologists and others in the assessment of swallowing mechanics. As noted previously, it should be coupled with the total evaluation of the oropharynx and esophagus. The MBS has also been called the video deglutition examination and videofluoroscopic study. The MBS is performed in the erect position. During this examination, tolerance of various consistencies of orally administered material is assessed. The MBS determines whether the patient can swallow safely without aspiration as well as helping to delineate the etiology of abnormal swallowing. As previously noted, this examination uses videorecording in order to minimize radiation dosage as well as to provide an opportunity to review the dynamics of swallowing. Comparisons from one examination to another are therefore quite easy.

Prior to the MBS, a bedside evaluation and review of the medical history and clinical status is performed. This includes a history of dietary limitations, behavior during ingestion of food, and the frequency of coughing or choking. Generally, significant cervical dysphagia with or without evidence of aspiration is evaluated prior to recommending an MBS.

Specially designed chairs are now available to accommodate the size restrictions for placement of the patient in a lateral and frontal position for videofluoroscopy. Swallowing mechanics are recorded utilizing barium as the contrast agent mixed with varying consistencies ranging from thin and thick liquids to paste consistencies and solid boluses such as bread or cookies. Videofluoroscopy includes visualization of the lips anteriorly, the soft palate superiorly, and the pharynx and airway. Postopera-

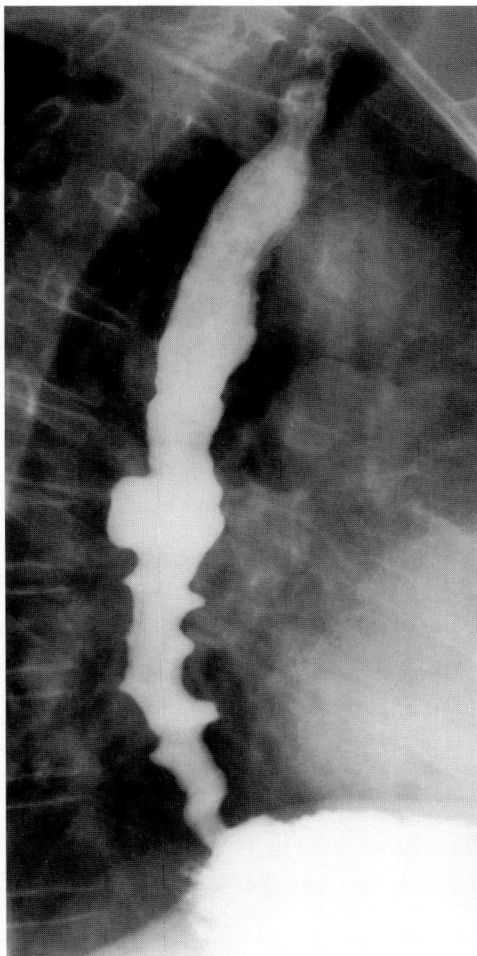

Fig. 5.6. Tertiary nonpropulsive contractions of the esophagus are displayed by this barium-filled esophagus. Tertiary contractions are to be differentiated from peristalsis since they are nonpropulsive, disorganized segmental contractions

tive patients are often evaluated with a water-soluble contrast when incomplete healing or extravasation of contrast may be expected. In the absence of a contraindication, barium sulfate is the contrast agent of choice. All phases of swallowing are recorded with each selected consistency. Penetration and aspiration as well as cough reflexes are noted. Abnormalities seen in the preparatory, oral, and pharyngeal phases of swallowing (Tables 5.1–5.3) are observed and a qualitative assessment is made. Of importance is the presence or absence of an adequate cough reflex when aspiration occurs. Cognition is an important and significant variable, especially in the neurologically impaired patients, and may make this study very difficult.

Generally, bolus size is limited to small amounts in the range of 3–4 cc which may be increased depending on the presence or absence of aspiration. Oftentimes, during the examination there is difficulty in one or more phases of swallowing, which may either shorten or terminate the examination. It is important to note whether aspiration occurs before, during, or after the swallow as the timing of aspiration will help direct the swallow rehabilitation program. Puddling of material in the vallecula or piriform sinuses which is incompletely cleared is often associated with overflow penetration and aspiration. Attempts at altering swallowing mechanics by head turning, chin tucking, or other maneuvers may be performed. These are used to assess whether or not such maneuvers may have therapeutic implications for the patient (LOGEMANN et al. 1989). The MBS is a qualitative examination of swallowing mechanics.

Dysphagic patients can be challenged with a solid bolus in an attempt to reproduce symptoms, particularly since subtle strictures of the esophagus often go undetected endoscopically. A convenient bolus is a marshmallow as it can be sized, is soft and tasty, and dissolves rapidly if impaction occurs. Swallowed as an unchewed bolus, impaction of the marshmallow at areas of narrowing will dramatically reproduce symptoms of dysphagia. Marshmallows or other solid bolus material should be used only in individuals with a normal cervical esophagus.

As a symptom, dysphagia spans the interest of radiologists, gastroenterologists, speech pathologists, and surgeons. Proper screening and selection of patients minimize the expenditure of valuable resources that may be unwarranted. Fluoroscopic observations of the mechanical events will continue to be the most sensitive technique available for the screening evaluation of these symptoms. The qualitative fluoroscopic observation of oropharyngeal and esophageal mechanics is the single most productive examination when motility is in question. Understanding normal physiology and identifying pathology is one of the real advantages in gastrointestinal radiology and continues to grow.

5.10
Perspectives on Esophageal Stents for Malignant Disease

In the United States, approximately 11 000 new cases of esophageal cancer are diagnosed yearly (BORING et al. 1993). The majority of these patients present

Table 5.4. Classification of esophageal motility disorders (from STEWART and DODDS 1994)

I. *Primary*	F. Neurologic disease
A. Achalasia	1. Parkinsonism
B. Diffuse esophageal spasm	2. Huntington's chorea
C. Intestinal pseudo-obstruction	3. Wilson's disease
D. Hypertensive peristalsis	4. Cerebrovascular disease
E. Presbyesophagus	5. Multiple sclerosis
F. Congenital tracheoesophageal fistula	6. Amyotrophic lateral sclerosis
G. Neonatal achalasia	7. Central nervous system neoplasm
	8. Bulbar poliomyelitis
II. *Secondary*	9. Pseudobulbar palsy
A. Connective tissue	10. Friedreich's hereditary spastic ataxia
B. Chemical or physical	11. Familial dysautonomia (Riley-Day syndrome)
1. Reflux (peptic) esophagitis	12. Stiff man's syndrome
2. Caustic esophagitis	13. Ganglioneuromatosis
3. Vagotomy	G. Muscular disease
4. Radiation	1. Myotonic dystrophy
C. Infection	2. Muscular dystrophy
1. Fungal: moniliasis	3. Oculopharyngeal dystrophy
2. Bacterial: tuberculosis, diphtheria	4. Myasthenia gravis (neuromotor end-plate)
3. Parasitic: Chagas' disease	H. Vascular
4. Viral: herpes simplex, cytomegalovirus	1. Varices (possibly)
D. Metabolic	2. Ischemia (possibly)
1. Diabetes	I. Neoplasm
2. Alcoholism	1. Obstruction
3. Amyloidosis	J. Pharmacologic
4. Serum pH and electrolyte disturbances (possibly)	1. Atropine, propantheline, curare, etc.
E. Endocrine	
1. Myxedema	
2. Thyrotoxicosis	

with dysphagia indicating significant narrowing of the esophageal lumen to usually more than 50%, or to less than 13 mm in diameter (GOLDSCHMID and NORD 1994). Around 90% of these patients are incurable. Options for palliation include peroral dilatations, plastic esophageal stents, surgery, radiotherapy, chemotherapy and tumor ablation with laser, thermocoagulation, photodynamic therapy, and alcohol injections. Most of these options either have significant morbidity/mortality rates or require repeated efforts to maintain luminal patency.

Esophageal stents have been used for palliation of malignant esophageal obstruction for more than 100 years. Early stents were made from ivory and boxwood, passed orally and fixed externally by various methods, including tying the stent to the moustache in one case (BOYCE 1993; EARLAM and CUNHA-MELO 1982). Blind peroral methods of stent insertion were replaced by surgical placement of Celestin tubes, but surgery was associated with high procedure-related complications. With the advent of flexible endoscopy the placement of rigid esophageal stents via the oral route became safer than the blind methods or surgical placement. Rigid stents

are made of latex or plastic and some physicians fashion their "homemade" stents using polyvinyl. They come in various lengths and most have an internal diameter of around 12 mm and an external diameter of 15–16 mm. To prevent migration, proximal funnels and distal flanges have been added. Some stents have an expandable foam cuff around the shaft to seal tracheoesophageal fistula. Unfortunately, these stents require preinsertion dilatation of the esophageal stricture 2–4 French sizes larger than the stent size and are not suitable for tortuous strictures. In a meta-analysis, procedure-related complications associated with these stents approached 20%, with death reported in 8.6% (KOZAREK 1994).

5.11
Self-expanding Metal Stents

Recently, several types of self-expanding esophageal metal stents (SEMS), similar to those used in the biliary, bronchial, and urinary tracts, have been approved by the Food and Drug Administration for palliation of malignant esophageal obstruction and tracheoesophageal fistula. The two main advantages of these stents are that the external diameter of the delivery system is smaller, which allows for easier insertion, even without preinsertion dilatation, and that, once deployed, they eventually expand to a diameter greater than plastic stents. Additionally, these stents are flexible, and can be used for angulated strictures.

5.11.1
Indications and Contraindications

Endoscopic and/or fluoroscopic placement of a SEMS should be considered in all cases of incurable esophageal/lung cancer for palliation of dysphagia. Although simple dilatation of a stricture may suffice in some cases, a stent is indicated when dilatation is ineffective, difficult, or required frequently. Stent insertion is the treatment of choice for patients with incessant coughing in the presence of a spontaneous or procedure-related tracheoesophageal fistula.

The decision to use a SEMS depends on the experience of the operator, the presence of alternative treatment modalities (e.g., Laser, Bicap), and tumor characteristics. Previously, tumors extending to within 2.0 cm of the UES have been avoided for possible stent insertion for fear of pulmonary aspiration, foreign body sensation, and proximal migration into the hypopharynx (KNYRIM et al. 1993; LIGHTDALE et al. 1987; TYTGAT 1980). Experience gained from plastic stents has shown that patients with proximal esophageal malignant strictures may benefit from stent placement, especially when a tracheoesophageal fistula is present (GOLDSCHMID et al. 1988; SPINELLI et al. 1991; LOIZOU et al. 1992). Stents can be placed across the LES in carcinomas involving the lower esophagus and/or gastric cardia. However, these patients will require lifelong antireflux measures. Submucosal, extrinsic compression (e.g., lung cancer) or noncircumferential tumors often provide insufficient anchorage and are therefore unsuitable for plastic stents. SEMS with uncovered wires at the ends can be used in these situations. Angulated strictures are no longer a contraindication for stent placement as SEMS are flexible. However, stents cannot be deployed in strictures that do not allow a guidewire to pass. Stent insertion is contraindicated in those unable to tolerate the procedure and is inappropriate in patients with very limited life expectancy (<1 month).

5.11.2
Stent Designs

Although differing in design, SEMS share a common principle of delivery system and deployment. All metallic stents are stretched out on a delivery catheter so as to reduce the diameter of the delivery system (6.0–12.7 mm). This limits the amount of preinsertion dilatation required, thereby potentially reducing the risks of perforation and bleeding. After deployment, the stent expands over a course of hours to days to its maximum diameter (16–18 mm). Thus, unlike the plastic stents, SEMS provide gradual progressive dilatation, which adds to their safety. Some of the other differences between the plastic and metals stents are shown in Table 5.5.

Metallic stents are made of a wire mesh or a metal coil. When the wires are bare, the stent is referred to as an uncovered stent. Once deployed, these stents expand in the esophagus, and over time, epithelial/malignant cells can grow through the gaps between the wires, integrating the stent into the esophageal

Table 5.5. Comparison of plastic and self-expandable esophageal metal stents

	Plastic Stents	Metal Stents
Diameter at insertion	15–16 mm	6–12.7 mm
Internal diameter	12 mm	16–18 mm
Prior dilatation	Required	Not required
Blockage	Frequent	Less frequent
Flexibility	Poor	Good
Can be removed	Yes	Only some types
Ideal tumor characteristics	Straight Circumferential	Can be angulated Noncircumferential also
Stent within stent	Not feasible	Feasible

wall (BETHGE et al. 1996a). These stents, therefore, rarely migrate and cannot be removed. Dysphagia can recur with tumor ingrowth. Uncovered stents cannot be used for sealing tracheoesophageal fistula. Stents are referred to as "covered" when silicon, polymer, or polyurethane is used to surround the wires. These stents prevent tumor ingrowth and are effective in sealing a tracheoesophageal fistula. Unfortunately, covered stents tend to migrate more frequently than uncovered stents. Measures to anchor these stents include flaring of the proximal and distal ends (e.g., Z-stent, Wilson-Cook, Winston-Salem, N.C.), bare wires at the proximal and distal ends (e.g., Wallstent, Schneider, Minneapolis, Minn.; Ultraflex, Microvasive, Boston, Mass.), and barbs (e.g., Z-stent, European design). Unlike the wire-mesh design, the EsophaCoil (Instent, Eden Prairie, Minn.) is a metal coil that, by its design, can be removed. Once fully expanded, close approximation of the coils prevents tumor ingrowth. Most of the SEMS shorten after release and this needs to be taken into account when selecting the correct length of the stent (the Z-stent shortens the least).

Characteristics of the various types of SEMS are shown in Table 5.6 (VAKIL and BETHGE 1996).

5.11.3
Technique of Stent Placement

Barium or endoscopic estimation of the tumor length is necessary to select the proper length of stent to be deployed. The stent should be long enough to bridge the malignant stricture and project 2–3 cm beyond the proximal and distal stricture margins. As bacteremia has been reported with stent insertion (SONG et al. 1991), appropriate antibiotic prophylaxis is recommended for patients with valvular heart disease, arteriovenous grafts, and recently placed foreign bodies.

Stent deployment requires endoscopic, fluoroscopic, or combined endoscopic and fluoroscopic guidance. In the combined approach (Fig. 5.7), endoscopy is initially performed to evaluate the stricture. For tight strictures, dilatation may be necessary using the wire-guided balloon or bougienage method to allow the endoscope to pass. Difficult strictures can be negotiated by using hydrophilic guidewire. With the guidewire in place, the endoscope is withdrawn to the lower margin of the stricture. Under fluoroscopic guidance, this lower end is marked externally by a radiopaque marker (e.g., a paper clip wire with adhesive tape). This procedure

Table 5.6. Self-expanding metal stents for the esophagus (from VAKIL and BETHGE 1996)

Characteristics	Covered Wallstent, US type	Covered Wallstent, European type	Ultraflex stent	Gianturco-Rösch Z-stent: with barbs (European type)	Z-stent: without barbs (US type)	EsophaCoil stent	Song stent
Stent material	Stainless steel	Stainless steel	Nickel titanium alloy (nitinol)	Stainless steel	Stainless steel	Nickel titanium alloy (nitinol)	Stainless steel
Diameter (mm) of insertion assembly	12.7	a) 6 b) 7.3	a) 8 b) 7	8	10.3	10.5	11
Stent diameter (mm) after full expansion	28[a]/18[b]	a) 29[a]/25[b] b) 24[a]/20[b]	18 mm	25[a]/16[b]	a) 21[a]/18[b] b) 25[a]/18[b]	a) 24[a]/18[b] b) 21[a]/16[b]	a) 22[a]/18[b] b) 20[a]/16[b]
Stent length after full expansion (mm)	40, 60, 90	110 mm	a) 70, 100, 150 mm b) 100, 150 mm	100, 120, 140	60, 80, 100, 120, 140	100, 150	60–180
Covered, uncovered, partially covered	Partially covered	Partially covered	a) Uncovered b) Partially covered	Covered	Covered	Uncovered	Covered
Covering material	Polymer	Polyurethane	a) None b) Polyurethane	Polyethlene	Polyurethane	None	Nylon mesh with silicone coating
FDA approval	Yes	No	Yes	No	Yes	Yes	No

[a] Diameter of the proximal and distal portions of the stent.
[b] Diameter of the mid-portion of the stent.

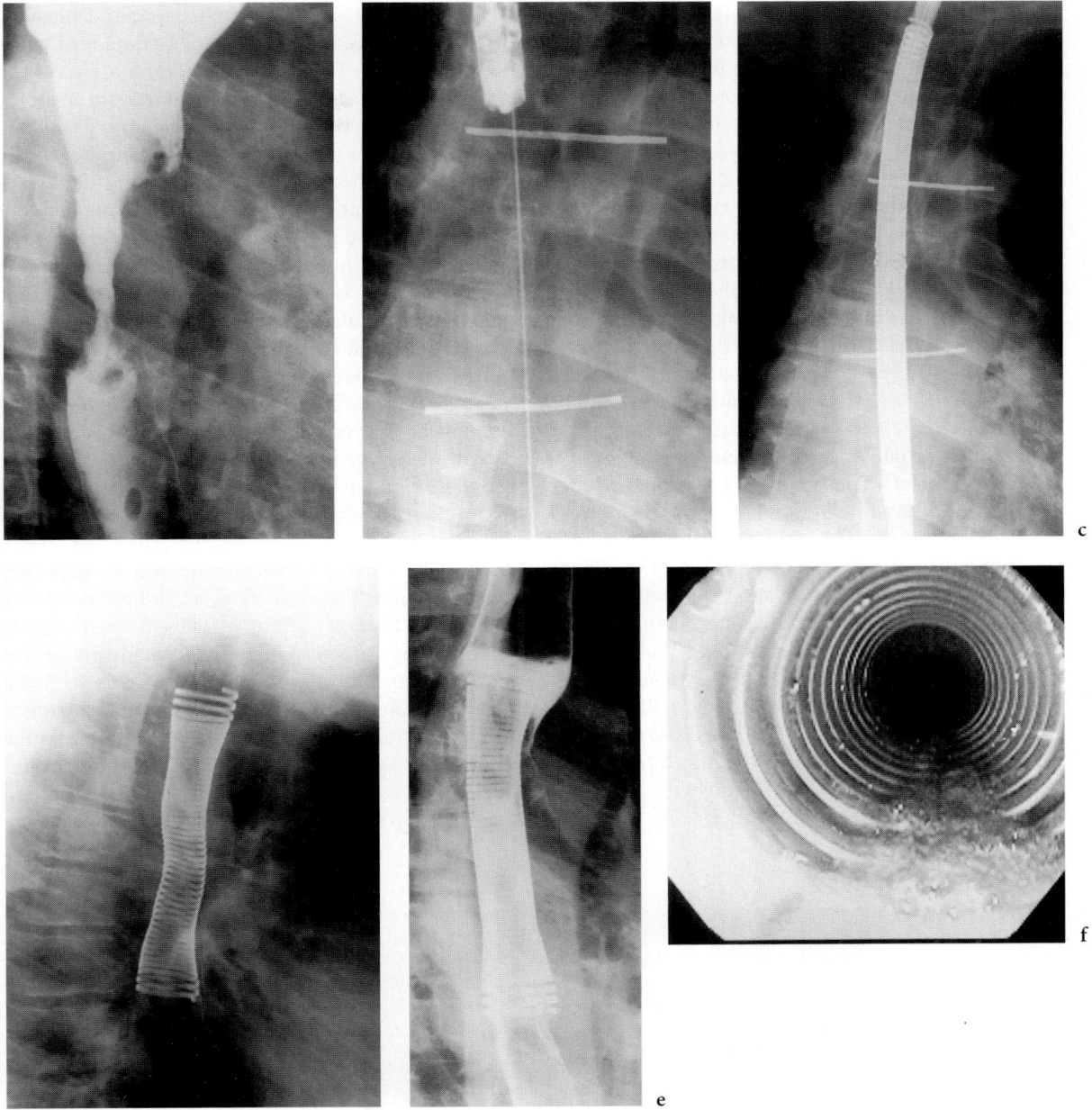

Fig. 5.7a–f. Steps in the deployment of a self-expanding esophageal metal stent (EsophaCoil). **a** Esophagram showing malignant esophageal stricture. **b** External radiopaque markers are placed at the upper and lower margins of the stricture using endoscopic and fluoroscopic guidance. **c** Delivery catheter with the collapsed stent is passed over the guide wire and positioned across the stricture. **d** Stent is deployed and expansion monitored fluoroscopically. **e** Esophagram post-stent deployment. **f** Endoscopic view of the upper end of the deployed stent

is repeated for the upper edge of the stricture (Fig. 5.7b). The relationship between the external markers and the stricture edges can change with body movement, as can be expected with a restless patient. As an alternative, internal markers can be used in the form of clips (DE BOER et al. 1995) or Lipidol injection (CHAN et al. 1994). After removal of the endoscope, the delivery system with the radiopaque collapsed stent is passed over the guidewire and fluoroscopically negotiated through the stricture. Because wires of some collapsed stents may not be easily visible on fluoroscopy, the delivery catheter has radiopaque markers indicating the length of the stent after deployment. Using these markers, the collapsed stent is positioned across the stricture to allow the deployed stent to project 2–3 cm beyond the stricture margins. For those delivery catheters without markers, the radiopaque collapsed stent can be fluoroscopically manipulated to position the endoscopically marked segment of the stricture in the middle of the nondeployed stent (Fig. 5.7c). The stent is then deployed and the progress of deployment monitored fluoroscopically. Minor adjustments can be made before full deployment. Although most of the SEMS are deployed distally first, some (e.g., EsophaCoil) can be deployed from either end first. To reduce the risk of proximal migration after deployment, it is important to wait a few minutes to allow for adequate expansion before removing the delivery catheter. The stent should be monitored fluoroscopically while removing the catheter (Fig. 5.7d). Immediately after deployment, the stent can be evaluated endoscopically (Fig. 5.7f), although one should be cautious about stent migration while pushing or withdrawing the scope. Examples of a deployed Z-stent, Ultraflex stent, and Wallstent are shown in Figs. 5.8, 5.9, and 5.10. Stents with strong radial force (e.g., covered Wallstent) will fully expand shortly after deployment while those with weak radial force (e.g., Ultraflex) may require a few days to expand or may require expansion with a balloon catheter.

Although the above combined method of stent insertion is preferable, stents can be deployed without fluoroscopy. The upper and lower margins of the stricture are measured in centimeters from the incisor teeth using an endoscope. The delivery catheter with centimeter markings is then appropriately positioned across the stricture and the stent deployed. An endoscope can be passed adjacent to the delivery catheter to visually monitor the upper end of the stricture during deployment and to make minor adjustments if required. Stent placement under fluoroscopic guidance alone is possible but is more "blind" and difficult than the above methods.

After stent placement, an esophagram is recommended (Fig. 5.7e). Leakage is carefully excluded and appropriate positioning confirmed. It is easier to reposition or remove some SEMS (e.g., Z-stent, EsophaCoil) soon after deployment. In certain situations (e.g., extension of tumor beyond the margins of the stent because of either tumor growth or wrong stent placement), a second SEMS can be deployed into a previously placed stent, as shown in Fig. 5.8 (Dua et al. 1997).

Follow-up care of patients with stent placement include instructions to properly chew food, avoid raw vegetables and grilled meats, drink adequate amount of fluids, and in those with stents across the gastroesophageal junction, follow standard antireflux measures. Medications preferably should be in the liquid form. Measures to disimpact food from a

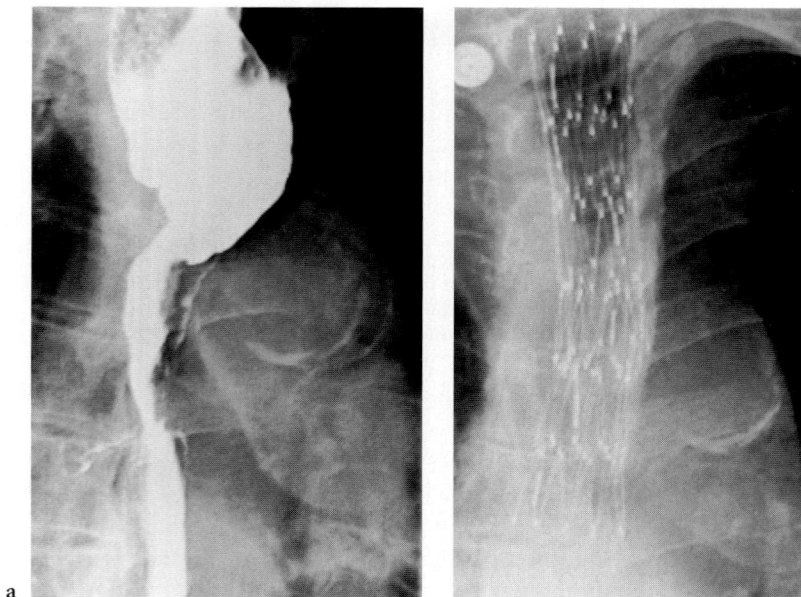

a

b

Fig. 5.8a,b. An example of a second Z-stent inserted into a previously misplaced Z-stent. **a** Esophagram showing a malignant esophageal stricture. **b** Two overlapping Z-stents

Fig. 5.9. a Esophagram showing malignant esophageal stricture. **b** Deployed Ultraflex stent

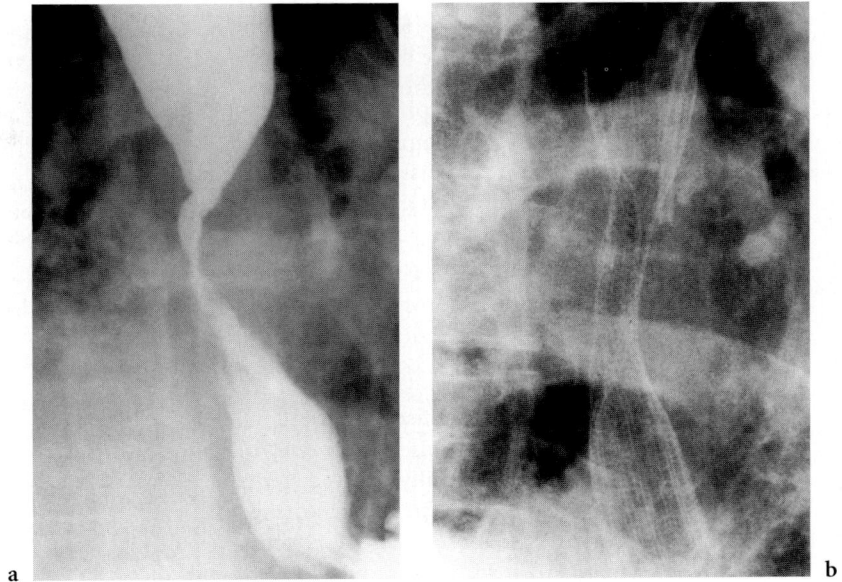

a

b

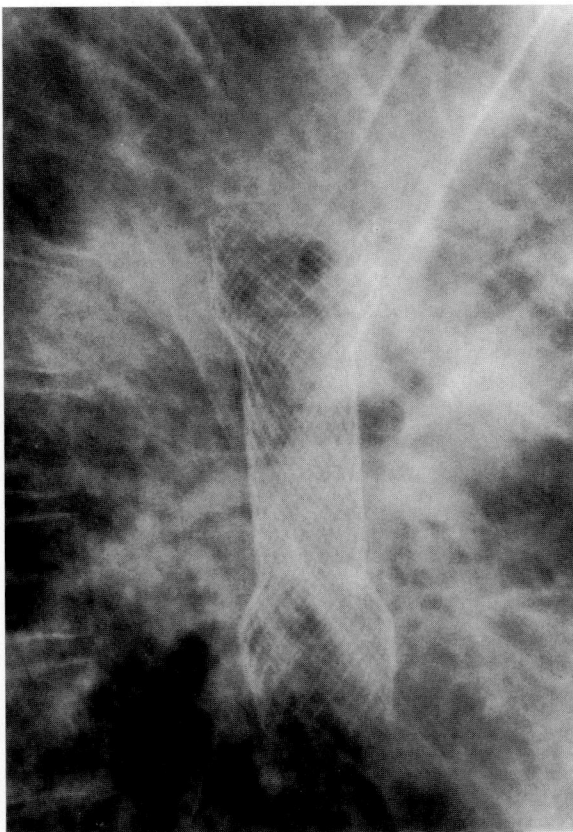

Fig. 5.10. Deployed Wallstent

blocked stent include drinking aerated liquids, passing a nasogastric tube, and endoscopy.

5.11.4
Results

Despite their expense, SEMS are safer and more cost-effective than plastic stents (DE PALMA et al. 1996; KNYRIM et al. 1993; WU et al. 1994). Although there are no major studies comparing the various types of SEMS, trials on individual stents have shown that they are highly effective in relieving dysphagia (83%–100%; ROCHLING et al. 1997; STRECKER et al. 1996; DE GREGORIO et al. 1996; ACUNAS et al. 1996; DE PALMA et al. 1995; GRUND et al. 1995; ELL et al. 1995; MAY et al. 1995; WATKINSON et al. 1995; SONG et al. 1994; WU et al. 1994; CWIKIEL et al. 1993). Similarly, SEMS have been shown to seal tracheoesophageal fistula in up to 100% of cases (ROCHLING et al. 1997; HAN et al. 1996; STRECKER et al. 1996; ELL et al. 1995; FIORINI et al. 1995; BETHGE et al. 1995; DO et al. 1993).

Complications reported with SEMS range from as low as 0% (DE PALMA et al. 1996) to as high as 31% (KOZAREK et al. 1995). Early complications include malposition, incomplete expansion, chest pain, perforation, bleeding, and tracheal compression.

Subacute complications include migration, erosion with perforation, bleeding, or tracheoesophageal fistula, tumor ingrowth and overgrowth, food impaction, reflux esophagitis, and aspiration. Serious stent-related complications were found to be significantly higher in those who previously received chemotherapy and/or radiotherapy (KINSMAN et al. 1996; BETHGE et al. 1996b).

5.11.5
Choice of Stent

Patients with tracheoesophageal fistula should be treated with covered stents. As these stents tend to migrate, it is advisable to use partially covered stents (e.g., Wallstent) for cancers with poor "anchoring" qualities. The bare wires of these partially covered stents become integrated into the esophageal wall, preventing migration. These stents cannot be removed. Fully covered stents (e.g., Z-stent) prevent tumor ingrowth, although they have a higher incidence of migration. Highly flexible stents such as the Ultraflex stent can be used for angulated strictures. EsophaCoil stents are potentially removable, although there are insufficient data to support this in patients who have had the stent in for longer than several weeks. Use of this stent for benign strictures is still not approved.

Self-expanding esophageal metal stents are now becoming popular in the palliation of malignant esophageal obstruction and tracheoesophageal fistula. The technology is evolving and will improve during the coming years. In the future, experience gained on removable SEMS may allow their use in benign esophageal strictures.

References

Acunas B, Rozanes I, Akpinar S, et al. (1996) Palliation of malignant esophageal strictures with self-expanding nitinol stents: drawbacks and complications. Radiology 199:-648–652

Bethge N, Sommer A, Vakil N (1995) Treatment of esophageal fistulas with a new polyurethane-covered, self-expanding mesh stent: a prospective study. Am J Gastroenterol 90:-2143–2146

Bethge N, Sommer A, Gross U, et al. (1996a) Human tissue responses to metal stents implanted in vivo for the palliation of malignant stenosis. Gastrointest Endosc 43:596–602

Bethge N, Sommer A, von Kleist D, et al. (1996b) A prospective trial of self-expanding metal stents in the palliation of malignant esophageal obstruction after failure of primary curative therapy. Gastrointest Endosc 44:283–286

Boring CC, Squires TS, Tong T (1993) Cancer statistics. CA Cancer J Clin 43:7–26

Boyce HW (1993) Stents for palliation of dysphagia due to esophageal cancer. N Engl J Med 329:1345–1346

Chan A, Leong H, Chung S, et al. (1994) Lipidol as a reliable marker for stenting in malignant esophageal stricture. Gastrointest Endosc 40:520–521

Cwikiel W, Stridbeck H, Tranberg K, et al. (1993) Malignant esophageal strictures: treatment with a self-expandable nitinol stent. Radiology 187:661–665

de Boer W, van Haren F, Driessen WMM (1995) Marking clips for the accurate positioning of self-expanding esophageal stents. Gastrointest Endosc 42:73–76

De Gregorio BT, Kinsman K, Katon RM, et al. (1996) Treatment of esophageal obstruction from mediastinal compressive tumors with covered, self-expanding metallic Z-stents. Gastrointest Endosc 43:483–489

De Palma GD, Galloro G, Sivero L, et al. (1995) Self-expanding metal stents for palliation of inoperable carcinoma of the esophagus and gastroesophageal junction. Am J Gastroenterol 90:2140–2142

De Palma G, di Matteo E, Romano G, et al. (1996) Plastic prosthesis versus expandable metal stents for palliation of inoperable thoracic carcinomas: a controlled prospective study. Gastrointest Endosc 43:478–482

Do YS, Song H, Lee BH, et al. (1993) Esophagorespiratory fistula associated with esophageal cancer: treatment with a Gianturco stent tube. Radiology 187:673–677

Dodds WJ, Stewart ET, Logemann JA (1990a) Physiology and radiology of the normal oral and pharyngeal phases of swallowing. AJR Am J Roentgenol 154:953–963

Dodds WJ, Logemann JA, Stewart ET (1990b) Radiologic assessment of abnormal oral and pharyngeal phases of swallowing. AJR Am J Roentgenol 154:965–974

Dua K, Rochling F, Saeian K, et al. (1997) Use of self-expanding metal stents (SEMS) for palliation of malignant esophageal obstruction/tracheo-esophageal (TE) fistula in patients with previously placed esophageal stents (abstract). Gastrointest Endosc 45:AB67

Earlam R, Cunha-Melo JR (1982) Malignant esophageal strictures: a review of techniques for palliative intubation. Br J Surg 69:61–68

Ell C, May A, Hahn EG (1995) Gianturco-Z stents in the palliative treatment of malignant esophageal obstruction and esophagotracheal fistulas. Endoscopy 27:495–500

Fiorini AB, Goldin E, Valero JL, et al. (1995) Expandable metal coil stent for treatment of broncho-esophageal fistula. Gastrointest Endosc 42:81–83

Goldschmid S, Nord HJ (1994) Endoscopic diagnosis and treatment of esophageal cancer. In: Van Dam J (ed) Gastrointestinal endoscopy. Clinics of North America, vol 4. Saunders, Philadelphia

Goldschmid S, Boyce HW, Nord HJ, et al. (1988) Treatment of pharyngoesophageal stenosis by polyvinyl prosthesis. Am J Gastroenterol 83:513–518

Grund KE, Storek D, Becker HD (1995) Highly flexible self-expanding meshed metal stents for palliation of malignant esophagogastric obstruction. Endoscopy 27:486–494

Han Y, Song H, Lee J, et al. (1996) Esophagorespiratory fistulae due to esophageal carcinoma: palliation with a covered Gianturco stent. Radiology 199:65–70

Kinsman K, DeGregorio B, Katon R, et al. (1996) Prior radiation and chemotherapy increases the risk of life-threatening complications after insertion of metallic stents for esophagogastric malignancy. Gastrointest Endosc 43:-196–203

Knyrim J, Wagner HJ, Bethge N, et al. (1993) A controlled trial of an expandable metal stent for palliation of esophageal obstruction due to inoperable cancer. N Engl J Med 329:1302–1307

Kozarek RA (1994) Use of expandable stents for esophageal and biliary stenosis. Gastroenterology 2:264–272

Kozarek R, Raltz S, Brugge W, et al. (1995) Prospective multicenter trial utilizing esophageal Z stent for dysphagia and TE fistula. Gastrointest Endosc 41:353–357

Lightdale CJ, Zimbalist E, Winawer SJ (1987) Outpatient management of esophageal cancer with endoscopic Nd: YAG laser. Am J Gastroenterol 82:46–56

Logemann JA (1983) Manual for the videofluorographic study of swallowing. College Hill Press, San Diego

Logemann JA, Kahrilas PJ, Kobara M, et al. (1989) The benefit of head rotation on pharyngoesophageal dysphagia. Arch Phys Med Rehab 70:767–771

Loizou LA, Rampton D, Brown SG (1992) Treatment of malignant strictures of the cervical esophagus by endoscopic intubation using modified endoprosthesis. Gastrointest Endosc 38:158–164

May A, Selmaier M, Hochberger J, et al. (1995) Memory metal stents for palliation of malignant obstruction of the oesophagus and cardia. Gut 37:309–313

Rochling FA, Dua K, Saeian K, et al. (1997) Treatment of malignant esophageal stricture and tracheoesophageal fistula with self-expanding metal stents (abstract). Gastrointest Endosc 45:AB80

Song HY, Choi KC, Cho BH, et al. (1991) Esophagogastric neoplasms: palliation with a modified Gianturco stent. Radiology 180:349–354

Song H, Do Y, Han Y, et al. (1994) Covered, expandable esophageal metallic stent tubes: experience in 119 patients. Radiology 193:689–695

Spinelli P, Cerrai FG, Meroni E (1991) Pharyngo-esophageal prostheses in malignancies of the cervical esophagus. Endoscopy 23:213–214

Stewart ET, Dodds WJ (1994) Radiology of the esophagus. In: Freeny PC, Stevenson GW (eds) Margulis and Burhenne's alimentary tract radiology, 5th edn. Mosby-Year Book, St. Louis, pp 192–263

Strecker E, Boos I, Vetter S, et al. (1996) Nitinol esophageal stents: new designs and clinical indications. Cardiovasc Intervent Radiol 19:15–20

Tytgat GN (1980) Endoscopic methods of treatment of gastrointestinal stenosis. Endoscopy 12 (Suppl):57–68

Vakil N, Bethge N (1996) Metal stents for malignant esophageal obstruction. Am J Gastroenterol 91:2471–2476

Watkinson AF, Ellul J, Entwisle K, et al. (1995) Esophageal carcinoma: initial results of palliative treatment with covered self-expanding endoprostheses. Radiology 195:821–827

Wu W, Katon R, Saxon R, et al. (1994) Silicone-covered self-expanding metallic stents for the palliation of malignant esophageal obstruction and esophagorespiratory fistula: experience in 32 patients and a review of the literature. Gastrointest Endosc 44:22–33

6 Stomach

R.M. Gore

R.M. Gore, MD, Professor and Vice Chairman, Department of
Diagnostic Radiology, Evanston Hospital-McGaw Medical
Center of Northwestern University, 2650 Ridge Avenue,
Evanston, IL 60201, USA

6.1
Introduction

The development and refinement of the double-contrast upper gastrointestinal (GI) series has dramatically improved the radiologist's ability to detect a variety of benign and malignant disorders of the stomach. Paradoxically, these advances have been accompanied by a gradual and steady decline in the number of radiologic upper GI studies performed in the United States over the past two decades (Levine and Laufer 1993). This trend can be attributed in part to the fact that patients with upper GI symptoms are treated empirically with H_2 blockers before undergoing additional diagnostic evaluation. The second major factor is the widespread use of endoscopy rather than barium studies as the initial diagnostic test in these symptomatic patients (Levine and Laufer 1993).

Although endoscopy is more sensitive for diagnosing mild inflammatory diseases of the stomach, it has not been proven that the ability to detect these lesions has had any significant impact on the management or eventual outcome of affected patients. Endoscopy is also an invasive procedure that has a small but significant morbidity related to the use of sedation and the risk of perforation. Additionally, endoscopy is 4–5 times more expensive than the barium study. The double-contrast upper GI examination is the cost-effective alternative to endoscopy (Levine 1995).

In this chapter, the double-contrast barium manifestations of the most important gastric disorders are highlighted with CT correlation where appropriate. Meticulous performance and interpretation of barium studies is essential if this technique is to remain a valuable examination, the results of which are regarded with confidence by our clinical colleagues.

6.2
Technical Considerations

The stomach is a capacious and complex organ that is predisposed to often very subtle pathology. To maximize the diagnostic accuracy of the upper GI examination, a biphasic study employing double-contrast views should be supplemented with single-contrast compression and barium-filled views (LAUFER 1994a; GELFAND et al. 1987).

Gastric evaluation is combined with the esophageal study in most patients. Double-contrast views of the esophagus are obtained in the upright position after the ingestion of effervescent granules and high-density barium. The patient is quickly lowered into the supine recumbent position to avoid excessive spillage of contrast into the duodenum. The patient is then rotated to achieve mucosal coating. The barium must wash away the surface layer of gastric mucus to achieve this coating. Residual food, secretions, or inadequate rotation and barium washing will degrade mucosal detail and thus the accuracy of the entire study (LAUFER 1994b). After adequate mucosal coating has been achieved, the patient is turned into the left posterior oblique position to thin out the barium pool in the gastric antrum. As the barium exits the antrum into the proximal stomach, spot films are obtained – the so-called flow technique (KIKUCHI et al. 1986). This is an excellent means of demonstrating subtle antral mucosal pathology. The patient is turned further to the left and air-contrast views of the antrum and duodenal bulb are obtained. The patient is then turned into the right lateral decubitus position, at which time air-contrast views of the fundus and cardia (FREENY 1979) are taken and a solid-column image of the duodenal bulb and proximal sweep obtained.

The patient is then turned into a recumbent right anterior oblique position and low-density barium is ingested. At this time oropharyngeal dynamics and esophageal motility are evaluated and barium distended views of the esophagus and gastroesophageal junction obtained (GELFAND 1994). With the stomach sufficiently distended with barium, prone or right anterior oblique compression views of the antrum and duodenal bulb are taken. Then a film with the patient in the prone position is obtained to include the proximal small bowel. The patient is then turned into the left decubitus and supine left posterior oblique position, during which the presence of spontaneous reflux is assessed and air-contrast views of the duodenal bulb and antrum are again taken. Finally, an upright film with gas distention of the fundus and cardia is taken, often with the patient rotated towards their left (HERLINGER et al. 1980). At this time the duodenal bulb can be reassessed, particularly if it lies posterior to the antrum, making its compression in the prone position difficult.

This biphasic technique allows air- and barium-filled evaluation of all parts of the stomach, and provides for compression views of the antrum and duodenal bulb (LAUFER and KRESSEL 1992; LEVINE et al. 1988).

6.3
The Gastric Mucosa

6.3.1
Areae Gastricae

Careful inspection of the surface mucosal pattern of the normal stomach reveals a fine reticular network of interlacing lines on double-contrast barium studies (Fig. 6.1a–c). This network is produced by barium trapped in a system of interconnecting grooves or furrows (*sulci gastricae*) that subdivide the surface of the mucosa into small (2–4 mm), slightly bulging, polygonal islands of mucosa called the *areae gastricae*. They have also been referred to as the fine relief or micromucosal pattern of the stomach, as opposed to the gross or macromucosal pattern formed by the gastric rugae. Unlike gastric rugae, areae gastricae are visible regardless of whether the stomach is distended or nondistended (MCINTOSH and KREEL 1977).

The areae gastricae are seen in 50%–75% of properly performed double-contrast studies of the stomach and are most commonly visualized in the antrum and body (RUBESIN and HERLINGER 1986). Areae gastricae can only be seen endoscopically if either blood or methylene blue fills the sulci gastricae. Radiographic visualization of the areae gastricae is of more than mere academic interest. It acts as a guide to the physiologic status of the gastric mucosa and serves as a helpful sign of pathologic alteration. Enlargement (>4 mm) or prominence of the areae gastricae is a sign of gastritis (Fig. 6.1d) and should prompt a search for erosions or ulcerations in the mucosa (GORE et al. 1995). The presence of a normal areae gastricae pattern excludes the presence of diffuse atrophic gastritis with a probability of 90%, far better than relying on the macromucosal (rugal) pattern. When the areae gastricae are distorted or absent focally in an otherwise regular surface pattern, there is often associated peptic ulcer disease or tumor (GORE and LICHTENSTEIN 1994).

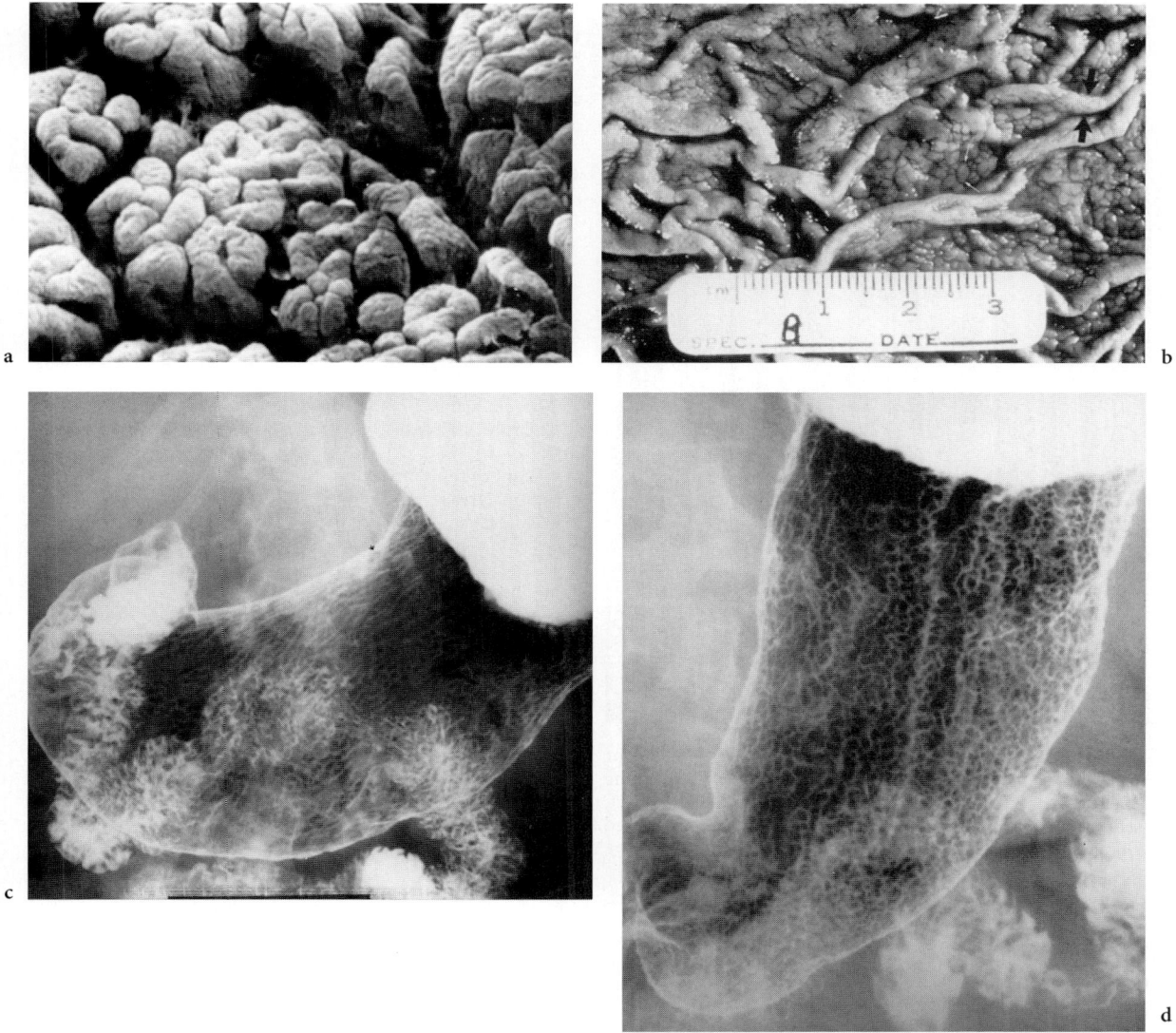

Fig. 6.1a–d. Normal mucosal surface pattern of stomach: areae gastricae. **a** Low-power (original magnification ×20) scanning electron micrograph showing the sulci gastricae that surround the areae gastricae. **b** Gross specimen of the stomach shows the macromucosal surface pattern (rugal folds) (*black arrows*) and the micromucosal surface pattern (areae gastricae) (*white arrows*). **c** These sulci fill with barium, forming the lacelike micromucosal pattern of the stomach on double-contrast studies – the areae gastricae. **d** Enlargement of the areae gastricae often signifies gastritis. (**a** and **b** courtesy of Gerald D. Dodd, MD, Jr. Houston, Texas and Harvey M. Goldstein, MD, San Antonio, Texas)

6.3.2
Gastric Antral Striations

Contraction of the muscularis mucosae of the gastric antrum can produce transverse fold-linear striations (Fig. 6.2) similar to the feline esophagus pattern. These are seen occasionally in patients with gastritis, antral erosions, or ulcers. Gastric antral striae tend to be more persistent than folds of the feline esophagus (CHO et al. 1987).

6.4
Gastritis

Gastritis is a very common disease that has a variety of causes, histologic findings, and radiologic manifestations (FURTH et al. 1995). The pathologic classification of gastritis has shifted from merely the descriptive to analyzing the cause of gastritis (TABLE 6.1).

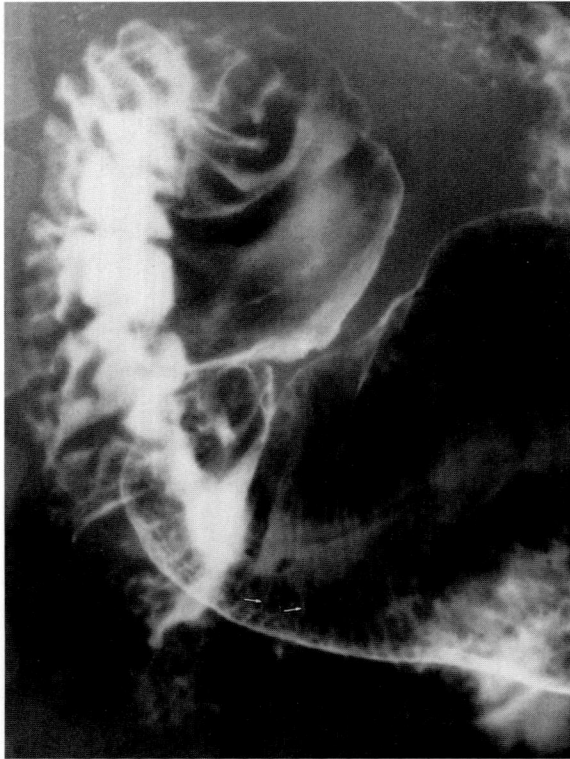

Fig. 6.2. Gastric striations. Fine transverse folds (*arrows*) or striae similar to the feline esophagus may be visualized in the gastric antrum. Unlike their transient esophageal counterpart, gastric striations are more persistent and have been associated with gastritis

Table 6.1. Simplified classification of gastritis (from FURTH et al. 1995)

Type of gastritis	Comments
Acute	
Erosive, hemorrhagic	NSAIDs, alcohol, steroids
Chronic	
H. pylori	Associated duodenal ulcer, gastric ulcer, cancer, lymphoma
Chemical	NSAIDs, bile reflux
Autoimmune atrophic (type A)	Body mucosa
Nonautoimmune atrophic (type B)	Multifocal, environmental, antrum, and lesser curve
Lymphocytic	Sprue-like
Miscellaneous	
Crohn's disease	Associated small-bowel disease
Other granulomatous gastritis	Isolated, sarcoid
Allergic	Immunoglobulin E eosinophilia
Zollinger-Ellison syndrome	Gastrinoma
Ménétrier's disease	Foveolar hyperplasia

NSAIDs, Nonsteroidal anti-inflammatory drugs.

6.4.1
Erosive Gastritis

Gastric erosions are superficial mucosal defects that do not penetrate beyond the muscularis mucosae (GORE and LICHTENSTEIN 1994). These erosions are often multiple, producing the disorder known as erosive gastritis. Predisposing factors for erosive gastritis include alcohol, aspirin, other nonsteroidal anti-inflammatory agents (NSAIDs), stress, potassium chloride, reserpine, trauma, burns, corticosteroids, Crohn's disease, viral (e.g., cytomegalovirus, herpesvirus) or fungal infection, and *Helicobacter pylori* infection (LEVINE 1994a). About 50% of cases are idiopathic. Patients with erosive gastritis may be asymptomatic or present with dyspepsia, epigastric pain, or upper gastrointestinal hemorrhage (LEVINE 1994b). Indeed, hemorrhagic erosive gastritis is responsible for between 10% and 20% of upper GI bleeding (LEVINE 1994c).

Erosive gastritis, while seldom visualized on single-contrast barium studies, is being observed with increasing frequency on double-contrast studies, with an overall prevalence of 0.5%–2.0% (LEVINE 1994a). An integral part of the double-contrast barium examination consists in washing barium over portions of the stomach likely to harbor erosions and obtaining barium pool images sufficiently thin to demonstrate erosions. Erosive gastritis usually manifests as "complete" or "varioliform" erosions that appear as punctate or slit-like collections of barium surrounded by radiolucent halos of edematous mucosa (Fig. 6.3a). Erosions that have the small lucent halo are called "complete" erosions. When the halo is not present the erosion is called incomplete. Varioliform erosions most often develop in the antrum and are often aligned with antral folds (LEVINE 1994a).

Aspirin and other NSAIDs tend to produce linear (Fig. 6.3b) and serpiginous erosions that tend to cluster in the gastric body, on or near the greater curvature (LEVINE et al. 1986). Perhaps erosions result from localized mucosal injury as the dissolving NSAID tablets or capsules lodge in the most dependent portion of the stomach. Chronic NSAID-related gastropathy is characterized by subtle flattening and stiffening of the adjacent greater curvature resulting

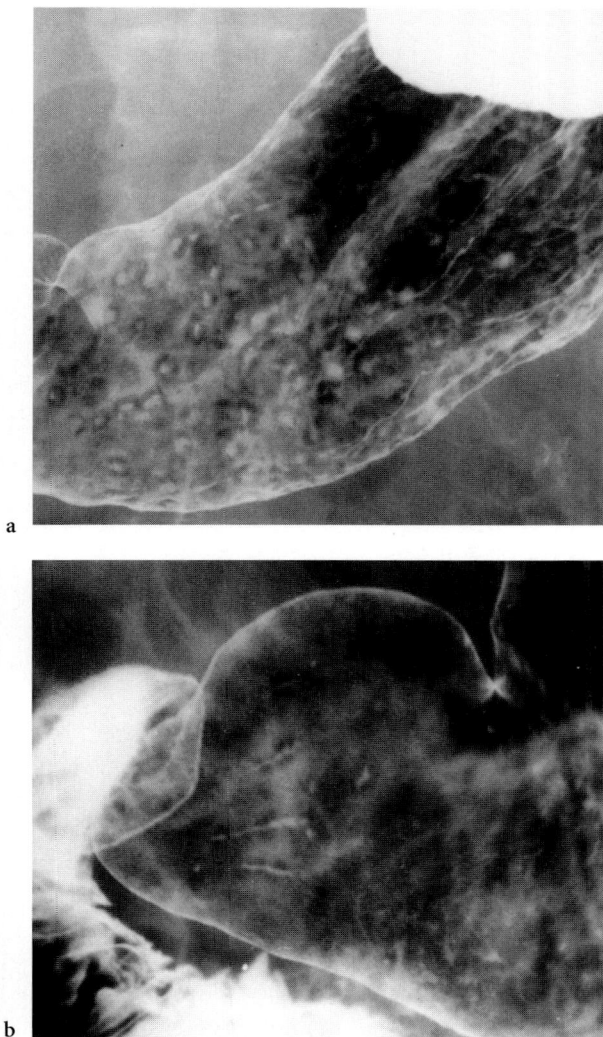

Fig. 6.3a,b. Erosive gastritis. a Multiple varioliform erosions in the antrum appear as tiny punctate and slit-like barium collections with surrounding halos of edematous mucosa. b Multiple linear erosions are present in the gastric antrum in this patient taking nonsteroidal anti-inflammatory drugs

from recurrent cycles of erosion formation and healing (LAVERAN-STIEBAR et al. 1994).

6.4.2
Helcobacter Gastritis

Helicobacter pylori is a gram-negative, short, slightly curved bacillus that infects the stomach of a large portion of the world's population (CELLO 1995). Gastric infection increases with patient age, is more common in men, and is more prevalent in lower socioeconomic populations. Although most infected people are asymptomatic, they almost always have an associated gastritis. Since first isolated from endoscopic biopsy specimens in 1982, *H. pylori* infection has come to be recognized as a major factor in the development of peptic ulcer disease (MARSHALL 1994). Indeed, *Helicobacter* gastritis is identified in essentially every patient with duodenal ulcer and nearly 80% of patients with gastric ulcers (PARSONNET et al. 1994). In many cases, gastric carcinoma and lymphoma are caused by *Helicobacter* gastritis (LEVINE et al. 1996; HANSSON et al. 1996).

Helicobacter pylori has a unique ability to survive the hostile gastric environment due in part to the ammonia and carbon dioxide released from urea by its active enzyme, urease. The urea breath test can be used to establish the presence of *H. pylori*; C^{13}- or C^{14}-radiolabeled urea is given by mouth and the amount of exhaled radioactive CO_2 is measured. More recently, serologic tests for the bacterium or its urease have been developed. It is important to establish this diagnosis because eradication of *H. pylori* with triple therapy (i.e. bismuth, metronidazole, and tetracycline or amoxicillin) in conjunction with H_2 blockers significantly lowers the rate of recurrence when compared with the use of histamine blockers alone (SOLL 1996).

Gastritis with thickened folds is the best radiologic sign of *H. pylori*. These enlarged folds are caused by mucosal and submucosal edema and inflammation and secondary hypertrophy or hyperplasia of the mucosa. The gastric antrum is the most common site of involvement; however, the proximal half of the stomach (Fig. 6.4a) or the entire stomach is often involved by this disease. Enlarged areae gastricae are a common concomitant finding in *H. pylori* gastritis (SOHN et al. 1995). Some 70% of patients with *H. pylori* have enlarged areae gastricae and thick gastric folds (Fig. 6.4b) so that this combination of findings should suggest the possibility of *H. pylori* gastritis (LEVINE and RUBESIN 1995). Although fold thickening is a nonspecific radiologic finding that can be caused by a variety of inflammatory disorders, *H. pylori* gastritis should be the primary consideration in the differential diagnosis of thick gastric folds in patients with epigastric pain, dyspepsia, and other upper GI symptoms (LEVINE 1994c).

Polypoid, lobulated folds difficult to distinguish from gastric carcinoma and lymphoma are another, less common radiologic manifestation of *H. pylori* gastritis on both double-contrast barium studies and CT (GORE et al. 1994).

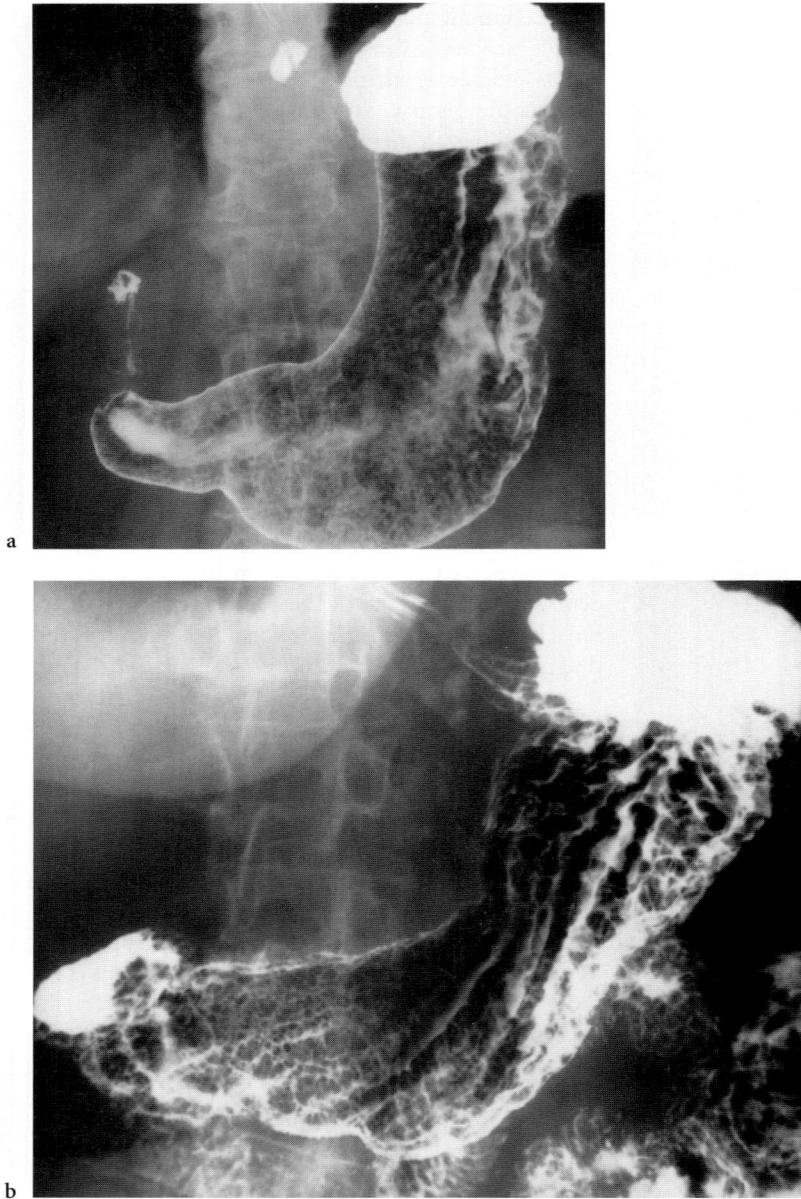

Fig. 6.4a,b. *Helicobacter pylori* gastritis. **a** Double-contrast radiograph demonstrates thickened, lobulated folds in the gastric body and fundus in this patient with *H. pylori* gastritis. **b** Enlarged areae gastricae accompany thick rugal folds in a different patient with *H. pylori* gastritis

Helicobacter pylori gastritis is a major public health issue and in the future, the combination of a barium study and serum *H. pylori* test could replace endoscopy and biopsy as the primary method of evaluating patients with dyspepsia and other upper GI symptoms (HEATLY and WYATT 1995).

6.4.3
Atrophic Gastritis

Patients with chronic atrophic gastritis and intestinal metaplasia are at increased risk for developing pernicious anemia, gastric polyps, and most significantly gastric cancer (HSING et al. 1993). Two types of chronic atrophic gastritis occur (WEINSTEIN 1993). Type A involves the body and fundus and is associated with antiparietal antibodies, achlorhydria, intestinal metaplasia, and pernicious anemia. Type B shows predominantly central involvement and is related to mucosal injury by infectious (*H. pylori*), toxic, and dietary agents, and previous surgery with chronic bile reflux into the stomach (KAWAGUCHI et al. 1996). About 10% of patients with type B gastritis and 1%–10% of patients with type A-related pernicious anemia will eventually develop gastric cancer

(LANZA 1995). Cancer risk is directly proportional to the severity of gastritis and is confined to the intestinal form of gastric cancer. The postulated mechanisms include bacterial overgrowth in the achlorhydric stomach, luminal pH changes, the trophic effects of gastrin, and the neoplastic potential of proliferating cells in the presence of chronic inflammation (BOLAND and SCHIEMAN 1995).

Clinically, patients may present with epigastric pain and early satiety. With pernicious anemia, patients may initially manifest with neurologic symptoms as a result of long-standing vitamin B_{12} deficiency (WEINSTEIN 1993).

On single-contrast barium studies, atrophic gastritis is characterized by the presence of a narrowed, tubular stomach with absent or decreased mucosal folds, predominantly in the body and fundus – the so-called bald fundus (GELFAND 1994; LEVINE 1994c). On double-contrast studies, atrophic gastritis manifests with absent folds in the fundus and body (Fig. 6.5), a fundal diameter of 8 cm or less, and small (1–2 mm in diameter) or absent areae gastricae (LEVINE et al. 1990b).

6.4.4
Eosinophilic Gastritis

Eosinophilic gastritis is an uncommon disorder in which there is eosinophilic infiltration of the stom-

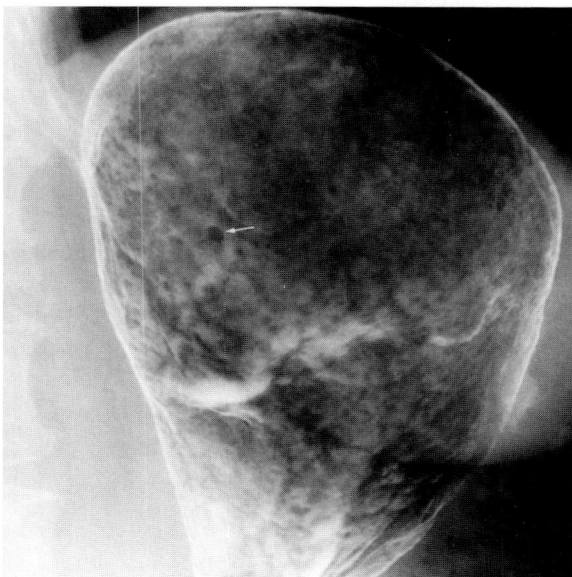

Fig. 6.5. Atrophic gastritis. Double-contrast view of the gastric fundus shows a paucity of rugal folds and absence of discernible areae gastricae. Note the hyperplastic polyp (*arrow*)

ach and small bowel associated with peripheral eosinophilia and history of allergies. Patients with eosinophilic gastritis typically present with epigastric pain, nausea and vomiting, or upper GI bleeding. Diarrhea, malabsorption, and protein-losing enteropathy are the major clinical manifestations of small bowel involvement (MacCARTY and TALLEY 1990).

Mucosal nodularity, fold thickening, or narrowing and rigidity of the distal half of the stomach are the typical radiologic findings in eosinophilic gastritis (BUCK and PANTONGRAG-BROWN 1994). Occasionally, gastric outlet obstruction may result from the severe antral narrowing. Coexistent small bowel involvement characterized by diffuse fold thickening and nodularity is seen in about 50% of patients with eosinophilic gastritis (VITELLAS et al. 1995).

6.4.5
Crohn's Disease

Gastroduodenal involvement occurs in a substantial minority of patients with Crohn's disease. Upper GI involvement usually coincides but occasionally precedes the more symptomatic and diagnostic ileocolic disease. Clinically, patients with gastric Crohn's disease may have epigastric pain, vomiting, and weight loss and occasionally acute or chronic upper GI hemorrhage. Antral or duodenal narrowing may cause gastric outlet obstruction with intractable nausea and vomiting (LEVINE 1994c).

Aphthoid ulcerations of the stomach (Fig. 6.6a) can be detected in more than 20% of patients with Crohn's disease (LEVINE 1994c). These lesions cluster in the antrum or antrum and body of the stomach and appear as punctate or slit-like collections of barium surrounded by radiolucent mounds of edema. These lesions may be indistinguishable from varioliform gastric erosions due to a variety of other causes; however, Crohn's disease should be suspected in patients who also have crampy abdominal pain and diarrhea (SIMPKINS and GORE 1994).

With progression of gastroduodenal Crohn's disease, one or more larger ulcers, thickened folds, and a nodular or cobblestone mucosa may develop in the gastric antrum or body. Scarring and fibrosis may eventually lead to the development of a tubular, funnel-shaped, and narrowed gastric antrum (Fig. 6.6b). In some patients, combined gastroduodenal cicatrization may produce a single, continuous tubular structure involving the antrum and duodenum with obliteration of normal landmarks at the pylorus

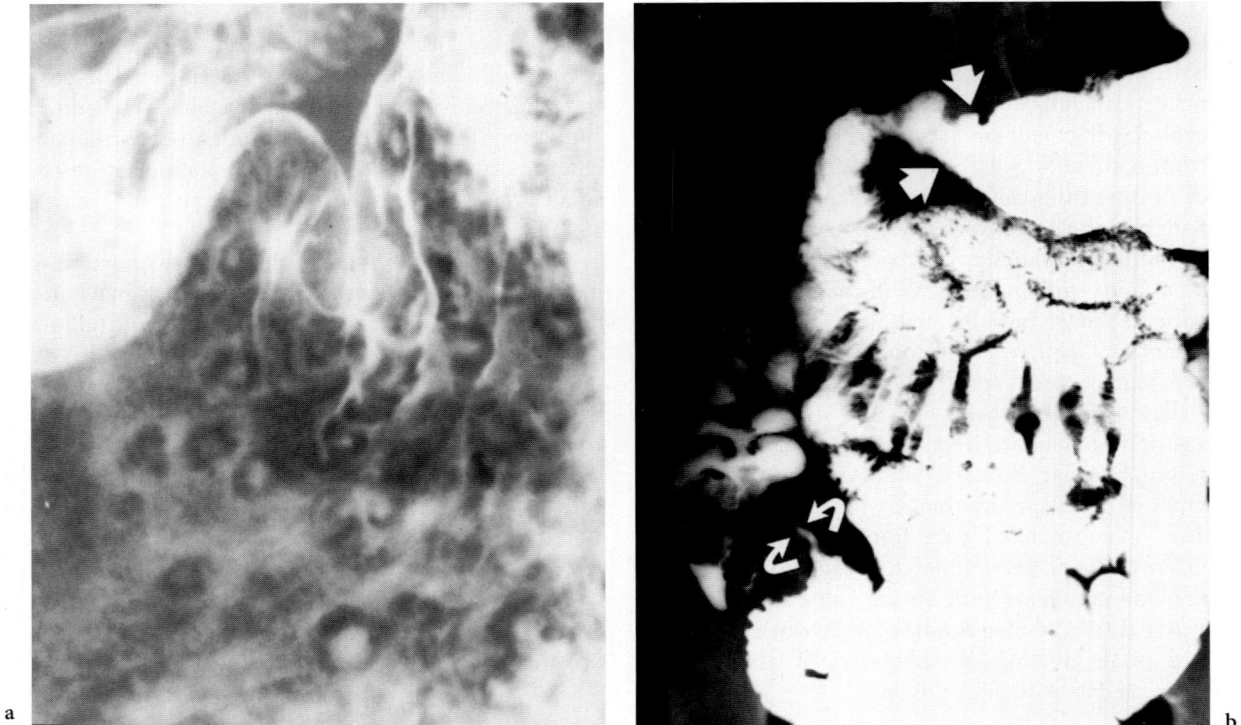

a

b

Fig. 6.6a,b. Crohn's disease. **a** Aphthoid ulcerations are present in the antrum of this patient with early gastric Crohn's disease. **b** There is antral narrowing associated with fold thick- ening (*straight arrows*) in the gastric antrum. Note the con- comitant ileal strictures (*curved arrows*) in this patient with long-standing Crohn's disease

– the "pseudo-Billroth I" sign (GORE and GHAHREMANI 1986). Rarely, postinflammatory pseudopolyps may be visualized or a gastrocolic fistula can develop.

6.4.6
Amyloidosis

Gastric infiltration can occur in primary or second- ary amyloidosis and is usually asymptomatic. Some patients present with nausea, vomiting, pain, and gastrointestinal hemorrhage (CARLSON and BREEN 1986).

Radiologically, amyloid deposition in the submu- cosa or lamina propria usually produces marked thickening of the rugal folds and a granular ap- pearance to the mucosa (TADA et al. 1994). When focal, amyloidosis may present as a submucosal polypoid mass (EISENBERG 1994). Antral narrow- ing and rigidity may occur, simulating linitis plastica. When the muscularis propria is involved, delayed gastric emptying may develop (MENKE et al. 1993).

6.4.7
Corrosive Gastritis

Intentional or accidental ingestion of acid produces a superficial necrosis of the mucosa. The distal stomach is most severely involved because the acid pools in the antrum if the patient is upright. The duodenum is often spared because the acid usually provokes an intense pylorospasm (SUGAWA and LUCAS 1989).

Acutely there is mucosal ulceration and thicken- ing of folds due to submucosal edema. Muscle spasm may cause narrowing of the gastric lumen. Gastric emphysema may develop. After 1–2 months, stenosis of the gastric lumen with marked deformity may de- velop due to submucosal fibrosis (MUHLETALER et al. 1980).

6.4.8
Ménétrier's Disease

Ménétrier's disease is a rare, idiopathic condition characterized by hyperplasia of the superficial (foveolar) layer of the mucosa associated with protein loss through the loose junctions between cells of the hyperplastic epithelium. Hypochlorhydria due to glandular atrophy is often present. The disease is usually limited to the proximal two-thirds of the stomach, is most marked along the greater curvature, and usually but not always stops abruptly at the antrum (EOLGADREN et al. 1993).

Ménétrier's disease occurs most commonly in middle life, more often in men than women, and in whites more frequently than in African-Americans. Patients present with epigastric pain, nausea, vomiting, and gastrointestinal bleeding (WEINSTEIN 1993).

On barium studies, Ménétrier's disease is classically manifested by grossly thickened lobulated folds in the gastric fundus and body with relative antral sparing (LEVINE 1994c). The greatest degree of fold thickening occurs on or near the greater curvature. Focally enlarged folds can be mistaken radiologically for polypoid carcinomas. In some patients, excessive gastric mucus may dilute the barium and compromise mucosal coating (LICHTENSTEIN 1993). On CT, Ménétrier's disease is characterized by a markedly thickened gastric wall with mass-like elevations representing giant, heaped-up folds protruding into the lumen (GORE et al. 1994).

6.4.9
Zollinger-Ellison Syndrome

In this disorder, there is hyperplasia of the glandular level of the epithelium, particularly the parietal cells, which is secondary to the hypergastrinemia caused by a pancreatic or duodenal gastrinoma (FURTH et al. 1995). Patients with Zollinger-Ellison syndrome present with gastric and/or duodenal ulcers. Although these ulcers were classically described as multifocal and postbulbar in location, most patients now present with solitary ulcers in the usual locations. Nearly 50% of patients also have diarrhea and/or steatorrhea due to the toxic effect of excess acid on the small bowel and deconjugation of bile salts. Diarrhea is the presenting complaint in up to one-third of cases (MCGUIGAN 1993).

Radiologically, there is thickening of the rugal folds caused by mucosal hyperplasia, but the folds are only mildly thickened and are much more regular than in Ménétrier's disease (BUCK and PANTONGRAG-BROWN 1994). The antrum may be involved as the excess serum gastrin causes conversion of the antral mucosa into a fundic type mucosa

(LICHTENSTEIN 1993). Increased gastric secretions may lead to dilution of the barium; however, the stomach may appear normal. Fold thickening is often observed in the duodenum and to a lesser extent the proximal jejunum, and the esophagus may show strictures, ulcers, and other signs of Barrett's esophagus (LEVINE 1994c).

6.5
Gastric Ulcers

A gastric ulcer is a mucosal defect that reaches the muscularis mucosae and beyond. Ulcers are usually single. An erosion is a defect limited to the superficial layer of the mucosa and is generally smaller than an ulcer. Erosions typically are multiple (LEVINE 1994b).

Gastric ulcers, unlike duodenal ulcers, are associated with normal or even decreased acid secretion. They form secondary to altered mucosal resistance due to weakening of the gel structure of the gastric mucosal layer (LAM et al. 1995).

The etiology of gastric ulcer disease is multifactorial. In addition to hereditary and environmental factors, a number of specific etiologic agents have been implicated: *H. pylori* infection, aspirin and other NSAIDs, alcohol, coffee, corticosteroids, stress, and tobacco (LAM 1995). *H. pylori* has been cultured in the stomach of 70%–95% of patients with antral gastritis and 60%–80% of patients with gastric ulcers (CELLO 1995). However, gastric ulcers can develop in the absence of *H. pylori* infection and *H. pylori* gastritis often occurs in the absence of gastric ulcers (MARSHALL 1994).

Aspirin and NSAIDs inhibit synthesis of prostaglandins that contribute to the integrity of the gastric mucosal barrier and favor back diffusion of H$^+$ions into the gastric cells. Nearly 20% of patients on high-dose aspirin therapy for longer than 3 months develop gastric ulcers (LAM et al. 1995). Indomethacin, butazolidin, ibuprofen, naproxen, and tolmetin produce both gastric erosions and gastric ulcers.

Gastric ulcers occur primarily in individuals older than 60 years with a slight female predominance due to the greater use of aspirin and NSAIDs in this segment of the population. For this reason hospital admissions for gastric ulcers with clinically significant hemorrhage have doubled in frequency since 1978 and perforations have become more prevalent (LAM et al. 1995).

Epigastric pain is the major symptom of gastric ulcer disease, often described as a burning discomfort, gnawing, or feeling of emptiness. It usually occurs 1–3 h postprandially but often awakens the patient at night. It is relieved by food or antacids and often aggravated by stress. Other symptoms include: right upper quadrant, back, or chest pain, belching, bloating, dyspepsia, nausea, vomiting, anorexia, and weight loss. Some patients present with symptoms and signs related to complications of their ulcers such as hemorrhage, obstruction, and perforation. Hemorrhage may be massive and life threatening or manifest by guaiac-positive stools or iron deficiency anemia (LAM et al. 1995).

Radiologically, gastric ulcers classically manifest as smooth, round, or ovoid barium collections. They may, however, appear linear, rod-shaped, star-shaped, rectangular, serpiginous, flamed-shaped, or as geographic lesions (LEVINE 1994b). The majority of ulcers seen on barium studies are small (<1 cm) due to the medical therapy these patients receive before their barium examination (LEVINE 1994a). Small ulcers are far more reliably detected with the double-contrast technique due to its ability to distend the stomach and coat the mucosa with a fine layer of barium (LEVINE et al. 1987).

The vast majority (90%) of gastric ulcers develop along the lesser curvature or posterior wall of the gastric antrum or body of the stomach (LAM et al. 1995). Posterior wall ulcers usually fill with barium on double-contrast films obtained in the supine or supine oblique position (KOGA et al. 1982). If barium only coats the rim of an unfilled crater, it will appear as a ring shadow on routine double-contrast views (LAUFER 1994b). In these cases, flow technique is employed to manipulate a thin pool of barium over the posterior gastric wall, filling these shallow posterior ulcers (KIKUCHI et al. 1986).

Less than 5% of gastric ulcers occur on the anterior wall (LEVINE 1994b). On double-contrast supine views these ulcers cast a ring shadow as barium coats the rim of the unfilled, nondependent ulcer crater. When these ring shadows are encountered, the patient should be turned 180° into the prone position and prone compression views should be obtained. This technique almost always demonstrates filling of these anterior wall ulcers. Thus, shallow posterior and anterior wall ulcers that produce ring shadows can be differentiated by a combination of prone compression views and flow technique.

Ulcers caused by ingestion of aspirin or other NSAIDs are responsible for the majority of gastric ulcers that are located along the greater curvature (LEVINE 1994b). This location accounts for only 5% of all gastric ulcers and is related to the effect of gravity as the tablets collect on or near the greater curvature (LEVINE et al. 1986). Giant NSAID-related greater curvature ulcers may eventually penetrate through the gastrocolic ligament into the superior border of the transverse colon leading to the development of gastrocolic fistula. Indeed, NSAID-related gastric ulcers are now the most common cause of these fistula (LEVINE et al. 1993).

Nearly 20% of patients with gastric ulcers have multiple lesions on double-contrast studies and the majority of these patients have a history of aspirin ingestion (LEVINE 1994b). Accordingly, whenever multiple ulcers are detected in the stomach, particularly in the greater curvature, NSAID use should be suspected (LEVINE 1994a).

6.5.1
Differentiation of Benign and Malignant Ulcers

It is essential for radiologists to differentiate benign from malignant gastric ulcers (Table 6.2; Fig. 6.7). With double-contrast techniques and meticulous attention to mucosal features such as mass effect and mucosal nodularity and destruction, barium studies can be very accurate in this differentiation (NELSON 1969; OTT et al. 1982). In one large series of 221 radiologically benign-appearing gastric ulcers, no

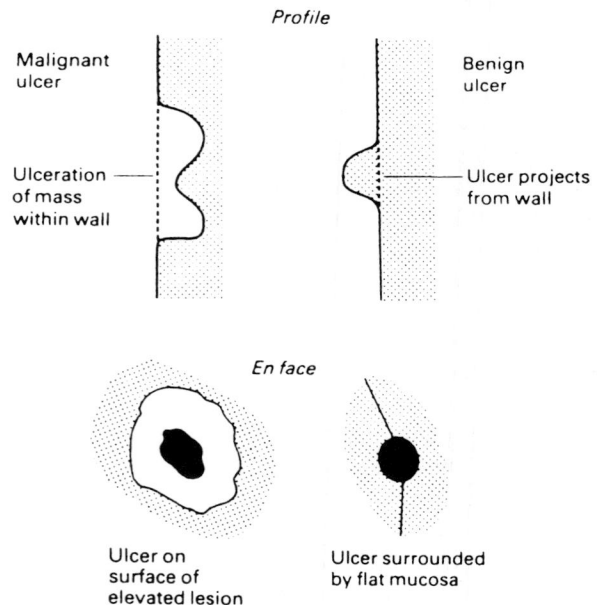

Fig. 6.7. Benign versus malignant gastric ulcers. This diagram depicts differentiating radiologic features on double-contrast barium studies. (From BARTRAM and KUMAR 1981)

Table 6.2. Benign versus malignant gastric ulcers: differential radiologic features (modified from HALPERT and GOODMAN 1993)

Features	Benign	Malignant
Hampton's line	Yes	No
Carman-Kirklin complex	No	Yes
Crescent sing	Yes	No
Project beyond gastric wall	Yes	No
Convergence of folds	To edge of crater	Stop short of crater
Radiating folds	Smooth	Thickened, irregular, club shaped
Ulcer shape	Linear, round, oval	Irregular
Position of ulcer mound	Central	Eccentric
Depth	Considerable depth in relation to size at mucosal surface	Shallow in relation to overall size
Ulcer collar	Smooth, symmetric	Eccentric
Margin	Smooth	Nodular, irregular
Peristalsis	Preserved	diminished or absent
Healing	Complete in 8 weeks	Very rare
Multiplicity	10%–30%	20%
Associated duodenal ulcer	50%–60%	Uncommon
Location	Rarely in fundus or proximal greater curvature	Anywhere

cases of carcinoma were detected endoscopically (THOMPSON et al. 1983). Thus when an ulcer is demonstrated as unequivocally benign on double-contrast studies, endoscopy can be avoided. This has enormous cost-saving implications.

6.5.2
Benign Gastric Ulcers

When viewed en face, unequivocally benign gastric ulcers are manifested by a round or oval ulcer crater that is surrounded by either a smooth mound of edema or symmetric, regular folds that radiate to the edge of the crater (Fig. 6.8a). The surrounding areae gastricae may be enlarged secondary to edema and inflammation and can often be seen extending to the edge of the ulcer crater without evidence of mass effect, nodularity, or tumor infiltration (BARTRAM and KUMAR 1981). In profile, benign gastric ulcers project beyond the gastric lumen (Fig. 6.8b) and are typically associated with a smooth, symmetric ulcer mound or collar or with smooth, straight mucosal folds that radiate to the edge of the ulcer crater (Fig. 6.9) (LEVINE 1994b).

There are three radiographic features seen on profile views that suggest a benign gastric ulcer: Hampton's line, an ulcer collar, and an ulcer mound (Fig. 6.10). These signs relate to undermining of the

mucosa due to the relative resistance of the mucosal layer to peptic digestion when compared to the submucosa (LEVINE 1994b). The more acid-peptic resistant mucosa appears to overhang the more readily destroyed submucosa. This undermining occurs in the presence of gastric acid whereas most gastric cancers occur in patients with achlorhydria. With minimal edema of the overhanging mucosa, a thin, sharply demarcated lucent line (Hampton's line) with parallel straight margins at the base of the crater may be seen tangentially (Fig 6.11). With progressive mucosal edema, a larger lucent ulcer collar can be seen separating the ulcer from the gastric lumen. An ulcer mound is created by extensive mucosal edema and may extend considerably beyond the limits of the ulcer (Fig. 6.12). In some ulcers, the rim of the undermined mucosa surrounding the orifice of the crater may become more edematous, producing a wide radiolucent band or ulcer collar. Other benign ulcers may have sufficient edema and inflammation to create an ulcer mound that projects into the lumen as a smooth, bilobed hemispheric mass when viewed in profile. Benign ulcer mounds typically have poorly defined outer borders that form obtuse, gently sloping angles with the adjacent gastric wall (LEVINE 1994a; GELFAND 1984).

Benign lesser curvature gastric ulcers can cause contraction of the adjacent gastric wall leading to the development of smooth, symmetric folds that radi-

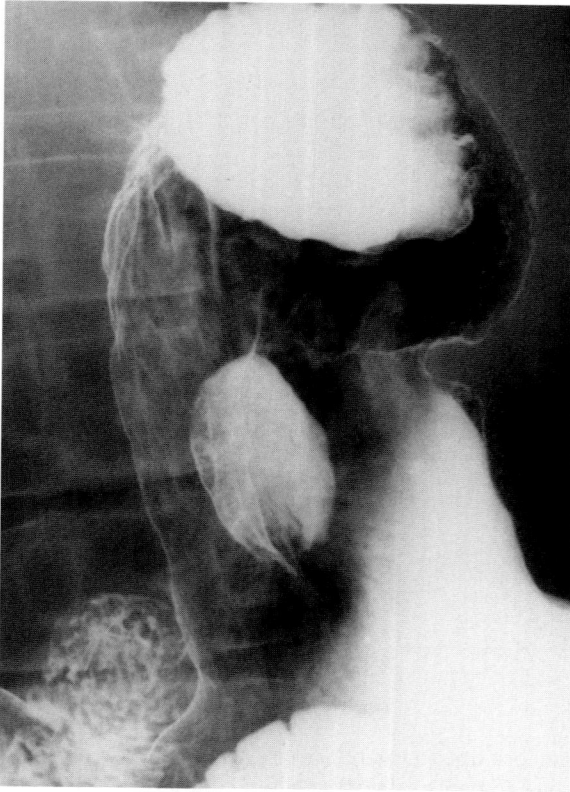
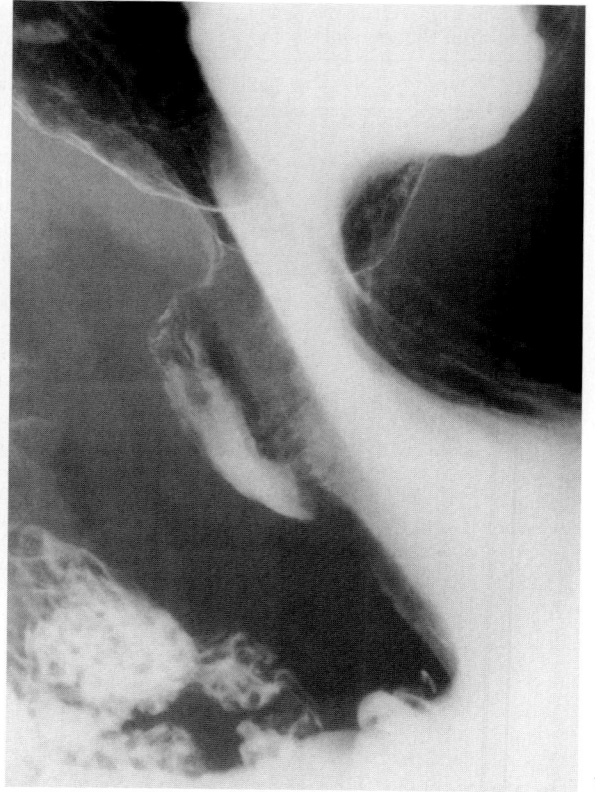

a

b

Fig. 6.8a,b. Benign gastric ulcer: penetration. **a** En face, this large posterior ulcer crater fills with barium. **b** Viewed tangentially, the ulcer projects beyond the expected confines of the gastric wall

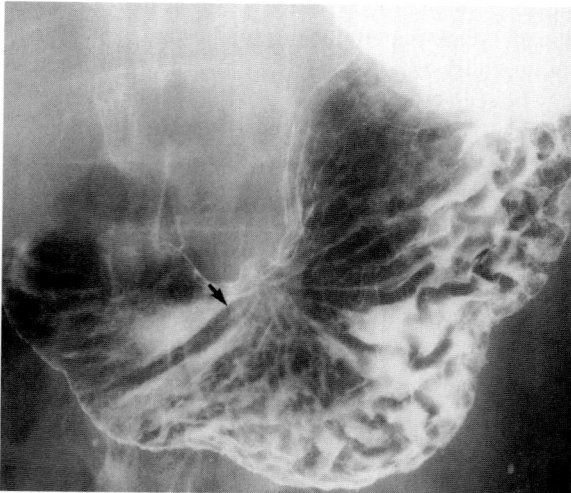
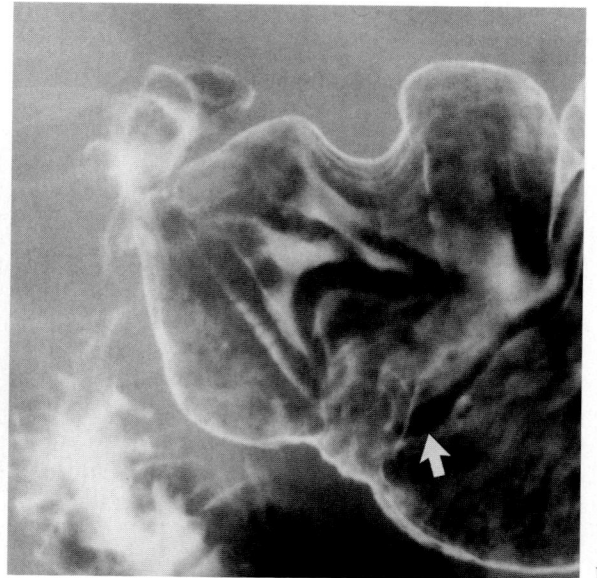

a

b

Fig. 6.9a,b. Benign versus malignant gastric ulcer. **a** Smooth, tapering folds are seen extending to the edge of the ulcer crater (*arrow*), indicating its benign nature. **b** By contrast, the folds leading to this ulcerated carcinoma are irregular and blunted (*arrow*)

ate to the edge of the ulcer crater. An incisura may also develop along the greater curvature (WOLF 1971). Ulcers may also be associated with enlarged areae gastricae because of edema and in-

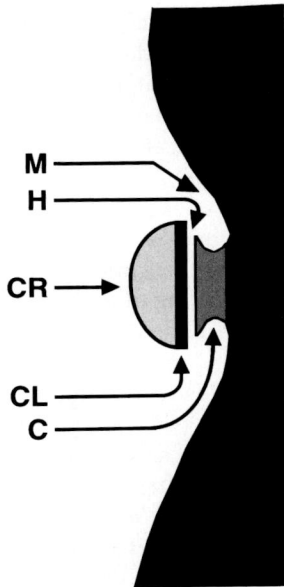

Fig. 6.10. Profile of a benign gastric ulcer. The crater (*CR*) is globular, sharp, and distinct. The neck is surrounded by a collar (*C*) which joins the crater to the lumen. The collar is parallel to the long axis of the stomach and does not project transversely into the lumen. A lucent or Hampton's line (*H*) intervenes between the collar and crater and marks the mucosa at the entrance to the ulcer. Deep to the Hampton's line there may also be a parallel slit-like cleft (*CL*) which fills with barium. The ulcer is located in the center of a symmetrical mound (*M*) which projects into the lumen but merges gradually with the adjacent, normally distensible, gastric wall. (From WOLF 1971)

flammation of the surrounding mucosa (LEVINE 1994b).

Almost all benign greater curvature ulcers are located on the distal half of the greater curvature, and the vast majority are caused by ingestion of aspirin or nonsteroidal anti-inflammatory drugs (LEVINE et al. 1986). These ulcers often appear to have an intraluminal location because of circular muscle spasm and retraction of the adjacent gastric wall. They are often associated with considerable mass effect with thickened, irregular folds due to marked edema and inflammation surrounding the ulcer. The inner margin of the ulcer may be concave toward the lumen due to a large mass of overhanging, edematous tissue producing the "quarter moon" or "crescent" sign (ZBORALSKE et al. 1978; HAN and WITTEN 1974). The orifice of the crater may be partially occluded due to this edematous tissue, leading to incomplete filling of the crater. As a result, benign greater curvature ulcers often have a suspicious radiographic appearance so that the usual criteria for differentiating benign and malignant ulcers elsewhere in the stomach are often unreliable in this location (LEVINE 1994b).

The location of an ulcer has little significance in terms of whether it is benign or malignant with the exception of the gastric fundus and the proximal half of the greater curvature. Benign ulcers are rarely found in these portions of the stomach, so that any ulcer in the fundus or proximal half of the greater curvature should be considered suspicious for malignancy until proven otherwise (LEVINE 1994b).

At one time, multiplicity of gastric ulcers was felt to be a sign of benignancy but up to 20% of patients

Fig. 6.11. Benign gastric ulcer: Hampton's line. The more acid-peptic resistant mucosa appears to overhang the more readily destroyed submucosa. This produces a thin, sharply demarcated lucent line (*arrows*) with parallel straight margins at the base of the crater

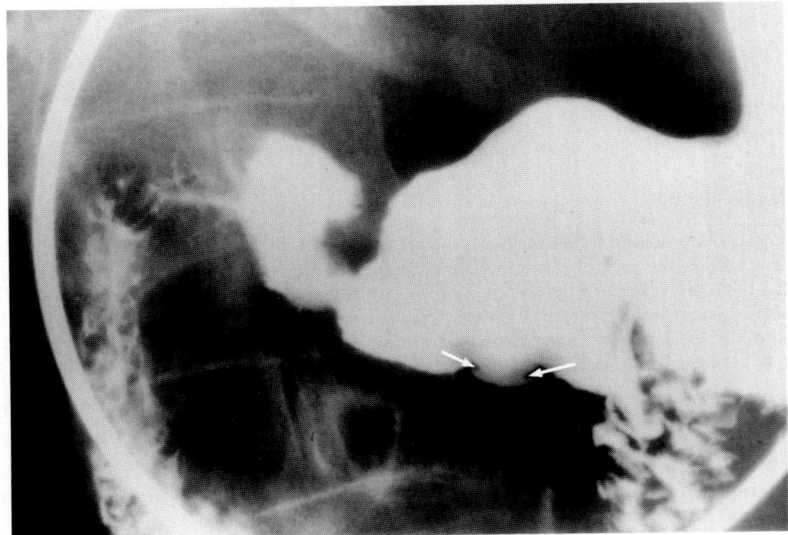

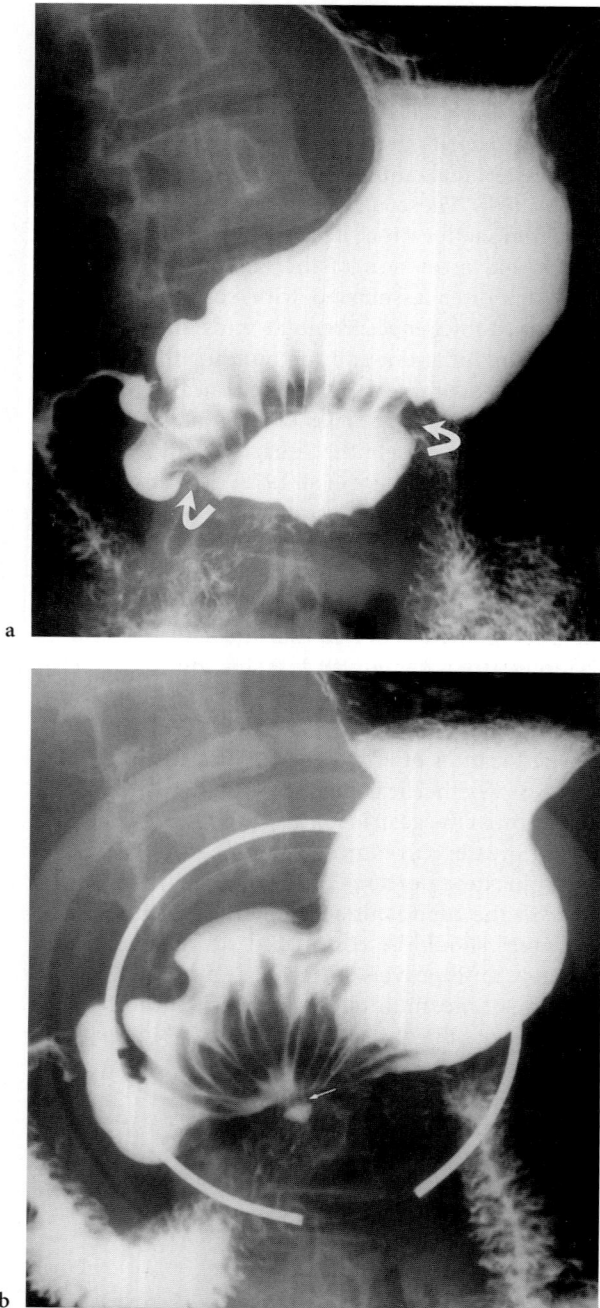

Fig. 6.12a,b. Benign gastric ulcer-healing. a There is a huge ulcer along the greater curvature. Note the radiating folds to the edge of the crater (*arrows*). b Follow-up study in 2 months shows considerable healing, smooth tapered radiating folds, and a smooth ulcer collar (*arrow*) separating the ulcer crater from the gastric lumen

with multiple ulcers have a malignant lesion (BLOOM et al. 1977; DAGRADI et al. 1975). Also, the size and shape of gastric ulcers were believed to be useful predictors of benign versus malignant disease; how-

ever, these signs have proven to be of little practical value.

Complete radiologic healing of a gastric ulcer is a fairly reliable sign of benignancy (KELLER et al. 1970). Benign ulcers usually respond dramatically to H_2 receptor antagonists; follow-up studies should be performed in 8 weeks to document healing. If the base of the ulcer crater contains poorly vascularized fibrous tissue, healing may be delayed. Complete healing of malignant ulcers may very rarely occur with medical therapy, however (KAGAN and STECKEL 1977).

Healing of a benign gastric ulcer can result in the production of bizarre deformities with mural retraction and stiffening, leading to residual deformity and stenosis. On double-contrast examinations, the gastric ulcer scar appears as a central pit, a depression, or a collection of folds converging toward the site of the healing ulcer (GELFAND and OTT 1981). Nodularity of the ulcer scar or irregularity, clubbing, or amputation of radiating folds should suggest a malignancy. Therefore, the surrounding gastric mucosa must be carefully assessed after ulcer healing has occurred. Endoscopy and biopsy are required if suspicious findings persist.

6.5.3
Malignant Gastric Ulcers

En face, malignant gastric ulcers classically appear as an irregular ulcer crater that is eccentrically located within an irregular mass with distortion or obliteration of the adjacent areae gastricae (LEVINE and MEGIBOW 1994b). Radiating folds may be present, but they tend to be nodular and irregular with fused, clubbed, or amputated tips that stop short of the ulcer crater. Radiating folds to a benign ulcer are smooth, slender, and appear to extend to the edge of the crater. When viewed tangentially, malignant gastric ulcers do not project beyond the expected outer gastric contour. A discrete tumor mass is often present and it forms acute angles with the gastric wall rather than the obtuse, gentle, sloping angles expected for a benign mound of edema. The adjacent mucosa may also be nodular or have thickened, lobulated folds that radiate to the ulcer because of infiltration of tumor (MARUYAMA and BABA 1994).

The Carman-Kirklin meniscus sign of a malignant gastric ulcer is created by a cancer that straddles the lesser curvature of the gastric antrum or body in which the tumor is a broad-based, flat lesion with central ulceration and elevated margins (KIRKLIN 1934). Compression of the lesion at fluoroscopy

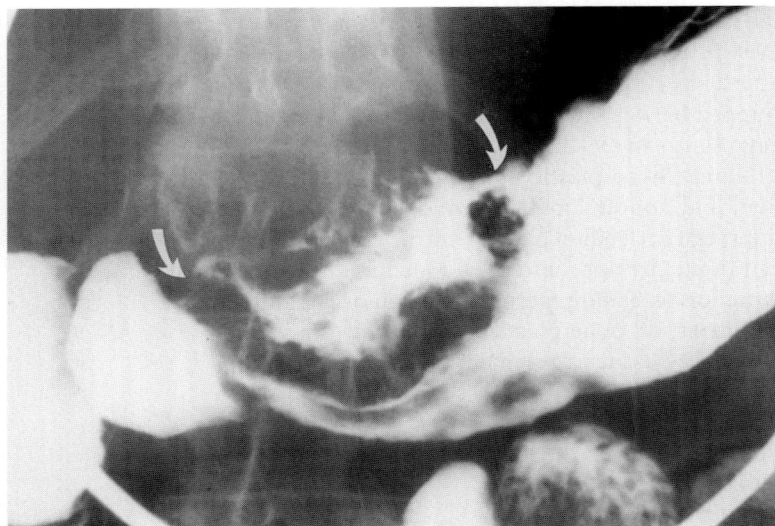

Fig. 6.13. Malignant gastric ulcer – the Carman-Kirklin meniscus sign. This ulcer, when viewed in profile and with compression, has a semicircular (meniscoid) appearance. The inner margin of the ulcer of this mass is convex towards the lumen. The radiolucent shadow (*curved arrows*) of the elevated ridge of neoplastic tissue is called the Carman-Kirklin complex

may demonstrate a discrete ulcer crater that has a meniscoid configuration. The convex inner border of the meniscus may be quite irregular and is directed towards the gastric lumen. The concave outer border of the meniscus represents the base of the broad, shallow ulcer and tends to be smoother and usually does not project beyond the expected gastric contour (Fig. 6.13). While the Carman-Kirklin meniscus complex is a reliable radiologic sign of malignancy, it is seen in only a small minority of malignant gastric ulcers (LEVINE 1994b).

Gastric ulcers that have an equivocal or suspicious appearance should undergo endoscopy with biopsy for further evaluation. Unequivocally benign-appearing gastric ulcers on double-contrast series can be followed to complete healing without endoscopy. After 8–10 weeks of medical management, a repeat barium study should be obtained to document ulcer healing (LEVINE et al. 1987). If the follow-up study shows a residual ulcer that has an equivocal or suspicious appearance, endoscopy should be performed. This approach avoids the need for endoscoping every gastric ulcer detected radiologically (LEVINE and LAUFER 1993).

6.6
Gastric Polyps

6.6.1
Hyperplastic Polyps

Hyperplastic polyps account for 75%–90% of all gastric polyps (FECZKO et al. 1985). They consist histologically of elongated, branching, cystically dilated glandular structures lined by a single layer of tall epithelial cells with abundant cytoplasm and small basal nuclei. Grossly, hyperplastic polyps appear as one or more sessile nodules that have a smooth, dome-shaped contour (LANZA 1995).

Hyperplastic polyps are often seen in the setting of chronic gastritis, atrophic gastritis, or bile reflux gastritis. They are not true neoplasms but are thought to result from excessive regenerative hyperplasia in areas of chronic gastritis (HEATLY and WYATT 1995). Although these polyps have no malignant potential, patients with hyperplastic polyps are at increased risk for harboring separate, coexisting gastric carcinomas. Between 8% and 28% of patients with hyperplastic polyps have a synchronous gastric carcinoma (ELDER 1995). Underlying atrophic gastritis, which predisposes to the development of cancer and polyps, is probably responsible for this association.

Although the risk of coexisting carcinoma is considerable, the role of endoscopic surveillance in patients with hyperplastic polyps alone has not been established. Most hyperplastic polyps are small, asymptomatic, and discovered as incidental findings on radiologic or endoscopic examinations. Polyps with a friable or ulcerated surface may bleed (LANZA 1995).

Radiologically, most hyperplastic gastric polyps are smooth, sessile, round, or oval lesions, ranging from 5 to 10 mm in size. They are usually multiple and they tend to be clustered in the gastric body or fundus. When multiple, hyperplastic polyps tend to be the same size (LEVINE 1994d).

Hyperplastic polyps located on the posterior gastric wall appear as smooth, round filling defects in the barium pool on double-ontrast studies (Levine 1994d). Polyps on the anterior, nondependent wall appear as ring shadows etched in white by barium trapped between the adjacent mucosa and the polyp edge (Laufer 1994b).

Rarely, hyperplastic polyps can be as large as 2–6 cm and appear lobulated, villous-like, and/or pedunculated. Pedunculated antral gastric polyps can rarely prolapse into the duodenum, causing obstruction. A giant hyperplastic polyp or conglomerate mass of hyperplastic polyps can simulate a polypoid gastric carcinoma radiologically (Glick et al. 1990).

6.6.2
Fundic Gland Polyposis

Fundic gland polyps are a variant of hyperplastic gastric polyps. These lesions are derived from hyperplastic fundic glands and as such have no malignant potential and are seen only in the proximal two-thirds of the stomach. These polyps are usually multiple so this entity has been called *fundic gland polyposis* (Marcial et al. 1993). There is no clear association of fundic gland polyposis with chronic nonspecific gastritis and no reported risk for adenocarcinoma. These lesions were first described in patients with familial adenomatous polyposis syndrome. Indeed about 40% of these patients have gastric polyps (Iida et al. 1985). These polyps are now more commonly seen in the general population, especially in middle-aged women (Fig. 6.14). These sporadically occurring cases usually have an average of four polyps (range 1–11) and they may remain stable for years or sometimes disappear spontaneously (Hizawa et al. 1993).

6.6.3
Cronkhite-Canada Syndrome

Cronkhite-Canada syndrome is a nonfamilial GI polyposis associated with a triad of ectodermal pathology: alopecia, onychodystrophy, and hyperpigmentation. These polyps are inflammatory or juvenile-type hamartomatous polyps that have little or no malignant potential. Patients are middle-aged or elderly and present with severe vomiting, diarrhea, weight loss, and electrolyte depletion (Lanza 1995).

Radiologically, patients with Cronkhite-Canada syndrome present with innumerable tiny (3–10 mm)

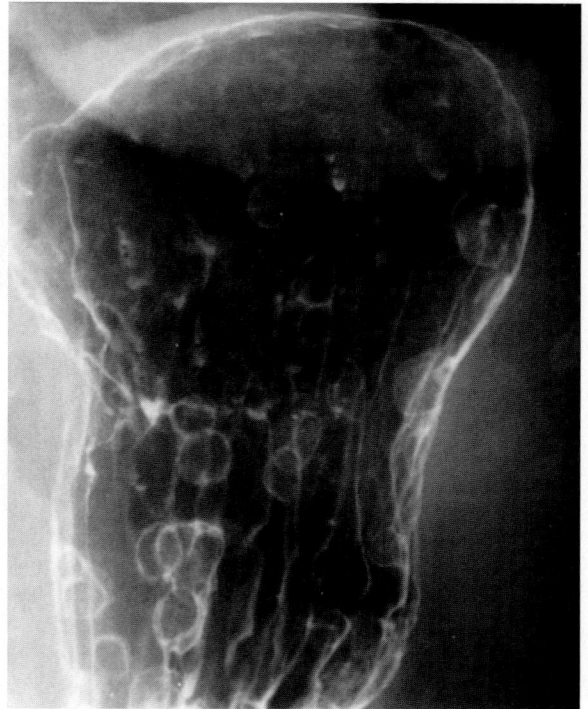

Fig. 6.14. Fundic gland polyposis. Multiple, uniform sized polyps are present in the fundus on this double-contrast barium study

sessile polyps in the stomach and colon. On double-contrast studies, a distinctive "whiskering" effect may be observed along the gastric margin as barium is trapped between these tiny mucosal excrescences and/or enlarged areae gastricae. Thickened rugal folds may be observed in some patients (Levine 1994d).

6.6.4
Adenomatous Polyps

While common in the colon, adenomatous polyps are rare in the stomach of the general population, constituting fewer than 20% of all gastric polyps (Feczko et al. 1985). Adenomatous polyps are larger and more commonly pedunculated than hyperplastic polyps. Adenomatous polyps are usually smaller than 2 cm; those that are larger harbor carcinomatous foci in approximately 40% of cases (Ginsburg et al. 1996). Some 11% of adenomas will develop carcinomatous foci within 4 years (Ming 1976). Adenomatous polyps develop in the duodenum of some 35%–100% of patients with familial adenomatous polyposis (Buck and Pantongrag-Brown 1994). They are usually small, multiple, and can undergo malignant change. Thus, surveillance and resection are indicated given the risk of benign and malignant neoplasms in this disorder (ORLOWSKA et al. 1995).

Clinically, patients with adenomatous polyps may present with epigastric pain or bloating, upper gastrointestinal bleeding, and rarely gastric outlet obstruction caused by the ball valve effect of polyps arising near the pylorus or prolapse of pedunculated antral polyps into the duodenum. Atrophic gastritis and achlorhydria are present in 85%–90% of these patients (DAVIS 1993).

Most adenomatous polyps visualized radiologically are greater than 1 cm in size, solitary, and located in the antrum. They may appear sessile or pedunculated and tend to have a more lobulated appearance than hyperplastic polyps (LEVINE 1994d). When pedunculated, the stalk may be seen en face as an inner ring shadow overlying the head of the polyp, producing the "Mexican hat" sign on double-contrast studies (LAUFER 1994b).

6.7
Benign Gastric Stromal Tumors

6.7.1
Leiomyoma

Leiomyomas are the most common benign gastric neoplasms. They arise from the smooth muscle layer of the gastric wall and approximately 80% are endogastric lesions that remain intramural but grow towards the lumen. Another 15% of leiomyomas are exogastric tumors that remain subserosal but grow outward from the stomach toward the peritoneal cavity. The remaining 5% of tumors have both endogastric and exogastric components, having a "dumbbell" shape (LANZA 1995).

Leiomyomas are usually asymptomatic when less than 3 cm in size. When larger, these tumors present with gastrointestinal hemorrhage as a result of ulceration or nausea and vomiting secondary to mass effect or intermittent gastric outlet obstruction. It is often difficult to differentiate leiomyomas from leiomyosarcomas on the basis of radiologic, endoscopic, or even histopathologic criteria. Their classification ultimately depends on the biologic behavior of the lesion (DAVIS 1993).

Most gastric leiomyomas appear as discrete submucosal lesions that have a smooth surface that is etched in white on double-contrast barium studies (Fig. 6.15). When viewed in profile, the borders of

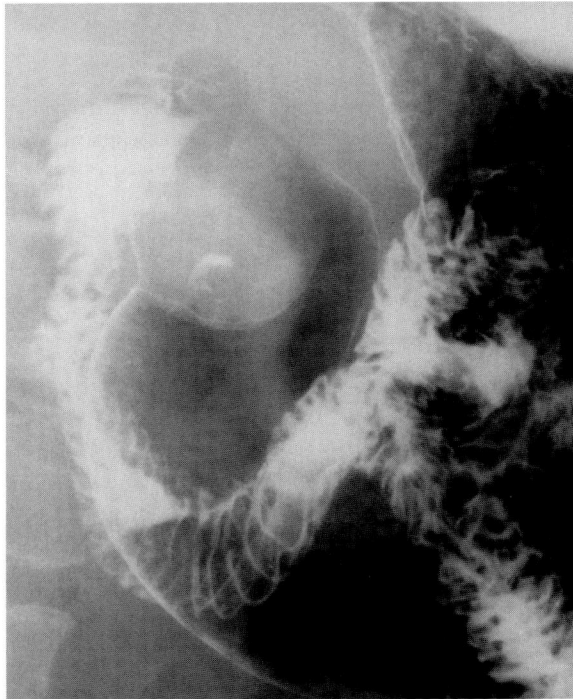

Fig. 6.15. Leiomyoma. A centrally ulcerated submucosal mass is present in the gastric antrum. This lesion encroaches significantly on the gastric lumen

these tumors form either right angles or slightly obtuse angles with the adjacent gastric wall. En face, the intraluminal surface of these tumors has distinct, abrupt, well-defined borders. The overlying mucosa is usually intact so that a normal areae gastricae pattern is often seen over these lesions. Leiomyomas vary greatly in size and tumors larger than 2 cm in diameter often contain ulceration that is manifested radiologically by a central barium collection 0.2–2 cm in size the so-called bull's-eye or target lesion (LEVINE 1994d).

On CT, gastric leiomyomas present as smooth masses of uniform soft tissue attenuation with a density similar to skeletal muscle (MEGIBOW et al. 1985). These masses usually project into the gastric lumen with a broad mural attachment but occasionally may appear primarily exogastric in location (GORE and GHAHREMANI 1994). Leiomyomas may contain irregular streaks or clumps of mottled calcification and are the most commonly calcified benign gastric tumors (THOENI and MOSS 1992). Although surface ulceration may be present, the outer borders of the leiomyoma are smooth, with preservation of the fat plane between the tumor and adjacent organs (GORE et al. 1994).

6.7.2
Leiomyoblastoma

Leiomyoblastomas are uncommon smooth muscle tumors that usually occur in the gastric antrum. They appear identical to leiomyomas radiographically and on gross inspection. Histologically they consist of round, polygonal, or epithelioid cells with eccentric nuclei, peripheral vacuolization, and a clear or acidophilic cytoplasm. Most leiomyo-

blastomas are benign; however, metastases to the liver and other structures occur in 10% of patients (DAVIS 1993). Size is a major factor in predicting biologic behavior as metastases seldom occur with lesions less than 6 cm in size (LANZA 1995).

Radiologically, these tumors are usually solitary and appear as smooth submucosal masses often with a central area of ulceration necrosis (LEVINE 1994d). Endogastric lesions can be pedunculated. Exogastric lesions can grow quite large and simulate extrinsic masses involving the stomach (Fig. 6.16a). On CT (Fig. 6.16b), leiomyoblastomas appear as a large spherical or elliptical exogastric mass of variable attenuation (CHOI et al. 1988). Density differences are a reflection of variable tumor growth rate and the presence of necrosis within the tumor (GORE and GHAHREMANI 1994; GORE et al. 1994).

6.7.3
Lipoma

Lipomas account for 2.3% of all benign gastric tumors (DAVIS 1993). They are usually solitary lesions that are asymptomatic unless large enough to bleed, ulcerate, or cause obstruction. Nearly 75% of lipomas are located in the gastric antrum. Approximately 95% are endogastric lesions that arise from submucosal fat and grow toward the lumen, whereas the remaining 5% are exogastric lesions that arise in the subserosal fat and grow outward from the stom-

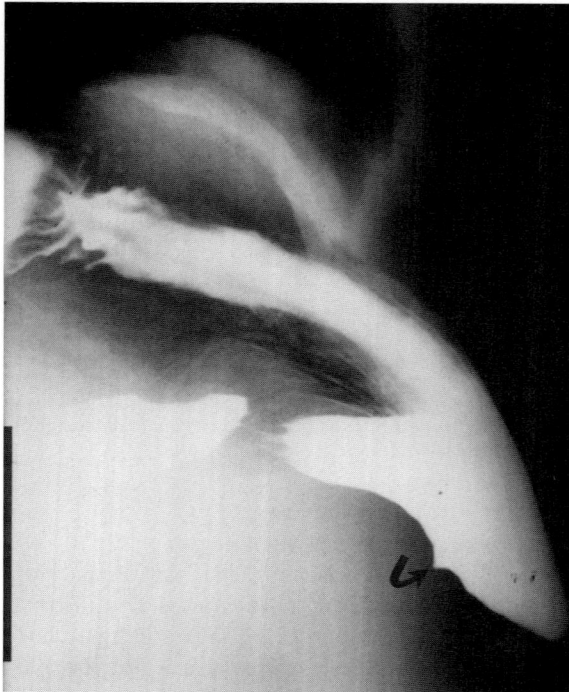

a

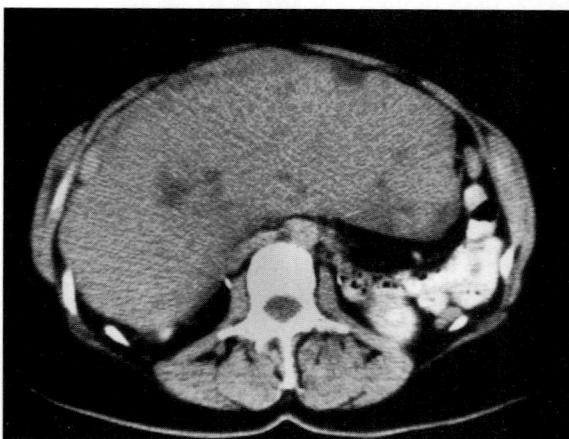

b

Fig. 6.16a,b. Giant leiomyoblastoma: CT–GI correlation. **a** Lateral spot film from an upper GI series demonstrates a large mass displacing the gastric antrum, tethering the wall (Curved *arrow*) along the greater curvature. **b** CT scan shows a huge, elliptical exogastric mass of variable attenuation

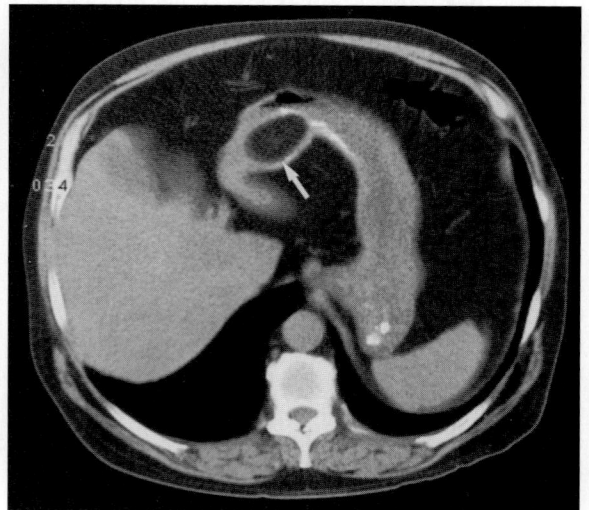

Fig. 6.17. Gastric lipoma. CT scan shows a smooth, well-marginated, homogeneous, fatty density mass in the antrum (*arrow*). (Case courtesy of Jay P. Heiken, St. Louis, Missouri)

ach (LANZA 1995). Large lesions develop areas of superficial ulceration due to pressure necrosis of the overlying mucosa.

On barium studies, lipomas present as a smooth submucosal mass or ulcerated bull's eye lesion that is identical to a leiomyoma or other mesenchymal tumor. Because of their soft consistency, the correct diagnosis can be suggested if these masses change in size and shape with peristalsis or manual palpation at fluoroscopy (LEVINE 1994d). CT can confirm the diagnosis (GORE and GHAHREMANI 1994; GORE et al. 1994) by showing a well-circumscribed mass of uniform fatty density with an attenuation of −80 to −120 Hounsfield units (Fig. 6.17). When these features are present, endoscopy or surgery can be avoided (HEIKEN et al. 1982).

6.8
Adenocarcinoma

Gastric adenocarcinoma is responsible for approximately 650 000 deaths worldwide each year and is probably second only to lung cancer as an overall cause of cancer-related mortality (FUCHS and MAYER 1995). Its incidence varies greatly from country to country, being particularly high in Japan (160 cases per 100 000 people per year) (LANZA 1995). As recently as the 1940s, gastric cancer was the most common malignant disease in the United States. Since then, there has been a dramatic decrease in the annual incidence and mortality from gastric cancer – currently ten cases and six cases per 100 000 population, respectively (FUCHS and MAYER 1995). Nevertheless, gastric cancer remains a deadly disease, accounting for nearly 23 000 new cases and 14 000 deaths per year in the United States (PARKER et al. 1996; SALVON-HARMON et al. 1995). The clinical diagnosis of gastric cancer is difficult due to the insidious onset of symptoms and their similarity in the early stages to benign causes of dyspepsia.

6.8.1
Barium Studies Versus Endoscopy in Gastric Cancer Detection

There is considerable debate in the medical community on how best to diagnose gastric cancer and other mucosal lesions of the upper GI tract: upper GI endoscopy or barium radiography. Citing outdated, pre-1970s radiology literature, some gastroenterolo-

gists have advocated performing endoscopy as the initial diagnostic procedure in all patients with upper GI symptoms. It is true that up to 25% of gastric cancers were missed on single-contrast barium studies and that this technique designated malignant gastric ulcers as benign in 6%–16% of cases (STRANDJORD 1960). The development and refinement of double-contrast techniques over the past two decades, however, have dramatically improved the radiologist's ability to detect gastric cancer and characterize gastric ulcers (DEKKER and OP DEN ORTH 1988; THOMPSON et al. 1983).

In a recent review of a large series of gastric cancers, these neoplasms were detected on double-contrast upper GI examinations in 99% of cases, and malignant tumor was diagnosed or suspected in 96% of cases (LOW et al. 1994). This is comparable to the reported sensitivity of endoscopy and biopsy of 94%–99%. In this series, the high sensitivity of barium radiology was accompanied by reasonably high specificity; endoscopy was recommended to rule out malignant tumor in only 3.5% of all patients who had double-contrast examinations. Thus, a high sensitivity in the detection of gastric carcinoma was achieved without exposing a large number of patients to unnecessary endoscopy. In Japan, double-contrast examinations are considered sufficiently sensitive and specific to serve as the primary screening examination for early gastric cancer (KOGA et al. 1982).

6.8.2
Early Gastric Cancer

Early gastric cancer (EGC) is defined as carcinoma limited to the mucosa and submucosa (Fig. 6.18), regardless of the presence or absence of lymph node involvement (DUPONT and COHN 1980). This term clinically suggests a lesion that is early, confined, and asymptomatic, but in some cases EGC may be symptomatic, large, and have lymph node involvement (WHITE et al. 1985). In Japan, the incidence of EGC is 25%–46% compared to an incidence of only 5%–25% in Western countries (ELDER 1995). This high incidence of EGC in Japan has led to mass screening of the adult population for gastric cancer, with nearly one-third of detected lesions being EGC (MARUYAMA 1992). Radiologists and endoscopists in the West are unlikely to encounter many early gastric cancers as long as these examinations are performed only on symptomatic patients and not as part of a screening program (MONTESI et al. 1982).

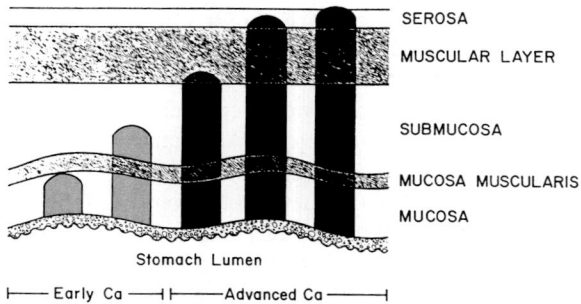

Fig. 6.18. Early versus advanced gastric cancer. In early gastric cancer the disease is limited to the mucosa and submucosa. The tumor penetrates beyond the submucosa in advanced gastric cancer. (From DUPONT and COHN 1980)

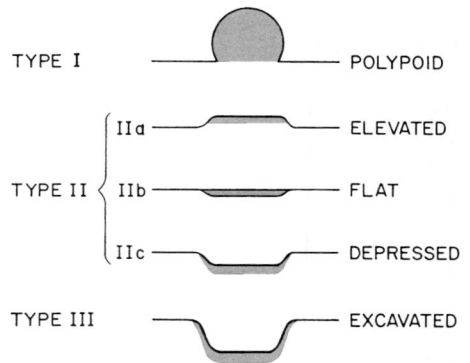

Fig. 6.19. Macroscopic classification of early gastric cancer. (From DAVIS 1993)

However, such screening programs do not appear to be warranted in the West because of the lower incidence of gastric cancer.

The Japanese Research Society for Gastric Cancer has divided EGC lesions into three main types and three main subtypes (Fig. 6.19). Type I EGCs are elevated lesions that protrude more than 5 mm into the lumen (Fig. 6.20). Radiographically they appear as small elevated lesions in the stomach. Adenomatous polyps can undergo malignant degeneration, so that any sessile or pedunculated gastric polyps greater than 1 cm in size should be viewed with suspicion for EGC (GOLD et al. 1984). Some polypoid EGCs may be quite large and symptomatic without penetrating the muscularis propria. Type I tumors are generally larger than 2 cm and only rarely pedunculated (MARUYAMA and BABA 1994).

Type II EGCs are also superficial lesions with elevated (IIa), flat (IIb), or depressed components (IIc). These tumors present radiologically as plaque-like elevations, mucosal nodularity, and/or shallow areas of ulceration. type IIa and IIb lesions usually involve the antrum; Type IIc lesions more often involve the angulus (MARUYAMA and BABA 1994). Type II lesions occasionally can be quite extensive, involving a large portion of the surface area of the stomach. Type I and IIa lesions are most frequently seen in the elderly population and constitute 25.4% of all cases of gastric cancer that occur in Japan (MARUYAMA and HAMADA 1994).

Type III EGCs are excavated lesions resembling gastric ulcers but with irregular ulcer craters, clubbing, fusion, or amputation of radiating folds (Fig. 6.21), and nodularity of the adjacent mucosa. Meticulous analysis of the radiographic findings of these lesions usually permits differentiation from benign gastric ulcers. If there is any doubt about the radiologic findings, then endoscopy with biopsy

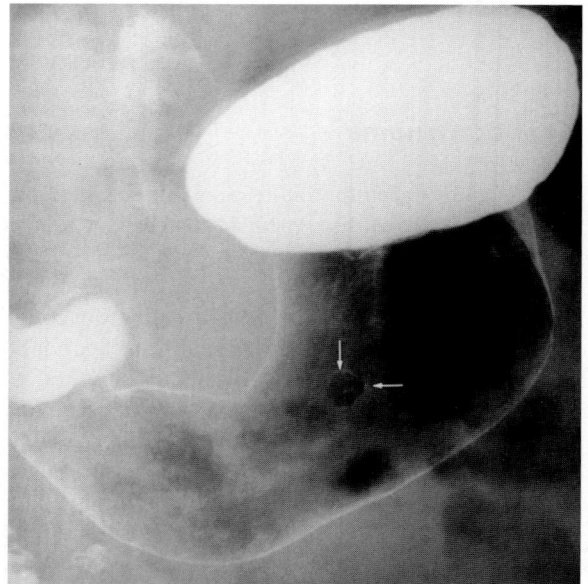

Fig. 6.20. Type I early gastric cancer. An adenomatous polyp (arrows) that has undergone malignant degeneration is present in the gastric body. Note the gastric atrophy

should be performed (LEVINE and MEGIBOW 1994a).

In one study, double-contrast upper GI examinations were fairly accurate in predicting the depth of invasion and histologic type of EGC (HARUMA et al. 1991). A lesion 20 mm or more in size with coarse, enlarged areae gastricae or a granular surface pattern was considered cancer limited to the mucosa. A lesion larger than 20 mm with an irregular nodular surface pattern was diagnosed as cancer that had invaded the submucosa. For depressed lesions, invasion limited to the mucosa was suggested by disappearance of the barium collection upon mild compression, a smooth and sharply defined granular surface, tapered converging mucosal folds, and wall rigidity within 1 cm Cancer invading the submucosa was suggested by a lesion that had a rigid or partial fusion of converging mucosal folds, and wall rigidity over 1 cm. Differentiated lesions were suggested by: (a) a smooth, fine, uniform surface; (b) gradual transition from normal surrounding mucosa; and (c) gradual tapering of converging mucosal folds. Undifferentiated cancers had: (a) an uneven, coarse surface with irregular granularities; (b) abrupt transition from normal surrounding mucosa; and (c) sudden interruption, tapering, clubbing, and fusion of converging mucosal folds. Using these criteria, the depth of tumor invasion was correctly predicted as being limited to the mucosa in 65.3% and to the submucosa in 59.1%, and the histologic type was correctly predicted in 78.9% of differentiated and 73.1% of undifferentiated carcinomas (HARUMA et al. 1991).

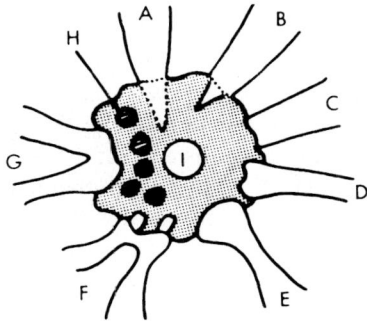

Fig. 6.21. Various appearances of converging fold terminations and central mucosa in excavated early gastric cancer. *A*, Gradual tapering; *B*, abrupt tapering; *C*, abrupt termination; *D* and *E*, clubbing; *F*, fusion with abrupt tapering; *G*, fusion (with V-shaped deformity); *H*, uneven base with nodules or depressions; *I*, smoother regenerative epithelium. Radiating folds in benign gastric ulcers are tapered, smooth, and extend to the edge of the ulcer. (From MARUYAMA and HAMADA 1994)

Synchronous EGCs occur in approximately 9% of patients. Careful preoperative radiography and endoscopy can depict nearly 70% of these lesions (BRANDT et al. 1989).

6.8.3
Advanced Gastric Cancer

Most symptomatic patients have advanced gastric cancer at the time of presentation. This is the type of gastric cancer that is usually found in the United States and Europe (OHMAN et al. 1980). Advanced gastric cancer denotes tumor that has penetrated the muscularis propria and is typically associated with distant or contiguous disease. As a result, advanced lesions are rarely curable (DAVIS 1993). This tumor is identified by the radiologist, pathologist, and endoscopist in patterns that were originally described by Borman (Fig. 6.22). The classification is based solely on gross appearances: polypoid, ulcerated, infiltrating. There is considerable overlap in this classification because many lesions have mixed morphologic features. The Kajitani classification is more simplified and allows easy recognition of the infiltrating pattern of advanced cancer (MARUYAMA and HAMADA 1994).

6.8.3.1
Borman Type 1: Polypoid–Fungating

Borman type 1 lesions are large polypoid (Fig. 6.23a) or fungating lesions (Fig. 6.23b) that have irregular lobulation and measure 3 cm or larger in greatest diameter. Radiographically, these tumors produce large, irregular filling defects in the barium pool and cast an irregular tumor shadow with coarse lobula-

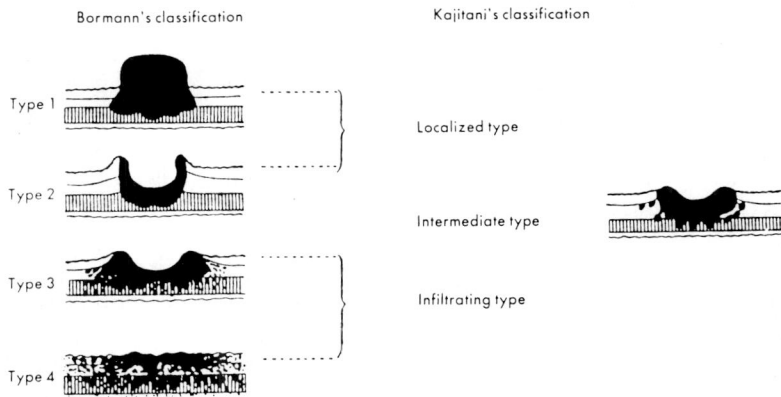

Fig. 6.22. Gross classification of advanced gastric cancer. (From MARUYAMA and HAMADA 1994)

a

b

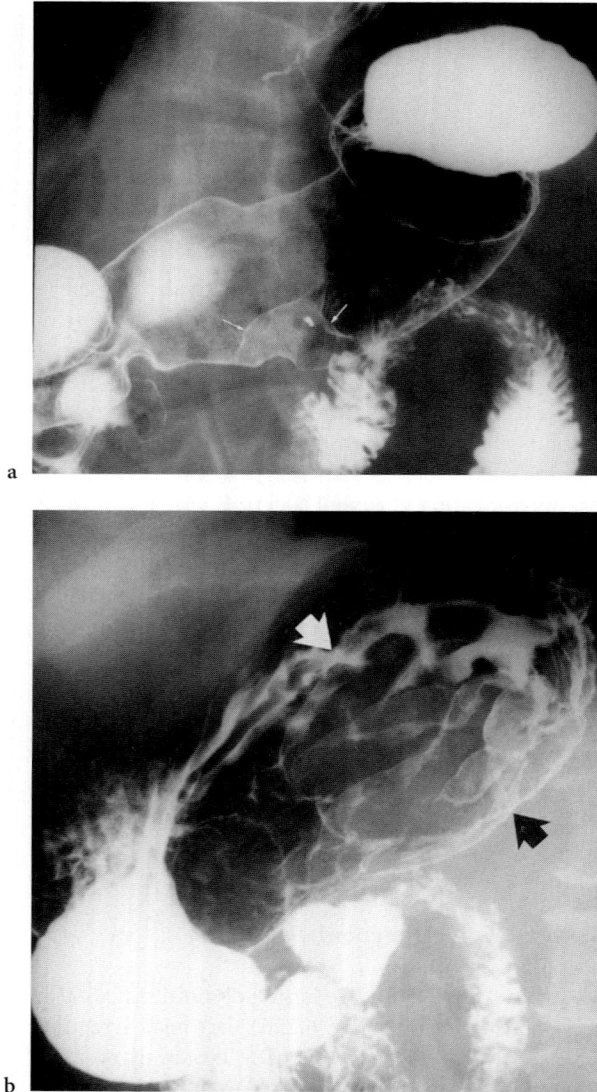

Fig. 6.23a,b. Advanced gastric carcinoma: polypoid–fungating. **a** A rather smooth, polypoid mass (*arrows*) is present along the greater curvature of the stomach. There is gastric atrophy and the patient has pernicious anemia. **b** A fungating Borman type 1 carcinoma presents as a large mass (*arrows*) in the posterior aspect of the proximal gastric body

tion on double-contrast and compression radiographs (LEVINE and MEGIBOW 1994a). On the nondependent surface of the stomach, these lesions, when viewed en face, are etched in white by a thin layer of barium trapped between the edge of the mass and the adjacent mucosa (LAUFER and KRESSEL 1992). Bulky lesions may significantly encroach upon the lumen but gastric outlet obstruction is uncommon. Polypoid antral tumors can prolapse through the pylorus into the duodenum and present as a mass at the base of the duodenal bulb.

6.8.3.2
Borman Type 2: Ulcerated

In Borman type 2 lesions, the bulk of tumor has been replaced by ulceration. These tumors have discrete, sharply defined borders so that the ulcer crater is clearly delineated from normal surrounding mucosa. These lesions typically exceed 3 cm in greatest diameter. When smaller, they may be difficult to differentiate from type IIc EGC on double-contrast studies (MARUYAMA 1992). The primary site may appear as an erosion or ulceration which, with progressive disease, replaces the mucosal surface. En face, these malignant ulcers are characterized by an irregular ulcer crater that is eccentrically located in a rind of neoplastic tissue. Discrete tumor nodules may be present in the adjacent mucosa and these ulcers may also have scalloped, angular, or stellate borders. If there are radiating folds converging to the edge of the ulcer, they are typically blunted, nodular, clubbed, or fused as a result of tumor infiltration (LEVINE and MEGIBOW 1994a). On double-contrast studies, ulcerated carcinomas (Fig. 6.24a) on the anterior or nondependent wall may be etched in white, producing a double ring shadow with the outer ring delineating the edge of the tumor and the inner ring indicating the edge of the ulcer (LAUFER 1994b). On prone compression views, the ulcer crater within the tumor mass fills with barium (Fig. 6.24b).

6.8.3.3
Borman Type 3: Infiltrative–Ulcerated

Borman type 3 lesions have a mixed morphology with both infiltrative and ulcerated components. The ulceration does not have discrete borders, however. The mass is usually more prominent than the ulcer (Fig. 6.25). Compression films show a large irregular crater and a surrounding radiolucent defect. Barium pool films demonstrate a filling defect and stiffening of the gastric wall. Because there is diffuse mural infiltration, stiffening of the gastric wall extends beyond the cancer ulcer crater (LEVINE and MEGIBOW 1994a).

6.8.3.4
Borman Type 4: Linitis Plastica

Scirrhous tumors of the stomach are diffusely infiltrating lesions that are associated with marked pro-

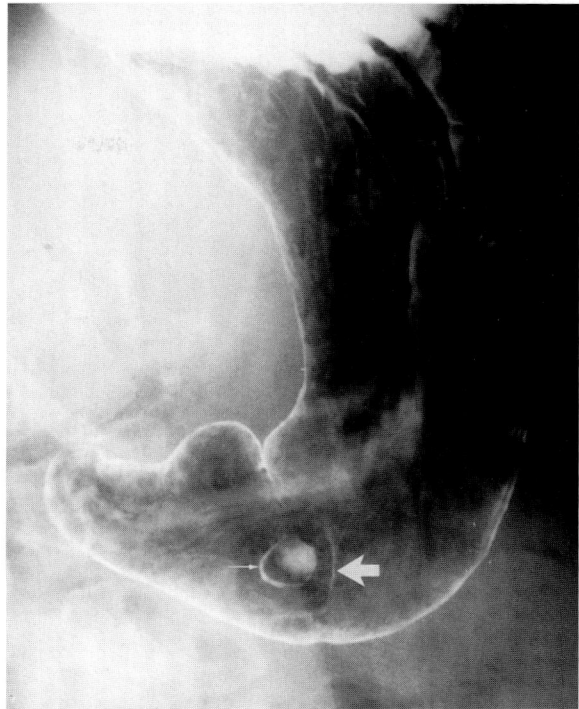

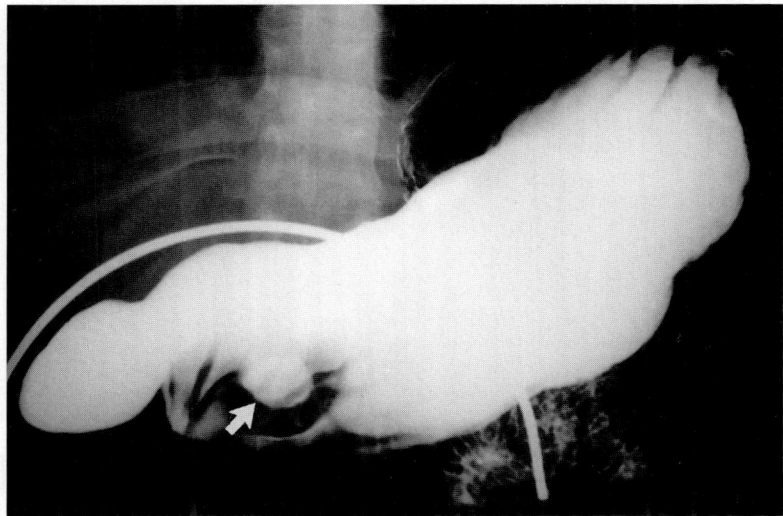

Fig. 6.24a,b. Advanced gastric cancer: ulcerated. **a** This Borman type 2 lesion along the anterior wall of the gastric antrum is etched in white, producing a double ring shadow with the outer ring (*large arrow*) delineating the edge of the tumor and the inner ring (*small arrow*) indicating the edge of the ulcer. **b** On prone compression view, the ulcer crater within the tumor mass fills with barium (*arrow*)

liferation of fibrotic tissue and desmoplasia (RASKIN 1976). This results in a grossly thickened stomach, with a shrunken lumen that has been likened to a leather bottle (Fig. 6.26a). The distal one-half of the stomach is most commonly involved and is severely narrowed (BALTHAZAR et al. 1980). In advanced cases, the entire stomach is infiltrated by tumor. More localized tumors may be confined to the prepyloric antrum and appear as short, annular le-

sions, with shelf-like proximal borders (Fig. 6.26b). Nearly 40% of these patients have localized lesions in the gastric fundus or body with antral sparing. This fact was not appreciated until double-contrast barium techniques afforded adequate distention of the proximal stomach (LEVINE et al. 1983).

Scirrhous carcinomas typically demonstrate gastric narrowing and rigidity; however, some lesions may cause only mild loss of distensibility. Instead,

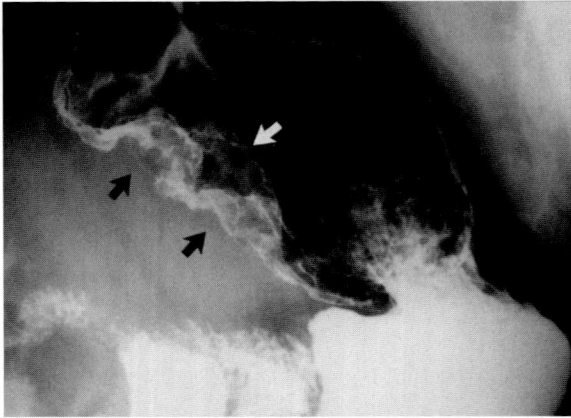

Fig. 6.25. Advanced gastric cancer: infiltrated–ulcerated. In this Borman type 3 lesion, the mass (*arrows*) is more prominent than the ulcer and the edge of the tumor is less well defined than the Borman type 2 lesion

these tumors cause distortion of the normal surface pattern on the stomach with mucosal nodularity, spiculation, ulceration, or thickened irregular folds (LEVINE and MEGIBOW 1994a). Thus, if too much reliance is placed upon gastric narrowing as the major criterion for diagnosing these tumors, they are likely to be missed (LEVINE et al. 1990a).

Primary gastric carcinomas may have several appearances on CT: a focal area of mural thickening with (Fig. 6.26c) or without ulceration; an exophytic intraluminal mass; or diffuse wall thickening with luminal narrowing characteristic of linitis plastica (GORE et al. 1994). The thickened wall usually has a density similar to that of skeletal muscle. In cases of

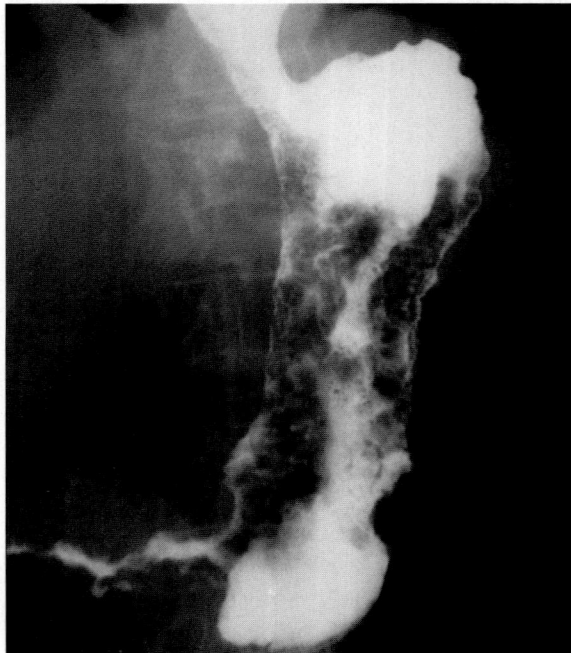

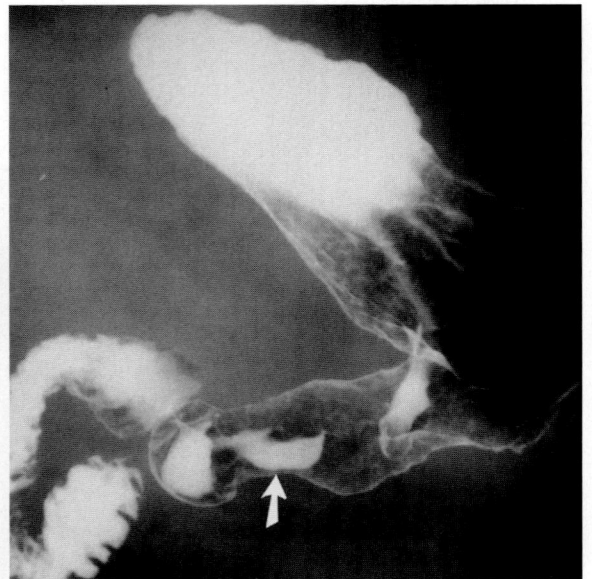

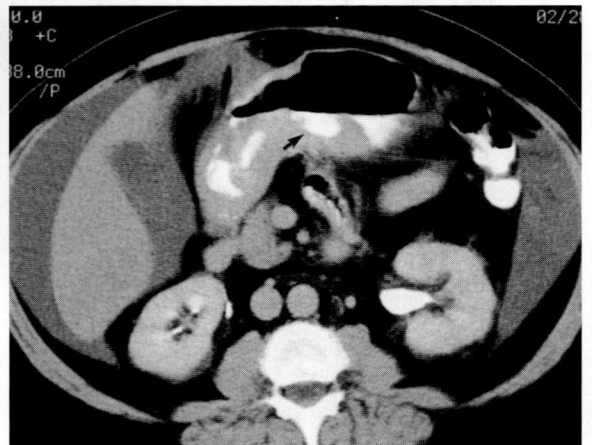

Fig. 6.26a–c. Advanced gastric cancer: scirrhous type – linitis plastica. **a** There is marked narrowing and rigidity of the gastric wall due to mural infiltration by tumor. **b, c** In this patient there is mural thickening with encasement of the gastric antrum associated with deep ulcerations (*arrows*) seen on both a double-contrast barium study and CT

mucin-producing adenocarcinomas, the tumor may contain stippled calcifications. Mural thickening in gastric cancer usually ranges between 6.0 mm and 4.0 cm (BOTET et al. 1991). The probability of transmural extension of tumor is directly correlated with mural thickness and is quite common when the wall is greater than 2 cm thick (GORE and GHAHREMANI 1994).

Scirrhous carcinomas may demonstrate significant contrast enhancement on dynamic CT scans (CHO et al. 1994). Infiltrating neoplasms can be recognized by the loss of the normal rugal fold pattern when the stomach is distended with a negative contrast agent. Polypoid gastric carcinomas present as soft tissue masses protruding into the lumen (GORE et al. 1994).

Carcinomas of the gastric cardia are notoriously difficult to appreciate on CT because of the soft tissue thickening often normally present at the gastroesophageal junction. Also, sliding hiatal hernias that are reduced beneath the diaphragm or that prolapse into the fundus may also simulate a mass in this region. Scanning the patient in the prone position following administration of an effervescent agent can help to differentiate a tumor from such a pseudolesion (GORE and GHAHREMANI 1994).

The primary role of CT in patients with gastric cancer is to assess the presence and extent of transmural or extragastric spread of tumor (Fig. 6.27), thereby assisting in the selection of surgical or conservative therapy (MILLER et al. 1997). If CT shows transmural extension with peritoneal tumor spread, or distant metastases, only palliative surgery or chemotherapy will be planned (TRENKNER et al. 1994). If the CT findings indicate a localized tumor, then staging laparotomy and curative surgery will be attempted (FUKUYA et al. 1995). Although initial reports were most optimistic about the preoperative CT staging of this neoplasm, more recent studies have been less sanguine (GORE and GHAHREMANI 1994).

When the gastric wall is infiltrated by tumor, the serosal contour becomes blurred and strand-like densities may be seen extending into the perigastric fat (HORI et al. 1992). Proximal gastric cancers may directly invade the adjacent esophagus via the gastrophrenic ligament, the left lobe of the liver via the gastrohepatic ligament, or reach the spleen via the gastrosplenic ligament. Distal gastric tumors can invade the neighboring duodenum, pancreas, and periaortic nodes via the inferior aspect of the lesser omentum – the hepatoduodenal ligament. The transverse colon can be invaded via the gastrocolic liga-

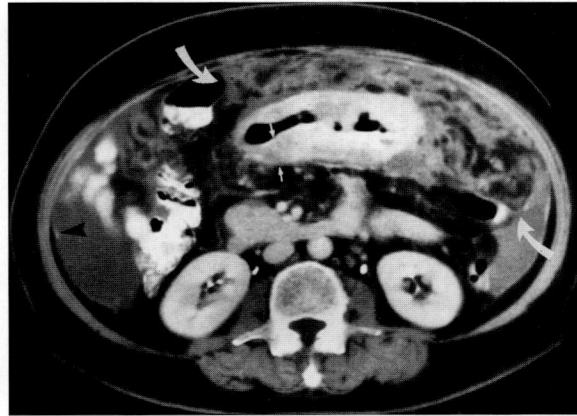

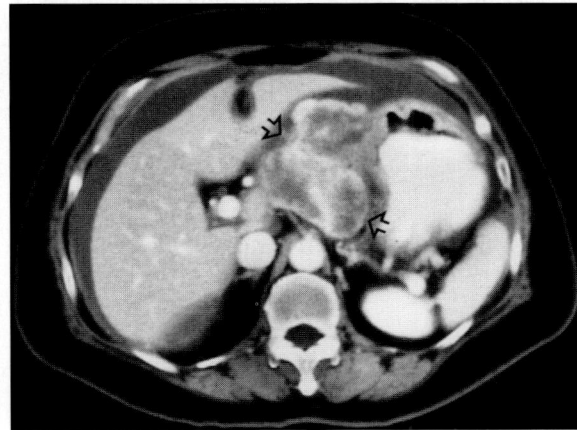

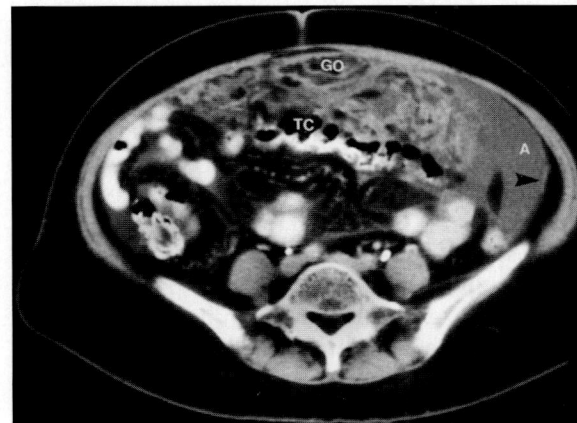

Fig. 6.27a–c. Disseminated gastric cancer: CT findings. **a** Mural thickening of the gastric antrum is present (*small arrows*). There is tumor spread to the gastrocolic ligament (*curved arrows*), ascites, and peritoneal implants (*arrowhead*). **b** The tumor has spread to the lymph nodes in the gastrohepatic ligament (*arrows*). **c** Tumor also involves the greater omentum (*GO*) and the transverse colon (*TC*). *A*, Ascites; *arrowhead*, peritoneal implant

ment, possibly resulting in colonic obstruction or gastrocolic fistula. Metastases to lymph nodes occur frequently in the gastrohepatic ligament (lesser omentum) and along the attachments of omental folds to the greater curvature. Carcinomatosis with diffuse peritoneal seeding and metastases to the ovaries or other pelvic organs are also well depicted on CT (LEVINE and MEGIBOW 1994b).

In one study comparing CT and surgical staging in 75 patients, 31% of gastric adenocarcinomas were understaged and 16% were overstaged by CT. False-negative results were primarily found in determining direct organ invasion, lymph node involvement, and peritoneal carcinomatosis. CT was 27% sensitive in predicting pancreatic invasion, and regional lymph node metastases were detected with a sensitivity of 67% and a specificity of 61% (SUSSMAN et al. 1988). Similar findings have been reported by other authors (MINAMI et al. 1992).

6.9
Other Gastric Malignancies

6.9.1
Lymphoma

Gastric lymphoma accounts for 50% of all gastrointestinal lymphomas, 25% of all extranodal lymphomas, and 3%–5% of all malignant neoplasms of the stomach. Lymphoma localized to the stomach and regional lymph nodes constitutes more than 50% of cases and is called primary gastric lymphoma. Secondary gastric lymphoma signifies gastric involvement in generalized lymphoma and is usually of the lymphocytic or histiocytic type. Gastric Hodgkin's disease is rare.

Most patients are in the sixth or seventh decade of life and there is a 1.5–2.0:1.0 male preponderance. Abdominal pain, nausea, vomiting, weight loss, anorexia, a palpable epigastric mass, and upper GI bleeding are the most common presenting clinical findings.

The specific radiological diagnosis of gastric lymphoma is seldom made because of its resemblance to gastric carcinoma. Abnormalities are seen in 90%–95% of cases on barium studies, however. Early gastric lymphoma is a lesion that is confined to the mucosa and submucosa and can occasionally be detected on double-contrast studies. It usually manifests as a depressed lesions showing irregular, shallow areas of ulceration accompanied by a nodular surrounding mucosa due to lymphomatous infiltra-

tion of the gastric wall (LEVINE and MEGIBOW 1994b). Early gastric lymphomas can occasionally present as small nodules, ulcerated submucosal masses, or enlarged rugal folds (SATO et al. 1986). Deep endoscopic biopsies are required for definitive diagnosis.

At the time of diagnosis, gastric lymphomas are usually advanced lesions with a mean diameter of 10 cm (LANZA 1995). Most cases involve the antrum and body although the entire stomach can be involved. Transpyloric spread of tumor into the duodenum occurs in some 30% of patients (CHO et al. 1996). Since gastric cancer invades the duodenum in only 5%–13% of patients, it has been argued that concomitant involvement of the stomach and duodenum by tumor should suggest lymphoma. Since adenocarcinoma is so much more common than lymphoma, it still is the most likely diagnosis on a statistical basis. In 10% of patients with gastric lymphoma, there is contiguous transcardiac spread of tumor from the gastric fundus into the distal esophagus (HRICAK 1980).

There are four gross pathologic types of gastric lymphoma and each has a radiologic correlate: infiltrative, ulcerative, polypoid, and nodular (FISCHBACK et al. 1992).

Infiltrative gastric lymphomas manifest as focal or diffuse enlargement of rugal folds (Fig. 6.28a) due to submucosal spread of tumor. The folds are often massively enlarged and have a distorted, nodular contour that can be confused for polypoid masses. Despite extensive lymphomatous infiltration, the stomach usually remains pliable and distensible without significant luminal narrowing (LEVINE and MEGIBOW 1994b).

One or more ulcerated lesions characterize *ulcerative* gastric lymphoma. These ulcers usually have an irregular configuration associated with nodularity of the surrounding mucosa or irregular, thickened folds due to lymphomatous infiltration of the gastric wall. Occasionally, the ulcers may be surrounded by a smooth mound of tumor or symmetric, radiating folds simulating the appearance of benign gastric ulcers. Uncommonly, gastric lymphomas present as giant cavitated lesions that result from tumor necrosis and excavation (LEVINE and MEGIBOW 1994b).

Polypoid gastric lymphomas are characterized by intraluminal masses that may simulate polypoid carcinomas. Multiple submucosal nodules ranging in size between several millimeters and several centimeters characterize the *nodular* form of gastric lymphoma (Fig. 6.28b).

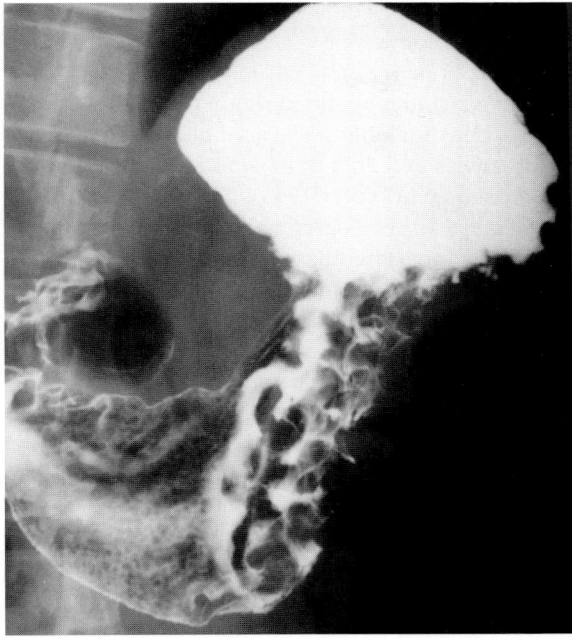

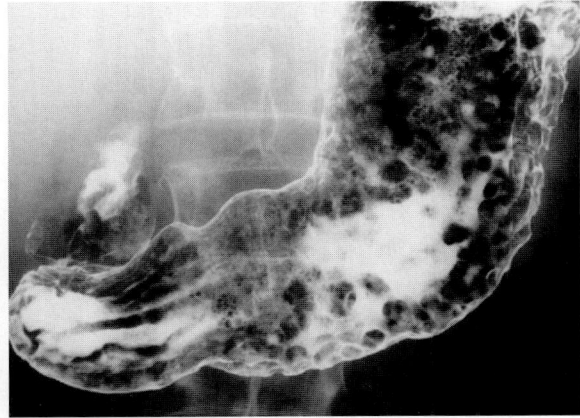

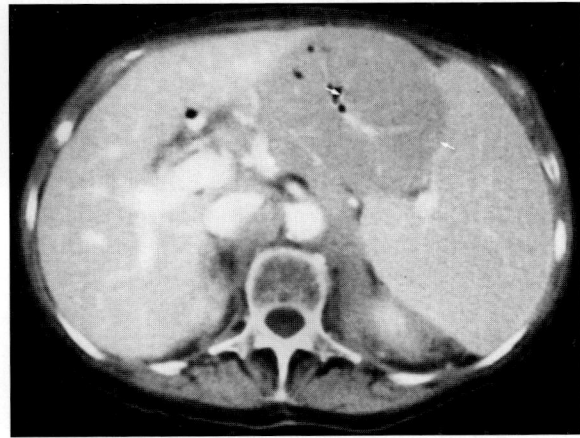

Fig. 6.28a–c. Gastric lymphoma. a There are diffusely thickened folds along the greater curvature of the body due to lymphomatous infiltration of the gastric wall. b Multiple polypoid masses are demonstrated in this patient with gastric lymphoma. c Massive mural thickening (4.2 cm) compresses the gastric lumen in this patient with histiocytic lymphoma (*arrows*). Note the splenomegaly and para-aortic adenopathy

Gastric lymphoma is usually histiocytic or lymphocytic (90%–95%) cell type, rather than Hodgkin's disease (5%–10%) (FISCHBACK et al. 1992). Patients with gastric lymphoma tend to be younger than those with adenocarcinoma and to have a more favorable prognosis. The lymphomatous process generally extends submucosally, producing thickening of the gastric wall and rugal fold pattern without mucosal abnormalities until ulceration occurs. Consequently barium studies may reveal only thickened folds and endoscopy with biopsy may be nondiagnostic due to the submucosal location of disease (LEVINE and MEGIBOW 1994b). Because CT can directly image the entire gastric wall and surrounding structures, it has proven very accurate in diagnosing and determining the extent of spread of gastric lymphoma (GORE et al. 1994).

Although the CT manifestations of gastric lymphoma and adenocarcinoma are similar, there are several differentiating features which can be

Table 6.3. Gastric lymphoma versus gastric adenocarcinoma: CT features (from THOENI and MASS 1992)

CT features	Lymphoma	Carcinoma
Mural thickness		
Mean	4.0 cm	1.8 cm
Range	1.1–7.7 cm	1.1–3.2 cm
Inhomogeneous wall	Uncommon	Common
Contour	Regular: 42%	Regular: 27%
	Irregular: 58%	Irregular: 73%
Extent	Diffuse: 83%	Focal: 91%
Direct spread to adjacent organs	42%	73%
Lymphadenopathy above and below level of renal hilum	42%	0

critical to patient management (Table 6.3). Mural thickening is quite prominent in lymphoma, with a mean thickness of 4–5 cm. It also tends to be more homogeneous, often involving the entire circumference of the stomach. The thickened folds have a club-like appearance as they project into the contrast-filled lumen. The outer contour of the gastric wall is usually smooth or lobulated in lymphoma and the perigastric fat plane is more likely to be completely preserved (GORE and GHAHREMANI 1994).

Three forms of gastric lymphoma have been described on CT: polypoid, infiltrating, and hypertrophic (THOENI and MOSS 1992). Any portion of the stomach can be involved and transpyloric spread of lymphoma into the duodenum is common. Diffuse gastric involvement is also more common in lymphoma than in adenocarcinoma. However, luminal narrowing is typically seen with carcinomas due to desmoplastic fibrosis and is seldom observed in patients with non-Hodgkin's lymphoma of the stomach (GORE et al. 1994).

Gastric lymphoma can extend directly into the spleen (via the gastrosplenic ligament), liver (via the gastrohepatic ligament), or colon (via the gastrocolic ligament), involve regional lymphnodes, or disseminate into the peritoneal cavity producing malignant ascites and omental masses. Although regional adenopathy is common in gastric cancer and lymphoma, adenopathy beneath the level of the renal veins without perigastric adenopathy may occur in lymphoma but is almost never seen in gastric adenocarcinoma. Adenopathy tends to be bulkier in lymphoma as well (CASTELLINO 1991).

6.9.2
Gastric Carcinoids

Gastric carcinoids have a spectrum of radiographic findings. Most patients present with one or more submucosal-appearing masses that range between 1 and 4 cm in size (LEVINE and MEGIBOW 1994b). If the central portion of the tumor becomes ulcerated it may have a "bull's-eye" appearance. Multiple gastric carcinoids must be differentiated from Kaposi's sarcoma, lymphoma, and metastases (BUCK and SOBIN 1990).

Gastric carcinoids may also present as one or more sessile or pedunculated polyps that are indistinguishable from hyperplastic or adenomatous polyps. Other patients may present with benign- or malignant-appearing gastric ulcers, which tend to be located on or near the lesser curvature. Advanced gastric carcinoid tumors may appear as polypoid intraluminal masses that simulate gastric carcinomas (BALTHAZAR et al. 1982).

6.9.3
Leiomyosarcoma

Leiomyosarcomas are uncommon gastric neoplasms that account for only 1%–3% of all primary gastric malignancies and 20% of all smooth muscle tumors of the stomach (DAVIS 1993). The majority of gastrointestinal leiomyosarcomas arise in the stomach. Gastric leiomyosarcomas involve the fundus and body in 90% of cases and the remaining 10% involve the antrum (LANZA 1995). These tumors can become quite large and it is difficult to accurately assess their size by endoscopy and barium studies since a major portion of the tumor may extend into the peritoneal cavity. CT is useful in this regard. Histologically, leiomyosarcomas can be difficult to differentiate from leiomyomas. As a rule, malignancy correlates with size; tumors large than 6 cm are almost always malignant; lesions smaller than 4 cm are usually benign (LANZA 1995).

Most patients present with gastrointestinal hemorrhage and less commonly anorexia, weight loss, pain, nausea, and vomiting.

Double-contrast barium studies are abnormal in more than 90% of patients with leiomyosarcomas: 50% are intramural lesions, 35% are exogastric lesions, and 15% are endogastric in location (LEVINE and MEGIBOW 1994b). Intramural lesions appear as large, lobulated submucosal masses in the gastric fundus or body. Exogastric tumors may present as giant soft tissue masses that cause extrinsic compression of the adjacent gastric wall (Fig. 6.29a). These exogastric lesions characteristically produce a central dimple or spicule at the site of attachment or pedicle of the mass.

The CT findings of gastric leiomyosarcomas are quite distinctive and usually can be distinguished from those of adenocarcinoma and lymphoma (SCATARIGE et al. 1985). The primary tumor is large and may be spherical or ellipsoid in shape. Deep ulceration (Fig. 6.29b), cavitation, and air-fluid levels may be present within the mass. There is no adjacent mural thickening, although attachment of the mass to the gastric wall may be visualized. If this connection is not visualized it may be difficult to identify the organ of origin of the tumor mass (McLEOD et al. 1984).

On contrast-enhanced helical CT scans, leiomyosarcomas often have a heterogeneous appearance with prominent low-density areas that represent extensive tumor necrosis. This finding is usually helpful in differentiating leiomyosarcomas from lymphoma,

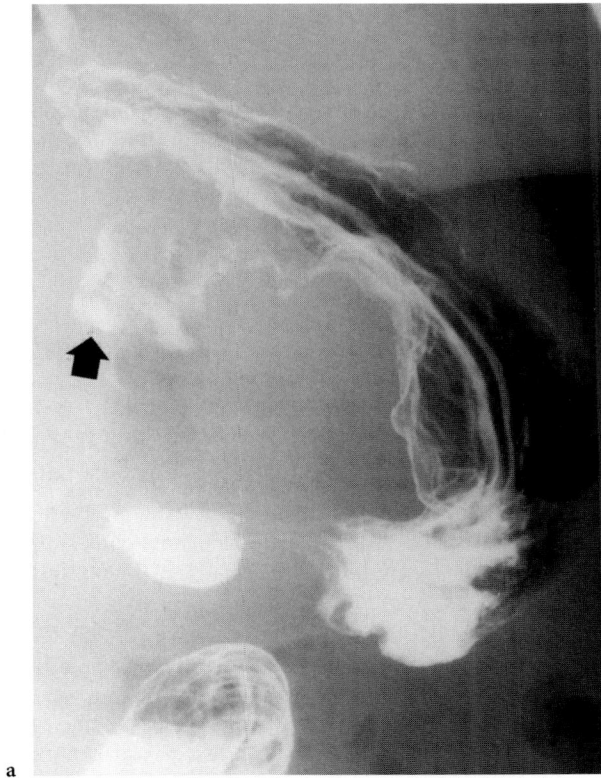

a

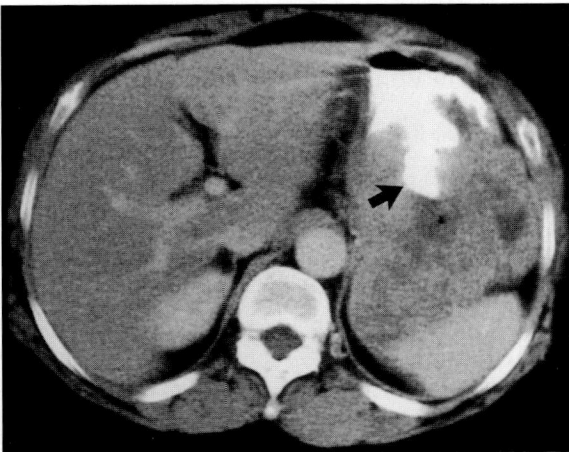

b

Fig. 6.29a,b. Leiomyosarcoma. CT-GI correlation. **a** Spot film from a double-contrast barium study of the stomach shows a large ulcerating (*arrow*) mass along the posterior aspect of the stomach. **b** CT documents a large, inhomogeneous, ulcerating (*arrow*) mass filling the left upper quadrant

because the latter tumor tends to have a more homogeneous appearance (GORE et al. 1994).

Computed tomography may demonstrate metastases to the liver, peritoneal cavity, and adjacent organs in advanced disease.

6.9.4
Kaposi's Sarcoma

Kaposi's sarcoma is a vascular endothelial tumor that develops in approximately 35% of patients with AIDS (YEE and WALL 1995). Cutaneous involvement is most common; the gastrointestinal tract is affected in nearly 50% of cases. The GI lesions, for reasons that are unclear, develop in homosexual men rather than intravenous drug abusers or transfusion recipients.

On double-contrast barium studies, Kaposi's sarcoma lesions manifest as one or more submucosal masses, ranging from 0.5 to 3.0 cm in size (LEVINE and MEGIBOW 1994b). As these masses enlarge, they often undergo central necrosis and ulceration producing a "bull's-eye" or "target" appearance (Fig. 6.30). Other radiologic presentations include thickened, nodular folds or polypoid gastric masses, and an infiltrative pattern indistinguishable from that of a primary scirrhous carcinoma (YEE and WALL 1995). Since these appearances are nonspecific, a CT can be helpful in detecting retroperitoneal adenopathy, splenomegaly, or other evidence of abdominal Kaposi's sarcoma.

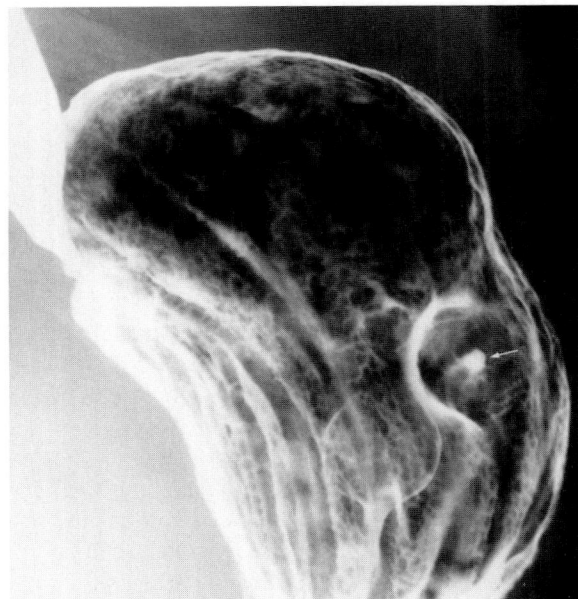

Fig. 6.30. Kaposi's sarcoma. Two submucosal masses are present in the proximal stomach in this patient with AIDS. One of the lesions has undergone central ulceration (*arrow*) producing a "bull's-eye" appearance

6.9.5
Gastric Metastases

Metastatic disease to the stomach is occurring with greater frequency as patients with disseminated tumors are living longer. Nearly 10% of patients who die from carcinoma of the breast and lung and from malignant melanoma (Fig. 6.31) have gastric involvement at autopsy (DAVIS 1993). The majority of lesions are hematogenous metastasis. Less frequent forms of metastases include: lymphatic spread; tumor spread by direct extension from neighboring structures or mesenteric reflections such as the gastrocolic ligament, transverse mesocolon, or greater omentum; and tumor seeding secondary to carcinomatosis (GLICK et al. 1986).

Radiologically, hematogenous metastases appear as one or more discrete submucosal masses (LEVINE and MEGIBOW 1994b). When there are multiple lesions, they tend to be of varying size because of periodic showers of tumor emboli into the arterial blood supply of the stomach. These submucosal masses may undergo central ulceration and necrosis as they outgrow their blood supply, producing "bull's-eye" or "target" lesions. Hematogenous metastases from breast carcinoma occasionally can produce a linitis plastica appearance indistinguishable from a primary scirrhous carcinoma (FECZKO et al. 1993).

6.10
Structural Abnormalities

6.10.1
Pancreatic Rest

Ectopic pancreatic rests occur throughout the gut, but most commonly occur within the stomach. These small, usually asymptomatic lesions consist of all pancreatic elements including acini, ducts, and islet cells (LANZA 1995).

Radiologically, they are almost always solitary lesions ranging in size from 1 to 3 cm. They usually appear as smooth, broad-based, submucosal masses on the greater curvature of the antrum, 1–6 cm from the pyloric channel (Fig. 6.32). In approximately 50% of patients, a central dimple or umbilication is visualized, representing the orifice of a primitive ductal system. This orifice varies from 1 to 5 mm in diameter and 5 to 10 mm in depth (LEVINE 1994d).

6.10.2
Gastric Diverticulum

Gastric diverticula arise in two different locations. *True gastric diverticula* are the most common form and occur just below the gastroesophageal junction on the posterior aspect of the lesser curvature (Fig. 6.33). These diverticula, which contain all gastric layers including muscularis propria, are usually asymptomatic. Rarely they can become quite large, impair emptying, and stasis may result. Diagnosis is seldom difficult since the stream of barium leaving the esophagus tends to flow across the entrance of the diverticulum, filling it with barium. Fundal diverticula range in size from 1 to 10 cm and are believed to be congenital (HERRERA and SEEDOR 1995).

Antral diverticulum is a rare anomaly characterized by focal invagination of the mucosa into the muscularis propria of the gastric wall. They occur along the greature curvature of the distal antrum and are rarely more than a few millimeters in diameter.

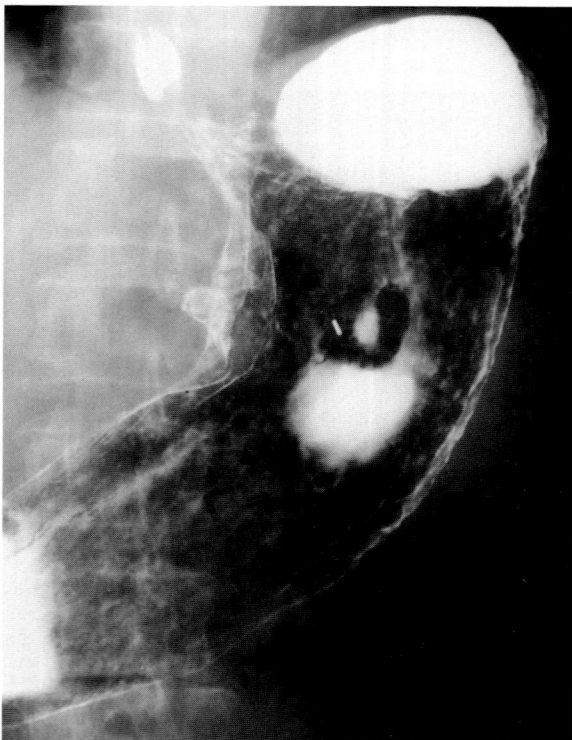

Fig. 6.31. Gastric metastases from malignant melanoma. Two large ulcerated masses are identified on this double-contrast study

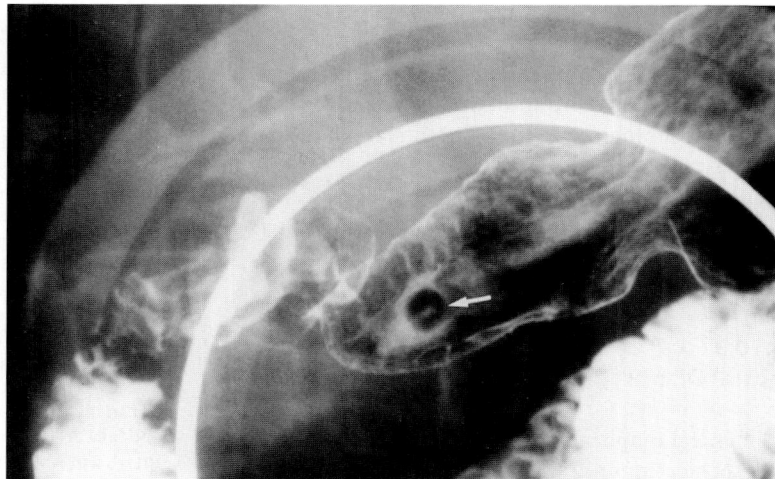

Fig. 6.32. Ectopic pancreatic rest. A submucosal mass (*arrow*) is present in the distal gastric antrum. The central umbilication or dimple represents the orifice of a primitive ductal system

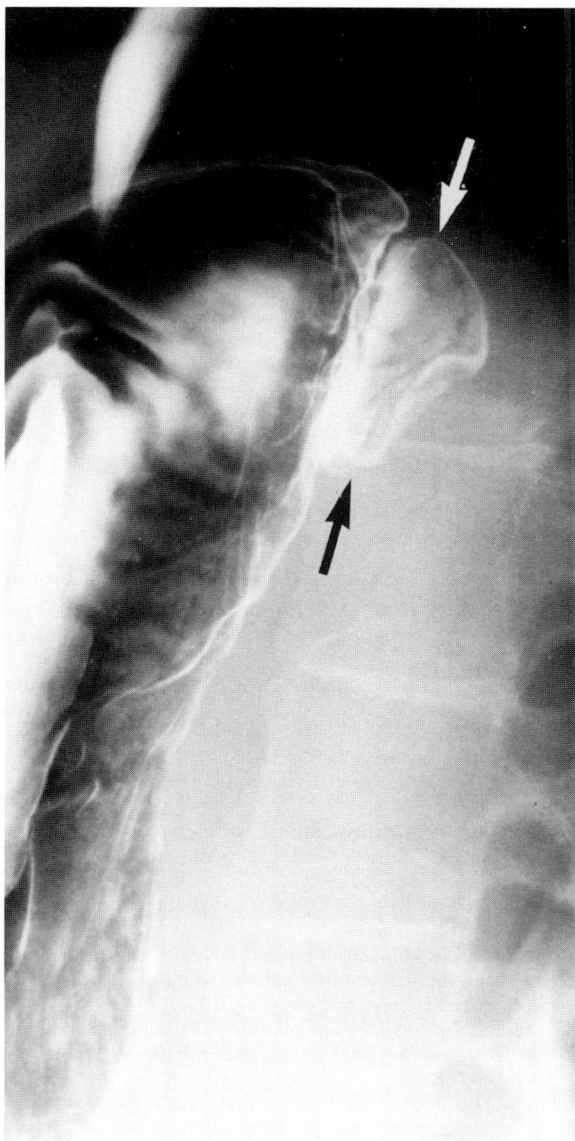

Fig. 6.33. Gastric diverticulum. A large diverticulum (*arrows*) is seen arising from the posterior wall of the fundus

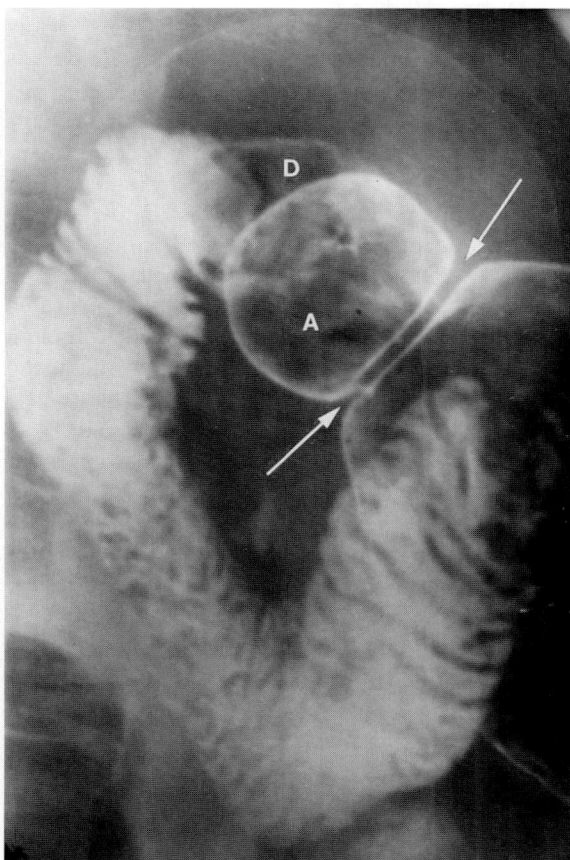

Fig. 6.34. Antral diaphragm. A symmetric annular mucosal ·ring (*arrows*) is seen on this double-contrast view of the gastric antrum. The distal antrum (*A*) together with the duodenal bulb (*D*) produce the characteristic "double-bulb" appearance

Being intramural, they do not significantly protrude from the normal contour of the stomach (EISENBERG 1994). Radiologically, their lenticular shape simulates a collar button ulcer and they are often misdiagnosed as a small greature curvature ulcer or an ectopic pancreatic rest (HERRERA and SEEDOR 1995).

6.10.3
Antral Diaphragm

The antral diaphragm or ring is a thin mucosal septum projecting into the gastric lumen perpendicular to its long axis. It is usually 2–4 mm in thickness and located 1.5–7 cm proximal to the pylorus. Histologically, these rings are composed of two layers of normal gastric mucosa covering a common muscularis mucosae and submucosa (EISENBERG 1994).

Radiographically, an antral diaphragm presents as a persistent, symmetric annular structure dividing the antrum (Fig. 6.34). The antral chamber distal to the ring may resemble the duodenal bulb itself, producing a "double bulb" configuration (GHAHREMANI 1973). As with esophageal mucosal rings, the antral diaphragm is best demonstrated when the lumen is maximally distended. Although most antral rings are asymptomatic and incidental findings, those with a small aperture can cause gastric outlet obstruction.

References

Balthazar EJ, Rosenberg H, Davidian MM (1980) Scirrhous carcinoma of the pyloric channel and distal antrum. AJR 134:669–673

Balthazar EJ, Megibow A, Bryk D, Cohen T (1982) Gastric carcinoid: radiographic features in eight cases. AJR 139:1123–1127

Bartram CJ, Kumar P (1981) Clinical radiology in gastroenterology. Blackwell, Oxford, pp 70–85

Bloom SM, Paul RE, Matsue H (1977) Improved radiologic detection of multiple gastric ulcers. AJR 128:949–952

Boland CR, Scheiman JM (1995) Tumors of the stomach. In: Yamada T (ed) Textbook of gastroenterology, 2nd edn. Lippincott, Philadelphia, pp 1494–1522

Botet JF, Lightdale CJ, Zauber AG (1991) Preoperative staging of gastric cancer: comparison of endoscopic, US, and dynamic CT. Radiology 181:426–432

Brandt D, Muramatsu Y, Ushio K (1989) Synchronous early gastric cancer. Radiology 173:649–652

Buck JL, Pantongrag-Brown L (1994) Gastritides, gastropathies, and polyps unique to the stomach. Radiol Clin North Am 32:1215–1231

Buck JL, Sobin LH (1990) Carcinoids of the gastrointestinal tract. Radiographics 10:1081–1095

Carlson HC, Breen JF (1986) Amyloidosis and plasma cell dyscrasias: gastrointestinal involvement. Semin Roentgenol 21:128–138

Castellino RA (1991) The non-Hodgkin lymphomas: practical concepts for the diagnostic radiologist. Radiology 178:315–321

Cello JP (1995) Helicobacter pylori and peptic ulcer disease. AJR 164:283–286

Cho J, Kim J, Rho S (1994) Preoperative assessment of gastric carcinoma value of the two-phase dynamic CT and mechanical IV injection of contrast material. AJR 163:69–75

Cho KC, Gold BM, Printz DA (1987) Multiple transverse folds in the gastric anturm. Radiology 164:339–341

Cho KC, Baker SR, Alterman DD, Fusco JM, Cho S (1996) Transpyloric spread of gastric tumor: comparison of adenocarcinoma and lymphoma. AJR 167:467–469

Choi BI, Ok ID, Im J (1988) Exogastric cystic leiomyoblastoma with unusual CT appearance. Gastrointest Radiol 13:109–111

Craanen ME, Dekker W, Ferwerda J (1991) Early gastric cancer: a clinicopathologic study. J Clin Gastroenterol 13:274–283

Dagradi AE, Falkner RE, Lee ER (1975) Multiple gastric ulcers: a radiographic sign of benignity? Radiology 114:23–27

Davis GR (1993) Neoplasms of the stomach. In: Sleisenger MH, Fordtran JS (eds) Gastrointestinal disease, 5th edn. Saunders, Philadelphia, pp 763–792

Dekker W, Op den Orth JO (1988) Biphasic radiologic examination and endoscopy of the upper gastrointestinal tract: a comparative study. J Clin Gastroenterol 10:461–465

Dupont GJ, Cohn I (1980) Gastric adenocarcinoma. Curr Probl Cancer 4:15–30

Eisenberg RL (1994) Miscellaneous abnormalities. In: Gore RM, Levine MS, Laufer I (eds) Textbook of gastrointestinal radiology. Saunders, Philadelphia, pp 717–741

Eisenberg RL (1996) Gastric ulcers. In: Eisenberg RL (ed) Gastrointestinal radiology: a pattern approach, 3rd edn. Lippincott-Raven, Philadelphia, pp 181–207

Elder JB (1995) Carcinoma of the stomach. In: Haubrich WS, Schaffner F (eds) Bockus gastroenterology, 5th edn. Saunders, Philadelphia, pp 854–874

Eolgadren HC, Carpenter HA, Talley NJ (1993) Ménétrier disease: a form of hypertrophic gastropathy or gastritis? Gastroenterology 104:1310–1319

Feczko PJ, Halpert RD, Ackerman LV (1985) Gastric polyps: radiological evaluation and clinical significance. Radiology 155:581–584

Feczko PJ, Collins DD, Mezwa DG (1993) Metastatic disease involving the gastrointestinal tract. Radiol Clin North Am 31:1359–1373

Fischback W, Kestel W, Kirchner DH (1992) Malignant lymphoma of the gastrointestinal tract. Cancer 70:1075–1082

Freeny PC (1979) Double-contrast gastrography of the fundus and cardia: normal landmarks and their pathologic changes. AJR 133:481–487

Fuchs CS, Mayer RJ (1995) Gastric carcinoma. N Engl J Med 333:32–41

Fukuya T, Hiroshi H, Nayashi T (1995) Lymph node metastases: efficacy of detection with helical CT in patients with gastric cancer. Radiology 197:705–711

Furth EE, Rubesin SE, Levine MS (1995) Pathologic primer on gastritis: an illustrated sum and substance. Radiology 197:693–698

Gelfand DW (1984) Gastrointestinal radiology. Churchill-Livingstone, New York, pp 195–240

Gelfand DW (1994) Barium studies: single contrast. In: Gore RM, Levine MS, Laufer I (eds) Textbook of gastrointestinal radiology. Saunders, Philadelphia, pp 81–92

Gelfand DW, Ott DJ (1981) Gastric ulcer scars. Radiology 140: 37–43

Gelfand DW, Chen YM, Ott DJ (1987) Multiphasic examinations of the stomach: efficacy of individual techniques in detecting 153 lesions. Radiology 162:829–834

Ghahremani GG (1973) Nonobstructive mucosal diaphragnis or rings of the gastric antrum in adults. AJR 121:236–247

Ginsberg GG, Al-Kawas FH, Fleischer DE, et al. (1996) Gastric polyps: relationship of size and histology to cancer risk. Am J Gastroenterol 91:714–717

Glick SN, Teplick JK, Levine MS, et al. (1986) Gastric cardia metastasis in esophageal carcinoma. Radiology 160:627–630

Glick SN, Teplick SK, Amenta PS (1990) Giant hyperplastic polyps of the gastric remnant simulating carcinoma. Gastrointest Radiol 15:151–155

Gold RP, Green PH, O'Toole KM (1984) Early gastric cancer: radiographic experience. Radiology 152:283–290

Gore RM, Ghahremani GG (1986) Crohn's disease of the upper gastrointestinal tract. Crit Rev Diagn Imaging 25:305–331

Gore RM, Ghahremani GG (1994) CT evaluation of the stomach. In: Fishman EK, Federle MP (eds) Body CT categorical course syllabus. American Roentgen Ray Society, Reston, Va. pp 131–140

Gore RM, Lichtenstein JE (1994) The gastrointestinal tract: anatomic-pathologic basis of radiologic findings. In: Taveras JM, Ferrucci JT (eds) Radiology – diagnosis – imaging – intervention. Lippincott, Philadelphia, chapter 4, pp 1–42

Gore RM, White EM, Ghahremani GG (1994) CT evaluation of the stomach: current status. Radiologist 1:345–356

Gore RM, Ghahremani GG, Miller FH (1995) Mucosal features of the alimentary tract on double-contrast barium studies. Radiologist 2:283–296

Gross Fisher S, Davis F, Nelson R (1993) A cohort study of stomach cancer risk in men after gastric surgery for benign disease. J Natl Cancer Inst 85:1303–1320

Halpert RD, Goodman P (1993) Gastrointestinal radiology – the requisites. Mosby, St. Louis, pp 33–82

Halvorsen RA, Illescas FF (1988) Gastric adenocarcinomas: CT versus surgical staging. Radiology 135:309–312

Han SY, Witten DM (1974) Benign gastric ulcer with crescent (quarter moon) sign. Radiology 113:573–575

Hansson L-E, Jerre R, Saunders SM, et al. (1996) The risk of adenocarcinoma of the stomach in patients with gastric or duodenal ulcer disease. N Engl J Med 335:242–249

Haruma K, Suzuki T, Tsuda T (1991) Evaluation of tumor growth rate in patients with early gastric carcinoma of the elevated type. Gastrointest Radiol 16:289–292

Heatly RV, Wyatt JI (1995) Gastritis and duodenitis. In: Haubrich WS, Schaffner F (eds) Bockus gastroenterology, 5th edn. Saunders, Philadelphia, pp 1410–1427

Heiken JP, Forde KA, Gold RP (1982) Computed tomography as a definitive method for diagnosing gastrointestinal lipomas. Radiology 142:409–414

Herlinger H, Grossman R, Laufer I (1980) The gastric cardia in double-contrast study: its dynamic image. AJR 135:21–29

Herrera AF, Seedor JW (1995) Diverticula of the stomach and duodenum. In: Haubrich WS, Schaffner F (eds) Bockus gastroenterology, 5th edn. Saunders, Philadelphia, pp 805–815

Hizawa K, Iida M, Matsumoto T, Aoyagi K, Yao T, Fujishima M (1993) Natural history of fundic gland polyposis without familial adenomatous coli; follow-up observation in 31 patients. Radiology 189:429–432

Hori S, Tsuda K, Murayama S (1992) CT of gastric carcinoma: preliminary results with a new scanning technique. Radiographics 12:257–268

Hricak H, Thoeni RF, Margulis AR (1980) Extension of gastric lymphoma into the esophagus and duodenum. Radiology 135:309–312

Hsing AW, Hansson LE, McLaughlin JK (1993) Pernicious anemia and subsequent cancer: a population-based cohort study. Cancer 71:745–750

Iida M, Tao T, Itoh H (1985) Natural history of fundic gland polyposis in patients with familial adenomatosis coli/Gardner's syndrome. Gastroenterology 89:1021–1025

Kagan RA, Steckel RJ (1977) Gastric ulcer in a young man with apparent healing. AJR 128:831–834

Kawaguchi H, Kogure T, Okuyama Y, et al. (1996) *Helicobacter pylori* infection is the major risk factor for atrophic gastritis. Am J Gastroenterol 91:959–963

Keller RJ, Wolf BS, Khilnani MT (1970) Roentgen features of healing and healed benign gastric ulcers. Radiology 97: 353–359

Kikuchi Y, Levine MS, Laufer I (1986) Value of flow technique for double-contrast examination of the stomach. AJR 147:1183–1184

Kirklin BR (1934) The value of the meniscus sign in the roentgenologic diagnosis of ulcerating gastric carcinoma. Radiology 22:131–135

Kodera Y, Yamamura Y, Torii A (1996) Gastric remnant carcinoma after partial gastrectomy for benign and malignant gastric lesions. J Am Coll Surg 182:1–6

Koga M, Nakata H, Kiyonari H (1982) Radiologic diagnosis of early gastric cancer by routine double-contrast examination. Gastrointest Radiol 7:205–215

Kottler RE, Tuft RJ (1981) Benign greater curve gastric ulcer: the "sump-ulcer". Br J Radiol 54:651–654

Lam SK, Hui WM, Ching CK (1995) Peptic ulcer disease: epidemiology, pathogenesis, and etiology. In: Haubrich WS, Schaffner F (eds) Bockus gastroenterology, 5th edn. Saunders, Philadelphia, pp 700–749

Lanza FL (1995) Benign and malignant tumors of the stomach other than carcinoma. In: Haubrich WS, Schaffner F (eds) Bockus gastroenterology, 5th edn. Saunders, Philadelphia, pp 841–858

Laufer I (1994a) Barium studies: upper gastrointestinal tract. In: Gore RM, Levine MS, Laufer I (eds) Textbook of gastrointestinal radiology. Saunders, Philadelphia, pp 292–303

Laufer I (1994b) Barium studies: principles of double-contrast diagnosis. In: Gore RM, Levine MS, Laufer I (eds) Textbook of gastrointestinal radiology. Saunders, Philadelphia, pp 38–49

Laufer I, Kressel HY (1992) Principles of double-contrast diagnosis. In: Laufer I, Levine MS (eds) Double contrast gastrointestinal radiology, 2nd edn. Saunders, Philadelphia, pp 9–54

Laveran-Stiebar RL, Laufer I, Levine MS (1994) Greater curvature antral flattening: a radiologic sign of NSAID-related gastropathy. Abdom Imaging 19:295–297

Levine MS (1994a) Erosive gastritis and gastric ulcers. Radiol Clin North Am 32:1203–1214

Levine MS (1994b) Peptic ulcers. In: Gore RM, Levine MS, Laufer I (eds) Textbook of gastrointestinal radiology. Saunders, Philadelphia, pp 562–597

Levine MS (1994c) Inflammatory conditions. In: Gore RM, Levine MS, Laufer I (eds) Textbook of gastrointestinal radiology. Saunders, Philadelphia, pp 598–627

Levine MS (1994d) Benign tumors. In: Gore RM, Levine MS, Laufer I (eds) Textbook of gastrointestinal radiology. Saunders, Philadelphia, pp 628–659

Levine MS (1995) Role of double-contrast upper gastrointestinal series in the 1990s. Gastroenterol Clin North Am 24:289–308

Levine MS, Laufer I (1993) The upper gastrointestinal series at a crossroads. AJR 161:1131–1134

Levine MS, Megibow AJ (1994a) Carcinoma. In: Gore RM, Levine MS, Laufer I (eds) Textbook of gastrointestinal radiology. Saunders, Philadelphia, pp 660–683

Levine MS, Megibow AJ (1994b) Other malignant tumors. In: Gore RM, Levine MS, Laufer I (eds) Textbook of gastrointestinal radiology. Saunders, Philadelphia, pp 684–716

Levine MS, Rubesin SE (1995) The *Helicobacter pylori* revolution: radiologic perspective. Radiology 195:593–596

Levine MS, Laufer I, Thompson JJ (1983) Carcinoma of the gastric cardia in young people. AJR 140:69–72

Levine MS, Verstandig A, Laufer I (1986) Serpiginous gastric erosions caused by aspirin and other nonsteroidal anti-inflammatory drugs. AJR 146:31–34

Levine MS, Creteur V, Kressel HY (1987) Benign gastric ulcers: diagnosis and follow-up with double-contrast radiography. Radiology 164:9–13

Levine MS, Rubesin SE, Herlinger H, Laufer I, et al. (1988) Double-contrast upper gastrointestinal examination: technique and interpretation. Radiology 168:593–602

Levine MS, Kong V, Rubesin SE, et al. (1990a) Scirrhous carcinoma of the stomach: radiologic and endoscopic diagnosis. Radiology 175:151–154

Levine MS, Palman CL, Rubesin SE (1990b) Atrophic gastritis in pernicious anemia: diagnosis by double-contrast radiography. Gastrointest Radiol 14:215–219

Levine MS, Kelly MR, Laufer I, Rubesin SE, Herlinger H (1993) Gastrocolic fistulas: the increasing role of aspirin. Radiology 187:359–361

Levine MS, Elmas N, Furth EE, Rubesin SE, Goldwein MI (1996) *Helicobacter pylori* and gastric MALT lymphoma. AJR 166:85–86

Lichtenstein JE (1993) Inflammatory conditions of the stomach and duodenum. Radiol Clin North Am 31:1359–1373

Low VHS, Levine MS, Rubesin SE, Laufer I (1994) Diagnosis of gastric carcinoma: sensitivity of double-contrast barium studies. AJR 162:329–334

MacCarty RL, Talley NJ (1990) Barium studies in diffuse eosinophilic gastroenteritis. Gastrointest Radiol 15:183–187

Marcial MA, Villaña M, Hernandez-Denton J, Colon-Pagan JR (1993) Fundic gland polyps: prevalence and clinicopathologic features. Am J Gastroenterol 88:1711–1713

Marshall BJ (1994) *Helicobacter pylori*. Am J Gastroenterol 89:5116–5128

Maruyama M (1992) Early diagnosis of gastrointestinal cancer. In: Laufer I, Levine MS (eds) Double contrast radiology, 2nd edn. Saunders, Philadelphia, pp 495–532

Maruyama M, Baba Y (1994) Gastric carcinoma. Radiol Clin North Am 32:1233–1252

Maruyama M, Hamada T (1994) Diagnosis of gastric cancer in Japan. In: Freeny PC, Stevenson GW (eds) Alimentary tract radiology, 5th edn. Mosby, St. Louis, pp 399–428

McGuigan JE (1993) Zollinger-Ellison syndrome and other hypersecretory states. In: Sleisenger MH, Fordtran JS (eds) Gastrointestinal disease, 5th edn. Saunders, Philadelphia, pp 679–697

McIntosh CE, Kreel L (1977) Anatomy and radiology of the areae gatricae. Gut 18:855–864

McLeod AJ, Zornoza J, Shirkhoda A (1984) Leiomyosarcoma: computed tomography findings. Radiology 152:133–136

Megibow AJ, Balthazar EJ, Hulnick DH, et al. (1985) CT evaluation of gastrointestinal leiomyomas and leiomyosarcomas. AJR 144:727–731

Menke DM, Kyle RA, Fleming CR, Wolfe JT, Kurtin PJ, Oldenburg WA (1993) Symptomatic gastric amyloidosis in patients with primary systemic amyloidosis. Mayo Clin Proc 68:763–767

Miller FH, Kochman ML, Talamonti MS, Ghahremani GG, Gore RM (1997) Gastric cancer: rediologic staging. Radiol Clin North Am 35:241–260

Minami M, Maeda H, Karauchi S (1992) Gastric tumors: radiologic-pathologic correlation and accuracy of T staging with dynamic CT. Radiology 185:173–175

Ming SC (1976) Malignant potential of gastric polyps. Gastrointest Radiol 1:121–125

Montesi A, Graziani L, Pesaresi A (1982) Radiologic diagnosis of early gastric cancer by routine double-contrast examination. Gastrointest Radiol 7:205–215

Muhletaler CA, Gerlock AJ, deSoto L, et al. (1980) Gastroduodenal lesions of ingested acids: radiographic findings. AJR 135:1247–1252

Nahrwold DL (1996) Gastric resection and reconstruction. In: Zuidema GD (ed) Shackelford's surgery of the alimentary tract, 4th edn. Saunders, Philadelphia, pp 152–165

Nelson SW (1969) The discovery of gastric ulcers and the differential diagnosis between benignancy and malignancy. Radiol Clin North Am 7:5–25

Ohman U, Emas S, Rubio C (1980) Relation between early and advanced gastric cancer. Am J Surg 140:351–355

Orlowska J, Jarosz D, Pachlewski J, Butruk E (1995) Malignant transformation of benign epithelial gastric polyps. Am J Gastroenterol 90:2152–2159

Ott DJ, Gelfand DW, Wu WC (1982) Detection of gastric ulcer: comparison of single- and double-examination. AJR 139:93–97

Parker SL, Tong T, Bolden S (1996) Cancer statistics, 1996. CA Cancer J Clin 46:5–27

Parsonnet J, Mendenhall WM, Stringer SP, et al. (1994) *Helicobacter pylori* infection and gastric lymphoma. N Engl J Med 330:1267–1271

Raskin MM (1976) Some specific radiological findings and considerations of linitis plastica of the gastrointestinal tract. Crit Rev Diagn Imaging 8:87–105

Rubesin SE, Herlinger H (1986) The effect of barium suspension viscosity on the delineation of areae gastricae. AJR 138:35–38

Salvon-Harman JC, Cady B, Nikulasson S (1995) Shifting proportions of gastric adenocarcinomas. Arch Surg 129:381–389

Sato T, Sakai Y, Ishiguro S (1986) Radiologic manifestations of early gastric lymphoma. AJR 146:513–517

Scatarige JA, Fishman EK, Jones B (1985) Gastric leiomyosarcoma: CT observations. J Comput Assist Tomogr 9:320–327

Simpkins KC, Gore RM (1994) Crohn's disease. In: Gore RM, Levine MS, Laufer I (eds) Textbook of gastrointestinal radiology. Saunders, Philadelphia, pp 2660–2682

Sohn J, Levine MS, Furth EE, et al. (1995) *Helicobacter pylori* gastritis: radiographic findings. Radiology 195:763–767

Soll AH (1996) Medical treatment of peptic ulcer disease. JAMA 275:622–629

Strandjord NM, Mosely RD, Schweinefus RL (1960) Gastric carcinoma: accuracy of radiologic diagnosis. Radiology 74:442–452

Sugawa C, Lucas CE (1989) Caustic injury of the upper gastrointestinal tract in adults: a clinical and endoscopic study. Surgery 106:802–807

Sussman SK, Halvorsen RA, Illescas FF, et al. (1988) Gastric adenocarcinoma: CT versus surgical staging. Radiology 167: 335–341

Tada S, Iida M, Yao T (1994) Gastrointestinal amyloidosis: radiologic features by chemical types. Radiology 190:37–42

Thoeni RF, Moss AA (1992) The gastrointestinal tract. In: Moss AA, Gamsu G, Genant HK (eds) Computed tomography of the body. Saunders, Philadelpia, pp 643–734

Thompson G, Somers S, Stevenson GW (1983) Benign gastric ulcer: a reliable radiologic diagnosis? AJR 141:331–333

Trenkner SW, Halvorsen RA, Thompson WM (1994) Neoplasms of the upper gastrointestinal tract. Radiol Clin North Am 32:1524

Vitellas KM, Bennett WF, Bova JG, Johnson JC, Greenson JK, Caldwell JH (1995) Radiographic manifestations of eosinophilic gastroenteritis. Abdom Imaging 20:406–413

Weinstein WM (1993) Gastritis and gastropathies. In: Sleisenger MH, Fordtran JS (eds) Gastrointestinal disease, 5th edn. Saunders, Philadelphia, pp 545–571

White RM, Levine MS, Enterline HT, Laufer I, Rubesin S, Herlinger H (1985) Early gastric cancer: recent experience. Radiology 155:25–27

Wolf BS (1971) Observations on roentgen features of benign and malignant ulcers. Semin Roentgenol 6:140–150

Yee J, Wall SD (1995) Gastrointestinal manifestations of AIDS. Gastroenterol Clin North Am 24:413–434

Zboralske FF, Stargardter FL, Harell GS (1978) Profile roentgenographic features of benign greater curvature ulcers. Radiology 127:63–67

7 Advances in Enteroclysis

J.C. Lappas and D.D.T. Maglinte

CONTENTS

7.1
Introduction

Diagnostic radiologists currently assume the primary responsibility for the imaging evaluation of the small bowel. While the modalities of ultrasonography, computed tomography, and magnetic resonance imaging are utilized to provide unique information, their role in small bowel evaluation remains complementary to the primary demonstration of small bowel details by barium contrast studies.

In medical centers particularly throughout Europe, the conventional barium methods for small bowel examination have been largely replaced by the enteroclysis procedure. This practice owes much to the work of Sellink and Miller (1982) and later

J.C. Lappas, MD, Professor of Radiology, Indiana University School of Medicine, Wishard Memorial Hospital, 1001 West Tenth Street, Indianapolis, IN 46202, USA
D.D.T. Maglinte, MD, FACR, Clinical Professor of Radiology, Indiana University School of Medicine, Methodist Hospital of Indiana, 1701 North Senate Boulevard, Indianapolis, IN 46206, USA

Nolan and Cadman (1987), who perfected and popularized the single-contrast enteroclysis methods. In the United States, enteroclysis was met with relative skepticism until the early 1980s, when the diagnosis of various focal lesions, including Meckel's diverticulum, could be made by the technique preoperatively and with reliability (Maglinte et al. 1980, 1984). Such reported experience stimulated interest in enteroclysis among North American radiologists.

The significant improvements in small bowel radiography are mainly attributable to the refinements in enteroclysis methods occurring during the course of the past 15 years. Advances in enteroclysis can be considered in two interrelated areas, beginning with the various technical details that improve the performance of enteroclysis, namely: patient premedication, modifications in enteroclysis catheters, contrast delivery systems, an understanding of infusion flow rates and intestinal response, and application of double-contrast methylcellulose forms of enteroclysis. Equipped with these improvements in technique, enthusiastic investigators continue to broaden the clinical application of the examination and the range of small bowel abnormalities amenable to radiologic diagnosis.

7.2
Methodologic Improvements

Improvements in technique are presented within the framework of the specific components of the enteroclysis examination.

7.2.1
Patient Preparation and Premedication

Adequate colon preparation for enteroclysis is advised as this allows for a faster examination with improved results (Maglinte et al. 1987). A full cecum retards intestinal flow through the ileum to the degree that more contrast medium is required to complete the procedure and patient comfort is compromised accordingly. Particulate material in the terminal ileum does not preclude a diagnostic examination, however, since these artifacts are removed by the luminal flow of contrast fluids. Satisfactory cleansing preparation is achieved with methods similar to those for barium enema studies: low-residue diet, ample fluids, and two laxatives on the day prior to examination and nothing by mouth on the day of examination. Administration of rectal enemas is discouraged because of the confusing small bowel patterns that may develop from admixing of refluxed enema fluid with the antegrade small bowel contrast media. Enteroclysis performed urgently for small bowel obstruction does not require bowel preparation.

Premedication for enteroclysis has received recent attention (MAGLINTE et al. 1987, 1988). Promotility agents that increase small bowel transit and thus reduce procedure time are recommended. Of the available drugs, metoclopramide hydrochloride (Reglan, A.H. Robins Co.) is preferred because of its combined stimulation of gastric and small bowel peristalsis and its infrequent association with side-effects. Specifically, administration of metoclopramide (10 mg, intravenously) immediately prior to the study facilitates the process of transpyloric intubation and also allows faster contrast infusion flow rates during enteroclysis (MAGLINTE et al. 1982). The dosage of metoclopramide should be increased accordingly if the patient has been taking medications that alter small bowel peristalsis, such as anticholinergic drugs, atropine, or narcotic analgesics and sedatives.

Efforts to improve patient comfort are an important consideration of current enteroclysis practice. In a clinical trial performed with and without mild sedation, the routine use of sedation was shown to improve patient tolerance and acceptance of enteroclysis without interfering in the quality of the examination or its duration (MAGLINTE et al. 1988). Intravenous premedication, preferably with 2–5 mg midazolam hydrochloride (Versed, Roche Laboratories) or 3–10 mg diazepam (Valium, Roche Laboratories), carefully titrated, is recommended. Some sedated patients may require a correspondingly appropriate increase in the dose of the promotility agent.

7.2.2
Enteroclysis Catheters and Intubation

Enteroclysis catheters are modifications of an original 14-F duodenal tube. Investigators have lengthened the catheter and provided various arrangements of infusion sideports. Nolan recently reduced its size to 10 F for increased flexibility (TRAILL and NOLAN 1995). Currently, the most significant adaptation to the enteroclysis catheter is that of a distal inflatable balloon that prevents duodenogastric reflux while allowing high infusion rates of the contrast media (Fig. 7.1) (MAGLINTE 1994). A multilumen small bowel tube for diagnostic enteroclysis and therapeutic gastrointestinal tract decompression also represents an innovative design (see Sect. 7.2.7) (MAGLINTE et al. 1992b).

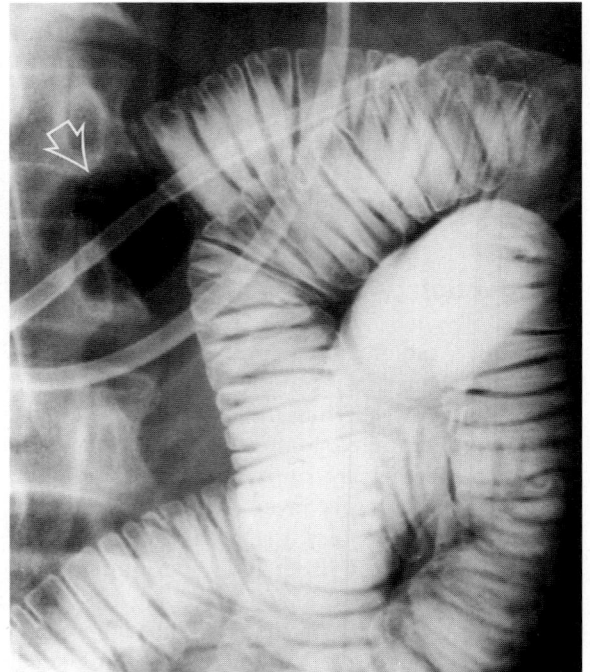

Fig. 7.1. Enteroclysis catheter (Maglinte Enteroclysis Catheter, Cook) made of radiopaque polymer with latex balloon and distal infusion sideports. Measuring 13 F in diameter and 155 cm long, the balloon distends to 2.5 cm with 15 ml injected air (*arrow*). A flexible, but rotationally rigid Teflon-coated guidewire (175 cm, 0.065 in. diameter) with a straight or angled guide tip is supplied to allow versatility during intubation maneuvers. The balloon (*arrow*) is ideally situated to the left of midline, with the catheter tip positioned in the distal duodenum or first few centimeters of jejunum for a satisfactory infusion. Note the prevention of duodenogastric reflux of contrast media during enteroclysis

Expertise in the technique of enteroclysis intubation is essential, particularly given that intubation is the main objection of patients to the diagnostic procedure. The transnasal intubation route, rather than a peroral approach, allows greater catheter control and faster intubation and has been preferred by patients who have undergone both forms of catheter insertion (MAGLINTE et al. 1986). The application of an anesthetic gel (2% viscous lidocaine hydrochloride) into the nasopharynx prior to transnasal intubation further aids in patient comfort. With experience, transpyloric intubation can be performed rapidly in most patients with successful positioning of the catheter at the duodenojejunal flexure reported within 1–4 min (TRAILL and NOLAN 1995; MAGLINTE et al. 1986).

Details of catheter manipulation to achieve a successful intubation have been aptly described in the literature and an understanding of the salient points is recommended for the serious practitioner (MAGLINTE and HERLINGER 1989a). Unique maneuvers can be applied to resolve the occasional difficulties in achieving a desired catheter position for enteroclysis. Among the techniques are the use of angled or curved tip guidewires for catheter deflection, torque rotation of catheters, and performance of the "double-back" maneuver (Fig. 7.2). The latter maneuver can obviate prolonged intubation in patients with an acute angulation between the fundus and the body of the stomach or in those with a large hiatus hernia (MAGLINTE and HERLINGER 1989a).

7.2.3
Contrast Delivery Systems

Catheter infusion for enteroclysis was initially achieved by the gravitational flow of the contrast media. This technique, as well as the use of hand-held syringes for direct catheter injection, has been replaced by mechanical infusion systems. An electric motor-driven pump for enteroclysis infusion is currently the most efficient delivery system, surpassing the performance of earlier hand-operated pump devices (Fig. 7.3) (ABU-YOUSEF et al. 1983; MAGLINTE and MILLER 1984). It allows the radiologist to precisely monitor and adjust infusion rates and markedly improves the uniformity of contrast flow into the small bowel during the procedure. In addition, its convenience allows for the removal of technical personnel from the immediate fluor-

oscopic environment, thus reducing radiation exposure to the support staff. These systems are very reliable and are associated with few mechanical problems.

7.2.4
Contrast Media Variations of Enteroclysis

Several enteroclysis methods based upon a varied use of contrast media are available for small bowel evaluation. The ease of infusion of low-density barium suspensions and the advantages of compression radiography are features in support of the *single-contrast* enteroclysis examination as performed initially by Sellink and currently by Nolan and others (SELLINK and MILLER 1982; NOLAN and CADMAN 1987; MAGLINTE and HERLINGER 1989b). The single-contrast examination may be modified by the additional infusion of water to provide a secondary double-contrast effect. Water may be infused during the final stages of examination either to maintain an uninterrupted flow of contrast through the terminal ileum or to improve the distension and visualization of the fold pattern of the distal small bowel. However, as a double-contrast agent, water provides only a brief effect since it readily diffuses with the barium suspension and degrades the surface coating of the small bowel mucosa.

Optimum mucosal surface pattern depiction and the ability to visualize through overlapping bowel loops support the advocates of *double-contrast* enteroclysis methods using air or methylcellulose. Air provides the greatest contrast between the mucosal barium and distended lumen and creates an unparalleled image of the small bowel surface pattern. Popular in Japan, this technique is highly dependent on examiner expertise and is difficult to reproduce (YAO 1994). Excessive density differences produced by air and the often vigorous stimulation of peristalsis can create difficulty in the diagnostic interpretation of the studies. Additionally, air passes rapidly through areas of luminal narrowing without inducing segments of prestenotic dilatation. The advantages of enteroclysis in the evaluation of small bowel obstruction are therefore negated and for similar reasons, the usefulness of this technique becomes limited in other clinical situations.

In comparing contrast methods, the use of aqueous methylcellulose has shown consistent advantages over other double-contrast agents (HERLINGER 1978; HERLINGER and MAGLINTE 1989). Methyl-

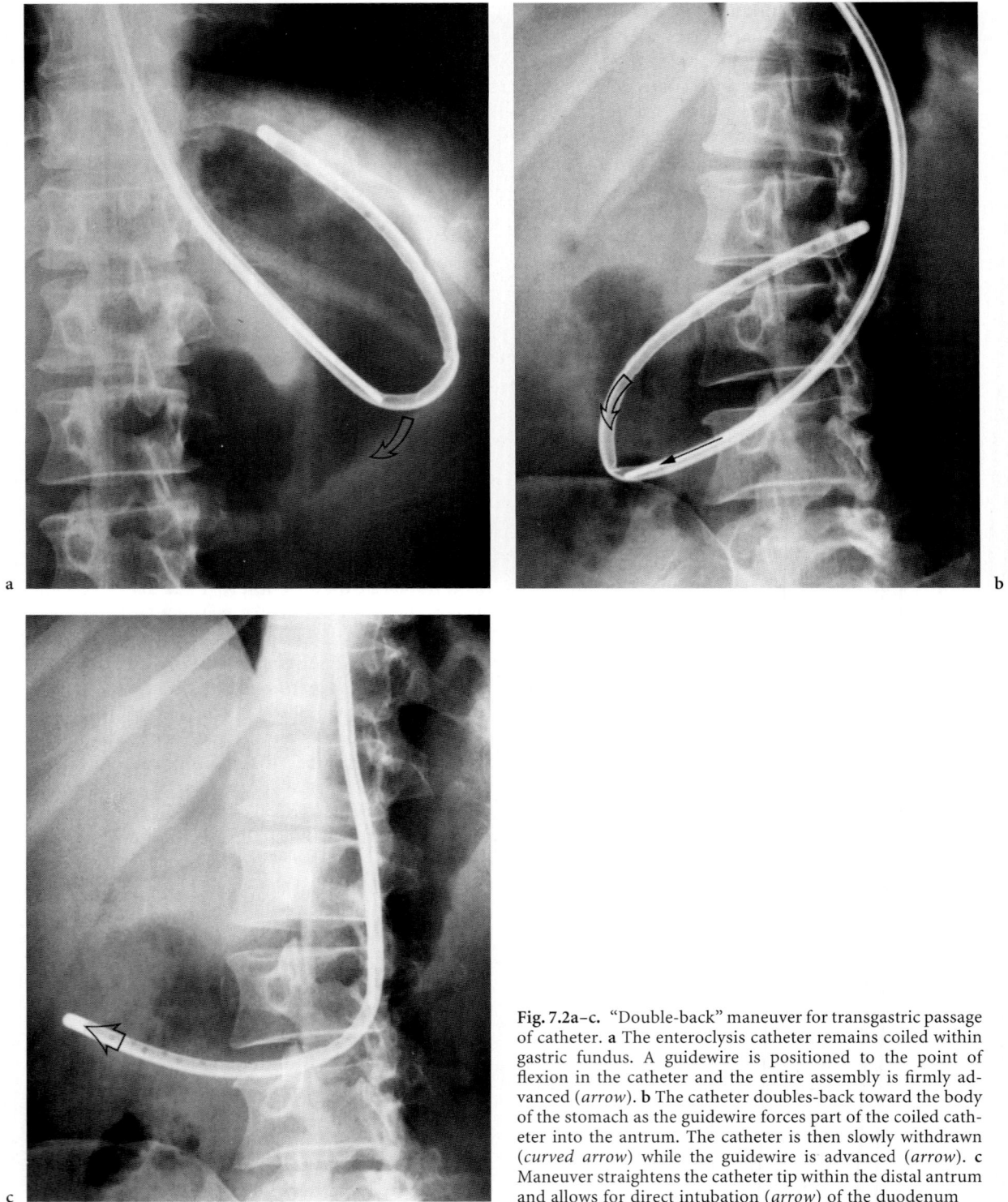

Fig. 7.2a–c. "Double-back" maneuver for transgastric passage of catheter. **a** The enteroclysis catheter remains coiled within gastric fundus. A guidewire is positioned to the point of flexion in the catheter and the entire assembly is firmly advanced (*arrow*). **b** The catheter doubles-back toward the body of the stomach as the guidewire forces part of the coiled catheter into the antrum. The catheter is then slowly withdrawn (*curved arrow*) while the guidewire is advanced (*arrow*). **c** Maneuver straightens the catheter tip within the distal antrum and allows for direct intubation (*arrow*) of the duodenum

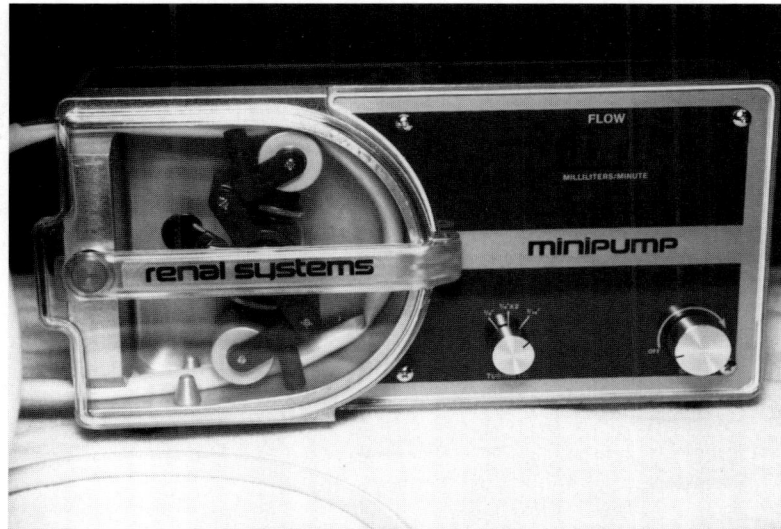

Fig. 7.3. Peristaltic tube pump (RS-7800 Minipump, Renal Systems, Inc.). This system achieves uniform delivery of contrast media throughout the entire range of infusion flow rates required for an ideal enteroclysis. Flow rates are displayed in real-time (ml/min) and are adjustable by dial in 1 ml/min increments

cellulose acts to propel the barium column through the small bowel and produces an interface of contrast between the density of the barium coating the mucosa and the water density of the methylcellulose distending the lumen (Fig. 7.4) (HERLINGER and MAGLINTE 1989). Double-contrast effect persists for sufficient duration because of the minimal diffusion between the methylcellulose and compatible barium suspensions. Excessive barium density within pelvic loops of small bowel can be avoided and surface features in overlapping loops are evident. In addition, methylcellulose promotes the evacuation of barium following the procedure.

A recent survey of members of the Society of Gastrointestinal Radiologists has shown that the double-contrast enteroclysis methods using methylcellulose are the most commonly used methods of enteroclysis examination in North America (BARLOON et al. 1988). Two methods of enteroclysis using methylcellulose have been popularized by Maglinte and Herlinger, with the differences between these two methods having lessened in recent years. The Herlinger technique primarily relies on the double-contrast effect of methylcellulose following an infusion of a small amount of high-density barium media, usually 180–220 ml of an 80% w/v suspension of barium (Entero H, E-Z-EM, Inc.) (HERLINGER and MAGLINTE 1989). Radiography with compression during the double-contrast phase is emphasized, since the barium is of higher density than ideally suited for single-contrast examination. In the Maglinte *biphasic* enteroclysis method, a greater volume of less-dense barium

is used and methylcellulose double-contrast serves to augment the initial single-contrast phase information.

7.2.5
Maglinte Biphasic Enteroclysis

By the use of an amount (350–500 ml depending on bowel length) and density of barium suspension satisfactory for single-contrast radiography and infusion of a methylcellulose solution, a complete single-contrast and double-contrast small bowel evaluation can be performed in a single examination (MAGLINTE and HERLINGER 1989b; MAGLINTE 1994). This method combines the value of fluoroscopy and compression radiography of the entire small bowel during the single-contrast phase with the advantages of double-contrast surface pattern depiction produced by methylcellulose.

A 50% w/v barium suspension, specifically formulated for the biphasic method with agents to prolong mucosal coating (Entrobar, Lafayette Pharmaceuticals, Inc.), is infused and followed by up to 2 l of 0.5% hydroxypropyl methylcellulose solution (Entrocel, Lafayette Pharmaceuticals, Inc.). Infusion of methylcellulose results in adequate amounts of barium being pushed distally to enable continuation of the single-contrast evaluation of the distal small bowel while a double-contrast effect is being produced in the more proximal segments. This volume and timing of infusion eliminates the need for adjunct techniques to visualize the distal ileum and

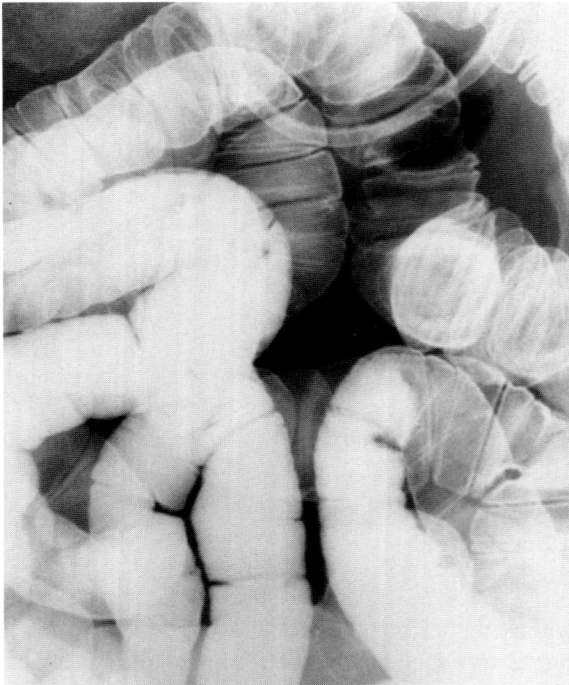

Fig. 7.4. Double-contrast phase of biphasic enteroclysis. Lumen translucency from methylcellulose infusion allows optimal imaging of the mucosal surface features. Note the continuation of single contrast in the distal bowel loops as the more proximal loops become transradient. Double contrast is valuable in imaging segments of overlapping bowel, especially within the pelvis

also allows an additional view of every segment of the small bowel to confirm diagnostic findings. In cases where the single-contrast phase shows all bowel loops normally distensible and the folds clearly defined, the examination may be concluded. The biphasic method offers flexibility in small bowel examination and is a reproducible alternative to the many enteroclysis methods described. It can be used routinely for all clinical indications of enteroclysis.

In the biphasic method, some lesions are better defined during the single-contrast phase with compression (Fig. 7.5), whereas the double-contrast phase excels in the demonstration of folds and more subtle surface abnormalities (Fig. 7.6). During contrast infusion, progress of the barium column is observed with frequent fluoroscopy and the lead portion is intermittently compressed using various obliquities and tube angulations allowed by the use of remote-controlled radiographic equipment. A routine filming sequence includes:

Single-contrast phase:

1. Compression radiographs of the proximal jejunum in slight obliquity after infusion of 300 ml of barium, followed by similar films of the distal jejunum and proximal ileum. If the distal ileum has been outlined with barium using less than the full amount, the barium infusion is stopped and that of methylcellulose begins.
2. Compression radiographs of the distal ileum, including the terminal ileum, complete the single-contrast examination. Methylcellulose infusion continues until all of the loop segments are adequately distended and interpreted.

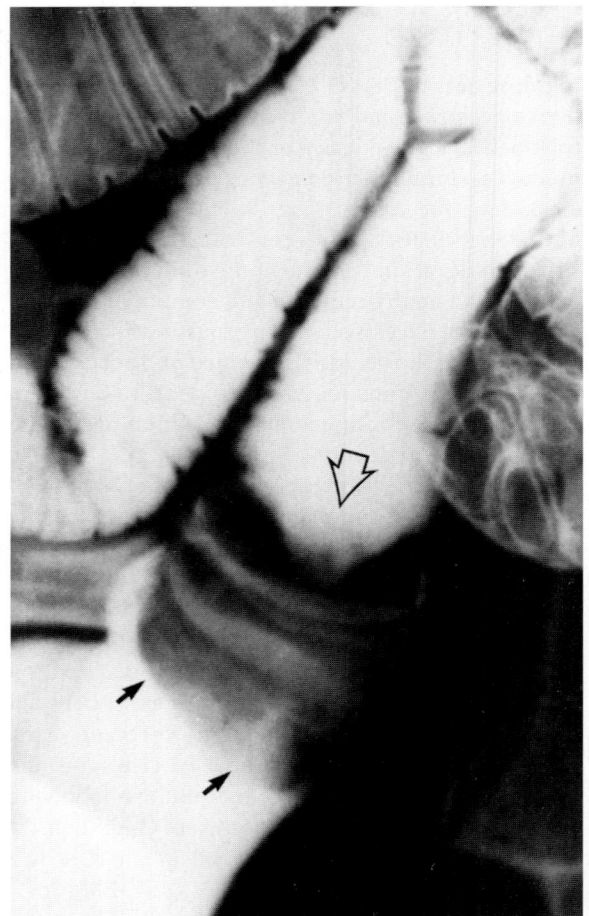

Fig. 7.5. Single-contrast during biphasic enteroclysis demonstrates luminal filling-defect (*arrows*) from metastatic melanoma. Tapering (*open arrow*) of the proximal loop indicates intussusception of the tumor. Single contrast excels at depicting contour abnormalities of the bowel, mass lesions, stricture, and fistulae

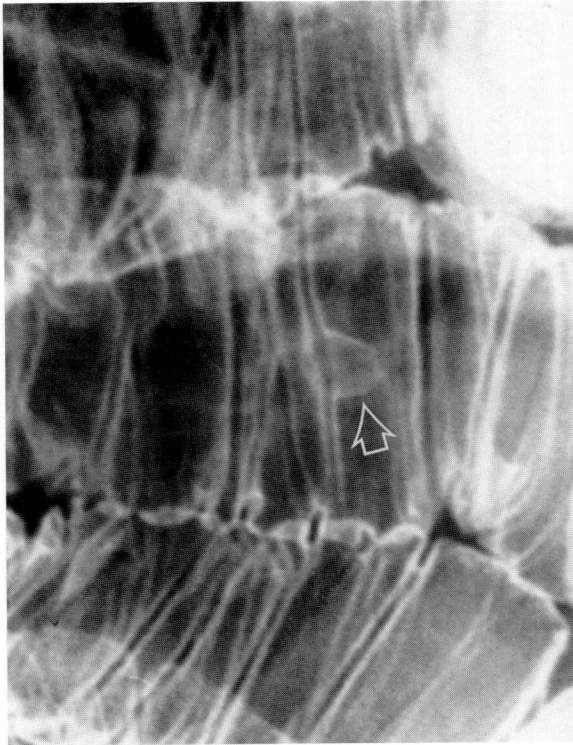

Fig. 7.6. Double contrast during biphasic enteroclysis accurately demonstrates an 8-mm polypoid lesion (*arrow*). Surgery confirmed a mucosal adenoma. Double contrast excels at depicting folds and more subtle surface abnormalities such as ulcerations and small tumors

Double-contrast phase:

1. Radiographs during mild compression are obtained from the proximal jejunal segments, progressing distally until all loop segments have been imaged in double contrast. One avoids excessive compression that results in dispersal of the barium coating. Lateral or steeply oblique radiographs are taken of the pelvic segments of ileum before contrast fills the descending colon.
2. Prone overhead radiographs complete routine filming. The need for a duodenal examination or further assessment of questionable abnormalities is determined prior to tube withdrawal.

7.2.6
Contrast Infusion Rates and Intestinal Response

The control of the flow of contrast media and the resulting distension and motility response of the small bowel is an important aspect of enteroclysis (Fig. 7.7). Lack of understanding these issues results in an unsatisfactory procedure and a prolonged examination which may yield questionable diagnostic results. For biphasic enteroclysis, a rate of infusion between 55 and 125 ml/min is recommended for the single-contrast phase and is continuously adjusted to give moderate distension without completely abolishing peristalsis (MAGLINTE 1994). Infusion at the higher rate is typically used if the metoclopramide dose has been increased to compensate for administration of a sedative. During the double-contrast phase, even higher flow rates (>125 ml/min) are often used to create hypotonia and greater degrees of distension in order to improve the demonstration of mucosal fold patterns.

It should be appreciated that the motility of the small bowel is variable in its response to different rates of infusion and is influenced by medications, including metoclopramide and sedatives, and certain pathologic conditions. Faster infusion rates produce increased dilatation of the bowel and are associated with hypotonia, whereas slower rates of infusion cause a more rapid passage of contrast media through the small bowel. Infusions administered too slowly produce inadequate lumen distension and a collapsed irregular fold pattern. Excessively fast rates of infusion abolish peristalsis and induce atony of the bowel. This precludes the assessment of motility, promotes duodenogastric reflux, and requires more barium to complete a prolonged examination. Continuation requires a brief reduction or cessation of the infusion until mild peristalsis resumes and contrast media infusion can then proceed at a newly adjusted flow rate. Alternatively, additional promotility agent may be given in extreme instances. In patients manifesting either an adynamic ileus or a hypermotility state, infusion rates may require dramatic adjustment to maintain uniform flow of contrast media, i.e., approximately 25–50 or 125–175 ml/min, respectively.

7.2.7
Adaptations of Enteroclysis for Specific Circumstances

7.2.7.1
Ileostomy Enteroclysis

Enteroclysis infusion can be safely performed in retrograde fashion in patients with an ileostomy (KAY and NOLAN 1989). Per ileostomy infusion is

a

b

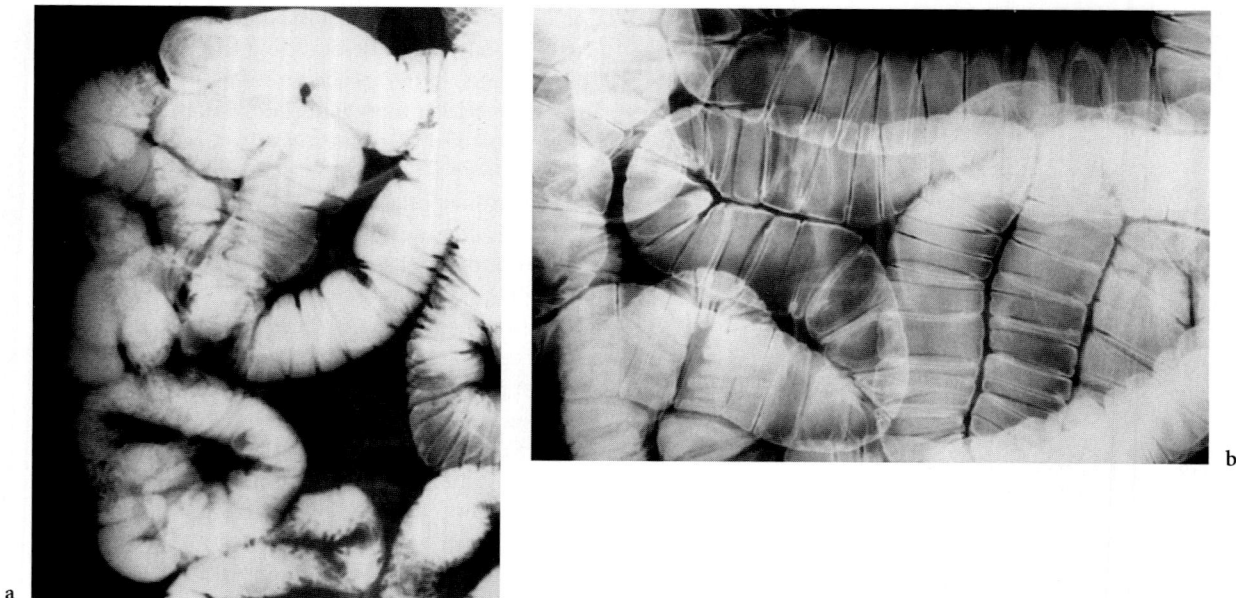

Fig. 7.7a,b. Biphasic enteroclysis. **a** Optimal rate of infusion (55–125 ml/min) during the single-contrast phase. Mild peristalsis remains present with a moderate distension of the small bowel loops. **b** Faster flow rates (>125 ml/min) during the double-contrast phase induce a desirable degree of hypotonia. This creates better lumen distension and separation of loops and improves the demonstration of mucosal fold patterns and surface defects. Applied compression is moderate so that the barium coating is not dispersed

better tolerated by patients and is preferred for the evaluation of ileostomy malfunction, recurrent inflammatory disease, or distal small bowel obstruction. Specific techniques for adapting various enteroclysis catheters for ileostomy intubation have been described, although the standard balloon catheter is preferred (MAGLINTE 1994). The catheter is introduced into the ostomy and the balloon gradually inflated during fluoroscopy and retracted until it is just beyond the peritoneal reflection. The purpose of the inflated balloon is not to occlude the bowel lumen proximal to the stoma, but to act as a seal from within against the usually narrower and nondistensible opening through the abdominal fascia. The balloon should be inflated slowly, using only enough air to produce a resistance to gentle withdrawal of the catheter. Before introducing contrast media, 0.5 mg glucagon intravenously should be given to abolish peristalsis. It is important to evaluate the prestomal portion of the ileostomy as fascial scarring can be a common cause of stomal malfunction. To avoid obscuring the prestomal area, the balloon catheter should be deflated near the end of the procedure and tangential spot films taken while some of the instilled barium overflows out of the stoma. A biphasic technique using less barium (350 ml) followed by methylcellulose allows evaluation of the entire small bowel. In patients with pelvic adhesions, severe discomfort may ensue during infusion and an analgesic, such as meperidine, may be required.

7.2.7.2
Enteroclysis in Partial Small Bowel Obstruction

The recent development of a special catheter to facilitate decompression of the high-grade partially obstructed small bowel and to perform enteroclysis has markedly improved the diagnosis and management of patients. This catheter eliminates the need either to replace a standard nasogastric tube (inappropriate for enteroclysis) with an enteroclysis catheter or to position an enteroclysis catheter in tandem with a nasogastric tube, thus making the procedure less complicated and easier for both patient and radiologist. The nasoenteric decompression enteroclysis catheter (Maglinte Decompression Sump/ Balloon Enteroclysis Catheter, Cook) is a modification of the balloon enteroclysis catheter (MAGLINTE et al. 1992b). It is a 14-F, 155 cm long, closed-end triple-lumen catheter (Fig. 7.8). The catheter tip is tapered to decrease irritation of the nasal passage and it is made of soft radiopaque polyvinyl chloride

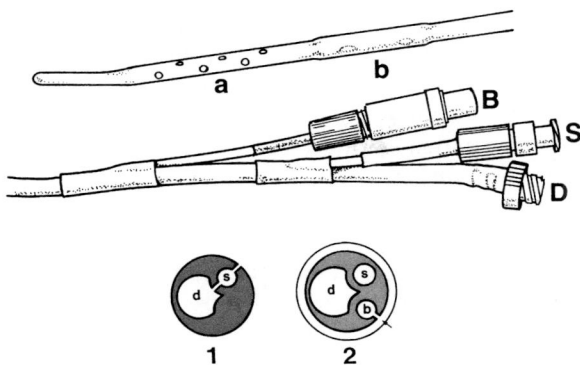

Fig. 7.8. Diagram of the construction of Maglinte decompression enteroclysis catheter. The *upper drawing* depicts the distal end of the catheter, the *middle drawing* depicts the proximal end, and the *bottom drawings* are cross-sections at the level of the distal sideports (*1*) and at the level of the balloon (*2*). The distal sideports in the upper drawing (*a*) allow continuity between the bowel lumen and the sump lumen (*s*), which in turn connects with the decompression (suction) lumen. The sump lumen (*s*) connects externally at *S* and the decompression lumen at *D*. Sideports communicating with the sump and suction lumens allow flushing of the catheter from the proximal attachment *S*, in order to prevent catheter blockage during decompression. The balloon lumen (*b*), which is provided with a one-way valve proximally at *B*, communicates with an inflatable balloon at level (*2*). For catheter placement in the small bowel, a 195-cm Teflon-coated stainless steel torque guidewire is provided with a straight tip to act as a stiffener and a 45° angled tip for directional control. Detailed instructions for nursing personnel accompany the catheter to ensure efficient suction and management

for patient comfort. The largest of three lumens, the decompression suction and contrast infusion lumen, continues distally to six catheter sideports that extend 2 cm proximal to the weighted distal tip. The medium-sized sump lumen is in continuity with the decompression lumen by a series of small holes which prevent the collapse of the main lumen during enteric suctioning. The third lumen, for balloon inflation, connects to a 2.5-cm silicone balloon positioned 8 cm from the distal tip. The balloon is used only if enteroclysis is performed and is deflated after infusion of the contrast media. The suction port is provided with an adapter to connect to electrical suction for gastric or enteric decompression.

A visual mark, 59 cm from the distal tip, indicates the catheter position within the stomach. The external landmark facilitates recognition of this level so that the catheter can be placed by clinicians in the emergency room or at the bedside for immediate gastric decompression. Subsequently, the catheter can be fluoroscopically positioned in the proximal jejunum for further small bowel decompression or enteroclysis if desired (MAGLINTE et al. 1994b). A

fluid-filled distended stomach should be decompressed before the catheter tip is positioned in the proximal jejunum, the ideal position of the nasoenteric decompression enteroclysis catheter. Because of the smaller size of the catheter (14 F) compared with the 16/18-F nasogastric tube, it is tolerated better by patients and is easier to maneuver into the duodenum and proximal jejunum (MAGLINTE et al. 1994b).

7.2.7.3
Enteroclysis in Occult Gastrointestinal Bleeding

Regardless of the report of a negative endoscopic examination performed for occult bleeding, the radiologist should examine the duodenum in detail, especially if the anatomic extent of the endoscopic assessment is unknown. The duodenum can be examined either simultaneously or after the routine radiographic evaluation of the jejunum and ileum (MAGLINTE 1994). By deflating the catheter's balloon during enteroclysis, some barium media refluxes into the duodenum. With the increased flow rate utilized for methylcellulose infusion, further reflux and distention of the duodenum results and morphologic assessment of the duodenum is then possible. Alternatively, the duodenum can be evaluated prior to catheter removal. After balloon deflation, the catheter tip is retracted into the proximal horizontal duodenum and barium infused (Fig. 7.9). Radiographs are then obtained in different projections. An ideal enteroclysis evaluation of the duodenum occurs before contrast opacification of the transverse colon.

7.2.7.4
Combined Enteroscopy and Enteroclysis

If proximal small bowel enteroscopy has been done in instances of malabsorption or evaluation of upper gastrointestinal bleeding, a recently described combined diagnostic procedure is available (McGOVERN and BARKIN 1990). For this purpose, an exchange wire with a flexible tip is introduced through the endoscope at the end of the examination and is advanced toward the jejunum. With the wire left in position, the sedated patient is transferred to Radiology for enteroclysis. An infusion catheter of reduced wall thickness and greater flexibility is threaded over the exchange wire and passed into the jejunum. The biphasic enteroclysis then proceeds in standard

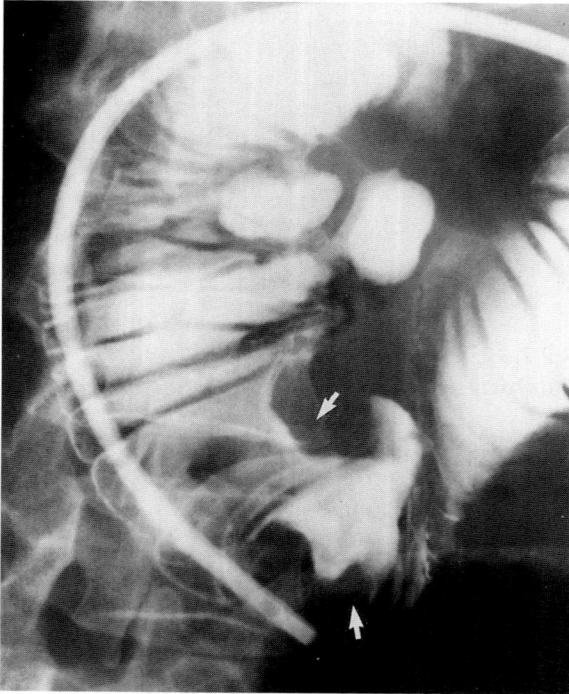

Fig. 7.9. Duodenal study after a normal enteroclysis evaluation of the jejunum and ileum for occult gastrointestinal bleed. Contrast infusion following repositioning of the catheter demonstrates a contour mass defect (*arrows*) secondary to an unsuspected lung carcinoma metastasis

al. 1994a). In one study, enteroclysis correctly predicted the presence of obstruction in 100%, the absence of obstruction in 80%, the level of obstruction in 89%, and the etiology of obstruction in 86% of operated patients (SHRAKE et al. 1991). Further, in a group of patients developing small bowel obstruction after laparotomy for malignancy, enteroclysis predicted the correct etiology of obstruction between adhesions, metastases, or radiation injury in 90% of cases (CAROLINE et al. 1984). Enteroclysis has shown considerable value in the often difficult assessment of obstruction in the early postoperative period (DEHN and NOLAN 1989). Recent descriptions of the diagnostic features of closed-loop obstruction on enteroclysis are an important contribution to prompt preoperative diagnosis and patient management (Fig. 7.10) (MAGLINTE et al. 1991a). In many radiologic practices, the predominant role for enteroclysis is its ability to detect symptomatic nonobstructing and partially obstructing adhesions (MAGLINTE et al. 1987, 1996).

fashion. For best results, the small bowel is insufflated with carbon dioxide rather than air during the enteroscopy.

7.3
Clinical Advances

The excellent results from the numerous studies that have dealt with the sensitivity of enteroclysis for most small bowel abnormalities support the authors' recommendation of utilizing enteroclysis as the initial small bowel examination in most clinical instances (MAGLINTE et al. 1996).

7.3.1
Small Bowel Obstruction

In the evaluation of partial, clinically intermittent, or suspected but uncertain cases of small bowel obstruction, enteroclysis is preferred to rapidly confirm obstruction and assess the cause (MAGLINTE et

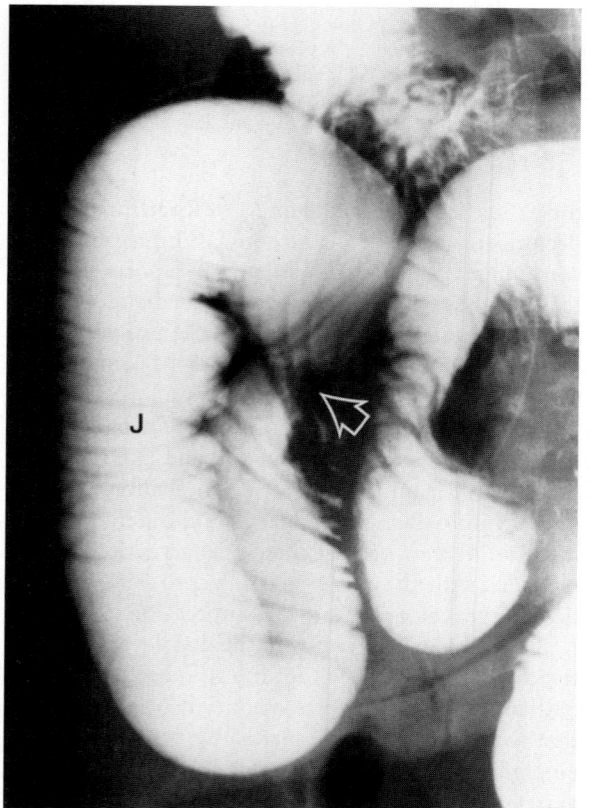

Fig. 7.10. Enteroclysis demonstration of a closed-loop, partial small bowel obstruction. An adhesive band (*arrow*) obstructs two segments of a single jejunal (*J*) loop

7.3.2
Neoplasms

Despite advances in both surgery and diagnostic imaging, the survival of patients with primary malignancies of the small bowel has not shown similar improvement. An analysis of patients with small bowel neoplasms has shown that the delay in establishing the diagnosis was often the result of relatively ineffective radiologic imaging (MAGLINTE et al. 1991b). In an American report comparing enteroclysis and the small bowel follow-through (SBFT) in 71 patients diagnosed with primary malignancy, the SBFT had a sensitivity of 61% and enteroclysis a sensitivity of 95% for the demonstration of jejunal or ileal tumors (BESSETTE et al. 1989). The actual neoplasm was only shown in 33% of conventional examinations whereas it was shown in 90% of biphasic enteroclysis studies (Fig. 7.11). European experience also supports the sensitivity of diagnosis of neoplasms by enteroclysis and in addition has shown the method to provide accurate

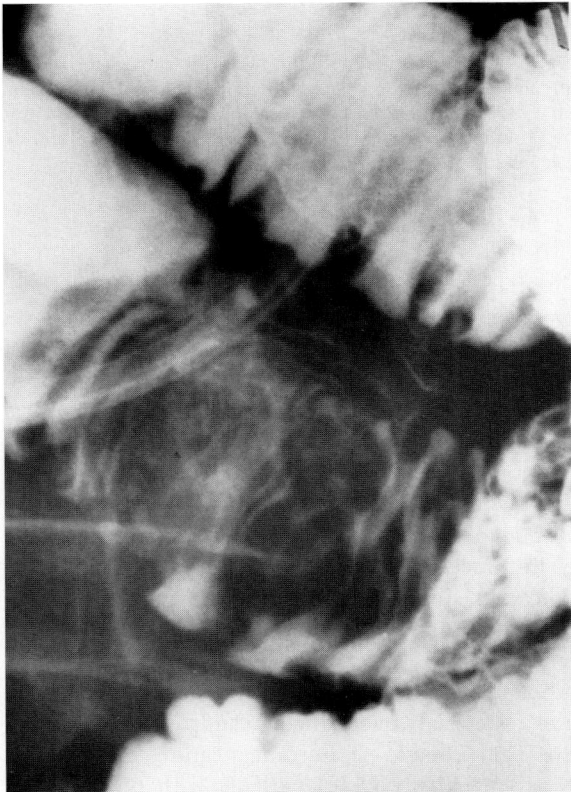

Fig. 7.11. Primary lymphoma. Enteroclysis depicts a short jejunal segment with disrupted folds and contour distortion of the loop by several small mural masses

preoperative differentiation among detected tumors (GOURTSOYIANNIS et al. 1993).

7.3.3
Crohn's Disease

An important indication for small bowel barium studies is the evaluation of Crohn's disease. The prospective accuracy and clinical relevance of enteroclysis in Crohn's disease was recently reported and the method was highly diagnostic, with a sensitivity, specificity, and accuracy of 100%, 98.3%, and 99.3% respectively (MAGLINTE et al. 1992a). Compared with SBFT, enteroclysis excels in demonstrating the extent of disease involvement, the presence of skip lesions or fistulae, and complications due to prior surgery. Enteroclysis provides detailed structural information relevant to the appropriate management of the disease (MAGLINTE et al. 1992a). In patients with Crohn's disease who present with findings of obstruction, the distinction between luminal narrowing caused by reversible edema and spasm, and narrowing due to fibrosis can be established. Detailed small bowel evaluation by enteroclysis is also appropriate in patients with severe clinical exacerbation, in preoperative patients undergoing planned resection, and in postsurgical patients developing clinical symptoms of recurrence (CHERNISH et al. 1992).

7.3.4
Occult Gastrointestinal Bleeding

Enteroclysis is indicated after all radiologic and endoscopic studies have been unrevealing in the evaluation of occult gastrointestinal bleeding. The diagnostic yield of enteroclysis in patients with occult bleeding is now established between 10% and 20% (REX et al. 1989; MOCH et al. 1994). In one series, benign and malignant neoplasms accounted for one-half of the abnormalities diagnosed, with Meckel diverticulum and a varied group of inflammatory processes also implicated as the cause of small bowel bleeding (Fig. 7.12) (REX et al. 1989). Collective experience from such clinical studies suggests that if enteroclysis fails to demonstrate a lesion as the likely source of bleeding, a vascular malformation (AVM) of the small bowel is the probable cause. Demonstrations of AVM by double-contrast enteroclysis have been reported, although the reliability of the method for this diagnosis appears mar-

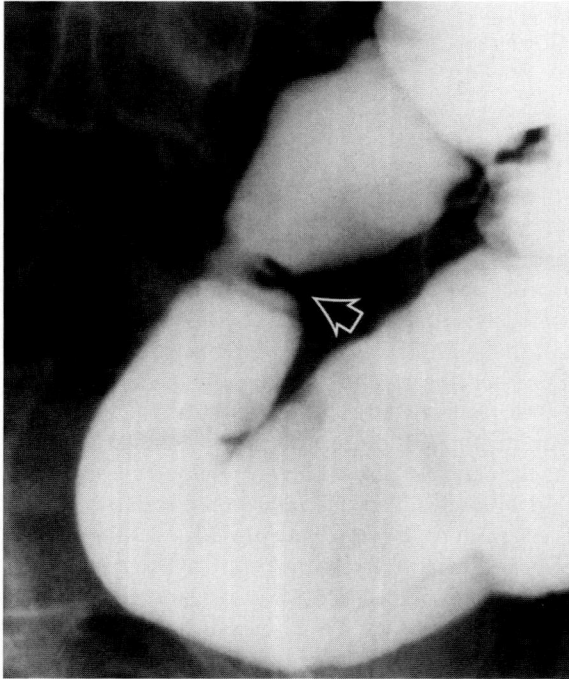

Fig. 7.12. Enteroclysis for evaluation of occult bleeding. Compression radiograph during single-contrast phase demonstrates a focal asymmetric narrowing (*arrow*) in the jejunum without an associated mass. Mild prestenotic dilatation is appreciated because of the controlled enteroclysis infusion rate. Because of the history of nonsteroidal antiinflammatory (NSAID) therapy for arthritis, a diaphragm-like stenosis with secondary ulcer and edema was diagnosed. NSAID enteropathy was confirmed at surgery

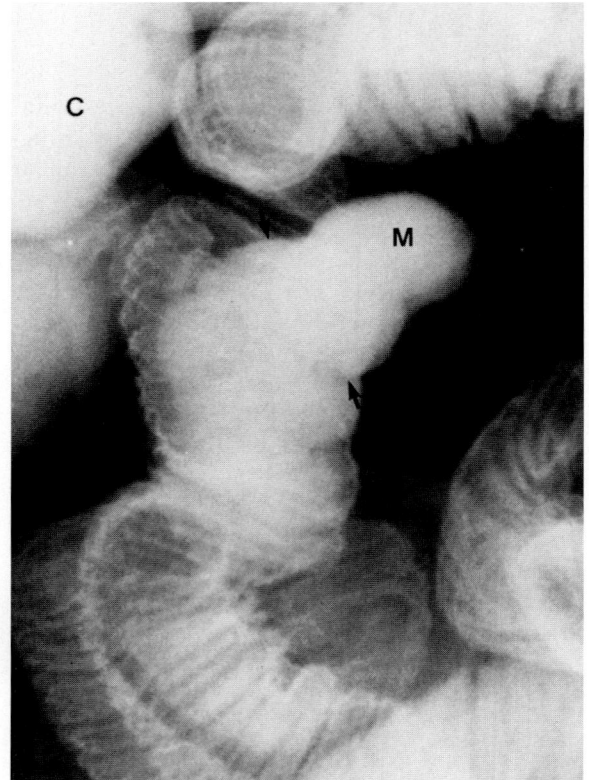

Fig. 7.13. Meckel's diverticulum (*M*) with a characteristic triangular plateau (*arrows*) and junctional fold pattern as seen on enteroclysis. A careful fluoroscopic evaluation, with compression, is necessary to detect Meckel's diverticulum. *C*, Cecum

ginal because of the lesion's inherent small size and pliability (HERLINGER et al. 1992). Meckel's diverticulum, regarded as an uncommon but important cause of unexplained bleeding in the adult, can be a difficult condition to diagnose preoperatively. In adults, enteroclysis demonstrates Meckel's and other small bowel diverticula more consistently than other diagnostic methods (Fig. 7.13) (MAGLINTE et al. 1980, 1985).

7.3.5
Malabsorption

Controlled enteroclysis infusion minimizes the adverse effects of intestinal hypersecretion on barium contrast images and makes it the preferred examination in malabsorptive states (HERLINGER 1993). In active celiac disease, enteroclysis demonstrates a reversal of the normal fold pattern that is specific for the diagnosis, i.e., reduced proximal jejunal (three or fewer folds per inch) and increased (four to six folds per inch) distal ileal folds (HERLINGER and MAGLINTE 1986). Although this pattern has been described with SBFT in long-standing nontropical sprue, enteroclysis has precisely determined the fold counts of the abnormal small bowel and can suggest the diagnosis of celiac disease, especially in cases with an atypical presentation (Fig. 7.14).

Enteroclysis is relevant in celiac disease in the following circumstances: (a) patients with atypical presentations, (b) patients in whom biopsy is consistent with celiac disease but the differentiation from other disorders with similar histology is indicated, e.g., bacterial overgrowth syndrome, giardiasis, Zollinger-Ellison syndrome, and eosinophilic gastroenteritis, and (c) patients with poor dietary response or clinical recurrence of celiac activity in order to identify possible complications, e.g., lymphoma or ulcerative jejunoileitis (HERLINGER

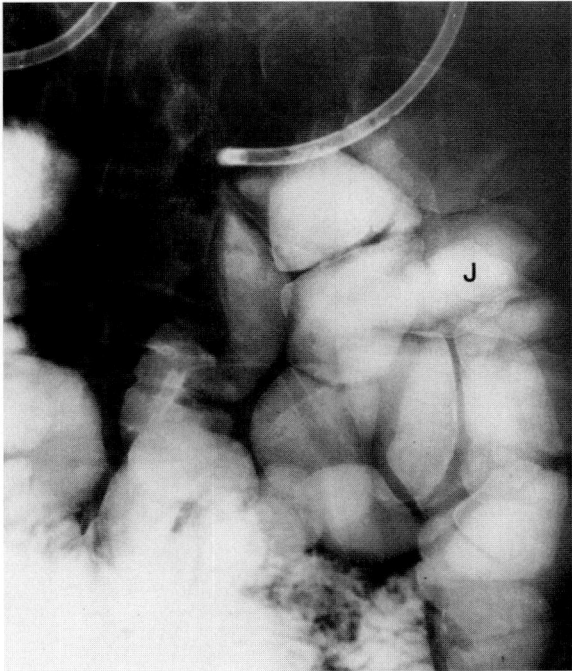

Fig. 7.14. Enteroclysis in atypical clinical presentation of celiac disease. Enteroclysis shows a near absence in the number of folds in the proximal jejunum (*J*). An increase in folds was evident in the more distal bowel, consistent with a reversal of the normal pattern. Fold changes in celiac disease are best appreciated during the methylcellulose double-contrast phase. Endoscopic biopsy confirmed the diagnosis

and MAGLINTE 1986). In patients with malabsorption from bacterial overgrowth, enteroclysis may show conditions that are associated with abnormal peristaltic function, e.g., scleroderma, amyloidosis, and pseudo-obstruction, or demonstrate predisposing structural abnormalities, e.g., jejunal diverticulosis, surgical blind loops.

References

Abu-Yousef MM, Benson CA, Lu CH, et al. (1983) Enteroclysis aided by an electric pump. Radiology 147:268–269

Barloon TJ, Lu CC, Franken EA Jr, et al. (1988) Small bowel enteroclysis survey. Gastrointest Radiol 13:203–206

Bessette JR, Maglinte DDT, Kelvin FM, Chernish SM (1989) Primary malignant tumors in the small-bowel: a comparison of the small-bowel enema and conventional follow-through examination. AJR 153:741–744

Caroline DF, Herlinger H, Laufer I, et al. (1984) Small bowel enema in the diagnosis of adhesive obstructions. AJR 142:1133–1139

Chernish SM, Maglinte DD, O'Connor K (1992) Evaluation of the small intestine by enteroclysis for Crohn's disease. Am J Gastroenterol 87:696–701

Dehn TCB, Nolan DJ (1989) Enteroclysis in the diagnosis of intestinal obstruction in the early postoperative period. Gastrointest Radiol 14:15–21

Gourtsoyiannis NC, Days D, Papaioannou N, et al. (1993) Benign tumors of the small intestine: preoperation evaluation with a barium infusion technique. Eur J Radiol 16:115–125

Herlinger H (1978) A modified technique for the double-contrast small bowel enema. Gastrointest Radiol 3:201–207

Herlinger H (1993) Enteroclysis in malabsorption: can it influence diagnosis and management? Radiology 33:335–342

Herlinger H, Maglinte DDT (1986) Jejunal fold separation in adult celiac disease: relevance of enteroclysis. Radiology 158:605–611

Herlinger H, Maglinte DDT (1989) The small bowel enema with methylcellulose. In: Herlinger H, Maglinte DDT (eds) Clinical radiology of the small intestine. Saunders, Philadelphia, pp 119–137

Herlinger H, Levine MS, Furth EE, et al. (1992) Arteriovenous malformation of the small bowel diagnosed with enteroclysis. AJR 159:1225–1226

Kay VJ, Nolan DJ (1989) The small bowel enema in the patient with an ileostomy. Clin Radiol 39:418–422

Maglinte DDT (1984) Balloon enteroclysis catheter. AJR 143:761–762

Maglinte DDT (1994) Biphasic enteroclysis with methylcellulose. In: Freeny PC, Stevenson GW (eds) Alimentary tract radiology, 5th edn. Mosby, St. Louis, pp 533–547

Maglinte DDT, Herlinger H (1989a) Enteroclysis catheters, intubation and infusion. In: Herlinger H, Maglinte DDT (eds) Clinical radiology of the small intestine. Saunders, Philadelphia, pp 85–106

Maglinte DDT, Herlinger H (1989b) Single contrast and biphasic enteroclysis. In: Herlinger H, Maglinte DDT (eds) Clinical radiology of the small intestine. Saunders, Philadelphia, pp 107–118

Maglinte DDT, Miller RE (1984) A comparison of pumps used for enteroclysis. Radiology 152:815

Maglinte DDT, Elmore MF, Dolan PA, et al. (1980) Meckel's diverticulum radiologic demonstration by enteroclysis. AJR 134:924–932

Maglinte DDT, Burney BT, Miller RE (1982) Technical factors for a more rapid enteroclysis. AJR 138:588–591

Maglinte DDT, Hall R, Miller RE, et al. (1984) Detection of surgical lesions of the small bowel by enteroclysis. Am J Surg 127:225–229

Maglinte DDT, Elmore MF, Chernish SM, et al. (1985) Enteroclysis in the diagnosis of chronic unexplained gastrointestinal bleeding. Dis Colon Rectum 28:403–405

Maglinte DDT, Lappas JC, Chernish SM, et al. (1986) Intubation routes for enteroclysis. Radiology 158:553–554

Maglinte DDT, Lappas JC, Kelvin FM, et al. (1987) Small bowel radiography: how, when, and why? Radiology 163:297–304

Maglinte DDT, Lappas JC, Chernish SM, et al. (1988) Improved tolerance of enteroclysis by use of sedation. AJR 151: 951–952

Maglinte DDT, Nolan DJ, Herlinger H (1991a) Preoperative diagnosis by enteroclysis of unsuspected closed loop obstruction in medically managed patients. J Clin Gastroenterol 13:308–312

Maglinte DDT, O'Connor K, Bessette J, et al. (1991b) The role of the physician in the late diagnosis of primary malignant tumors of the small intestine. Am J Gastroenterol 86:304–308

Maglinte DDT, Chernish SM, Kelvin FM, et al. (1992a) Crohn disease of the small intestine: accuracy and relevance of enteroclysis. Radiology 184:541–545

Maglinte DDT, Stevens LH, Hall RC, et al. (1992b) Dual-purpose tube for enteroclysis and nasogastric-nasoenteric decompression. Radiology 185:281–282

Maglinte DDT, Herlinger H, Turner WW Jr, Kelvin FM (1994a) Radiologic management of small-bowel obstruction: a practical approach. Emerg Radiol 1:138–149

Maglinte DDT, Kelvin FM, Micon LT, et al. (1994b) Nasointestinal tube for decompression or enteroclysis: experience with 150 patients. Abdom Imaging 19:108–112

Maglinte DDT, Kelvin FM, O'Connor K, et al. (1996) Current status of small bowel radiography. Abdom Imaging 2:247–257

McGovern R, Barkin JS (1990) Enteroscopy and enteroclysis: an improved method for combined procedure. Gastrointest Radiol 15:327–328

Moch A, Herlinger H, Kochman ML, et al. (1994) Enteroclysis in the evaluation of obscure gastrointestinal bleeding. AJR 163:1381–1384

Nolan DJ, Cadman PJ (1987) The small bowel enema made easy. Clin Radiol 38:295–301

Rex DK, Lappas JC, Maglinte DDT, et al. (1989) Enteroclysis in the evaluation of suspected small intestinal bleeding. Gastroenterology 97:58–60

Sellink JL, Miller RE (1982) Radiology of the small bowel: modern enteroclysis technique and atlas. Martinus Nijhoff, The Hague

Shrake PD, Rex DK, Lappas JC, et al. (1991) Radiographic evaluation of suspected small bowel obstruction. Am J Gastroenterol 86:175–178

Traill ZC, Nolan DJ (1995) Technical note: intubation fluoroscopy times using a new enteroclysis tube. Clin Radiol 50:339–340

Yao T (1994) Double-contrast enteroclysis with air. In: Freeny PC, Stevenson GW (eds) Alimentary tract radiology, 5th edn. Mosby, St. Louis, pp 548–551

8 Colon

C.I. Bartram

with contribution from N.M.deSouza

CONTENTS

8.1
Introduction

The first double-contrast barium enema (DCBE) is credited to Fischer in 1923. The technique was brought to prominence by Welin (WELIN 1967) in the 1960s, and became the primary examination for colonic investigation up to the mid 1980s. During the past decade there has been a major swing to colonoscopy, with new challenges from within radiology. The ability to acquire volume data easily and quickly with helical computed tomography (CT), coupled with developments in 3D software and fast processing, have opened up possibilities for CT colography (HARA et al. 1996). The impact of these developments has been to shift the emphasis in colonic radiology from primary mucosal diagnosis to functional abnormalities.

8.2
The Barium Enema Versus Endoscopy

The DCBE is a simple and safe procedure, but with a higher diagnostic threshold than endoscopy. The reason for this is that for an abnormality to be visible on the DCBE, the change in surface texture of the mucosa has to be sufficient to alter the thin layer of barium suspension coating the mucus surface, or a focal lesion must be present that is either sufficiently

C.I. BARTRAM, FRCP, FRCR, Intestinal Imaging 4V, St. Mark's Hospital, Northwick Park, Harrow HA1 3UJ, UK

depressed to create a barium pool or elevated to form a meniscus. Changes in mucosal vascularity are an earlier marker for colitis than surface erosion. Other vascular lesions, such as telangiectasia and angiomas, are easily visible endoscopically though not on DCBE as there is no surface change.

The DCBE is inadequate on its own to exclude colitis, though the likelihood of colitis being overlooked when DCBE, sigmoidoscopy and rectal biopsy are negative, is remote. A small group of patients, with chronic watery diarrhoea, may have microscopic or collagenous colitis. Diagnosis requires endoscopic biopsy, and although there is one report of radiological abnormality (GLICK et al. 1989), this is really a histological diagnosis. Suspected colitis has become an indication for primary endoscopy, with some justification, though in acute colitis the instant enema (DCBE without bowel preparation) (THOMAS 1979) is a safer examination yielding adequate diagnostic information. In chronic colitis a DCBE gives an excellent road map of the colitis, and is better than endoscopy at demonstrating strictures of fistula. Considerable endoscopic effort has been put into screening for cancer in ulcerative colitis, though its value is debated and interval cancers reported. The rational for screening is the histological detection of severe dysplasia from endoscopic biopsies. Macrodysplastic elevated lesions are a marker for early cancer, but may be difficult to diagnose endoscopically when all the mucosa is grossly abnormal. The DCBE has advantages in being able to show small elevated lesions in these circumstances, and particularly any irregular infiltration in the base of a dysplastic mass lesion that has become an early carcinoma. Endoscopic biopsy of such lesions may show only severe dysplasia.

There is also a diagnostic threshold for polyp diagnosis on DCBE. Using current techniques, polyps <5 mm are not diagnosed reliably. The double-contrast technique has the sensitivity to resolve minute polyps, but the distinction from retained residue is difficult. To avoid a step increase in false-positive diagnoses, it is common practice to report polyps <5 mm only when the radiographic signs are unequivocal. Colonoscopy has no such disadvantage, and with dye spray and video magnification the mucosal pattern may be examined in minute detail.

The detection and removal of diminutive polyps (<5 mm) has been considered important, as it was assumed that all adenomas, irrespective of size, had the same potential for growth and malignant change. Small rectal and duodenal polyps in familial adenomatous polyposis may regress, and a recent endoscopic study has shown that in the colon polyps 5–9 mm in size frequently regress (HOFSTAD et al. 1996). A Japanese study (NEYAMA et al. 1995), using high-quality DCBE to follow 125 polyps <6 mm in size for a mean of 24 months, showed that 86 did not change in size, 4 decreased by 1 mm, 27 increased by 1 mm, and 8 increased by 2–3 mm. A postulate is that adenomas are capable of spontaneous regression until oncogenic mutation has occurred. Mutation would seem to be present in polyps >10 mm, as malignancy is rare in smaller polyps, becoming frequent in larger ones. There is evidence that the cancer risk of diminutive adenomas has been over-emphasised,

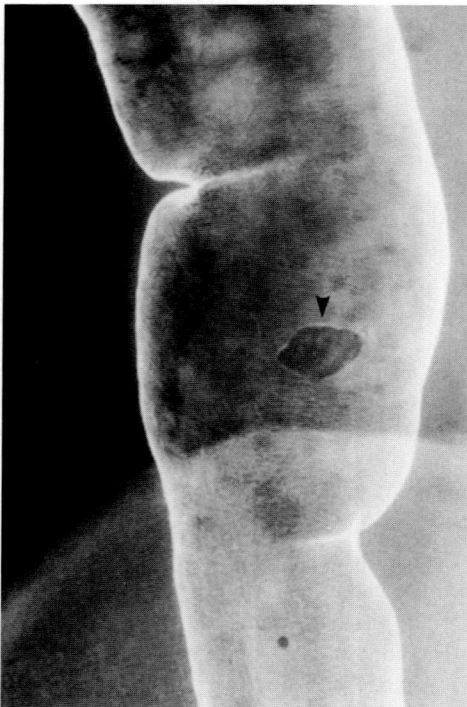

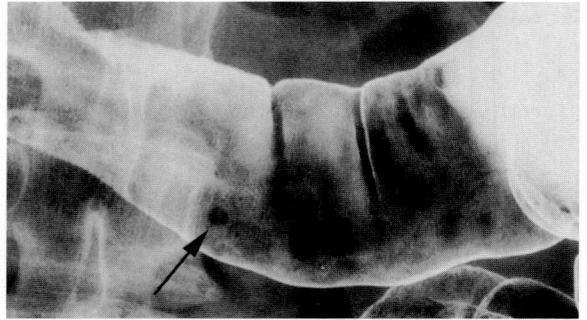

Fig. 8.2. Flat adenoma (3 mm in diameter) in the transverse colon with a central depression shown on close up (*arrowhead*). (Courtesy of Dr. Maruyama, Cancer Institute Hospital, Tokyo)

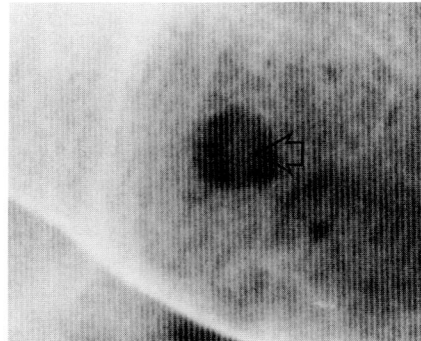

Fig. 8.1. Flat adenoma, 10 mm in diameter, in the descending colon showing a contour line (*arrowhead*). Note that the innominate groove pattern is visible. (Courtesy of Dr. Maruyama, Cancer Institute Hospital, Tokyo)

and endoscopic resection of all these is not obligatory. This strengthens the role of the DCBE in cancer surveillance, as the sensitivity for detection of polyps >9 mm is high.

Work from Japan, originally by Muto (MUTO et al. 1985), suggests that cancer may also develop for a flat, rather than polypoid adenoma as typically seen in the West. The significance of flat adenomas in Western populations has yet to be determined (BOND 1995). These lesions are difficult to detect. In one series (MATSUMOTO et al. 1993) only 11/21 were visible on DCBE. Of 1881 colorectal neoplasms measuring <10 mm in size, 66 were classified as depressed type II lesions (FUJIYA and MARUYAMA 1996) or "flat" adenomas. Of these, 38% were in the transverse colon. Radiographic features were a menisceal contour line (Fig. 8.1) in a small dot of barium in a depressed central area (Fig. 8.2) in about 60%. The key to diagnosis is moderate distension of the lumen (MARUYAMA 1992), so that the contour deformity of the lesion is retained (Fig. 8.3). This is easily effaced with overdistension.

A major change in clinical practice has been the replacement of rigid by flexible sigmoidoscopy.

Fig. 8.3. A 3-mm adenoma seen in profile (*arrowhead*), with close up showing central depression. Note that the colon is only moderately distended. All the cases illustrated were diagnosed radiographically prior to endoscopy. (Courtesy of Dr. Maruyama, Cancer Institute Hospital, Tokyo)

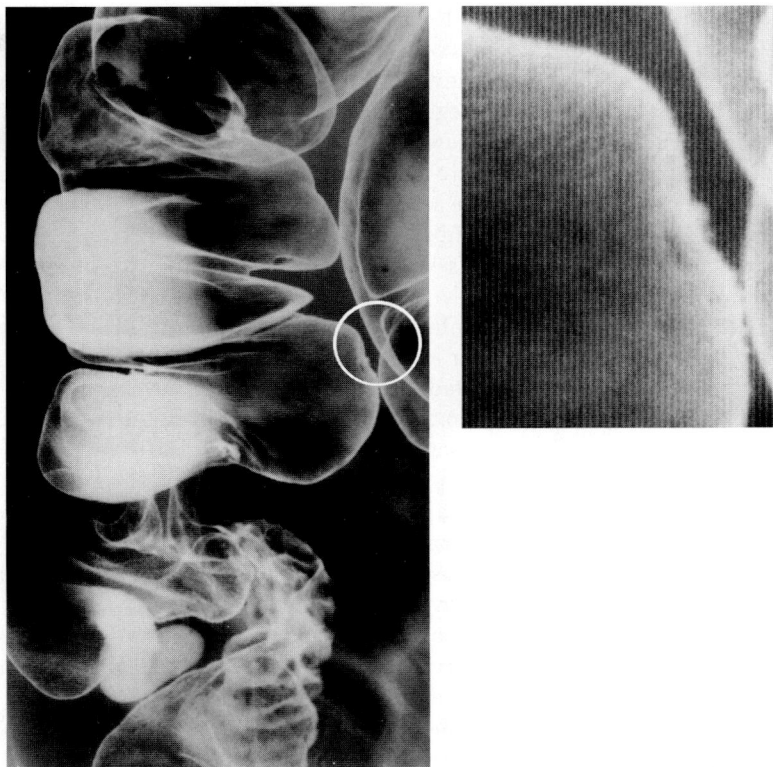

Rigid sigmoidoscopy is limited to the rectum and distal sigmoid. Flexible sigmoidoscopy examines the entire sigmoid, supporting a weak area in DCBE diagnosis. The argument for total colonoscopy after flexible sigmoidoscopy is less robust than for rigid sigmoidoscopy. If polyps have been found at sigmoidoscopy, total colonoscopy to perform polypectomy is the logical choice (STEVENSON 1991). However, if flexible sigmoidoscopy is negative, then considerations of total colonic examination, safety, ease and cost become more relevant. The DCBE provides a complete study, whereas colonoscopy is complete in only 75%–95% of cases. Barium enema is easier, cheaper and considerably safer. A recent survey (BLAKEBOROUGH et al. 1997) has shown a mortality of only 1 in 56786 for DCBE, 5 times safer than diagnostic total colonoscopy. Potential radiation hazards have also been reduced significantly with digital imaging. The combination of DCBE and flexible sigmoidoscopy has been shown to work well, with 100% sensitivity for detection of cancer and polyps >5mm in size (HOUGH et al. 1994).

The development of double-contrast techniques has depended on technical innovation. Fluoroscopy with simple fluorescent screens limited barium radiology to single contrast. It was not practical to perform double-contrast studies until image intensification enabled these images to be seen fluoroscopically. CT has been recommended as the primary examination in the frail elderly (DIXON et al. 1995), though its diagnostic capability is limited. Cross-sectional imaging of the prepared gas-distended bowel with 3D reconstruction offers considerable potential for the diagnosis of polypoid lesions in particular; it is, however, premature to suggest that this should replace DCBE. DCBE remains the examination of choice for fine mucosal detail. The diagnosis of flat adenomas represents a challenge to increase the sensitivity of DCBE in a comparable way to the double-contrast examinations of the stomach developed to diagnose early gastric cancer. DCBE is a very cost-effective procedure. Training technologists (MANNION et al. 1995; SOMERS et al. 1981) to perform DCBEs is a way of maintaining a low-cost examination that will be attractive to healthcare providers.

8.3
Colorectal Function

The colon is separated from the small bowel by the ileocaecal valves, a crescentic fold with sphincteric function (PELLIGRINI et al. 1995) that delivers a liquid chyme into the proximal colon. Water reabsorption in the colon converts this into semi-solid faeces. After a meal irregular non-propulsive segmental contractions associated with some higher amplitude contractions that are propulsive in either direction over a short distance are seen in the colon. About 4–5 times a day high-amplitude mass contractions move colonic contents distally. Distension of the distal rectum induces a desire to defaecate. The recto-anal reflex lowers internal sphincter tone, preparing the anorectum for defaecation (KAMM et al. 1992). If this is inhibited, increased tone in the rectum allows retrograde movement of faeces as the colon relaxes and the sensation to defaecate diminishes. If defaecation takes place, the left side of the colon may be emptied by a combination of colonic contraction moving faecal material into the rectum after each stool is passed. Defaecation is therefore a complex function involving physiological co-ordination between the rectum and the colon.

Constipation, defined as infrequent and/or excessive straining at defaecation, was originally thought to be solely colonic in origin. Slow transit constipation is associated with reduced mass colonic contractions (BASSOTTI et al. 1992), and typically affects young females. Symptoms of bloating and abdominal pain are secondary to faecal retention. However, radiographic and physiological studies suggested that an evacuatory problem might also be present (TURNBULL et al. 1988) in many of these patients, with paradoxical contraction of the pelvic floor instead of relaxation during defaecation. Anismus (PRESTON and LENNARD-JONES 1985) has become an accepted term for this. The investigation of chronic idiopathic constipation therefore involves assessment of colonic transit and evacuation.

Feacal incontinence is graded by loss of continence to gas, liquid or formed stool. Most incontinence was considered neurogenic in origin until endosonography revealed that in women incontinence was often secondary to obstetric trauma (BARTRAM and SULTAN 1995). Endo-anal sonography, and recently magnetic resonance imaging (MRI), have become essential investigations in patients presenting with faecal incontinence to ascertain whether there is sphincter damage amenable to surgical repair.

8.3.1
Colonic Transit Studies

The transit of an object through the gut may be assessed from the time it takes to appear in the stool, though a more convenient method is to measure the disappearance for a radio-opaque marker from the colon with a plain film. A number of variations of this basic technique are in use. The simplest is to give 20 markers on day 1, with a plain film on day 6, when >80% should have passed (HINTON et al. 1969), or put another way, four or less markers should remain. A problem with a single set of markers is that just one bowel action during the study period may mean that most of the markers are passed, in spite of reduced bowel frequency. Instead three different shaped markers (EVANS et al. 1992) may be given on days 1, 2 and 3 with a film on day 6. The normal range is <5 day 1 markers, <6 day 2 markers and <12 day 3 markers.

The concept of segmental transit was introduced by ARHAN et al. (1981), where the transit times in three colonic segments were calculated from multiple markers and films. A simplified technique (METCALF et al. 1987), using three sets of markers and only one abdominal film, allows assessment of total colonic transit time (35 ± 2.1 h), right colon (11.3 ± 1.1 h), left colon (11.4 ± 1.4 h) and rectosigmoid (12.4 ± 1.1 h). Comparison with scintigraphy has shown that the markers give an accurate representation of colonic transit (VAN DER SIJP et al. 1993). The problem is that although the concept of segmental transit may be valid with regular bowel function, changes in segmental transit in response to slow overall transit are not clearly understood. Transit studies give an overall assessment of bowel frequency. Retention of markers indicates reduced frequency, and classifies the patient as having "slow colonic transit".

8.3.2
Evacuation Proctography

Various terms are used to describe fluoroscopy of voluntary rectal voiding. Dynamic rectal examination (WIERSMA et al. 1994) and evacuation proctography (EP) (BARTRAM et al. 1988) suggest the functional nature of the examination, without implying simulation of defaecation. As has been discussed, defaecation involves integrated action between the colon and rectum. These elements are absent in EP, which is only a passive test of voluntary rectal emptying. Initial over-enthusiasm for EP has turned to criticism for lack of diagnostic specificity. This is as much a reflection of the clinical options for treatment as it is of the examination itself. There are specific EP parameters that allow patients to be placed within treatment-defined groups. However, as with functional abnormalities in general, management remains controversial.

Evacuation proctography may be standard or extended. The basic examination involves first cleansing the rectum, with either suppositories or a disposable enema, and opacifying the small bowel by giving an oral mixture of 200 ml water, 100 ml barium suspension (100% wt/vol) with 30 ml Gastrografin. Gastrointestinal transit of this is rapid with adequate radiographic density. After 30 min, 120–250 ml of a barium paste (Evacupaste, E-Z-EM Inc., Westbury, New York) is carefully injected into the rectum. The vagina may also be opacified, preferably using a contrast gel (ARCHER et al. 1992) rather than contrast gauze soaked as this may splint the vagina. The patient is seated on a commode, containing filtration equivalent to 4 mm of copper to prevent screen flare out, placed sideways on the footstep of the upright screening table. Lateral fluoroscopy of the rectum is performed during evacuation, and recorded using either video, cut film or digital imaging with a dose reduced programme and one film per second (Fig. 8.4). Extended EP involves additional opacification of the bladder (HOCK et al. 1993;

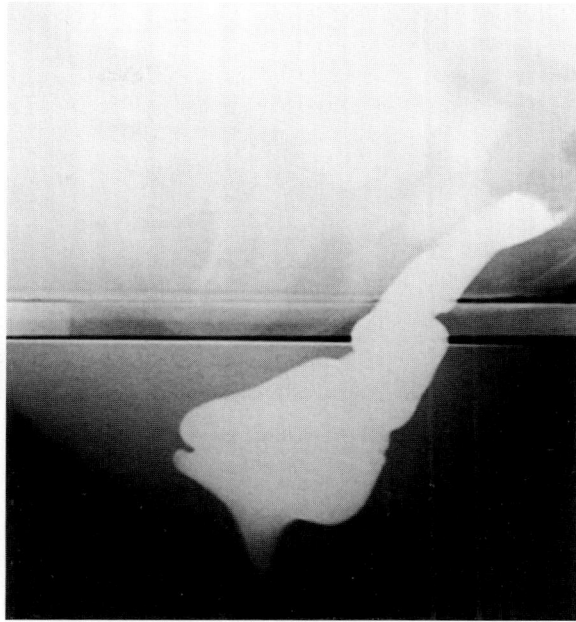

Fig. 8.5. There is marked pelvic floor descent with excessive straining in this 45-year-old female with anismus. After >30 s of evacuation, the rectum has only emptied a little and there is poor opening of the anal canal

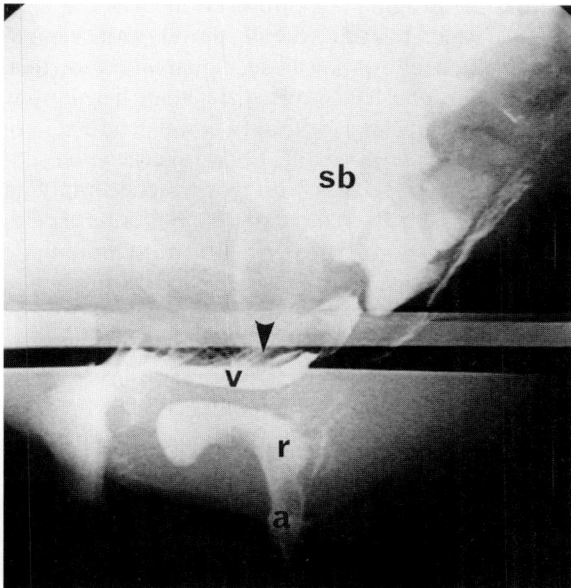

Fig. 8.4. Evacuation proctogram image from digital recording taken towards the end of evacuation. The opacified small bowel (*sb*) is seen extending down into the pouch of Douglas. The vagina (*v*) has also been opacified and is closely related to the rectum (*r*), where a small anterior rectocoele is present. There is no clear distinction from the anal canal (*a*) as the anorectal junction has become effaced during evacuation. The ischial tuberosity (*arrowhead*) is within the field of view and acts as a reference point for measurements of pelvic floor descent

ALTRINGER et al. 1995) so that cystocoele may also be diagnosed, and the entire pelvic floor assessed.

EP parameters related to clinical disorders are as follows:

1. *Time to evacuate and completeness of evacuation*: Normal emptying of the rectal ampulla (that part of the rectum below the main fold), taken from the time the anal canal starts to open to when emptying ceases, is rapid (<30 s) and complete. Delayed voiding and failure to empty >66% of the ampulla (Fig. 8.5) are good indicators of anismus (HALLIGAN et al. 1995a).

2. *Pelvic floor descent*: The anorectal junction should be at or just above the plane of the ischial tuberosities. If it is below this plane at rest, there may be pelvic floor weakness, and descent during evacuation of >3 cm suggests excessive straining and/or weakness. Though this defines the descending perineal syndrome, this is probably not a distinct clinical entity.

3. *Rectocoeles*: Anterior rectocoele <2 cm in depth, measured from the anterior border of the anal canal to the anterior wall of the rectocoele, is a normal variant in the female. Large rectocoeles are

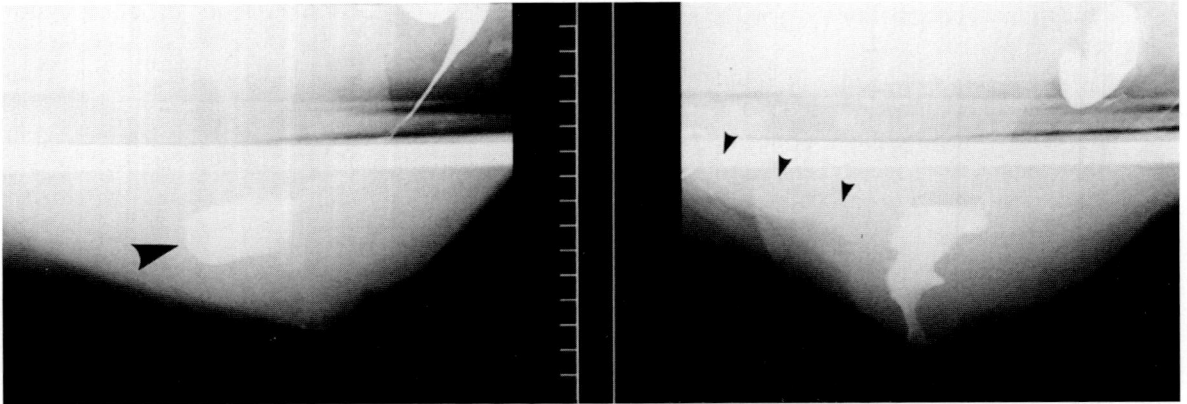

Fig. 8.6. At the end of evacuation there is a small anterior rectocoele (*large arrowhead* in left side view) that has not emptied of barium, though the distal rectum is empty. The patient felt that evacuation was incomplete. The right side view shows the patient digitating (*small arrowheads* outline her finger), pressing on the posterior wall of the rectum to collapse the rectocoele. She was then able to empty the rectum completely and did not experience any further feeling of incomplete evacuation

common in parous women, but seldom functionally significant. Trapping of contrast within the rectocoele at the end of evacuation is associated with a significant pressure drop within the rectocoele (HALLIGAN and BARTRAM 1995a). Although this does not impede rectal emptying, it often leads to a sense of incomplete evacuation, and it may necessitate vaginal digitation (Fig. 8.6) to empty the rectocoele (HALLIGAN et al. 1996).

4. *Rectal intussusception*: Internal prolapse is seen at the end of evacuation when the rectum is almost empty (Fig. 8.7). The distal wall of the rectum folds in on itself, prolapsing down into the anal canal, which is then splayed open by the intussusception. This is best appreciated in the postero-anterior (PA) plane, where the pattern of the collapsing rectum is seen and reveals how the prolapse develops (Fig. 8.8). In the lateral view the rectum is flattened against the levators and it is difficult to distinguish actual prolapse from just asymmetry during rectal collapse. Rectal intussusception has been classified as a normal finding (SHORVON et al. 1989). If there is doubt as to the presence of an intussusception, the patient should be screened in the PA plane during evacuation (McGEE and BARTRAM 1993), as prolongation of a rectal fold into the anal canal provides an unambiguous definition of intra-anal intussusception. Vaginal opacification may preclude PA screening, and should be omitted where prolapse is suspected. External rectal prolapse is not always diagnosed clinically, as patients are reticent to strain adequately. EP is useful to confirm external prolapse in suspected cases.

5. *Enterocoeles*: Separation between the vagina and the rectum during evacuation (Fig. 8.9) indicates filling of an abnormally deep pouch of Douglas with some viscus. Most enterocoeles are due to small bowel, although bladder, uterus or sigmoid colon may also prolapse into the pouch of Douglas. The normal rectovaginal septum is located at the level of the vaginal vault. Small bowel and vaginal opacification allows accurate demarcation of this. Peritoneography has shown that small herniations of the pelvic floor without bowel content are common (HALLIGAN et al. 1995b). Large enterocoeles are not associated with poor rectal emptying (HALLIGAN and BARTRAM 1995a), but enterocoeles extending down into the perineum are symptomatic (Fig. 8.10), causing a sensation of incomplete e vacuation.

Although the anorectal angle is often quoted, its measurement is subject to significant observer variation (PENNINCKX et al. 1990). The axis of the anal canal is clearly defined, but the axis of the posterior rectal wall is less precise. The anorectal angle attained prominence in early work on post anal repair, where static films of the anorectum demarcated by an opaque catheter provided clear definition of the angle. It is of less relevance in dynamic studies. The anorectal angle is related to the position of the pelvic floor: as this descends so the angle opens up. Conversely, if descent is minimal, so is the change in angle. Paradoxical contraction of the puborectalis produces a rounded filling defect in the posterior wall of the distal rectum (Fig. 8.11). This may be seen as part of anismus, but really makes assessment of

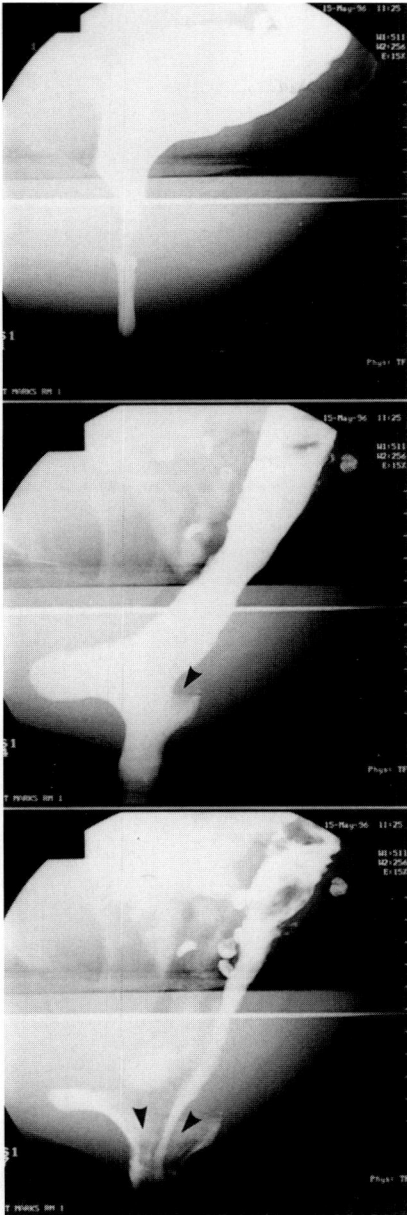

Fig. 8.7. Three views demonstrating the development of an intra-anal intussusception. In the upper view the rectum is at rest. The middle view, during rapid evacuation, reveals an initial infolding of the posterior wall of the rectum (*arrowhead*) leading to a circumferential intussusception (*small arrowheads* in lower view)

The extended proctogram, or dynamic cystoproctography, which incorporates cystography is tailored more for urogynaecological rather than coloproctological interests. Cystography shows a cystocoele and bladder configuration. Funnelling of the bladder neck at rest with absent bladder contraction is said to contraindicate urethropexy. A large undrained cystocoele entering a deep pouch of Douglas may prevent enterocoele, sigmoidocoele or possible rectocoele formation. Conversely, if the rectum is distended, this may stop a cystocoele developing (BENSON and KELVIN 1996). For this reason cystography should be performed prior to rectal opacification during dynamic cystoproctography. Weakness often involves all pelvic floor compartments (HALLIGAN et al. 1996), although a recent MRI study suggests that visceral prolapse at multiple sites is commoner in constipation than in faecal incontinence, where there is greater anorectal junction descent (HEALY et al. 1996).

Biofeedback to retrain pelvic floor co-ordination has proved successful in treating anismus. Surgery has a very limited role in refractory constipation, but repairs of symptomatic enterocoele and rectocoele with trapping, and various procedures for intussusception have proved beneficial. Treatment-defined groups do therefore exist, and using the proctographic parameters described above, patients may be allocated into the appropriate group. Acceptance of these confirms a clear role for EP in the management of pelvic floor disorders.

8.3.3
Endoluminal Imaging of the Anal Sphincters

Evacuation proctography has minimal value in faecal incontinence. An open anal canal at rest with involuntary loss of contrast indicates sphincter weakness. The rectum is often straight and vertical. The volume of contrast that may be retained and ability to close the anal canal give some indication of the degree of sphincter weakness. Abnormal rectal contractility leading to incontinence may be seen in colitis, but unless there is suspected rectal prolapse the examination seldom yields information that affects management. What is important in faecal incontinence is to image damage to the sphincteric mechanism.

The anatomy of the anal sphincters is complex. The circular muscle of the rectum is continuous with the internal sphincter, which is a specialised condensation of circular smooth muscle in the upper half of

the anorectal angle impossible. The anteroposterior diameter of the anal canal may also be measured, and relates to rate of evacuation. As with the anorectal angle, it has no diagnostic value as an isolated feature.

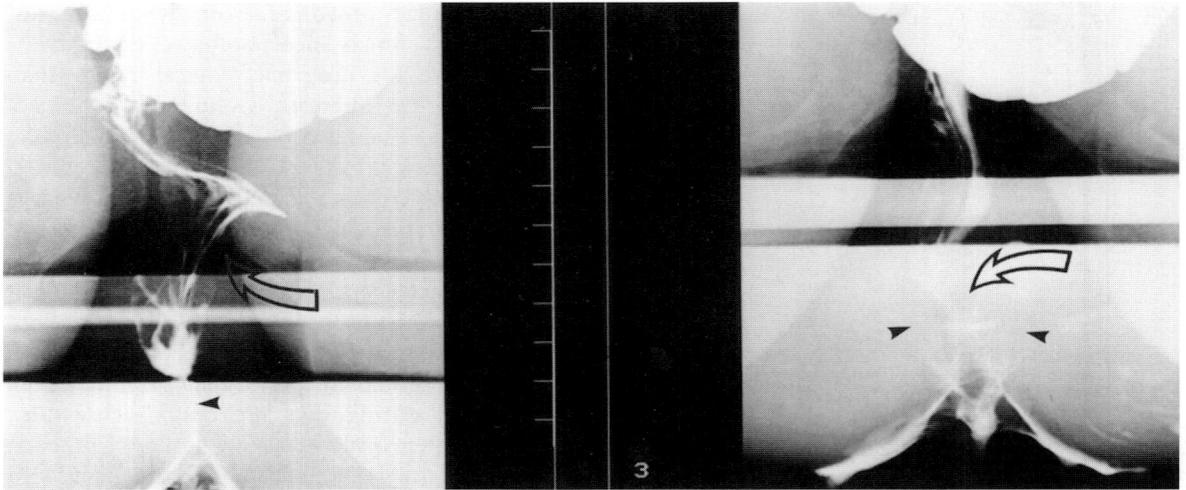

Fig. 8.8. Antero-posterior view of the collapsed rectum. On the left side the patient is at rest and the anal canal a narrow slit (*single arrowhead*). During attempted evacuation the dis-tal rectal fold (*open arrow*) prolapsed down into the anal canal, splaying this open (*arrowheads*)

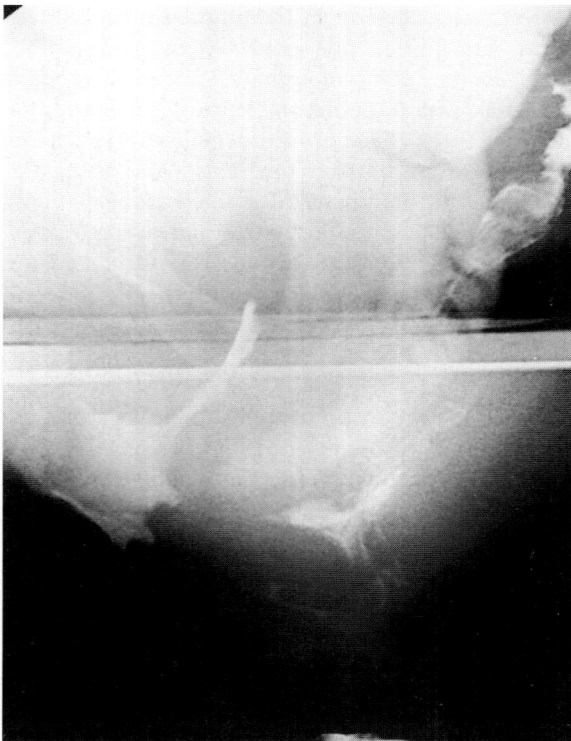

Fig. 8.9. Enterocoele causing marked separation between the rectum and vagina

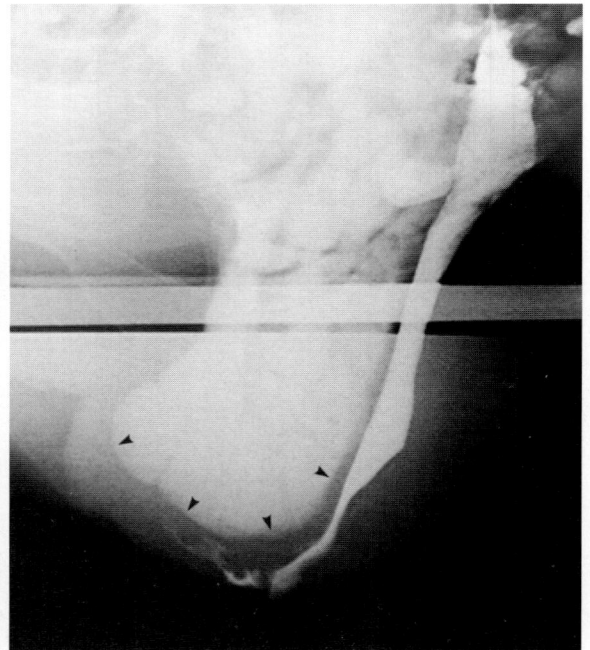

Fig. 8.10. Large enterocoele (*arrowheads*) extending down to the perineum. The presence of the enterocoele caused a sensation of incomplete emptying

the anal canal. This maintains a continuous tone, responsible for 85% of the resting pressure within the canal. It does not close the canal completely. The final seal is provided by the subepithelium and anal cushions, which are specialised subepithelial vascular spaces. The external sphincter is formed from a deep, a superficial and a subcutaneous part. The deep part is closely opposed to the puborectalis. The

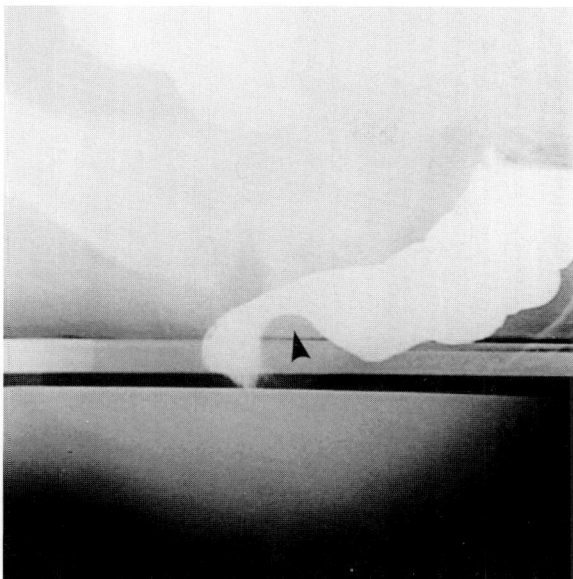

Fig. 8.11. Anismus with a prominent puborectalis impression (*arrowhead*) persisting throughout evacuation

sphincter is composed of striated type I tonic contracting muscle fibres. It is responsible for only about 15% of the resting pressure but all the squeeze pressure, being under voluntary control. The longitudinal muscle is a complex mesh of fibro-elastic tissue with some smooth muscle, permeating throughout the sphincter complex and terminating in the peri-anal skin. Its function is to bind the sphincter together and to the perianal structures.

8.3.3.1
Endosonography

Since its introduction in 1989 (LAW and BARTRAM 1989), anal endosonography has made a significant impact on the management of faecal incontinence. An axial image of the circular sphincteric muscles is optimal, and is provided by the B&K Medical Scanner (Sandtoften 9, Gentofote, Denmark) type 3535 or equivalent using the 1850 axial endoscopic probe with the 6004 type 10-MHz transducer with a hard plastic cone filled with degassed water. This transducer has a focal range of 5–45 mm with an axial resolution of <0.05 mm and lateral resolution of 0.5–1 mm. Transvaginal endosonography has been suggested as an alternative, but is not so accurate for detecting sphincter damage (FRUDINGER et al. 1997). Patients are examined prone to optimise the symmetry of the perineal structures (FRUDINGER

and BARTRAM 1996). The anatomy is complex (BARTRAM and FRUDINGER 1997). The reflectivity of the different layers – subepithelium (moderately reflective), internal sphincter (low reflectivity), longitudinal muscle (moderately reflective) and external sphincter (striated increased reflectivity in the deep part, often poor reflectivity in the superficial part and increased reflectivity in the subcutaneous part) – allows clear anatomic distinction (Fig. 8.12).

Abnormalities in the internal sphincter may be of thickness or integrity. The internal sphincter becomes thicker with age, as the ratio of collagen to smooth muscle increases. In the young adult it is 1–2 mm, in adults 2–3 mm and in the elderly up to 3.4 mm in thickness. Any measurement over 3.5 mm is abnormal, although in younger patients >3 mm would also be abnormal. Very thick sphincters (>5 mm) are found in the rare hereditary internal sphincter myopathy. Most thick internal sphincters in the 3–4.5 mm range seem to be associated with rectal prolapse (Fig. 8.13) and many of these patients have the solitary rectal ulcer syndrome (HALLIGAN et al. 1995b). A subgroup of patients with pas-

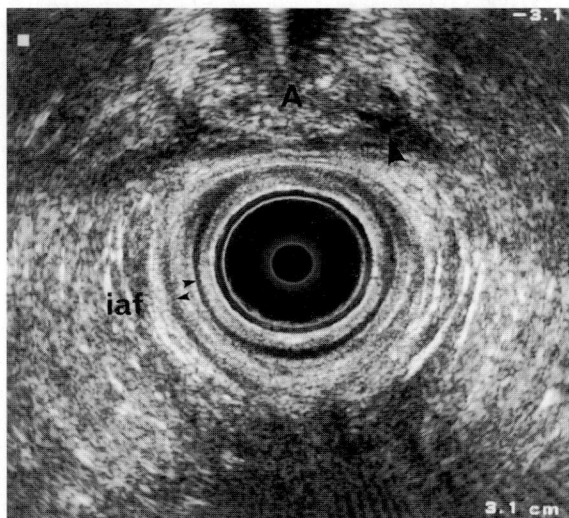

Fig. 8.12. Endosonography in mid canal level in a young female. Anteriorly (*A*) there is a broad moderately reflective arc of the bulbospongiosus. Posterior to this on either side is a triangular low reflective segment of the transverse perineii (*large arrowhead*). The cone creates two concentric bright interfaces. Outside this lies the subepithelium. The internal sphincter (*inner small arrowhead*) is a well-defined low reflective ring. The longitudinal muscle (between the *two small arrowheads*) is moderately reflective, and the external sphincter a thin ring of low reflectivity (*outer small arrowhead*). Outside the sphincter are patchy reflections from stroma and fat within the ischioanal fossa (*iaf*). Posteriorly there is a broad acoustic shadow from the ano-coccygeal ligament

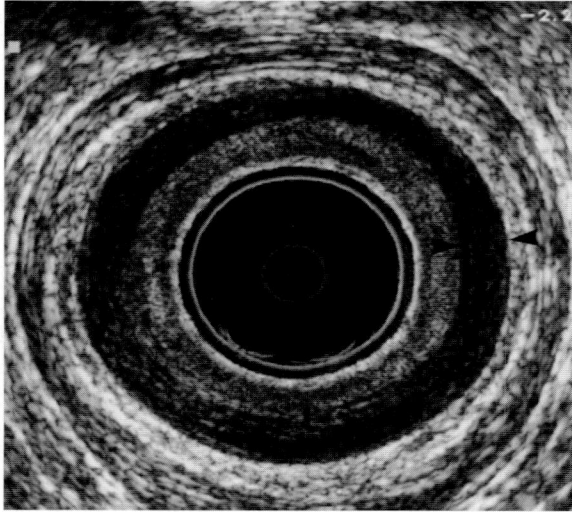

Fig. 8.13. A 27-year-old female patient with the solitary rectal ulcer syndrome. The internal sphincter is abnormally thick (3.8 mm between *arrowheads*) and the subepithelium also prominent

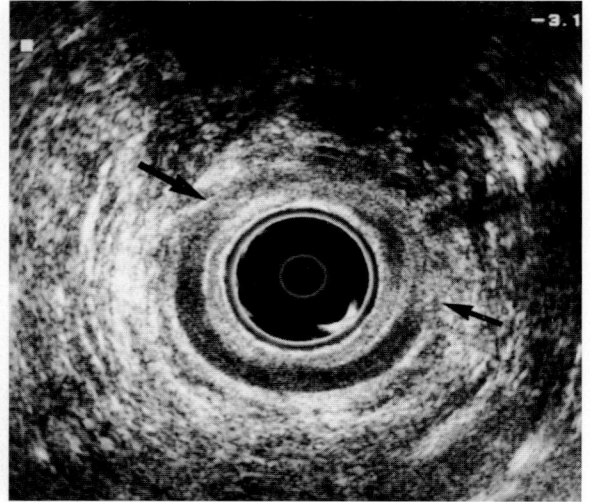

Fig. 8.15. Extensive anterior tear between 10 and 3 o'clock (*arrows*) involving the external and internal anal sphincters, in a 46-year-old female with incontinence following a forceps-assisted delivery some 17 years previously

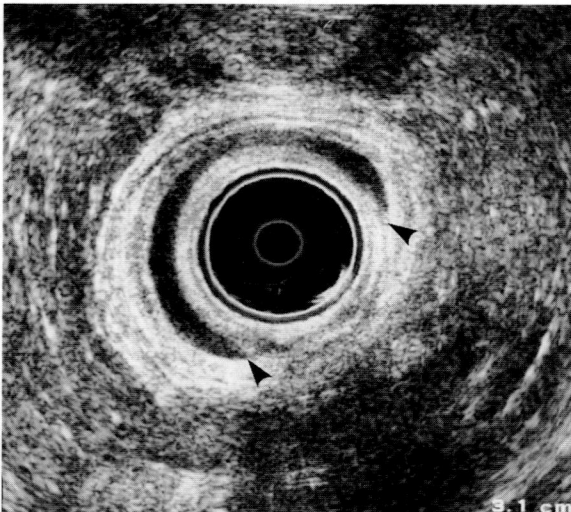

Fig. 8.14. Lateral internal anal sphincterotomy between 3 and 7 o'clock (*arrowheads*)

sive faecal incontinence have an abnormally thin sphincter (<2 mm over 55 years), possibly due to primary internal sphincter degeneration (VAIZEY et al. 1997).

The ring of the internal sphincter should always be intact. Localised thinning may result from abnormal stretching. Anal dilatation procedures can result in either single or multiple breaks in the ring. Fragmentation of the internal sphincter is diagnostic of

this procedure. Lateral sphincterotomy creates a well-defined defect in the lower third (Fig. 8.14). More extensive division may result in incontinence (BARTRAM and SULTAN 1995).

The anal sphincter is subjected to considerable stretching forces during vaginal delivery. These may tear the external, and often also the internal sphincter (Fig. 8.15). As with all tears in striated muscle, these heal with granulation tissue and fibrosis. Fibrous tissue is sonographically amorphous and of medium to low reflectivity, easily distinguishable from the moderately reflective fibrillated pattern of striated muscle. Endosonography has shown that about a third of all vaginal deliveries are associated with some sphincter disruption. Risk factors are forceps delivery, large foetal head and rapid delivery. Sphincter repair is inadequate (Fig. 8.16) unless the anterior ring is restored. An overlapping technique is recommended to achieve this.

Endosonography has been disappointing for anal fistula. The primary track (Fig. 8.17), secondary extension and internal opening may be demonstrated, but no better than by digital examination, although abscesses are detected better sonographically (DEEN et al. 1994). Reduced visualisation outside the sphincter limits the value of endosonography, as complex tracks are difficult to trace.

Malignancy is hyporeflective, and endosonography can accurately stage early disease and recurrence (HERZOG et al. 1994).

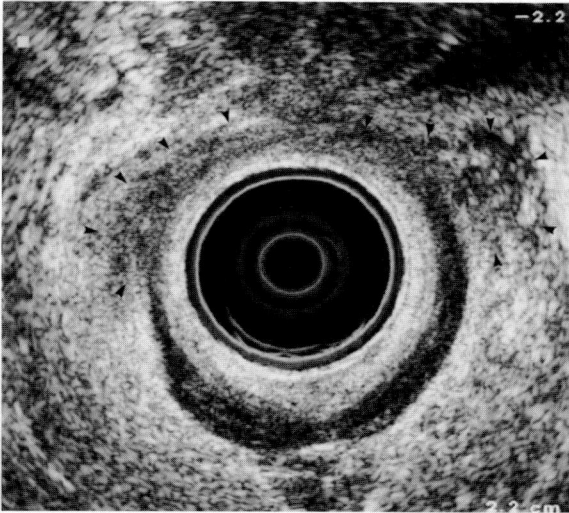

Fig. 8.16. Anterior scarring (*arrowheads*) with persisting external and internal sphincter defects in a 29-year-old female with faecal incontinence following a third degree tear with inadequate primary repair

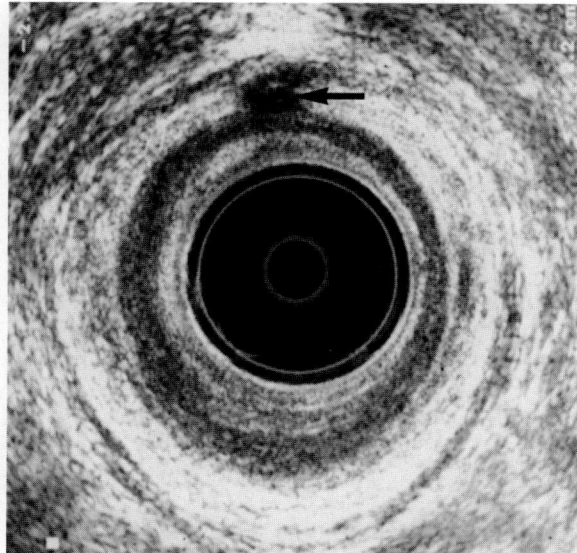

Fig. 8.17. Low reflective primary track running anteriorly in the longitudinal muscle (*arrow*)

8.3.3.2
Endoluminal Magnetic Resonance Imaging

Magnetic resonance imaging (MRI) of the anus has proved unsatisfactory using whole-body coils due to inadequate resolution (pixel size between 1 and 2 mm). At 0.5 T (LUNISS et al. 1994) and 1.5 T (TJANDRA and SISSONS 1994; SCHÄFER et al. 1994) it has not been possible to distinguish the sub-epithelium from the internal anal sphincter, and sometimes not even from the external sphincter.

Surface coils greatly improve signal-to-noise and resolution from adjacent issue. Unfortunately, the development of internal surface receiver coils has been slow. Imaging of the anal sphincter has been attempted with a rectal and an endovaginal coil (YANG et al. 1994). However, the sensitive volume of these coils was not suited to imaging the anus. Coils specifically designed for endo-anal use (DESOUZA et al. 1995a–c; HUSSAIN et al. 1995) have been developed. A cylindrical saddle geometry coil, 9 mm in diameter and 9 cm in length, has proved ideal. The coil is placed inside a rigid protective tube of external diameter 11 mm with a slightly bulbous proximal end. With the subject in the left lateral position the coil can be easily positioned within the canal following digital rectal examination. The subject is then turned supine, and the coil immobilised externally in a clamp (Fig. 8.18) to avoid image degradation from coil movement.

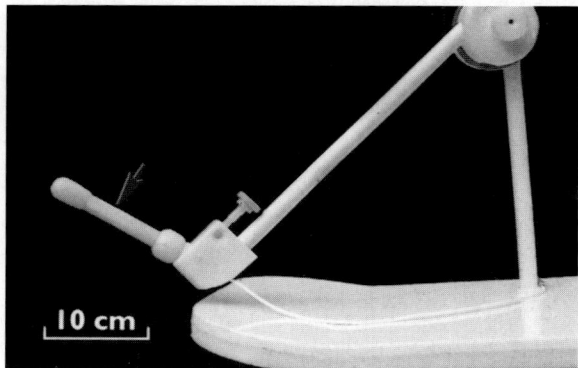

Fig. 8.18. Cylindrical 9-cm length surface coil (*arrow*) positioned in clamp for immobilisation

Standard imaging protocols are used to produce high-resolution images (pixel size ~0.6 mm) with good tissue contrast. Adequate information is usually obtained using T1-weighted spin-echo [SE 720/20 (TR/TE) ms], T2-weighted spin-echo [SE 2500/80 (TR/TE) ms] and short TI inversion recovery [STIR 2500/30/110–130 (TR/TE/TI) ms] sequences. Occasionally dynamic scanning after a bolus injection of 0.1 mmol/kg body weight of gadopentetate dimeglumine (Gd-DTPA) and post-contrast images may be helpful: this is particularly so if peri-anal sepsis is suspected.

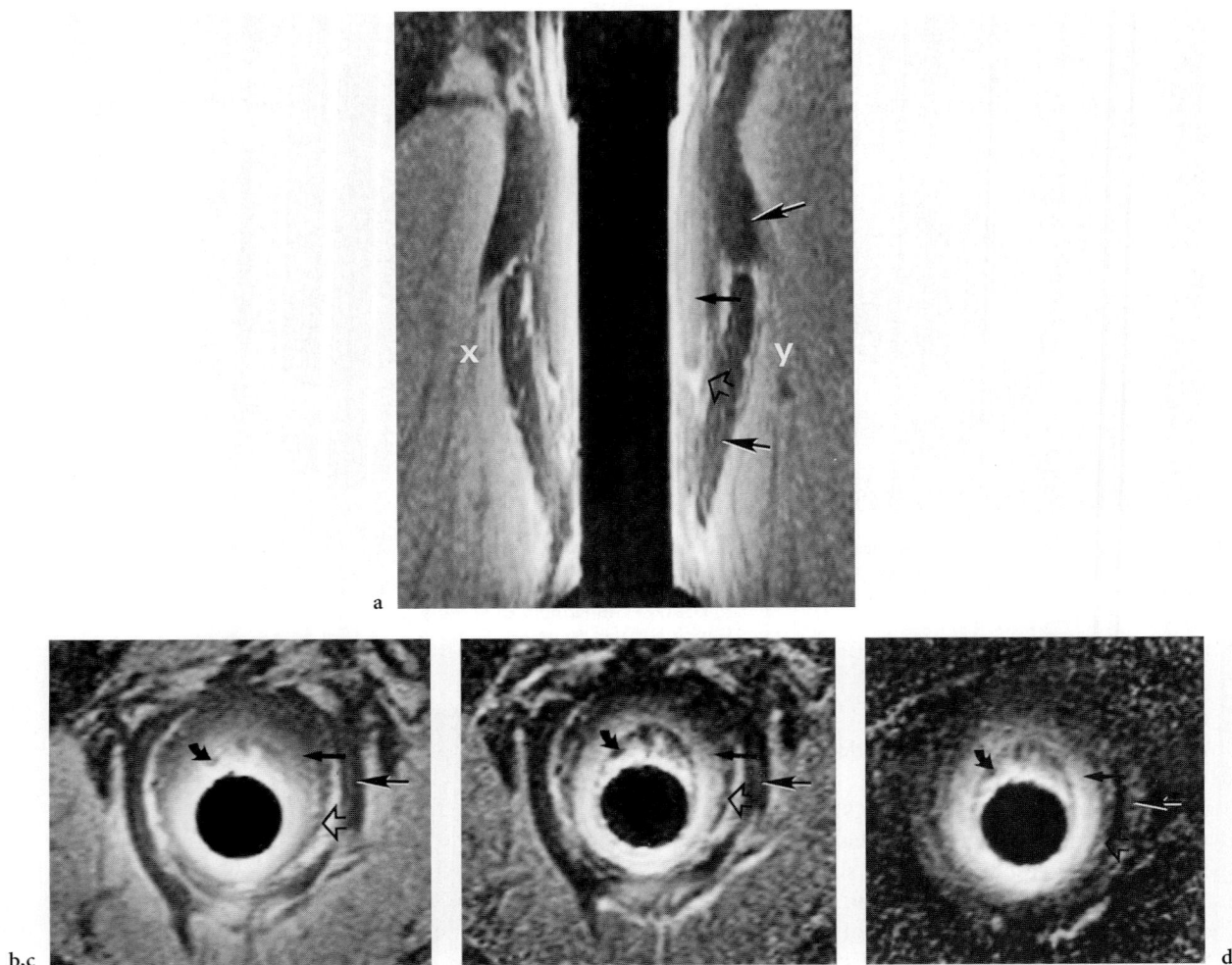

Fig. 8.19a–d. Normal male subject aged 33 years: coronal T1-weighted coronal spin-echo (SE800/20) (**a**) and transverse T1-weighted spin-echo (SE780/20) (**b**), T2-weighted spin-echo (SE2500/80) (**c**) and STIR (IR 2500/30/110 ms) (**d**) images through the mid-section of the anal sphincter at the level of *x* and *y* in **a**. (Anterior is upper and posterior is lower in this and subsequent transverse figures.) The low signal submucosa and adjacent subepithelial muscle (*curved black arrows*) are readily identified. The internal sphincter (*straight black arrows*) has a high signal on all sequences. The longitudinal muscle (*hollow black arrows*) separates the internal and external sphincter on the coronal image and has a low signal intensity beaded appearance on the transverse images. The medial and lateral intersphincteric layers have a high signal intensity in **b** and **c**. The external sphincter (*black and white arrows*) has a low signal on all sequences. Note that the total anal coil diameter is 12 mm, providing a scale for this and subsequent images

The anal sphincter complex is shown in coronal section in Fig. 8.19a with the transverse images in Fig. 8.19b–d. The layers seen from inside out are:

1. *Mucosa*: High signal stripe along the anal canal on all sequences.
2. *Subepithelial tissues*: Low signal smooth muscle and high signal fat (Fig. 8.19b–d); may be thick anteriorly (Fig. 8.19c). Encompasses linear high signal anteriorly from a venous plexus.
3. *Internal sphincter*: High signal on all sequences, particularly on T2-weighted and STIR sequences.
4. *Longitudinal muscle*: Low signal fibre bundles surrounded by high signal fat and fibro-elastic tissue are seen on transverse T1- and T2-weighted images.
5. *External sphincter*: Variable with intermediate to low signal intensity on intensity-corrected images.

The anatomy of the external sphincter is complex. The circular subcutaneous component lies medially and inferior to the internal sphincter with the superficial component contiguous and superior (Fig.

a

b

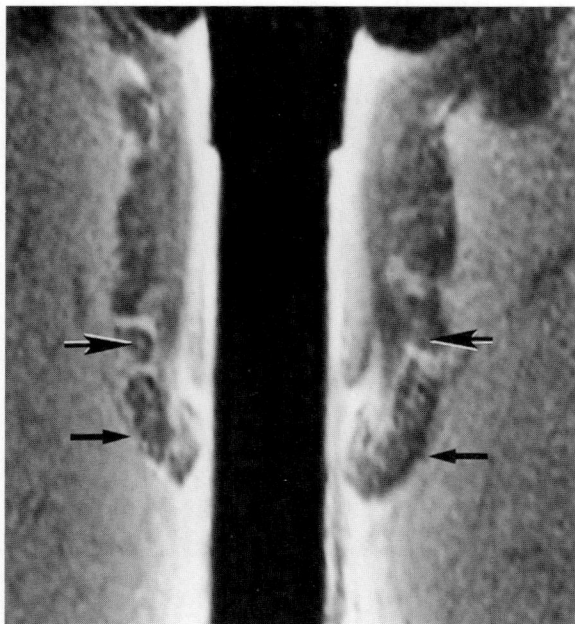

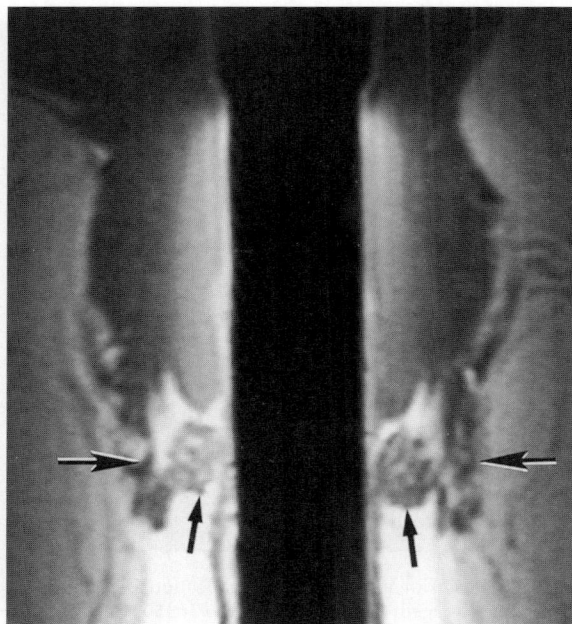

Fig. 8.20. Coronal T1-weighted images (SE800/20) in two normal females aged 41 years (**a**) and 31 years (**b**). The subcutaneous external sphincter (*small black arrows*) caps the internal and superficial external sphincter in **a**. The superficial external sphincter (*black and white arrows*) extends inferiorly and lateral to the subcutaneous sphincter in **b**

8.20a). However, the subcutaneous component sometimes lies medially and superior to the lower limit of the superficial component of the sphincter, which can extend inferior to it and surround it (Fig. 8.20b). The fibres of the superficial external sphincter abut the subcutaneous sphincter and extend superiorly and laterally. Superiorly the superficial sphincter is bound by a fascial plane which is relatively constant (Fig. 8.20a). The deep external sphincter appears continuous with puborectalis posteriorly and is well defined on sagittal images. Anteriorly it is circular and separated from puborectalis. As with endosonography, differences are seen in the perineum and external sphincter anteriorly. In males the superficial fibres insert anteriorly into the central perineum, whereas the sloping anterior aspect of the external sphincter appears incomplete higher in the anterior canal in females.

8.3.3.2.1
SIGNAL INTENSITIES WITH DIFFERENT
PULSE SEQUENCES

The internal sphincter has a high signal intensity for all sequences (Fig. 8.18b–d). There is little difference on T1-weighted intensity-corrected images, but the differences on the T2-weighted and STIR images are more marked. The high signal intensity reflects the smooth muscle content of the internal sphincter. In some cases a thin rim of lower signal at the periphery of the internal sphincter is discernible, which may represent an outer layer of collagen containing the neurovascular bundles.

8.3.3.2.2
CONTRAST ENHANCEMENT

The administration of 0.1 mmol/kg Gd-DTPA enhances the internal sphincter, beginning at 30 s after injection and peaking at 90 s. The external sphincter enhances more slowly and to a much lesser degree. Maximal differentiation between the internal and external sphincters is seen at about 90 s. Contrast enhancement is a feature of smooth muscle, but may also be related to increased metabolic from the tone maintained by the internal sphincter. Normal enhancement should not be mistaken for enhancement secondary to infection or other pathologic process.

8.3.3.2.3
PATHOLOGIC FEATURES

The good anatomic detail produced with endocoils (HUSSAIN et al. 1995) and multiplanar imaging provide an excellent basis for demonstration of disease. The increase signal in T1 and T2 associated with

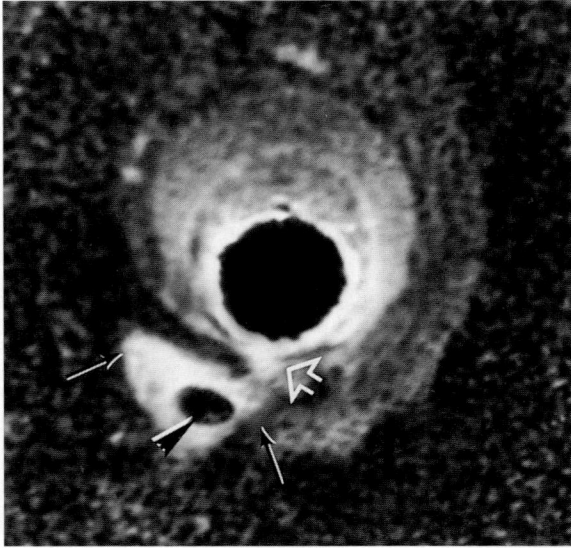

Fig. 8.21. Posterior intrasphincteric collection and fistula-in-ano in a male aged 49 years: transverse IR2500/32/110 scan. The abscess (*black and white arrows*) is highlighted and has a low signal within it (*arrowhead*) due to air. Communication with the anus is seen (*hollow arrow*)

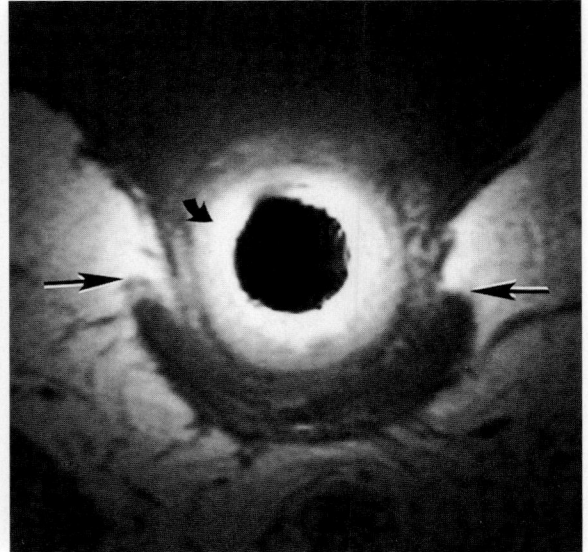

Fig. 8.22. Deep external sphincter tear in a female aged 60 years: transverse SE820/20 image. There is complete division of the external sphincter fibres bilaterally (*black and white arrows*). The internal sphincter remains intact (*curved arrow*)

infection produces high soft tissue contrast to facilitate demonstration of abscesses or fistulous tracks. Although previous studies using a conventional body coil have demonstrated the efficacy of MRI in diagnosing anal fistula (LUNISS et al. 1994) and changes in Crohn's disease (TJANDRA and SISSONS 1994), the greater resolution provided by an internal coil is likely to result in further diagnostic improvement. Contrast enhancement is seen in and around inflammatory lesions and must be distinguished from normal enhancement. Established scar has a low signal on both T1- and T2-weighted images, and is seen in close relation to normal sphincter and surrounding fat. Changes associated with hypertrophy and atrophy are also readily shown.

In peri-anal sepsis STIR images are most useful for highlighting fistulous tracks and fluid collections (Fig. 8.21). The T1-weighted contrast-enhanced scans serve to confirm the information available on STIR, and are particularly useful if the abscess is several centimetres away from the mucosa, when the signal-to-noise drop-off with distance from the coil combined with the lower signal-to-noise of the STIR sequences makes it difficult to define these lesions on STIR. Coronal and sagittal images, in addition to the axial plane, are used to assess the full extent of a fistula. Coronal images show the exact relationship

of the fistula to the levator ani, whereas anterior or posterior extensions are demonstrated best on sagittal images.

Sphincter disruption can be clearly identified with these high-resolution scans (Fig. 8.22). In particular the use of T2-weighted sequences provides tissue contrast between the lower signal external sphincter and the homogeneous higher signal of the circular internal sphincter. Loss of the normal homogeneous high signal intensity of the internal sphincter is easily recognised in internal sphincter disruption.

Magnetic resonance imaging allows clear delineation of tumour extent and invasion (Fig. 8.23) particularly in relation to the levators. The exact distance from each of the components of the external sphincter and the extent of internal sphincter involvement can be accurately assessed prior to surgery.

8.3.3.3
Endosonography Versus Magnetic Resonance Imaging

Magnetic resonance imaging is time consuming and expensive compared with endosonography, which takes less than 5 min. Endosonography is therefore

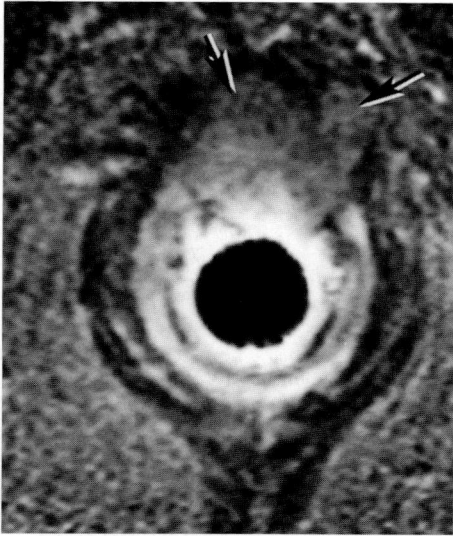

Fig. 8.23. Squamous cell carcinoma in a male aged 68 years: transverse SE2500/80 image. There is a lobulated homogeneous mass extending outside the sphincter (*black and white arrows*)

more suitable for high volume screening in faecal incontinence to detect sphincter abnormality. MRI is the examination of choice in complex anal fistula, though whether an endocoil is needed for this has yet to be proved. The added definition from the endocoil is helpful in patients with possible recurrent sepsis within the sphincter, but sepsis extending above the levators is well seen with just a body coil. MRI defines the external sphincter in greater detail, and endosonography the internal sphincter. Both demonstrate sphincter damage. MRI with an endocoil gives exquisite detail of the muscular structure of the external sphincter, which may be translated into improved interpretation of sonographic images. There is much that is complementary between these two methods, and the choice in a unit may well depend on the volume of patients to be examined.

References

Altringer WE, Saclarides TJ, Dominguez JM, Brubaker LT, Smith CS (1995) Four-contrast defecography: pelvic "flooroscopy". Dis Colon Rectum 38:695–699

Archer BD, Somers S, Stevenson GW (1992) Contrast medium gel for marking vaginal position during defecography. Radiology 182:278–279

Arhan P, Devroede G, Jehannin B, et al. (1981) Segmental colonic transit time. Dis Colon Rectum 24:625–629

Bartram CI, Frudinger A (1997) A handbook of anal endosonography. Wrightson Biomedical, Petersfield, UK and Bristol, Pa., USA

Bartram CI, Sultan AH (1995) Anal endosonography in faecal incontinence. Gut 37:4–6

Bartram CI, Turnbull GK, Lennard-Jones JE (1988) Evacuation proctography: an investigation of rectal expulsion in 20 subjects without defecatory disturbance. Gastrointest Radiol 13:72–80

Bassotti G, Imbimbo BP, Betti C, Dozzini G, Morelli A (1992) Impaired colonic motor response to eating in patients with slow-transit constipation. Am J Gastroenterol 87:504–508

Benson JT, Kelvin FM (1996) Dynamic cystoproctography. In: Blaivas J, Chancellor M (eds) Atlas of urodynamics. Williams and Wilkins, Baltimore, pp 126–144

Blakeborough A, Sheridan MB, Chapman AH (1997) Complications of barium enema examination: a survey of UK consultant radiologists 1992–4. Clin Radiol 52:142–148

Bond JH (1995) Small flat adenomas appear to have little clinical importance in Western countries. Gastrointest Endosc 42:184–187

Deen KI, Williams JG, Hutchinson F, Keighley MR, Kumar D (1994) Fistulas in ano: endoanal ultrasonographic assessment assists decision making for surgery. Gut 35:391–394

deSouza NM, Kmiot WA, Puni R, Hall AS, Bartram CI, Bydder GM (1995a) High resolution magnetic resonance imaging of the anal sphincter using an internal coil. Gut 37:284–287

deSouza NM, Puni R, Gilderdale DJ, Bydder GM (1995b) Magnetic resonance imaging of the anal sphincter using an internal coil. Magn Reson Q 11:45–46

deSouza NM, Puni R, Kmiot WA, Bartram CI, Hall AS, Bydder GM (1995c) MRI of the anal sphincter. J Comput Assist Tomogr 19:745–751

Dixon AK, Freeman AH, Coni NK (1995) CT of the colon in frail elderly patients. Clin Radiol 16:165–172

Evans RC, Kamm MA, Hinton JM, Lennard-Jones JE (1992) The normal range and a simple diagram for recording whole gut transit time. Int J Colorect Dis 7:15–17

Frudinger A, Bartram CI (1996) Patient position and manoeuvres during anal endosonography. Accepted in publication Abdom. Imaging.

Frudinger A, Bartram CI, Kamm MA (1997) Transvaginal endosonography compared to anal endosonography in the detection of anal sphincter defects. AJR 168:1435–1438

Fujiya M, Maruyama M (1997) Small depressed neoplasm of the large bowel; its radiographic visualisation and clinical significance. Adom. Imaging 22:325–331

Glick SN, Teplick SK, Amenta PS (1989) Microscopic (collagenous) colitis. AJR 153:955–996

Halligan S, Bartram CI (1995a) Is barium trapping in rectoceles significant? Dis Colon Rectum 38:764–768

Halligan MS, Bartram CI (1995b) Evacuation proctography combined with positive contrast peritoneography to demonstrate pelvic floor hernias. Abdom Imaging 20:442–445

Halligan MS, Bartram CI (1996) Is digitation associated with proctographic abnormality? Int J Colorect Dis 11:167–171

Halligan S, Bartram CI, Park HJ, Kamm MA (1995a) The proctographic features of anismus. Radiology 197:679–682

Halligan S, Sultan A, Rottenberg G, Bartram CI (1995b) Endosonography of the anal sphincters in solitary rectal ulcer syndrome. Int J Colorectal Dis 10:79–82

158   C.I. Bartram

Halligan MS, Spence-Jones C, Kamm MA, Bartram CI (1996) Dynamic cystoproctography and physiologal testing in women with urinary stress incontinence and urogenital prolapse. Clin Radiol 51:785–790

Hara AK, Johnson CD, Reed JE, Ehman RL, Ilstrup DM (1996) Colorectal polyp detection with CT colography: two- versus three-dimensional techniques. Radiology 200:49–54

Healy JC, Halligan MS, Reznek RH, Watson S, Phillips RK, Armstrong P (1997) Patterns of prolapse in female patients with symptoms of pelvic floor weakness. Assessment with MR Imaging

Herzog U, Boss M, Spichtin HP (1994) Endoanal ultra-sonography in the follow-up of anal carcinoma. Surg Endosc 8:1186–1189

Hinton JM, Lennard-Jones JE, Young AC (1969) A new method for studying gut transit times using radio-opapue markers. Gut 10:842–847

Hock D, Lombard R, Jehaes C, et al. (1993) Colpocy-stodefecography. Dis Colon Rectum 36:1015–1021

Hofstad B, Vatn MH, Andersen SN, et al. (1996) Growth of colorectal polyps: redetection and evaluation of unresected polyps for a period of three years. Gut 39:449–456

Hough DM, Malone DE, Rawlinson J, et al. (1994) Colon cancer detection: an algorithm using endoscopy and barium enema. Clin Radiol 49:170–175

Hussain SM, Stoker J, Lameris JS (1995) Anal sphincter complex: endoanal MR imaging of normal anatomy. Radiology 197:671–677

Kamm MA, van der Sijp JR, Lennard-Jones JE (1992) Observations on the characteristics of stimulated defaecation in severe idiopathic constipation. Int J Colorectal Dis 7:197–201

Law PJ, Bartram CI (1989) Anal endosonography: technique and normal anatomy. Gastrointest Radiol 14:349–353

Luniss PH, Barker PG, Sultan AH, et al. (1994) Magnetic resonance imaging of fistula-in-ano. Dis Colon Rectum 37:708–718

Mannion RA, Bewell J, Langan C, Robertson M, Chapman AH (1995) A barium enema training programme for radiographers: a pilot study. Clin Radiol 50:715–718

Maruyama M (1992) Early diagnosis of gastrointestinal cancer. In: Laufer I, Levine MS (eds) Double contrast gastrointestinal radiology, 2nd edn. Saunders, Philadelphia, pp 495–532

Matsumoto T, Iida M, Kohrogi N, et al. (1993) Minute nonpolypoid adenomas of the colon depicted with barium enema examination. Radiology 187:377–380

McGee SG, Bartram CI (1993) Intra-anal intussusception: diagnosis by posteroanterior stress proctography. Abdom Imaging 18:136–140

Metcalf AM, Phillips SF, Zinsmeister AR, MacCarty RL, Beart RW, Wolff BG (1987) Simplified assessment of segmental colonic transit. Gastroenterology 92:40–47

Muto T, Kamiya J, Sawada T, et al. (1985) Small "flat adenoma" of the large bowel with special reference to its clinicopathologic features. Dis Colon Rectum 28:847–851

Pelligrini MSF, Manneschi LI, Manneschi L (1995) The caecolonic junction in humans has a sphincteric anatomy and function. Gut 37:493–498

Penninckx F, Debruyne C, Lestar B, Kerremans R (1990) Observer variation in the radiological measurement of the anorectal angle. Int J Colorectal Dis 5:94–97

Preston DM, Lennard-Jones JE (1985) Anismus in chronic constipation. Dig Dis Sci 5:413–418

Schäfer A, Enck P, Fürst G, Kahn T, Frieling T, Lübke TJ (1994) Anatomy of the anal sphincters. Comparison of anal endosonography to magnetic resonance imaging. Dis Colon Rectum 37:777–781

Shorvon PJ, McHugh S, Diamant NE, Somers S, Stevenson GW (1989) Defecography in normal volunteers: results and implications. Gut 30:1737–1749

Somers S, Stevenson GW, Laufer I, Gledhill L, Nugent J (1981) Evaluation of double contrast barium enemas performed by radiographic technologists. J Can Assoc Radiol 32:227–228

Stevenson GW (1991) Medical imaging in the prevention, diagnosis, and management of colon cancer. In: Herlinger H, Megibow AJ (eds) Advances in gastrointestinal radiology. Mosby Year Book, St. Louis, pp 1–20

Thomas BM (1979) The instant enema in inflammatory disease of the colon. Clin Radiol 30:165–168

Tjandra JJ, Sissons GRJ (1994) Magnetic resonance imaging facilitates assessment of perianal Crohn's disease. Aust NZ J Surg 64:470–474

Turnbull GK, Bartram CI, Lennard-Jones JE (1988) Radiologic studies of rectal evacuation in adults with idiopathic constipation. Dis Colon Rectum 31:190–197

Neyama T, Kawamoto K, Iwashita I et al. (1995) Natural history of minute sessile colonie adenomas based on radiographic findings. Is endoscopic removal of every clonie adenoma necessary? Dis Colon Rectum 38:268–272

Vaizey CJ, Kamm MA, Bartram CI (1997) Primary internal sphincter degeneration – a newly recognised cause of passive faecal incontinence. Lancet 349:612–615

van der Sijp JR, Kamm MA, Nightingale JM, et al. (1993) Radioisotope determination of regional colonic transit in severe constipation: comparison with radio opaque markers. Gut 34:402–408

Wall LL, Helms M, Peattie AB, Pearce M, Stanton SL (1994) Bladder neck mobility and the outcome of surgery for genuine stress urinary incontinence. A logistic regression analysis of lateral bead-chain cystourethrograms. J Reprod Med 39:429–435

Welin S (1967) Results of the Malmo technique of colon examination. JAMA 199:369

Wiersma TG, Mulder CJ, Reeders JW, Tytgat GN, Van Waes PF (1994) Dynamic rectal examination (defecography). Baillieres Clin Gastroenterol 8:729–741

Yang A, Yang SS, Mostwin JL, Berg HK, Vachom DA, Genadry RR (1994) Anatomic and pathologic components of rectal continence and prolapse: demonstration with dynamic and high-resolution static MR imaging. Radiology 193p:438

9 Peritoneal Reflections, Ligaments, Recesses, and Mesenteries

M.A. Meyers and R.E. Mindelzun

CONTENTS

9.1
Introduction

The peritoneal cavity is the largest lumen in the body. It is lined by a serosal layer which reflects at multiple specific sites to constitute mesenteries and ligaments, extending to support and ensheath parenchymal organs and bowel. The scaffolds provided by the mesenteries and ligaments – conveying subserous connective tissue, nerves, blood vessels,

M.A. Meyers, MD, FACR, FACG, Professor of Radiology and Medicine, Department of Radiology, School of Medicine, Health Sciences Center, S.U.N.Y. at Stony Brook, Stony Brook, NY 11794-8460, USA
R.E. Mindelzun, MD, FACR, Associate Professor of Radiology, Department of Radiology, School of Medicine, Stanford University, 300 Pasteur Drive, Room H 1307, Stanford, CA 94305-5105, USA

and lymphatics – serve as pathways for the dissemination of disease between diverse sites. These same structures contribute to the formation of multiple recesses or compartments within the peritoneal cavity. Because of the dynamic circulation of intraperitoneal fluid related to physical and anatomic factors and local responses, these reflections and recesses serve as watershed areas and drainage basins for inflammatory, hemorrhagic, and malignant effusions. These modes of pathogenesis and the characteristic radiologic features have been firmly established and clearly documented (Meyers 1994, 1970a,b, 1973a,b, 1975, 1976, 1981a,b; Meyers and Whalen 1971, 1973; Meyers and McSweeney 1972; Meyers and Evans 1973; Meyers et al. 1973a,b, 1981, 1987; Churchill and Meyers 1986; Oliphant and Berne 1982; Oliphant et al. 1986, 1988, 1993a,b, 1994, 1995, 1996). It is fundamental that technological advances in imaging have both consistently confirmed these original insights regarding pathogenesis (Auh et al. 1994; Arenas et al. 1994; DeMeo et al. 1995) and further extended the clinical capabilities for diagnosis and determination of the most appropriate management options.

The mesenteries, furthermore, may themselves give rise to congenital disorders and primary tumors, and react to other regional or systemic conditions.

A brief review of key anatomic and dynamic considerations is basic to an understanding of the spread and localization of intraperitoneal abscesses, seeded metastases (peritoneal carcinomatosis), and planes of dissemination.

9.2
Anatomic and Dynamic Considerations

9.2.1
The Posterior Peritoneal Attachments and Peritoneal Spaces

Figure 9.1 indicates the peritoneal reflections from the posterior abdominal wall deep to the bowel, liver,

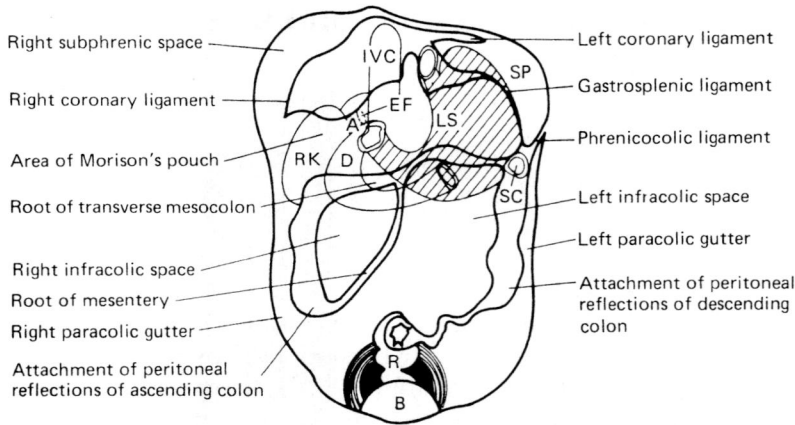

Fig. 9.1. Posterior peritoneal reflections and recesses. *SP*, spleen; *LS*, Lesser sac; *IVC*, inferior vena cava; *EF*, epiploic foramen of Winslow; *RK*, right kidney; *D*, duodenum; *A*, adrenal gland; *SC*, splenic flexure of colon; *R*, rectum; *B*, urinary bladder. The removed stomach is indicated. (Modified from MEYERS 1970a)

and spleen. The transverse mesocolon constitutes the major barrier dividing the abdominal cavity into supramesocolic and inframesocolic compartments. The obliquely oriented root of the small bowel mesentery further divides the inframesocolic compartment into a smaller right infracolic space and a larger left infracolic space, which is open anatomically toward the pelvis.

The pelvis is the most dependent part of the peritoneal cavity in either the supine or the erect position. Its compartments include the midline cul-de-sac or pouch of Douglas (rectovaginal pouch in the female and rectovesical pouch in the male) and the lateral paravesical recesses. It is anatomically continuous with both lateral paracolic gutters. The right paracolic gutter is wide and deep and is continuous superiorly with the right subhepatic space and its posterosuperior extension deep to the liver, Morison's pouch (MORISON 1894) (also known as the right posterior subhepatic space or as the hepatorenal fossa). Morison's pouch is of great significance in the spread and localization of intraperitoneal infections and seeded metastases since it is the lowest part of the right paravertebral groove when the body is in the supine position. Posteriorly and medially, the reflections of the right coronary ligament separate the right subhepatic and subphrenic spaces. The right subhepatic space is anatomically continuous with the right subphrenic space around the lateral edge of the right coronary ligament of the liver. The right subphrenic space is a large continuous compartment extending over the diaphragmatic surface of the right lobe of the liver to its margination posteriorly and inferiorly by the right coronary ligament. The falciform ligament separates the right and left subphrenic spaces. In contrast, the left paracolic gutter is narrow and shallow and is

interrrupted from continuity with the left subphrenic space (perisplenic or left perihepatic space) by the phrenicocolic ligament, which extends from the splenic flexure of the colon to the left diaphragm. The suspending coronary ligament of the left lobe of the liver, unlike the right, is attached superiorly and is quite small. The anatomic spaces surrounding the left lobe of the liver are thus freely communicating.

The lesser sac (omental bursa) (Fig. 9.2) is developmentally cut off from the rest of the peritoneal cavity except for the narrow inlet known as the epiploic foramen (foramen of Winslow). The lesser sac lies behind the lesser omentum, the stomach and duodenal bulb, and the gastrocolic ligament. It is bounded inferiorly by the transverse colon and the mesocolon. A prominent oblique fold of peritoneum, the gastropancreatic plica, is raised from the posterior abdominal wall by the left gastric artery. The plica is a fatty triangular structure measuring 2–3 cm in cross-section at its base and is inclined toward the posterior wall of the stomach (KUMPAN 1987). This fold often divides the lesser sac into two compartments: a smaller medial compartment to the right and a larger lateral compartment to the left inferiorly. The ultrasonographic features of the lesser sac have been described (WEILL et al. 1983), but it is computed tomography that clearly demonstrates the anatomic characteristics in vivo.

9.2.2
Pathways of Intraperitoneal Spread of Infection

Figure 9.3 summarizes the major pathways of spread of intraperitoneal infections. Given the source of contamination, an understanding of the dynamics of

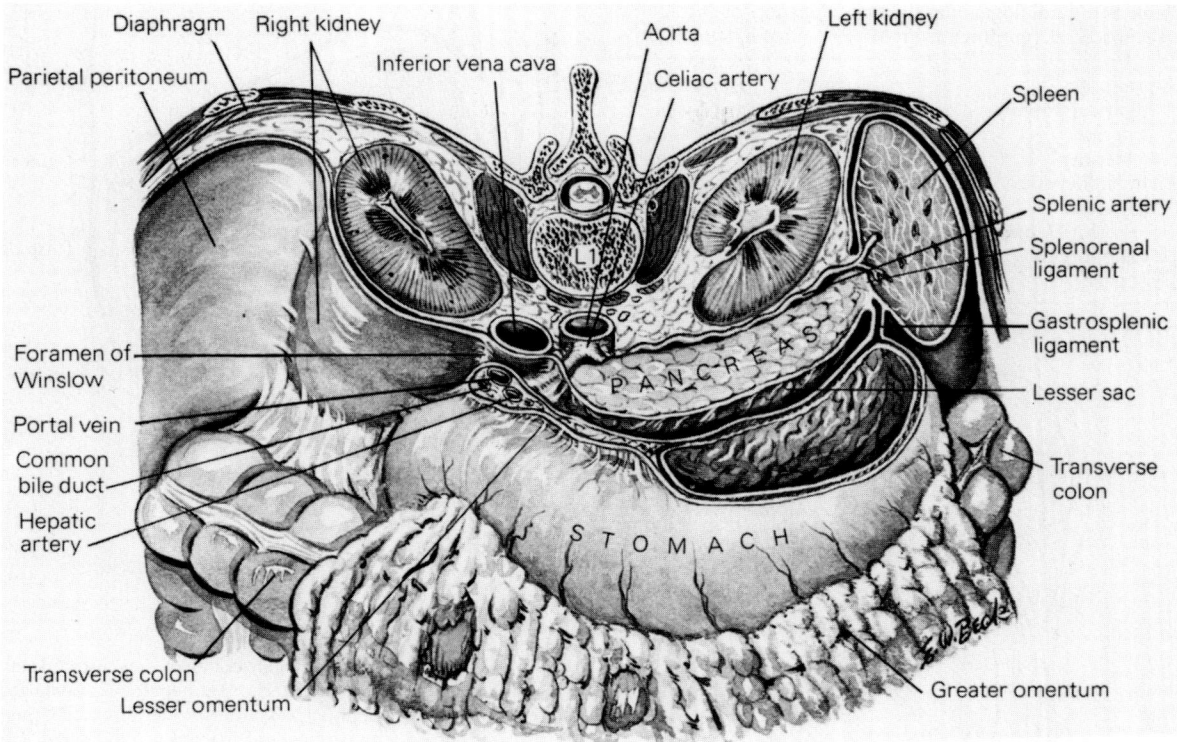

Fig. 9.2. The lesser sac and its relationships. The foramen of Winslow generally is wide enough to allow the introduction of one to two fingers, but in vivo it represents merely a potential communication between the greater and lesser peritoneal cavities. (From MEYERS 1994)

spread allows the anticipation of a remote abscess at a specific site. Conversely, in a distant infection occurring initially at clinical presentation, the occult primary site may be readily discovered.

9.3
Imaging Features of the Spread and Localization of Intraperitoneal Abscesses

The spread of infection within the peritoneal cavity is governed by (a) the site, nature, and rapidity of outflow of the escaping visceral contents, (b) mesenteric partitions and peritoneal recesses, (c) gravity, (d) intraperitoneal pressure gradients, and (e) the position of the body (MEYERS 1994, 1970a, 1973a; MEYERS and WHALEN 1971).

Intra-abdominal abscesses (Table 9.1) may be radiologically manifested by demonstrating (a) a soft tissue mass, (b) a collection or pattern of extraluminal gas, (c) viscus displacement, (d) loss of normally visualized structures, (e) fixation of a normally mobile organ, or (f) opacification of a commu-

nicating sinus or fistulous tract. Secondary signs include scoliosis, elevation or splinting of a diaphragm, localized or generalized ileus, and pulmonary basilar changes. These pathways and localizing features are not only evident when using conventional radiologic techniques; rather, they have also been confirmed by ultrasonography, isotopic studies, and computed tomography (CT). Knowledge of the preferential pathways of spread and subsequent compartmentalization permits the early diagnosis of abscess formation often remote from its site of origin.

9.3.1
Pelvic Abscesses

Fluid introduced into the inframesocolic compartment almost immediately seeks the pelvic cavity, first filling out the central pouch of Douglas and then the lateral paravesical fossae. This pathway is a function primarily of gravity and explains why the pelvis is the most common site of any residual abscess formation following generalized peritonitis.

Table 9.1. Radiologic-anatomic classification of intraperito-neal abscesses (modified from MEYERS and WHALEN 1971)

Supramesocolic	Inframesocolic
Right subphrenic	Pelvic
Anterior	Paracolic
Posterior	Right
Right subhepatic	Left
Anterior	Infracolic
Posterior (Morison's pouch)	Right
Left subphrenic	Left
Lesser sac	

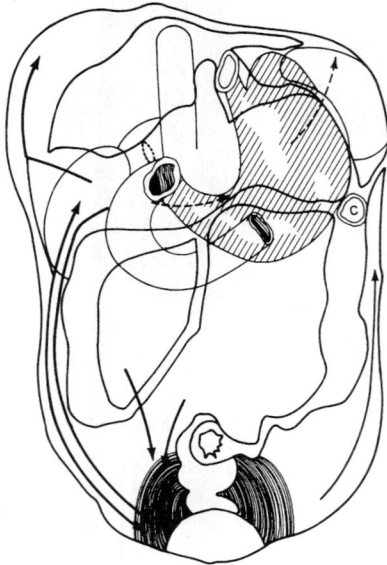

Fig. 9.3. Diagram of the pathways of flow of peritoneal exu-dates. Preferential flow from the infracolic spaces is to the dependent pelvic recesses. Flow up the narrow and shallow left paracolic gutter is weak and is impeded by the phrenicocolic ligament at the level of the anatomic splenic flexure of the colon (*C*). The right paracolic gutter is the major bidirectional conduit of fluid between the lower and upper abdominal recesses. Cephalad progression is to the dependent hepatorenal fossa (Morison's pouch) and then to the right subphrenic space. Fluid in the left upper quadrant, typically arising from contiguous organs, is drawn anterior to the stom-ach into the left subphrenic space. (Modified from MEYERS 1970a)

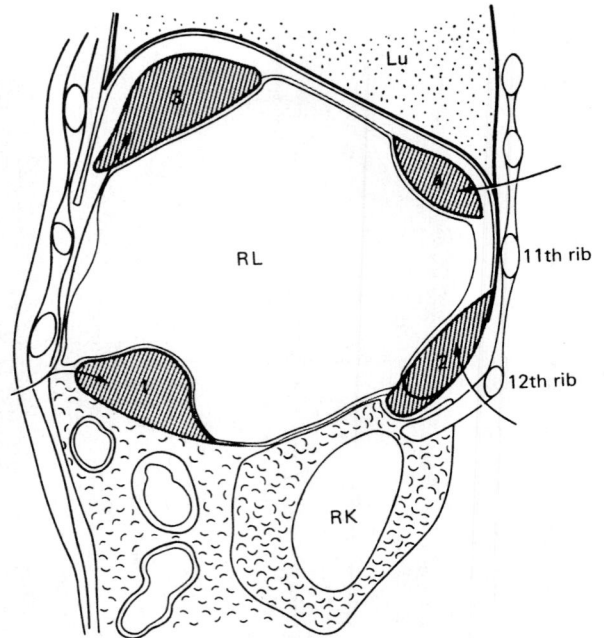

Fig. 9.4. The four sites of localized abscesses around the right lobe of the liver: *1*, Anterior subhepatic; *2*, posterior subhepatic (Morison's pouch); *3*, anterior subphrenic; *4*, pos-terior subphrenic. The surgical approaches are indicated. *Lu*, Lung; *RL*, right lobe of liver; *RK*, right kidney. (From MEYERS 1994)

taminated does the infected material reach the right subphrenic space (Fig. 9.4). Direct passage from the right subphrenic space across the midline to the left subphrenic space is prevented by the falciform liga-ment (Fig. 9.5).

These dynamics of flow explain the incidence and location of intraperitoneal abscesses reported em-pirically in large clinical series. The frequency of subphrenic and subhepatic abscesses is 2–3 times greater on the right than on the left and the most common site is Morison's pouch. Abscesses of Morison's pouch and the right subphrenic space often coexist.

9.3.2
Right Subhepatic and Subphrenic Abscesses

The major flow from the pelvis is up the right paracolic gutter (MEYERS 1970a). Ascent into the supramesocolic compartment is a response also to negative subdiaphragmatic pressure, which de-creases further with inspiration (MEYERS 1994). Fluid preferentially seeks the dependent recess of Morison's pouch. Only after Morison's pouch is con-

9.3.3
Lesser Sac Abscesses

Anatomically, Morison's pouch communicates with the lesser sac via the epiploic foramen. Noninfected intraperitoneal fluid originating within the greater peritoneal cavity may thus readily gain entrance to the lesser sac. However, this slitlike connection is easily sealed off by adhesions, so the lesser sac is not usually contaminated in generalized peritonitis un-

Fig. 9.5. Right subphrenic abscess. CT shows a gas-containing abscess (*A*) in the right subphrenic space demarcated anteriorly at the level of the falciform ligament. It extends posterior to the liver (*L*) as far as the attachment of the superior coronary ligament (*arrow*). This is separated by the diaphragm (*D*) from an associated pleural effusion (*E*) which extends into the medial costophrenic angle. (From MEYERS 1994)

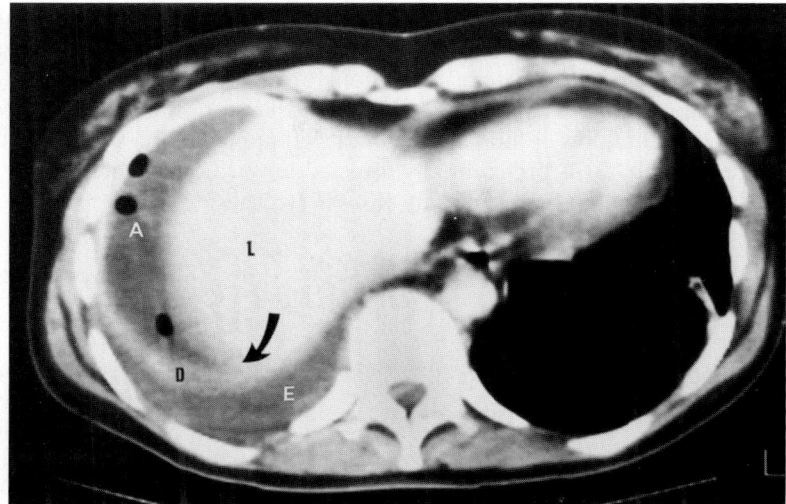

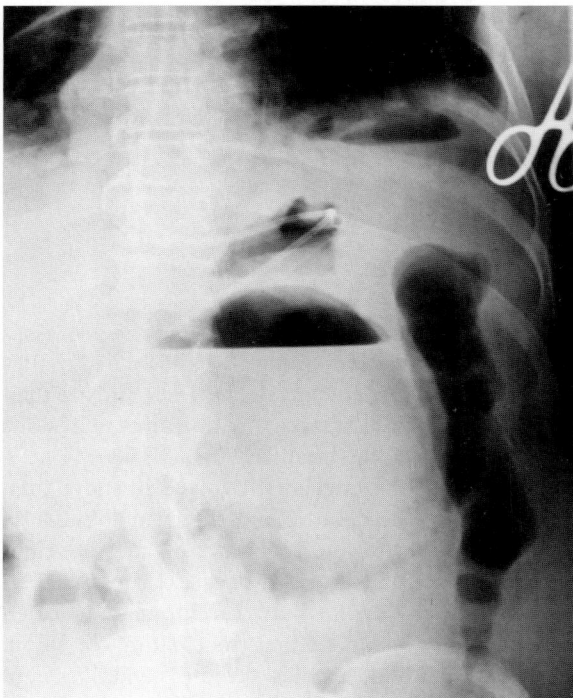

Fig. 9.7. Left subphrenic abscess secondary to anterior perforation of a gastric ulcer.CT demonstrates that the abscess (*A*) is bordered by the falciform ligament (*arrow*), the anterior peritoneal reflections of the stomach (*S*), and the liver (*L*). (From MEYERS 1994)

Fig. 9.6. Lesser sac abscess. Erect plain film of the abdomen demonstrates a large abscess with an air-fluid level in the lesser sac, bulging between the stomach and the transverse colon, which is displaced inferiorly. A component projects below the left diaphragm. These changes are secondary to a perforated ulcer of the posterior wall of the stomach

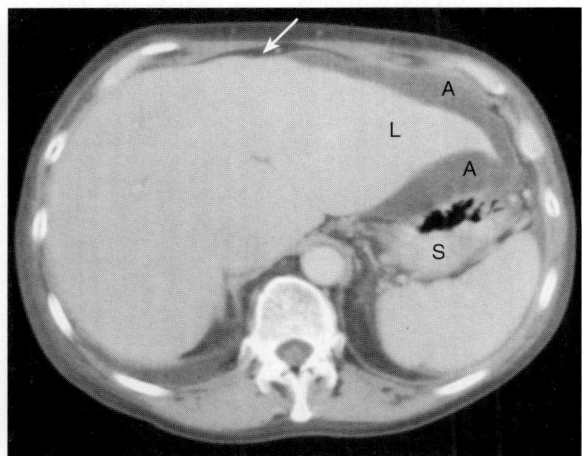

less the primary infection arises in the walls of the lesser sac itself. Abscesses here are therefore encountered most often following perforated posterior ulcers of the stomach or duodenal bulb and pancreatitis (Fig. 9.6). Lesser sac abscesses typically

displace the stomach anteriorly and the transverse colon inferiorly. Adhesions developing along the peritoneal fold raised by the left gastric artery often clearly partition an abscess to one of its two major compartments.

9.3.4
Left Subphrenic Abscesses

Abscesses in the left subphrenic space may result from perforated anterior ulcers of the stomach (Fig. 9.7) or duodenal bulb, but are seen particularly as complications of gastric or colonic surgery and of splenectomy. Anastomotic leaks are being increasingly recognized as a source of postoperative left subphrenic abscesses (MEYERS 1994). The most consistent aspect of flow of fluid arising in the left upper quadrant is that it is preferentially directed upward to the subphrenic area, where an abscess typically coalesces.

9.4
Intraperitoneal Seeding
(Peritoneal Carcinomatosis)

The deposition and growth of seeded neoplasms in the abdomen similarly depend on the natural flow of ascites within the peritoneal recesses (MEYERS 1973b). A primary neoplasm can shed cells into the ascitic fluid induced. The degree of ascites need not be great for the transportation and deposition of malignant cells. Intraperitoneal fluid, rather than being static, continually follows a circulation

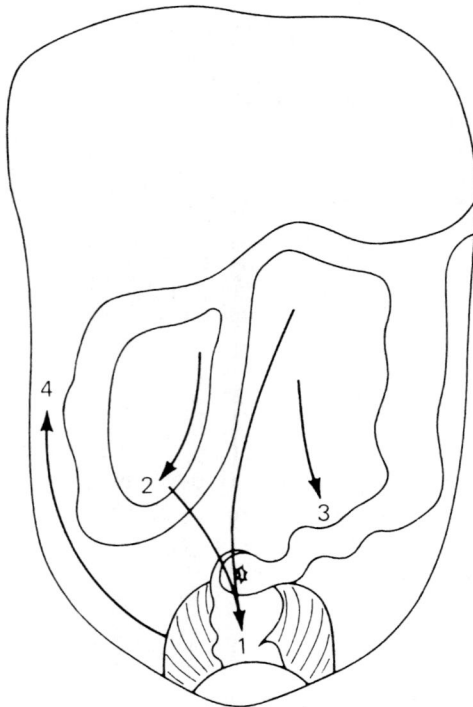

Fig. 9.8. The four predominant sites (*1–4*) in the lower abdomen for the lodgment and growth of seeded metastases as determined by the dynamic circulation of ascitic fluid. See text for further explanation. (From MEYERS 1994)

through the abdomen (MEYERS 1973b). These dynamic pathways of distribution and sequential spread depend particularly on mesenteric reflections and peritoneal recesses, as well as on the forces of gravity and negative subdiaphragmatic pressure.

9.4.1
Pathways of Ascitic Flow and Deposition of Seeded Cells

Four predominant sites in the lower abdomen are identified clearly as the sites of preferential, repeated, or arrested flow of ascitic fluid: (a) the pelvic cavity, particularly the pouch of Douglas; (b) the right lower quadrant at the termination of the small bowel mesentery; (c) the superior aspect of the sigmoid mesocolon; and (d) the right paracolic gutter. These pathways are illustrated in Fig. 9.8, and determine the most common sites of seeded metastases (peritoneal carcinomatosis) (MEYERS 1994, 1970a, 1973b, 1975, 1981b; MEYERS and McSWEENEY 1972).

9.4.2
Seeded Sites

Stasis or pooling of ascitic fluid favors the processes of deposition, fixation, and growth of seeded malignant cells. The seeded deposits coalesce and are then fixed to the serosal surfaces by fibrinous adhesions that quickly become organized.

The pouch of Douglas is involved in more than 50%, the lower small bowel mesentery in about 40%, the sigmoid mesocolon in about 20%, and the right paracolic gutter in about 20% of cases (MEYERS 1994, 1973b). In males, the primary carcinoma most often arises in the gastrointestinal tract (stomach, colon, pancreas), and in females, in the genital system (ovary).

9.4.2.1
Pouch of Douglas (Rectosigmoid Junction): Radiologic Features

Seeding at this site is most common. On barium enema study, this results in a characteristic pattern of fixed parallel folds or a nodular indentation on the anterior aspect of the rectosigmoid junction (Meyers 1973b) (Fig. 9.9). These changes reflect the coalescence of deposits with a dense fibrous reaction. This

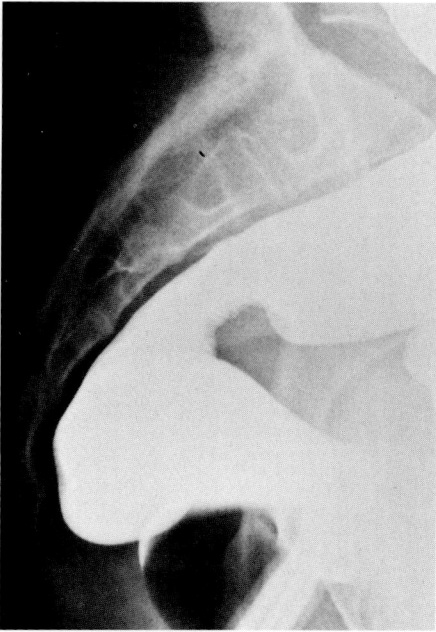

Fig. 9.9. Seeded ovarian metastasis in the pouch of Douglas. Barium enema study demonstrates nodular indentation upon the ventral aspect of the rectosigmoid junction, corresponding to a mass at the inferior peritoneal reflection constituting the pouch of Douglas. Characteristic tethering of mucosal folds is a consequence of the associated desmoplastic reaction

may be clinically palpable as the classic Blumer's shelf (MEYERS 1994).

9.4.2.2
Lower Small Bowel Mesentery (Terminal Ileum and Cecum): Radiologic Features

A series of peritoneal recesses is formed along the right side of the ruffled small bowel mesentery obliquely toward the right lower quadrant of the abdomen. These also serve to pool collections of ascitic fluid (MEYERS 1994, 1973b, 1975; MEYERS and McSWEENEY 1972). It is within the lower recesses that the most consistent pool of fluid forms before overflow into the pelvis occurs.

Seeded deposits lodging within the lower recesses of the small bowel mesentery in the right infracolic space are clinically identifiable in more than 40% of cases by their displacement of distal ileal loops, perhaps with pressure effects also upon the medial contour of the cecum and ascending colon. If the desmoplastic response to the seeded metastases is severe, marked fixation and angulation of ileal loops in the right lower quadrant result.

9.4.2.3
Sigmoid Colon: Radiologic Features

Lodgment and growth of deposits arrested along the barrier of the sigmoid mesocolon in the left lower quadrant result in changes characteristically localized to the superior border of the sigmoid colon. The associated desmoplastic reaction causes tethering of the mucosal folds, often toward a common point in the mesentery at the site of the secondary lesion. This localization occurs in more than 20% of cases of metastatic seeding.

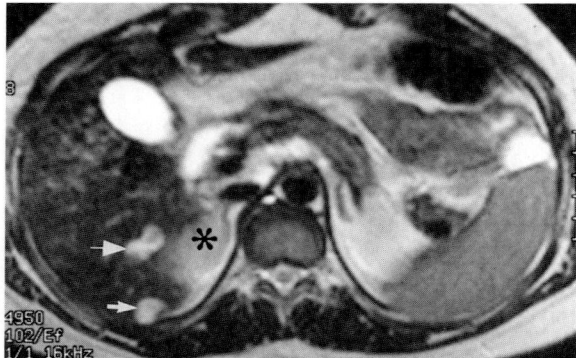

Fig. 9.10. Seeded ovarian implants in Morison's pouch. Transaxial T2-weighted MR image shows two seeded metastases (arrows) in Morison's pouch adjacent to the upper pole of the right kidney (asterisk). (From FORSTNER et al. 1995a)

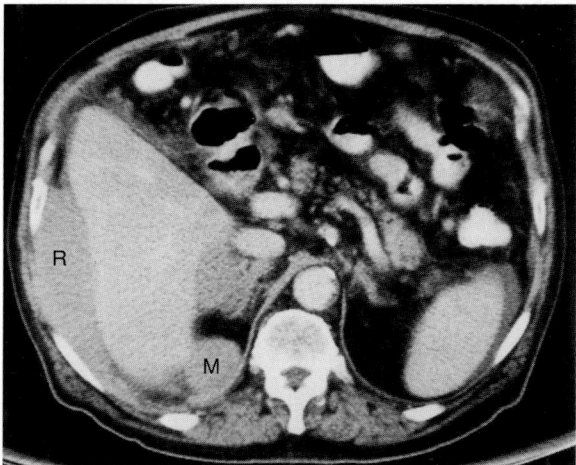

Fig. 9.11. Seeded implant in Morison's pouch and right subphrenic space. CT demonstrates seeded metastasis in Morison's pouch (M) and a separate larger one in the right subphrenic space (R). Note how these localize according to the boundaries of the right coronary ligament, above and below the bare area of the liver. (From DE MEO et al. 1995)

9.4.2.4
Right Paracolic Gutter (Cecum and Ascending Colon): Radiologic Features

Deposition and growth in this peritoneal recess are shown by mass changes lateral and posterior to the cecum and proximal ascending colon. Tethering of mucosal folds or angulated fixation of a small bowel loop in this area may occur as a consequence of an associated fibrous reaction. This localization in the right paracolic gutter occurs in 18% of cases. More cephalad seeding in the right subhepatic space may occasionally be identified (Figs. 9.10, 9.11).

9.4.2.5
Seeded Perihepatic and Subdiaphragmatic Metastases

Transcoelomic migration of fluid, particles, and cells cephalad toward the undersurface of the diaphragm is caused by changes in intraperitoneal pressure during breathing and the topographic arrangement of the peritoneal recesses (MEYERS 1994, 1973b). In ovarian carcinoma, shed tumor cells have been shown to be removed from the peritoneal cavity through lymphatic channels located in the diaphragm, a process more extensive on the right side, overlying the liver (FELDMAN et al. 1972; HIGGINS and GRAHAM 1929).

It is being increasingly recognized that metastatic ovarian implants along the right hemidiaphragm and liver capsule are frequent. Peritoneoscopic studies have shown metastatic diaphragmatic involvement in 61% of patients with ovarian carcinoma (ROSENOFF et al. 1975), and more significantly, that in 21%–34% of patients otherwise diagnosed as having stage I or stage II disease there is seeding on the undersurface of the diaphragm, particularly on the right (DAGNINI et al. 1987; YOUNG et al. 1983). These implants are generally only 2–3 mm in diameter, but may reach a size of several centimeters.

The perihepatic dissemination of ovarian carcinoma is now being increasingly detected by computed tomography. Peritoneal implants may be seen as nodular, plaquelike, or sheetlike masses (MEYERS 1994). Parietal peritoneal thickening with contrast enhancement of the peritoneum, making the peritoneum visible as a smooth or nodular line along the abdominal wall, representing confluent seeded deposits, may be conspicuous. In one series of patients with peritoneal tumor spread studied by CT, it was evident in 62% (WALKEY et al. 1988).

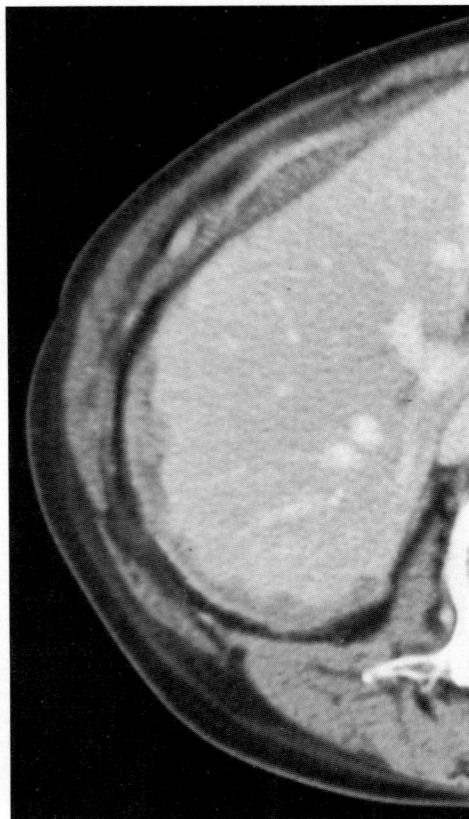

Fig. 9.12. Pseudomyxoma peritonei. CT shows seeded implants of mucinous cystadenocarcinoma of the ovary, producing scalloped indentations upon the surface of the liver. Posteriorly, the metastases are limited by the superior reflection of the right coronary ligament. Anteriorly, a larger implant extends toward the falciform ligament

Pseudomyxoma peritonei, when it occurs secondary to a mucinous carcinoma of the ovary or gastrointestinal tract, is characterized by a redistributed pattern of peritoneal carcinomatosis (SUGARBAKER 1996) which must be pathologically distinguished from the condition associated with an appendiceal mucinous adenoma (RONNETT et al. 1995). It may be displayed and evaluated by ultrasonography or magnetic resonance imaging (MRI), but CT is the modality most widely used (WALENSKY et al. 1996). Gelatinous perihepatic deposits produce characteristic scalloping of the liver contour (CHURCHILL and MEYERS 1986) (Fig. 9.12). Delineation by the falciform ligament is a characteristic landmark of the process of intraperitoneal seeding (Figs. 9.5, 9.7, 9.12).

In serous cystadenocarcinoma of the ovary, calcified perihepatic metastatic implants may be

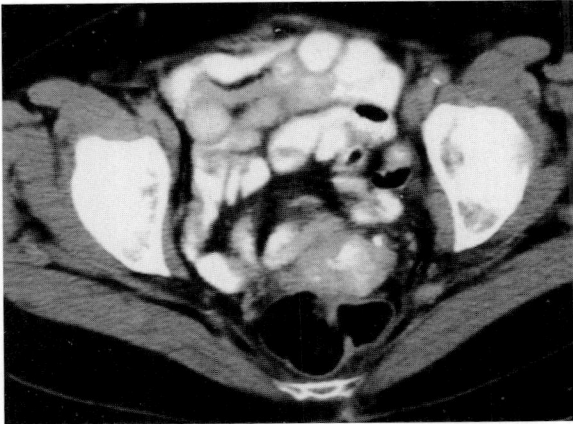

a

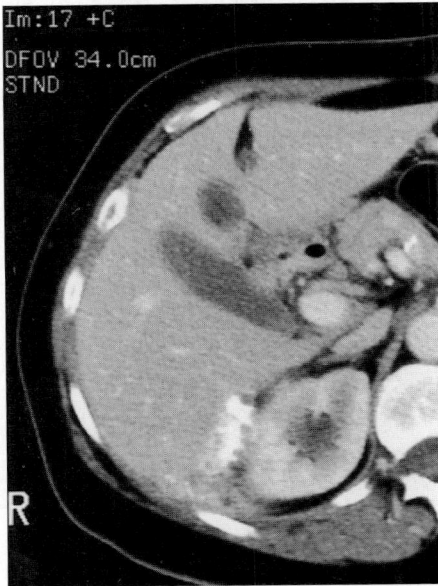

b

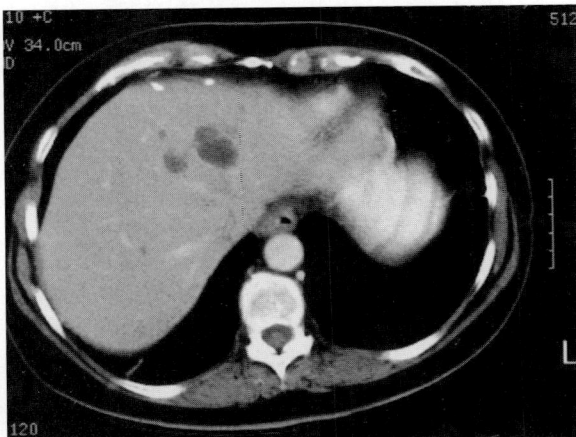

c

detected (Fig. 9.13) (Meyers 1994; Walkey et al. 1988; Mitchell et al. 1986; Solomon and Rubinstein 1984). This is the most common type of ovarian carcinoma and contains histologic calcification, psammoma bodies, in approximately 30% of cases (Ferenczy et al. 1977). The perihepatic calcifications are seen related to the right hemidiaphragm and liver surface even up to the immediate subphrenic region, as well as on the falciform ligament. Calcified implants may also be noted in the right paracolic gutter, in Morison's pouch, and adjacent to the spleen.

9.4.2.6
Two Unusual Sites of Peritoneal Carcinomatosis

9.4.2.6.1
SISTER MARY JOSEPH'S NODULE

A dramatic occurrence of metastatic spread is the umbilical lesion known as Sister Mary Joseph's nodule (Fig. 9.14). Named after the surgical assistant to Dr. William Mayo, who first called his attention to this sign of intra-abdominal malignancy, many hundreds of cases have now been reported secondary, most commonly, to carcinomas of the stomach, ovary, colon, and pancreas. Various modes of spread to the umbilicus have been proposed, ranging from lymphatic or hematogenous dissemination via the abdominal folds to seeded implants (Barrow 1966; Shetty 1990; Powell et al. 1984; Weiss et al. 1994).

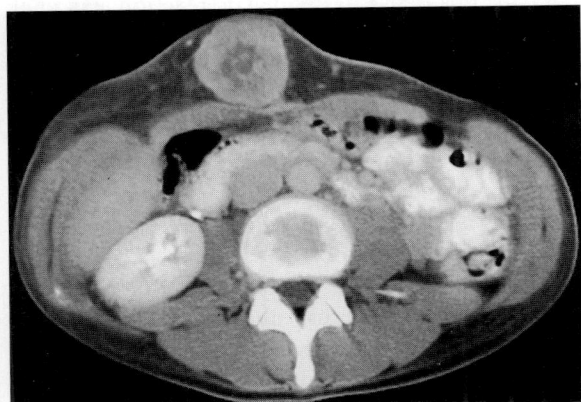

Fig. 9.13a–c. Calcified perihepatic implants from ovarian serous cystadenocarcinoma. Calcified seeded metastases are evident in (**a**) the pouch of Douglas, (**b**) Morison's pouch, and (**c**) the right subphrenic space on the liver surface up to the falciform ligament

Fig. 9.14. Sister Mary Joseph's nodule. CT demonstrates a large umbilical nodule with central necrosis. In this 33 year-old male with adenocarcinoma of the esophagogastric junction, carcinomatosis included a lesser omental mass (coronary lymphadenopathy) and bilateral adrenal metastases

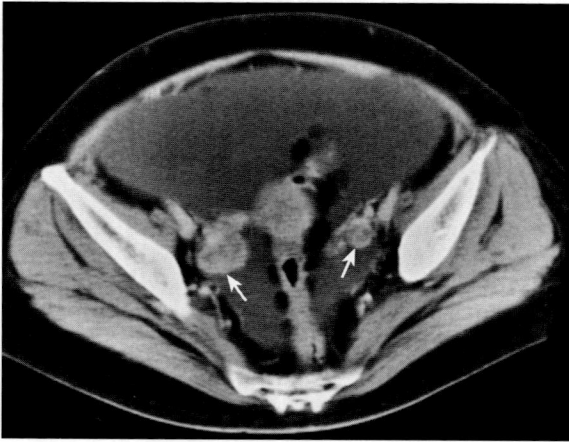

Fig. 9.15. Bilateral Krukenberg tumors of the ovaries. CT shows the ovarian masses (*arrows*) secondary to gastric carcinoma, highlighted by massive ascites

9.4.2.6.2

KRUKENBERG TUMORS

A striking targeted pathway of seeding is occasionally encountered as the entity of Krukenberg tumors of the ovaries (KRUKENBERG 1896; CHOI et al. 1988; MATA et al. 1988; HA et al. 1995). These are usually secondary to gastric or colon mucinous adenocarcinomas, are usually bilateral, and are associated with ascites (Fig. 9.15). Their likely pathogenesis has been recently elucidated as fixation and entrance of seeded cells at sites of ovarian follicular rupture and perigonadal fat milky spots (SUGARBAKER and AVERBACH 1996). In a recent study of Krukenberg tumors by MRI, most showed a characteristic finding of varied hypointense solid components from a dense desmoplastic reaction (HA et al. 1995).

Fig. 9.16a,b. Peritoneal carcinomatosis detected by ultrasonography. **a** Seeded implant on greater omentum is shown as a hypoechoic solid nodule (*between crosses*) surrounded by fat in an otherwise normal omentum (*between arrows*). **b** Seeded implant (*arrowheads*), 13 mm in length, on the ventral parietal peritoneum near the liver (*L*), shown as a focal hypoechoic linear interruption of the hyperechoic peritoneal line (*P*). (From RIOUX and MICHAUD 1995)

9.4.3
Current Developments and Advances

Multiple approaches are being applied in pursuit of refining the diagnostic accuracy of peritoneal carcinomatosis. Whereas CT may clearly demonstrate localized or diffuse involvement of the peritoneum and its reflections and recesses, it is not reliable for low-volume tumor on peritoneal surfaces and its greatest inaccuracies have been recorded in the pelvis (JACQUET et al. 1993). Positive-contrast peritoneography has been used in the demonstration of abdominal metastases (MEYERS 1973a, 1975). When coupled with CT (DUNNICK et al. 1979; ROUB et al. 1979; GIUNTA et al. 1990; HALVORSEN et al. 1991), it may further enhance the demonstration of

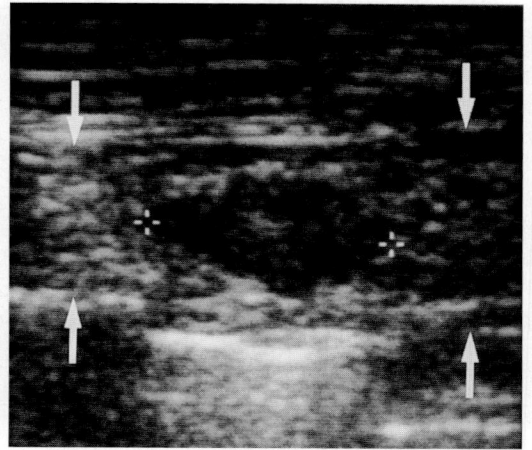

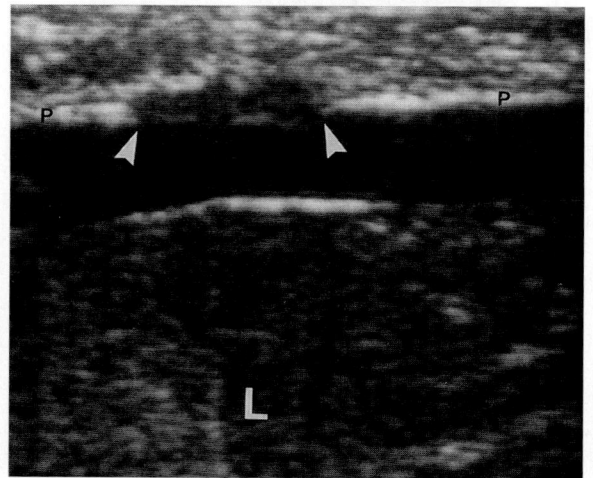

small peritoneal lesions, but small implants in curved recesses may be missed on axial sectional imaging. CT with induced pneumoperitoneum with CO_2 has been recently reported with disclosure of implants even <2 mm in size, but with significant limitations (CASIERO-ALVES et al. 1995). Abdominal ultrasonography has revealed signs for peritoneal carcinomatosis that account for malignant ascites in 78%–92% of cases (WEILL et al. 1990; DERCHI et al. 1987; GOERG and SCHWERK 1991). Using high-resolution ultrasonography, RIOUX and MICHAUD (1995) have recently documented omental, serosal, and peritoneal implants (Fig. 9.16). They describe a new finding of interruption of the anterior hyperechoic peritoneal line, representing tumor involvement of the anterior abdominal wall. Following early reports (CHOU et al. 1992, 1994), MRI of peritoneal implants has been accelerated with technological improvements. Seeded peritoneal metastases may be evident as discrete nodules (FORSTNER et al. 1995a,b,c,) (Fig. 9.10) or as peritoneal thickening and enhancement (LOW and SIGETI 1994).

9.5
The Subperitoneal Space

Recent insights have designated the anatomic continuum of the intraperitoneal and extraperitoneal tissues of the abdomen and pelvis as the subperitoneal space and established the clinical usefulness in identifying the bidirectional spread of disease between intraperitoneal and extraperitoneal sites and structures (MEYERS 1981b; MEYERS et al. 1987; OLIPHANT and BERNE 1982; OLIPHANT et al. 1986, 1988, 1993a,b, 1994, 1995, 1996). Recognizing that the mesenchyme beneath the peritoneum is a substrate in continuity throughout the body, this holistic paradigm explains many instances in which the sites of the presence or extension of disease states have previously appeared paradoxical. Central to this global context are the roots themselves of major abdominal and pelvis ligaments and mesenteries which provide the major avenues. These constitute an important natural pathway for extension of primary neoplasms to other sites that may not be in actual contiguity. In the upper abdomen, peritoneal reflections constitute nine major ligaments and mesenteries that provide continuity of anatomic planes for the spread of malignancies (Table 9.2). These not only connect intraperitoneal sites, but also extend between intraperitoneal and extraperitoneal sites. In the lower abdomen and pelvis, the sigmoid mesocolon and broad ligament are the major relevant structures. The ligaments and mesenteries

Table 9.2. Major upper abdominal peritoneal reflections

Gastrohepatic ligament
Hepatoduodenal ligament
Gastrocolic ligament
Transverse mesocolon
Duodenocolic ligament
Gastrosplenic ligament
Splenorenal ligament
Phrenicocolic ligament
Small bowel mesentery

are generally readily recognizable on CT and MRI by either their typical location and organ relationships or the landmarks provided by their major constituent vessels. The ventral portion of the mesenteric plane allows direct spread between the liver, gallbladder, pancreas, and proximal gastrointestinal tract. The dorsal portion provides subperitoneal continuity between the spleen, pancreas, left kidney, and gastrointestinal tract distal to the stomach. Female pelvis subperitoneal continuity is provided by the broad ligament. Other avenues of continuity include the posterior central plane delineated by the major blood vessels and their branches and the subperitoneal lateral planes.

9.6
The Mesenteries

9.6.1
Anatomy

The abdominal mesenteries represent membranous folds which extend from the retroperitoneum to the serosal surface of the bowel (MEYERS 1994; OLIPHANT et al. 1993a). They contain the superior or inferior mesenteric artery and their branches, the mesenteric veins and lymphatics, the autonomic nerve plexuses, connective tissues, and variable amounts of fat. Normal mesenteries can currently be visualized on CT in virtually all patients. They are identified because of their fat density (−100 to -160 HU), which is interlaced with multiple vessels and lymph nodes. Normal mesenteric lymph nodes measure less than 1 cm in their short axis. There are approximately 100–200 lymph nodes in the mesentery which are organized into three basic groups: (a) adjacent to the bowel wall, (b) paralleling the major branches of the mesenteric vessels, and (c) adjacent to the upper trunks of the superior and inferior mesenteric arteries. The mesenteric lymph nodes are predictably found anterior and posterior to the adjacent vessel (FRANK and HERN 1968).

9.6.2
Congenital or Developmental Disorders

9.6.2.1
Lymphangioma

Lymphangiomas represent the most common cystic tumors of the mesentery (TAKIFF et al. 1985; ROS 1987; ACKERMAN 1954). Most lesions are to some

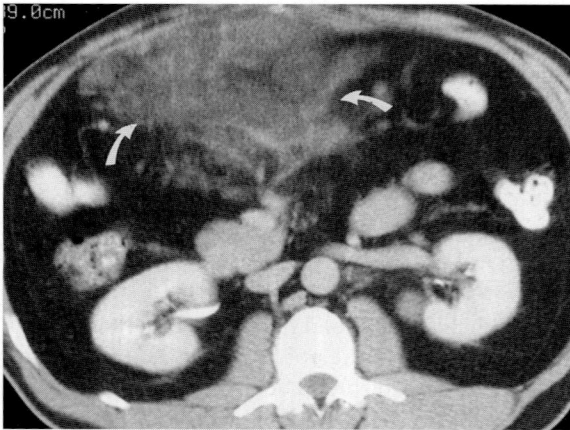

Fig. 9.17. Mesenteric lymphangioma. There is a large tumor mass (*arrows*) infiltrating the mesentery. It contains a low-density fatty matrix and was noted on the other sections to extend to the bowel wall. (From MINDELZUN 1995)

degree multilocular with a wall that merges imperceptibly with the wall of the adjacent bowel (Fig. 9.17). This close approximation makes surgical dissection difficult, often leading to resection of the adjacent intestine. Although mesenteric lymphangiomas are most likely to be found within the small bowel mesentery, they may occur in the omentum as well as the sigmoid mesocolon. The fluid within the lymphangioma can be quite variable and may be serous, chylous, or hemorrhagic. Identification of streaky low density within a multicystic lesion of the mesentery on either CT or MRI suggests the diagnosis of a lymphangioma. Occasionally, a simple lymphatic cyst of the mesentery can be diagnosed when a fat-fluid level is present within a cystic mass.

9.6.2.2
Mesenteric Pseudocyst/Hemorrhagic Cyst

Mesenteric pseudocysts, which are pathologically distinguished from the more common pancreatic pseudocysts, usually contain blood and are thought to evolve from prior hematomas or abscesses (ACKERMAN 1954). Their appearance can be variable from unilocular to multilocular and they can be generally differentiated from pancreatic pseudocysts by the lack of inflammation in the other retroperitoneal compartments. The wall tends to be thicker than that of a simple cyst and may readily enhance on CT. On ultrasonography, variable quantities of debris can be found within the cyst.

9.6.2.3
Enteric Duplication Cyst

Enteric duplication cysts are usually unilocular and can be diagnosed when a well-defined muscular wall with a characteristic echogenic submucosa is noted on ultrasonography (ROS 1987; ACKERMAN 1954). On CT, this wall commonly enhances. Serous fluid is typically found in the cyst, although blood may be present from prior hemorrhage. Gas or contrast material within an enteric duplication cyst indicates communication with the bowel.

9.6.2.4
Enteric Cyst

An enteric cyst, like a mesothelial cyst, has a thin wall and usually contains clear serous fluid which is readily identifiable on CT, MRI, or ultrasonography.

9.6.3
Inflammatory Processes

9.6.3.1
Pancreatitis

The small bowel mesentery provides a common pathway for the spread of pancreatitis. In acute pancreatitis, the mesentery is extensively infiltrated by pancreatic exudates which extend from the pancreas to the surface of the bowel. In chronic pancreatitis, this inflammation can appear very heterogeneous with regions of fluid accumulation and fibrosis making the process difficult to differentiate from inflammatory or neoplastic diseases of the mesentery. In that situation, prior pancreatitis is suggested by the presence of inflammation in the pancreas, in the retroperitoneum, and in the transverse mesocolon (Fig. 9.18) (MEYERS and EVANS 1973; MEYERS et al. 1987).

9.6.3.2
Infections

Many bowel infections lead to local adenopathy. On CT, these lymph nodes are mildly enlarged and streaky densities are present throughout the mesentery. A typical example would be mesenteric lymphadenitis secondary to an acute enteritis.

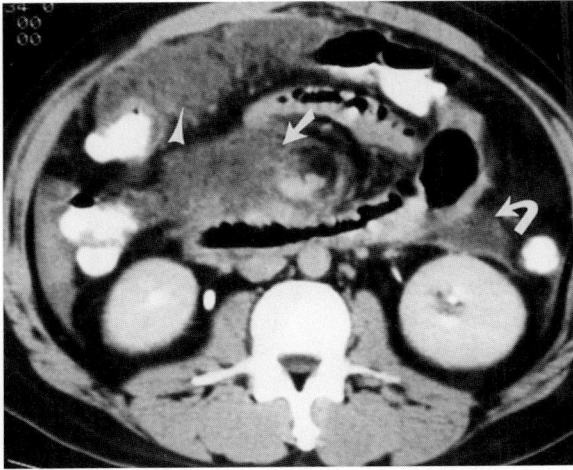

Fig. 9.18. Acute pancreatitis. Fluid is noted within the small bowel mesentery (*arrow*) with effacement of the mesenteric vessels and infiltration of the transverse portion of the duodenum. The correct diagnosis is suggested by the presence of fluid within the transverse mesocolon (*arrowhead*) and in the anterior pararenal space (*curved arrow*). (From MINDELZUN et al. 1996)

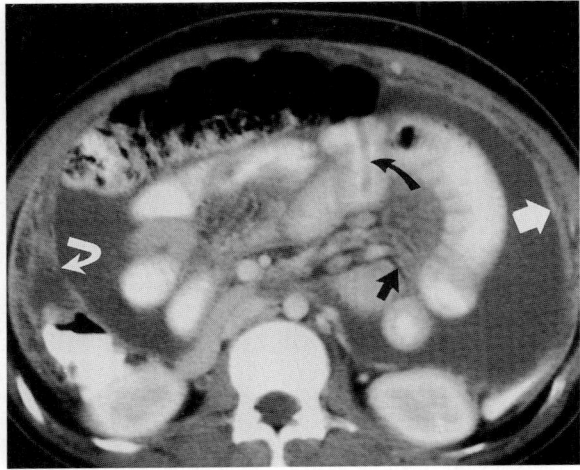

Fig. 9.19. Tuberculous peritonitis. Large amount of fluid present within the peritoneal cavity with a marked thickening of the peritoneum and transperitoneal permeation (*white arrow*). There is extensive infiltration of the mesentery (*black arrow*) and marked thickening of the omentum (*curved white arrow*). Multiple small lymph nodes are noted adjacent to the mesenteric vessels. There is an incidental ascarid in the small intestine (*curved black arrow*). (From MINDELZUN et al. 1996)

Similarly abdominal tuberculosis or *mycobacterium avium-intracellulare* (MAI) may lead to extensive mesenteric lymphadenopathy (LEDER and LOW 1995; HULNICK et al. 1985) (Fig. 9.19).

In appendicitis, the mesoappendix is commonly inflamed and appears as a linear or triangular area of increased density paralleling the ileocolic vessels in the right lower quadrant (Fig. 9.20) (LANE et al. 1996). The presence of an appendicolith or an appendix which measures more than 6 mm in its transverse diameter helps to differentiate appendicitis from other entities such as cecal diverticulitis. In diverticulitis, diverticular perforation commonly occurs into its adjacent mesentery (PADIDAR et al. 1994). This inflammation is manifested in the sigmoid mesentery as an area of increased density with engorgement of the vasa recta, which are especially prominent after contrast administration, creating a "centipede" sign (Fig. 9.21). Extension of the inflammation laterally thickens the margin of the sigmoid mesocolon, producing a "comma" sign (Fig. 9.22). The correct diagnosis is suggested by the presence of ectopic gas formation, a focal mass, or an abscess. Although sigmoid inflammation and vascular prominence suggest a diagnosis of diverticulitis, a perforated malignancy may have a similar appearance

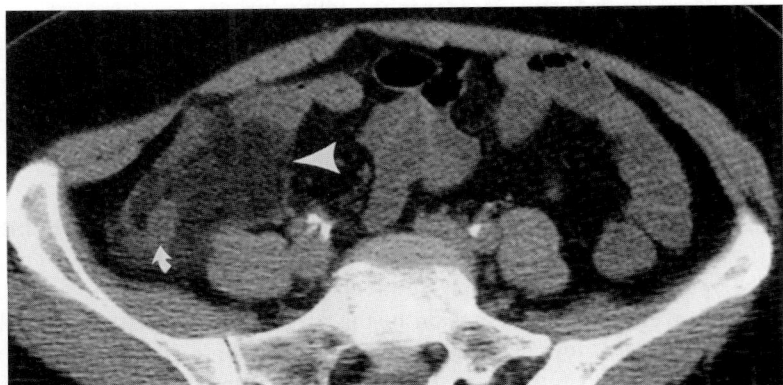

Fig. 9.20. Acute appendicitis. Noncontrast CT scan. The appendix (*arrow*) is enlarged, measuring more than 7 mm in its transverse diameter. The adjoining mesoappendix (*arrowhead*) is infiltrated with inflammatory cells and fluid, thus differentiating appendicitis from cecal diverticulitis

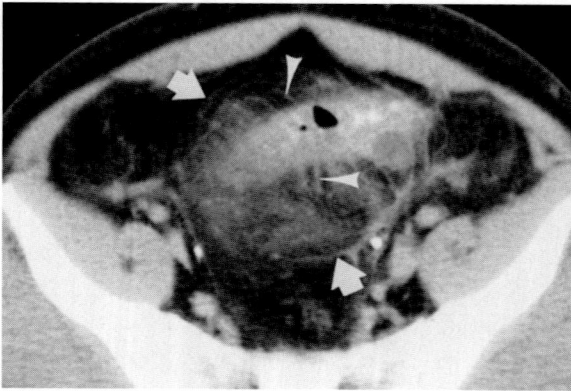

Fig. 9.21. Diverticulitis. Generalized infiltration of the sigmoid mesentery. The sigmoid vessels (*arrowheads*) are engorged, resulting in a "centipede" sign. The visceral margin of the sigmoid mesentery (*arrows*) is accentuated by the local inflammation. The colonic lumen is narrowed and there is considerable submucosal inflammation and edema. (From PADIDAR et al. 1994)

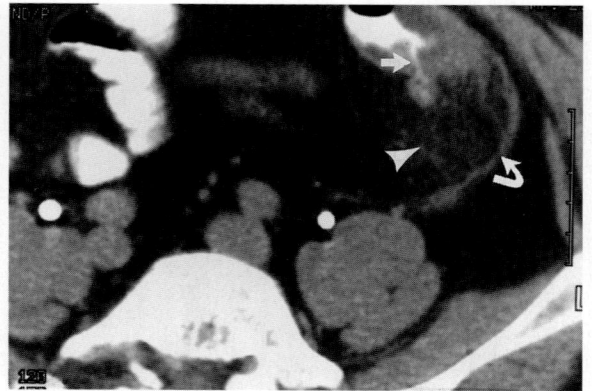

Fig. 9.22. Early diverticulitis. There is a focal diverticular perforation (*arrow*) resulting in inflammation of the sigmoid mesentery (*arrowhead*). Attention to this region of abnormality is drawn by the presence of a prominent "comma" sign (*curved arrow*), which represents thickening of the peritoneal covering of the mesentery and typically occurs on its lateral surface. (From PADIDAR et al. 1994)

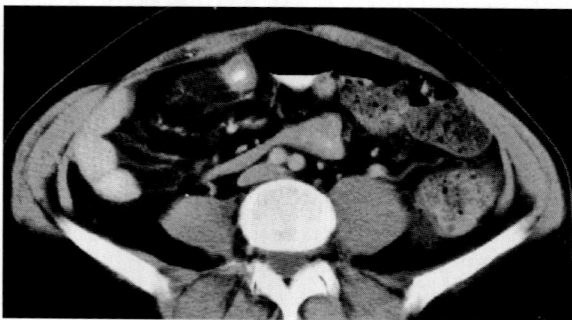

Fig. 9.23. Crohn's disease. Spiral CT demonstrates a distal ileal loop with considerable mural thickening, including a curvilinear zone of fluid. Increased mesenteric fat is present in the right lower quadrant, within which enhanced vessels show dilatation and tortuosity. The vasa recta approaching the mesenteric side of the diseased loop are spaced apart by the fatty proliferation, resulting in the "comb sign"

and close clinical and radiographic follow-up is indicated.

9.6.3.3
Crohn's Disease

Mesenteric fibrofatty proliferation ("creeping fat") is a common feature of Crohn's disease (GORE 1989). Transmural inflammation may result in thickening of the bowel wall and induration of the mesentery. Increased blood flow leads to vascular congestion and prominence of the vasa recta ("comb" sign)

(MEYERS and MCGUIRE 1995) (Fig. 9.23). Fistulae and abscesses are a common feature. Local adenopathy is often present although the nodes are rarely larger than 1 cm. Differentiation from diseases which may have a similar appearance such as lymphoma can be made on the basis of the presence of the above features and the lack of significant mesenteric and retroperitoneal adenopathy.

9.6.4
Neoplasms

Primary tumors arising in the mesentery are decidedly rare. They usually have a mesenchymal origin (ACKERMAN 1954). Primary cystic tumors are twice as common as primary solid tumors and even among solid tumors the benign variety is more common than the malignant type. Lesions which occur near the bowel wall or in the middle of the mesentery tend to be benign whereas those that arise near the root of the mesentery are more likely to be malignant.

9.6.4.1
Benign Neoplasms

9.6.4.1.1
DESMOID TUMOR
Mesenteric desmoids represent the most common primary tumor of the mesentery and usually occur at

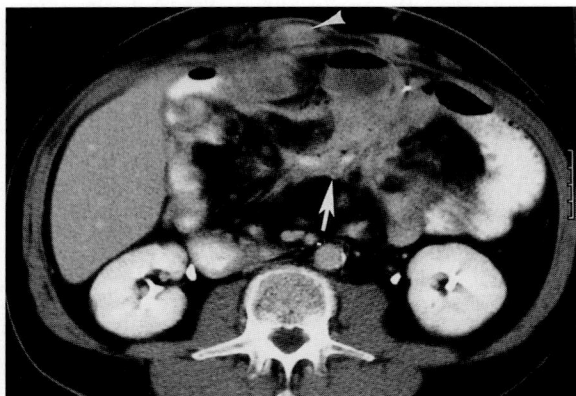

Fig. 9.24. Desmoid tumor of the mesentery in a patient with Gardner's syndrome. Extensive nodular infiltration of the mesentery (*arrow*), which extends to the serosal surface of the small bowel. The correct diagnosis is established with the identification of similar tumors within the anterior abdominal musculature (*arrowhead*). (From MINDELZUN et al. 1996)

the base of the mesentery (CASILLAS et al. 1991; MASUDA 1994; BARON and LEE 1981). They are benign lesions without neoplastic or inflammatory characteristics which are thought to arise from the aponeurosis or fascia of muscle groups. They most commonly occur in women and are generally associated with Gardner's syndrome (Fig. 9.24), pregnancy, and estrogen therapy. They are usually slow-growing tumors which, despite their benign histology, have a tendency to recur locally in half the patients. Desmoids can be divided into those that involve the abdominal wall and those that affect other regions (extra abdominal desmoids). Their high recurrence rate is probably related to their lack of a capsule and their infiltration of surrounding tissues.

The CT and MRI appearances of desmoids depend on the amount of fibroblast proliferation, collagen deposition, and intrinsic vascularity of the tumor. The lesions on CT are usually of a higher attenuation than adjacent muscle and enhance heterogeneously. On MRI, the lesions show low signal intensity on T1 images and variable intensity on T2 images.

When associated with Gardner's syndrome, mesenteric desmoids are usually seen several years after the patient's bowel surgery, although occasionally they may be noted prior to operation. In the postoperative state they are distinguished from postoperative fibrosis by their mass effect. They can be generally differentiated from low-grade fibrosarcomas by the presence of multiple lesions in and out of the abdominal cavity. Because they are clinically silent they tend to present as large masses

which compress adjacent organs. Mesenteric desmoids can usually be differentiated from non-Hodgkin's lymphoma by the presence of a single mass in the mesentery rather than adenopathy and by the absence of associated retroperitoneal adenopathy.

9.6.4.1.2
CYSTIC MESOTHELIOMA

Cystic mesotheliomas usually occur in young to middle aged women with a prior history of abdominal surgery, pelvic inflammatory disease, or endometriosis (O'NEIL et al. 1989). The tumor typically contains multiple tiny cysts with thin fibrous septae. This multiloculated appearance can be mistaken for a lymphangioma. Although they arise from mesothelial cells of the peritoneum they are not thought to have any association with asbestos exposure but rather may develop as inclusion cysts secondary to entrapment of mesothelial cells after laparotomy. At surgery they are often inadequately resected and often recur despite their benign nature.

9.6.4.1.3
MESENTERIC TERATOMA

Mesenteric teratomas tend to be complex lesions which have cystic and solid elements and may contain calcifications (BOWEN et al. 1987). They arise from all three germ layers and may demonstrate small amounts of fat which suggest their diagnosis.

9.6.4.1.4
LIPOMA

Lipomas are tumors containing fat which should be readily recognized on CT or MRI (WALGORE et al. 1981). They may occasionally demonstrate thin septations. If the tumor has a benign appearance without solid elements it can probably be safely followed with serial imaging studies.

9.6.4.2
Malignant Neoplasms (ACKERMAN 1954; HAMRICK-TURNER et al. 1992; SILVERMAN et al. 1987; WHITEHEAD 1995)

9.6.4.2.1
NON-HODGKIN'S LYMPHOMA

Non-Hodgkin's lymphoma is the most common malignant tumor of the small bowel mesentery (MUELLER et al. 1980). Fifty percent of newly

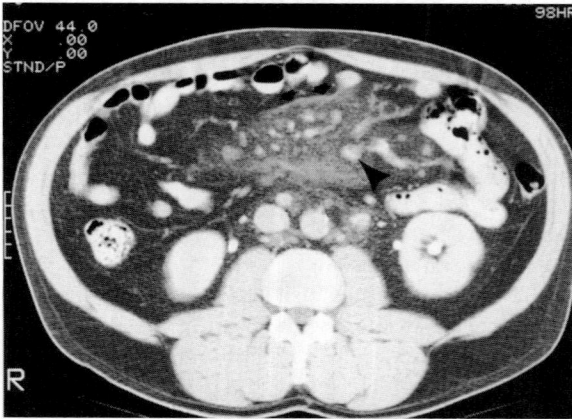

Fig. 9.25. Non-Hodgkin's lymphoma. The mesentery is increased in density and the visceral peritoneum (*arrows*) is highlighted by the lymphedema. Enhancing modestly enlarged lymph nodes are identified centrally (*arrowhead*) within the mesentery. (From MINDELZUN et al. 1996)

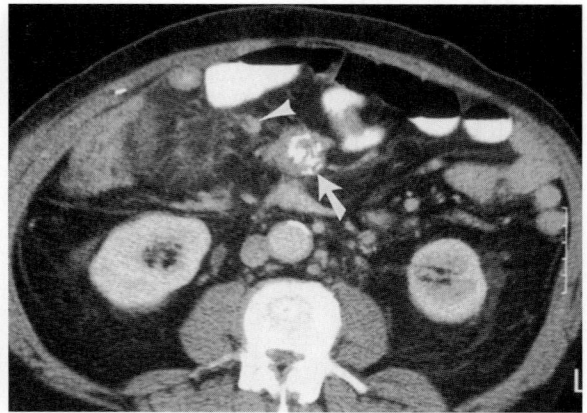

Fig. 9.26. Carcinoid tumor of the mesentery. There is a large central mesenteric lesion (*arrow*) with multiple calcifications. Radiating tumor nodules (*arrowhead*) are noted in the adjoining mesentery

diagnosed patients will exhibit mesenteric involvement (Fig. 9.25) (GOFFINET et al. 1973). Non-Hodgkin's lymphoma presents in the mesentery as multiple enlarged lymph nodes which occur anterior and posterior to the mesenteric vessels. When these nodules enlarge they present as conglomerate masses which encircle the contrast-enhanced vessels, creating a so-called sandwich sign (MUELLER et al. 1980). Although the small bowel mesentery is most commonly involved, the disease may involve the other mesenteries such as those of the transverse colon and the sigmoid colon. After treatment the tumor masses usually regress and a diffuse haziness is then seen throughout the mesentery, most likely representing diffuse lymphedema and fluid within the mesenteric interstitium. This appearance may persist for several years after the patient's original treatment and when there is no other evidence of active disease (MINDELZUN 1995). It has been suggested in the literature that mesenteric involvement in Hodgkin's disease occurs in approximately 5% of patients at the time of presentation but in our experience mesenteric Hodgkin's disease has been decidedly rare.

9.6.4.2.2
CARCINOID TUMORS

Carcinoid tumors usually present in the mesentery as central masses with radiating spicules which extend from the center of the tumor mass (Fig. 9.26) (ACKERMAN 1954; PENTONGRAG-BROWN et al. 1995). The actual tumor mass is often quite small but

is characterized by a large palpable lesion because of the associated fibrosis. Of all the carcinoids, one-fifth involve the small bowel and of these 90% arise in the ileum. At the time of presentation, more than half have nodal metastases. Eighty percent of lesions larger than 2 cm will have liver metastases. In addition to the characteristic infiltration along the neurovascular bundles, there is associated necrosis and secondary calcification. Seventy-percent of mesenteric carcinoids have sufficient calcification for CT visualization (PENTONGRAG-BROWN et al. 1995). The majority of these will be small stippled calcifications, although coarse and dense calcifications as well as diffuse calcifications can be seen throughout the lesion. Extension of the tumor to the adjacent bowel wall results in focal thickening. In the differential diagnosis, it is helpful to note that scirrhous carcinomas to the mesentery tend to be multiple and are rarely calcified.

9.6.4.2.3
LEIOMYOMA

Leiomyosarcomas are rare tumors in the mesentery and are usually characterized by stromal degeneration, hemorrhage, and necrosis (ACKERMAN 1954; WHITEHEAD 1995). On CT, the presence of blood elements and fluid levels may suggest this diagnosis.

9.6.4.2.4
LIPOSARCOMA

Liposarcomas of the mesentery are unusual. Typically these tumors originate in the retroperitoneum.

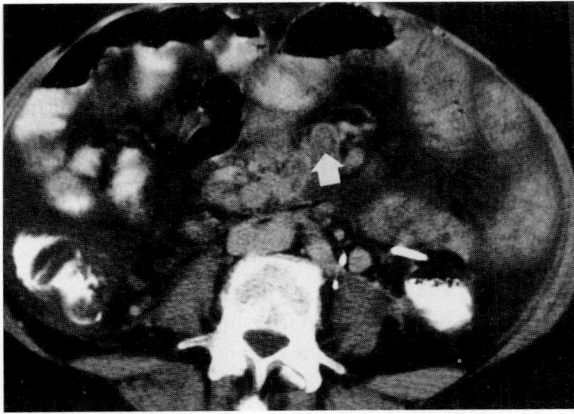

Fig. 9.27. Metastatic adenocarcinoma of unknown primary. Multiple necrotic lymph nodes (*arrow*) are noted within the mesentery adjacent to the central mesenteric vessels

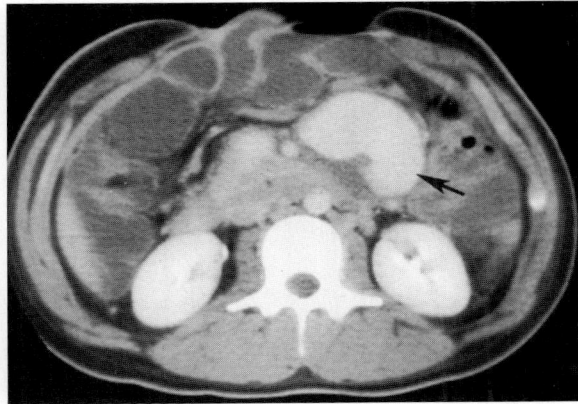

Fig. 9.28. Mesenteric artery aneurysm and arteriovenous communication. Young man who was shot in the abdomen and developed a large aneurysm (*arrow*) which arose from the superior mesenteric artery near the first jejunal branch and communicated with the superior mesenteric vein. This was confirmed angiographically and surgically repaired

In contrast to simple lipomas, liposarcomas usually contain a mixture of tissues resulting in masses with heterogeneous characteristics and contrast enhancement (WALGORE et al. 1981). Lipogenic liposarcomas contain a greater amount of fat than the myxoid variety. Infiltration of surrounding tissues tends to be very variable as the lesions are characteristically pleomorphic.

9.6.4.2.5
METASTATIC DISEASE

Metastatic disease to the mesenteries can result from: (a) hematogenous spread, (b) lymphatic spread, (c) extension along mesenteric surfaces, and (d) peritoneal seeding (LEVITT et al. 1982). In differentiating those diseases which spread on the surface of the mesentery from those which occur within the mesentery itself, an important clue lies in the appearance of the mesenteric vessels and the surrounding fat. Those diseases which spread along the surface of the mesentery compress the fat whereas diseases which spread within the mesentery replace the fat and efface the mesenteric vessels (MINDELZUN 1995). Aside from the lymphomas, metastases to the peripheral lymph nodes of the mesentery usually originate from the contiguous intestines and tend to spread centripetally. These masses are often quite large when first recognized (Fig. 9.27). The most common central lymph node metastases originate in the colon, stomach, pancreas, breast, and ovary (LEVITT et al. 1982).

9.6.5
Vascular Abnormalities

Vascular abnormalities of the mesenteries are readily identifiable after contrast enhancement and possess features typical of these lesions at other sites. The most common lesions are aneurysms, pseudoaneurysms, arteriovenous malformations (Fig. 9.28), and mesenteric varices.

9.6.6
Idiopathic Disease

9.6.6.1
Retractile Mesenteritis

Retractile mesenteritis is characterized by a progressive fibrotic reaction associated with nonenzymatic necrosis. It may occur as a manifestation of a systemic disease or may be primary in the mesentery and omentum (MATA et al. 1987). Numerous names have been given to this disease such as mesenteric lipodystrophy when there is predominent inflammation and retractile mesenteritis when it is primarily fibrotic. It may represent a form of Weber-Christian Disease (relapsing febrile nodular nonsuppurative panniculitis). The rare cases described have been very pleomorphic, reflecting the varying degrees of inflammation and fibrosis. Characteristically, increased density is noted throughout the mesentery,

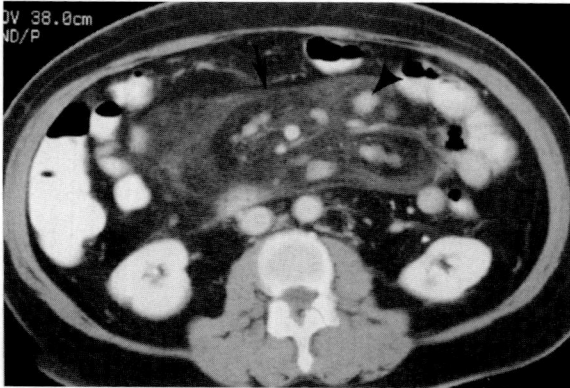

Fig. 9.29. Mesenteric panniculitis. Misty mesentery (*arrow*) with a prominent halo of fat around the enhancing lymph nodes (*arrowhead*) and the mesenteric vessels. (From MINDELZUN et al. 1996)

from the central vessels to the bowel wall. Peripheral radiolucencies may be seen around the blood vessels and the lymph nodes ("halo" sign) (Fig. 9.29). As the disease extends centrally, it tends to surround the central blood vessels without displacing or occluding them ("cloaking" sign). Microcalcifications are identified pathologically but they are usually not visible radiographically. The MRI characteristics are that of a low signal lesion on T1 and on T2 images. Retractile mesenteritis is typically seen in middle-aged men and may show complete regression after steroid therapy.

9.6.6.2
Castleman's Disease (Angiofollicular Lymph Node Hyperplasia)

Castleman's disease is a disease of unknown etiology which generally affects the thorax (FRIZZERA 1988). When the abdomen is involved, it results in enlarged retroperitoneal and mesenteric lymph nodes which characteristically enhance densely on dynamic CT. Enhancing lymph nodes have also been reported in angioimmunoblastic lymphadenopathy; in vascular metastases from renal cell carcinoma, papillary thyroid carcinoma, and small cell carcinoma; and in sarcoid, lymphoma, and Kaposi sarcoma. The multiplicity of enhancing lymph nodes should be helpful in differentiating these from primariy hypervascular lesions of the mesentery such as hemangiopericytoma, hemangioma, hemangiosarcoma, fibrous histiocytoma, and liposarcoma.

9.6.6.3
Whipple's Disease

Whipple's disease is characterized by an abnormal proliferation of macrophages in the intestinal submucosa of the proximal small bowel which may be caused by a bacterium related to the streptococci. On CT, low-density lymph nodes, containing fatty acids, can be identified in the mesentery (RIJKE 1983). The associated lymphatic stasis and lymphadenopathy are probably responsible for the markedly thickened mucosal folds of the proximal intestine. The differential diagnosis of low-density lymph nodes in the mesentery includes tuberculosis, AIDS, squamous carcinomas, ovarian carcinoma, lymphoma, and testicular carcinomas.

9.6.6.4
Acquired Immunodeficiency Syndrome

Mesenteric lymphadenopathy is commonly seen in acquired immune deficiency syndrome (AIDS), although the visualized lymph nodes are usually only modestly enlarged. When the lymph nodes are larger than 1.5 cm, diseases such as MAI (Fig. 9.30), lymphoma, and Kaposi sarcoma need to be considered and biopsy performed. When lymphadenopathy is present in association with splenomegaly and perirectal inflammation, it has been referred to as "lymphadenopathy" syndrome.

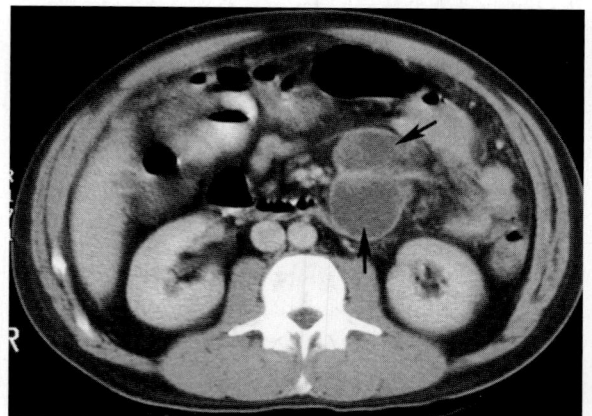

Fig. 9.30. Lymphadenopathy secondary to MAI. Young man with AIDS who developed abdominal pain. There are multiple enlarged low-density lymph nodes (*arrows*) in the mesentery, creating a "sandwich" sign

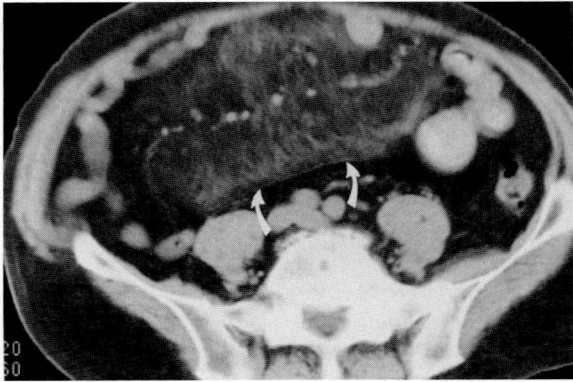

Fig. 9.31. Misty mesentery after treatment for non-Hodgkin's lymphoma. This CT scan was obtained after 1 year of chemotherapy, when the patient was felt to be free of disease. Prior to this, he had extensive retroperitoneal and mesenteric adenopathy. The mesentery is extensively infiltrated (*curved arrows*), probably secondary to lymphedema. (From MINDELZUN 1995)

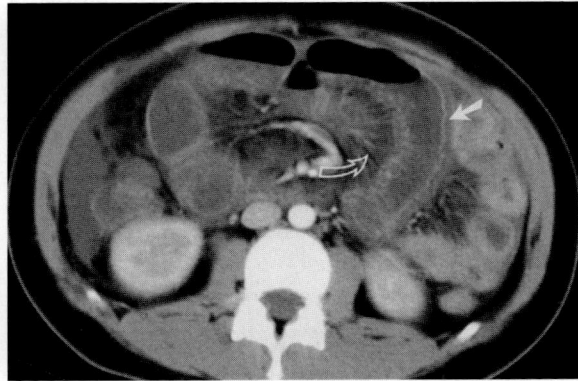

Fig. 9.32. Systemic lupus erythematosus with extensive small bowel vasculitis. Marked thickening of the wall of the small bowel (*arrow*) and considerable fluid within the small bowel mesentery (*open arrow*) are present. Prominent enhancement of the small bowel mucosa is seen in addition to fluid within the right and left paracolic gutters. (From MINDELZUN et al. 1996)

9.6.7
"Misty" Mesentery

The abdominal mesenteries are composed primarily of fat interlaced with the major vessels to the intestines. Disease of the intestines and of the mesentery is often recognized by infiltration of this fat and an increase in its density on CT (TAKANO et al. 1990). Infiltration of the fat by cells, fluid (edema, lymph, and blood), tumor, or fibrosis has been termed the "misty" mesentery (Fig. 9.31) (MINDELZUN et al. 1996). The normal mesentery has a density of −100 to −160 HU. Infiltration by fluid or cells increases its density to −40 to −60 HU, upon which it becomes readily discernible from other abdominal fat tissues. Because of the presence of increased density, the vessels become effaced and are only recognizable when contrast material is administered. In addition to increased density, one can recognize the misty mesentery by the highlighting of the visceral peritoneum which occurs when fluid is deposited in the intramesenteric compartment.

9.6.7.1
Mesenteric Edema

Mesenteric edema has many etiologies such as hypoalbuminemia, cirrhosis, heart failure, constrictive pericarditis, tricuspid disease, portal hypertension, portal vein thrombosis, hepatic vein thrombosis, mesenteric arterial and venous thrombosis, nephrosis, vasculitis (Fig. 9.32), Budd-Chiari syndrome, inferior vena caval obstruction, and trauma (SILVERMAN et al. 1987). Mesenteric edema secondary to a systemic process is usually associated with generalized subcutaneous edema and with ascites. Subcutaneous edema is recognized because of the deposition of a crescentic region of increased density, usually in a dependent position, representing extracellular water. The misty mesentery of mesenteric edema is often diffuse and extends from the serosal surface of the bowel to the central superior mesenteric artery and vein. In cirrhosis, portal hypertension has been shown to increase the density of the mesentery secondary to edema (TYRREL et al. 1990). In contradistinction to systemic edema, mesenteric edema secondary to arterial or venous thrombosis (Fig. 9.33) tends to be more focal and can be suggested by the presence of clots or an actual reduction in the lumen of the involved mesenteric vessels. Other findings which suggest the diagnosis of ischemia include thickening of the bowel wall, intraneural blood (Fig. 9.34), a "target" sign, pneumatosis intestinalis, gas within the mesenteric venous radicles, gas in the portal venous system, and segmental edema (ROSEN et al. 1984; NGHIEM et al. 1993).

9.6.7.2
Inflammation

Inflammatory processes are a common cause of infiltration of the mesentery. Typically in pancreatitis there is inflammation of the small bowel mesentery and the transverse mesocolon (JEFFREY et al. 1983). The correct diagnosis is suggested by the presence of pancreatic disease as well as infiltration of the retroperitoneal compartments. Similarly, processes such as diverticulitis, appendicitis, and inflammatory bowel disease result in local mesenteric inflammation. The mesenteries are commonly involved in abdominal tuberculosis manifested as tuberculous mesenteric lymphadenopathy (LEDER and LOW 1995). Infiltration of the mesentery in abdominal tuberculosis is usually patchy and the mesentery becomes heterogeneous with an increase in a number of visualized lymph nodes (Fig. 9.19). The correct diagnosis is suggested by the presence of high-density ascites, peritoneal thickening, peritoneal enhancement, omental infiltration, bowel wall thickening, cecal amputation, peripherally enhancing lymph nodes typically with low-density centers, transperitoneal inflammation, and an enhancing peritoneal "line" (HA et al. 1996; MEHTA et al. 1985).

9.6.7.3
Hemorrhage

Blood in the mesentery can originate from arteries and veins supplying the mesentery, the bowel wall, the retroperitoneum or the pelvis (Fig. 9.35). Clotted blood is recognized by its high CT numbers (50–70 HU) (NGHIEM et al. 1993). In addition after trauma, fluid from the lacerated bowel can intravasate into the mesentery (Fig. 9.36) along with oral contrast material and gas. In traumatic lacerations of the small bowel, the findings in the mesentery are often more readily identifiable than abnormalities in the bowel wall itself, which usually consist in local bowel wall thickening.

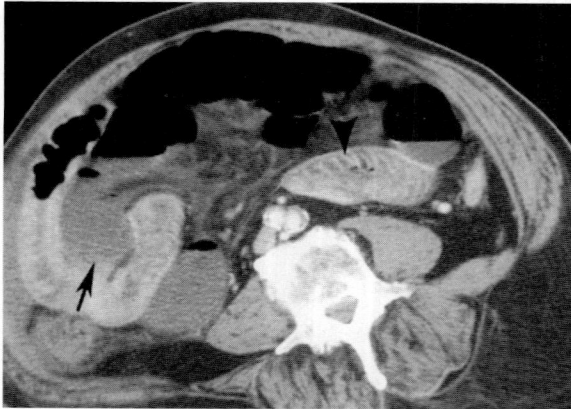

Fig. 9.33. Mesenteric artery thrombosis. Considerable fluid is present within the mesentery (*arrow*), resulting in a misty mesentery. There is prominent enhancement of the small bowel mucosa (*arrowhead*), probably representing rebound hyperemia. Thrombosis of the superior mesenteric artery was identified on CT sections at higher levels. (From MINDELZUN et al. 1996)

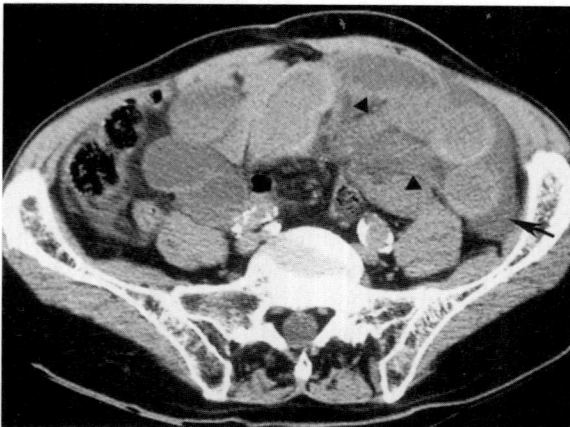

Fig. 9.34. Intestinal hemorrhage associated with ischemia. No oral or intravenous contrast was administered. High-density fluid, representing blood, is present within the mesentery (*arrowheads*). The bowel wall is increased in density because of the presence of intramural blood. In addition, high-density fluid is noted in the left paracolic gutter (*arrow*). (From MINDELZUN et al. 1996)

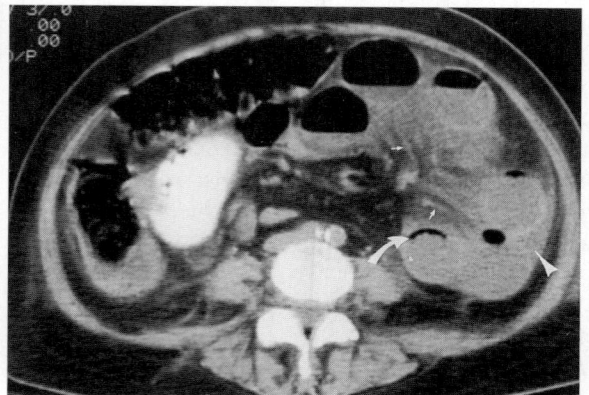

Fig. 9.35. Jejunal injury after blunt trauma. The mesentery to the jejunum is infiltrated with blood with loss of definition of the segmental vessels (*small arrows*). Blood is present within the peritoneal cavity (*arrowhead*). Transmural disruption has also resulted in focal jejunal pneumatosis (*curved arrow*). (From MINDELZUN et al. 1996)

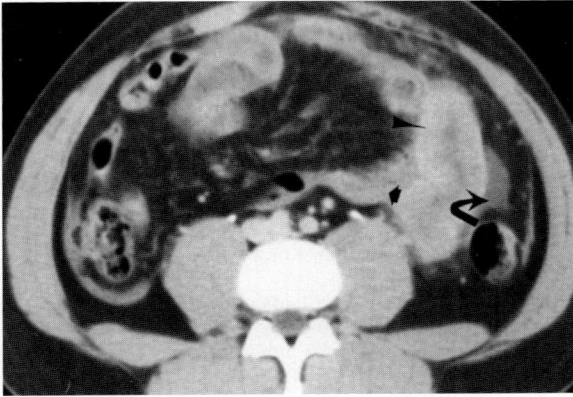

Fig. 9.36. Traumatic laceration of the jejunum. The CT scan was performed with intravenous but without oral contrast. Free fluid is present within the peritoneal cavity (*curved arrow*) under the greater omentum. The jejunum is markedly thickened (*arrowhead*) and intramural blood is present. In addition, a hematoma is noted to extend along the small bowel mesentery (*black arrow*). (From MINDELZUN et al. 1996)

9.6.7.4
Lymphedema

Lymphedema of the mesentery occurs after obstruction of the lymphatics leads to permeation of fluid into the interstitium of the mesentery. Possible etiologies include congenital anomalies, inflammation, neoplasms, surgery, and radiation therapy. Congenital malformations of the lymphatic system may result in collateral flow through the mesenteries with development of secondary lymphedema. In intestinal lymphangiectasia, there is lymphatic stasis with development of mesenteric lymphedema and chylous ascites (BASHIR et al. 1992).

Non-Hodgkin's lymphoma is a common cause of an isolated misty mesentery. At the time of presentation the patient may exhibit numerous enlarged lymph nodes in the mesentery (sandwich sign) and lymphedema which is recognized as an area of increased tissue density between the enlarged lymph nodes and the visceral peritoneum. After chemotherapy, the involved lymph nodes generally shrink and the underlying infiltration of the mesenteries becomes more obvious. This misty mesentery has been noted to persist for several years (Fig. 9.31) (MINDELZUN et al. 1996). Chylous ascites has occasionally been identified with mesenteric lymphadenopathy (BASHIR et al. 1992). Mesenteric involvement in Hodgkin's disease is quite rare. In addition to the lymphomas, metastatic

disease to the mesentery from carcinoma of the pancreas, carcinoma of the colon, carcinoma of the breast, carcinoid melanoma, leukemia, gastrointestinal stromal tumor, mesothelioma, and ovarian cancer may occasionally cause mesenteric edema secondary to lymphatic obstruction. In these processes the lymph nodes are usually quite large and readily identifiable (LEVITT et al. 1982).

Mesenteric panniculitis may result in mesenteric infiltration which appears very similar to non-Hodgkin's lymphoma, especially after chemotherapeutic treatment of the lymphoma. Typically there is a "halo" of fat around the lymph nodes and the vessels of the mesentery in association with perivascular "cloaking". A misty mesentery may also be simulated by a combination of tumor fibrosis and lymphedema such as one sees with a carcinoid of the mesentery. The frequent central calcifications which occur in up to three-quarters of these patients should suggest this diagnosis (Fig. 9.26). Similarly, desmoid tumors can occasionally diffusely infiltrate the mesentery but are recognized by their mass effect and the presence of abdominal wall desmoids or fibromas (Fig. 9.24).

References

Ackerman LV (1954) Tumors of the retroperitoneum, mesentery and peritoneum, Armed Forces Institute of Pathology, Washington, DC

Arenas AP, Sanchez LV, Albillos JM, et al. (1994) Direct dissemination of pathologic abdominal processes through perihepatic ligaments: identification with CT. Radiographics 14:515–527

Auh YH, Lim JH, Kim KW, et al. (1994) Loculated fluid collections in hepatic fissures and recesses: CT appearance and potential pitfalls. Radiographics 14:529–540

Baron RL, Lee JKT (1981) Mesenteric desmoid tumors: sonographic and computed tomographic appearance. Radiology 140:777–779

Barrow MV (1966) Metastatic tumors of the umbilicus. J Chron Dis 19:1113–1117

Bashir NL, Wilson NM, Russo F, al-Hassan H, Allen DR (1992) Aetiology and treatment of chylous ascites. Br J Surg 79: 1145–1150

Bowen B, Ros PR, McCarthy MJ, et al. (1987) Gastrointestinal teratomas: CT and MR appearance with pathologic correlation. Radiology 162:431–433

Casiero-Alves G, Goncalo M, Abraul E, et al. (1995) Induced pneumoperitoneum in CT evaluation of peritoneal carcinomatosis. Abdom Imaging 20:52–55

Casillas J, Sais GJ, Greve JL, Ipparraguire MC, Morillo G (1991) Imaging of intra- and extra-abdominal desmoid tumors. Radiographics 11:959–968

Choi BI, Choo IW, Han MC, et al. (1988) Sonographic appearance of Kruckenberg tumor from gastric carcinoma. Gastrointest Radiol 13:15–18

Chou CK, Liu GC, Chen LT, et al. (1992) MRI manifestations of peritoneal carcinomatosis. Gastrointest Radiol 17:336–338

Chou CK, Liu GC, Su JH, et al. (1994) MRI demonstration of peritoneal implants. Abdom Imaging 19:95–101

Churchill R, Meyers MA (1986) Intraperitoneal fluid collections. In: Meyers MA (ed) Computed tomography of the gastrointestinal tract: including the peritoneal cavity and mesentery. Springer, Berlin Heidelberg New York, chapter 7

Dagnini G, Marin G, Caldironi MW, et al. (1987) Laparoscopy in staging, follow-up, and restaging of ovarian carcinoma. Gastrointest Endosc 33:80–83

DeMeo JH, Fulcher AS, Austin RF Jr (1995) Anatomic CT demonstration of the peritoneal spaces, ligaments and mesenteries: normal and pathologic processes. Radiographics 15:755–770

Derchi LE, Solbiati L, Rizzatto G, et al. (1987) Normal anatomy and pathologic changes of the small bowel mesentery: US appearance. Radiology 164:649–652

Dunnick NR, Jones RB, Doppman JL, et al. (1979) Intraperitoneal contrast infusion for assessment of intraperitoneal fluid dynamics. AJR 133:221–223

Feldman GB, Knapp RC, Order SE (1972) The role of lymphatic obstruction in the formation of ascites in a murine ovarian carcinoma. Cancer Res 32:1663–1666

Ferenczy A, Talens M, Zoghby M, et al. (1977) Ultrastructural studies on the morphogenesis of psammoma bodies in ovarian serous neoplasia. Cancer 39:2451–2459

Forstner R, Hricak H, Powell CB, et al. (1995a) Ovarian cancer recurrence: value of MR imaging. Radiology 196:715–720

Forstner R, Hricak H, Occhipinti KA, et al. (1995b) Ovarian cancer: staging with CT and MR imaging. Radiology 197:619–626

Forstner R, Hricak H, White S (1995c) CT and MRI of ovarian cancer. Abdom Imaging 20:2–8

Frank BW, Hern F Jr (1968) Intestinal and liver lymph and lymphatics. Gastroenterology 55:408–422

Frizzera G (1988) Castleman's disease and related disorders. Semin Diagn Pathol 5:346–364

Giunta S, Tipaldi L, Diotellevi F, et al. (1990) CT demonstration of peritoneal metastases after intraperitoneal injection of contrast media. Clin Imaging 14:31–34

Goerg C, Schwerk W-B (1991) Malignant ascites: sonographic signs of peritoneal carcinomatosis. Eur J Cancer 27:720–723

Goffinet DR, Castellino RA, Kim H, et al. (1973) Staging laparotomies in unselected previously untreated patients with non-Hodgkin's lymphomas. Cancer 32:672–681

Gore RM (1989) CT of inflammatory bowel disease. Radiol Clin North Am 27:717–729

Ha HK, Baek SY, Kim SH, et al. (1995) Krukenberg's tumor of the ovary: MR imaging features. AJR 164:1435–1439

Ha HK, Jung JI, Lee MS, et al. (1996) CT differentiation of tuberculous peritonitis and peritoneal carcinomatosis. AJR 167:743–748

Halvorsen RA, Panushka C, Oaklet GJ, et al. (1991) Intraperitoneal contrast material improves the CT detection of peritoneal metastases. AJR 157:37–40

Hamrick-Turner JE, Chiechi MV, Abbitt PL, Ros PR (1992) Neoplastic and inflammatory processes of the peritoneum omentum and mesentery; diagnosis with CT. Radiographics 12:1051–1068

Higgins GM, Graham AS (1929) Lymphatic drainage from the peritoneal cavity in the dog. Arch Surg 19:453–465

Hulnick DH, Megibow AJ, Naidich DP, et al. (1985) Abdominal tuberculosis: CT evaluation. Radiology 157:199–204

Jacquet P, Jelinek JS, Steves MA (1993) Evaluation of computed tomography in patients with peritoneal carcinomatosis. Cancer 72:1631–1636

Jeffrey RB, Federle MP, Laing FC (1983) Computed tomography of mesenteric involvement in fulminant pancreatitis. Radiology 147:185–188

Krukenberg F (1896) Ueber das Fibrosarcoma ovarii mucocellular (Carcinomatodes). Arch Gynecol 50:287–321

Kumpan W (1987) Computertomographische Analyse postoperativer abdomineller Kompartments. Radiologie 27:203–215

Lane MJ, Katz DS, Ross BA, Clautice-Engle TL, Mindelzun RE, Jeffrey RB (1996) Unenhanced Helical CT for suspected appendicitis. Accepted for publication in AJR

Leder RA, Low VH (1995) Tuberculosis of the abdomen. Radiol Clin North Am 33:691–705

Levitt RG, Koehler RE, Sagel SS, Lee JK (1982) Metastatic disease of the mesentery and omentum. Radiol Clin North Am 20:501–510

Low RN, Sigeti JS (1994) MR imaging of peritoneal disease: comparison of contrast-enhanced fast multiplanar spoiled gradient-recalled and spin-echo imaging. AJR 163:1131–1140

Masuda K (1994) CT of intraabdominal desmoid tumors: is the tumor different in patients with Gardner's disease? AJR 162:339–342

Mata JM, Inaraja L, Martin J, et al. (1987) CT features of mesenteric panniculitis. J Comput Assist Tomogr 11:1021–1023

Mata JM, Inaraja L, Rams A, et al. (1988) CT findings in metastatic ovarian tumors from gastrointestinal tract neoplasms (Krukenberg tumors). Gastrointest Radiol 13:242–246

Mehta JB, Eapen T, Gubler R, et al. (1985) Abdominal tuberculosis mimicking neoplasia on computed tomography. South Med J 78:1385–1386

Meyers MA (1970a) The spread and localization of acute intraperitoneal effusions. Radiology 95:547–554

Meyers MA (1970b) Roentgen significance of the phrenicocolic ligament. Radiology 95:539–545

Meyers MA (1973a) Peritoneography: normal and pathologic anatomy. AJR 117:353–365

Meyers MA (1973b) Distribution of intra-abdominal malignant seeding: dependency on dynamics of flow of ascitic fluid. AJR 119:198–206

Meyers MA (1975) Metastatic seeding along small bowel mesentery: roentgen features. AJR 123:67–73

Meyers MA (1976) Clinical report: a new view of the peritoneal cavity. Mod Med 44:51–56

Meyers MA (1981a) Abdominal abscesses. In: Donner MW, Heuck FHW (eds) Radiology today. Springer, Berlin Heidelberg New York, pp 186–190

Meyers MA (1981b) Intraperitoneal spread of malignancies and its effect on the bowel. Second Annual Leeds Lecture. Clin Radiol 32:129–146

Meyers MA (1994) Dynamic radiology of the abdomen: normal and pathologic anatomy, 4th edn. Springer, Berlin Heidelberg New York

Meyers MA, Evans JA (1973) Effects of pancreatitis on the small bowel and colon: spread along mesenteric planes. AJR 119:151–165

Meyers MA, McGuire PV (1995) Spiral CT demonstration of hypervascularity in Crohn disease: "vascular jejunization of the ileum" or the "comb sign". Abdom Imaging 20:327–332

Meyers MA, McSweeney J (1972) Secondary neoplasms of the bowel. Radiology 105:1–11

Meyers MA, Whalen JP (1971) Radiologic aspects of intraabdominal abscesses. In: Ariel I, Kazarian K (eds) The diagnosis and treatment of intraabdominal abscesses. Williams & Wilkins, Baltimore

Meyers MA, Whalen JP (1973) Roentgen significance of the duodenocolic relationships: an anatomic approach. AJR 117:263–274

Meyers MA, Volberg F, Katzen B, et al. (1973a) Haustral anatomy and pathology: a new look. I. Roentgen identification of normal pattern and relationships. Radiology 108:-497–504

Meyers MA, Volberg F, Katzen B, et al. (1973b) Haustral anatomy and pathology: a new look. II. Roentgen interpretation of pathologic alterations. Radiology 108:505–512

Meyers MA, Ghahremani GG, Gold BM (1981) Post-operative abdominal abscesses. In: Meyers MA, Ghahremani GG (eds) Iatrogenic gastrointestinal complications. Springer, Berlin Heidelberg New York, chapter 10

Meyers MA, Oliphant M, Berne AS, et al. (1987) The peritoneal ligaments and mesenteries: pathways of intra-abdominal spread of disease. Annual oration. Radiology 163:593–604

Mindelzun RE (1995) The abdominal mesenteries: anatomy and diseases. Contemp Diagn Radiol 18:1–6

Mindelzun RE, Jeffrey RB, Lane MJ, Silverman PM (1996) The misty mesentery on CT: differential diagnosis. AJR 167:61–65

Mitchell DG, Hill MC, Hill S, et al. (1986) Serous carcinoma of the ovary: CT identification of metastatic calcified implants. Radiology 158:649–652

Morison R (1984) The anatomy of the right hypochondrium relating especially to operations for gallstones. BMJ 2:968

Mueller PR, Ferrucci JT, Harbin WP, et al. (1980) Appearance of lymphatous involvement of the mesentery by ultrasonography and body computed tomography: the "sandwich sign." Radiology 134:467–473

Nghiem HV, Jeffrey RB Jr, Mindelzun RE (1993) CT of blunt trauma to the bowel and mesentery. AJR 160:53–58

Oliphant M, Berne AS (1982) Computed tomography of the subperitoneal space: demonstration of direct spread of intraabdominal disease. J Comput Assist Tomogr 6:1127–1137

Oliphant M, Berne AS, Meyers MA (1986) Subperitoneal spread of intraabdominal disease. In: Meyers MA (ed) Computed tomography of the gastrointestinal tract: including the peritoneal cavity and mesenteries. Springer, Berlin Heidelberg New York, pp 95–136

Oliphant M, Berne AS, Meyers MA (1988) Imaging the direct bidirectional spread of disease between the abdomen and female pelvis via the subperitoneal space. Gastrointest Radiol 13:285–298

Oliphant M, Berne AS, Meyers MA (1993a) Spread of disease via the subperitoneal space: the small bowel mesentery. Abdom Imaging 18:108–116

Oliphant M, Berne AS, Meyers MA (1993b) Bidirectional spread of disease via the subperitoneal space: the lower abdomen and left pelvis. Abdom Imaging 18:117–125

Oliphant M, Berne AS, Meyers MA (1994) The subperitoneal space: normal and pathologic anatomy. In: Meyers MA (ed) Dynamic radiology of the abdomen: normal and pathologic anatomy, 4th edn. Springer, Berlin Heidelberg New York, pp 431–453

Oliphant M, Berne AS, Meyers MA (1995) Direct spread of subperitoneal disease into solid organs: radiologic diagnosis. Abdom Imaging 20:141–147

Oliphant M, Berne AS, Meyers MA (1996) The subperitoneal space of the abdomen and pelvis: planes of continuity AJR 167:1433–1439

O'Neil JD, Ross PR, Storm BJ, et al. (1989) Cystic mesothelioma of the peritoneum. Radiology 170:333–337

Padidar AM, Jeffrey RB, Mindelzun RE, Dolph JF (1994) Differentiating sigmoid diverticulitis from carcinoma on CT scans: mesenteric inflammation suggests diverticulitis, AJR 163:81–83

Pentongrag-Brown L, Buetow PC, Carr NJ, et al. (1995) Calcification and fibrosis in mesenteric carcinoid tumor: CT findings and pathologic correlation. AJR 164:387–391

Powell FC, Cooper AJ, Massa MC, et al. (1984) Sister Mary Joseph's nodule: a clinical and histologic study. J Am Acad Dermatol 10:610–615

Rijke AM, Falke THM, de Vries RRP (1983) Computed tomography in Whipple disease. J Comput Assist Tomogr 7:1101–1102

Rioux M, Michaud C (1995) Sonographic detection of peritoneal carcinomatosis: a prospective study of 37 cases. Abdom Imaging 20:47–51

Ronnett BM, Zahn CM, Kurman RJ, et al. (1995) Disseminated peritoneal adenomucinosis and peritoneal mucinous carcinomatosis: a clinicopathologic analysis of 109 cases with emphasis on distinguishing pathologic features, site of origin, prognosis, and relationship to "pseudomyxoma peritonei". Am J Surg Pathol 19:1390–1408

Ros PR (1987) Mesenteric and omental cysts: histologic classification with imaging correlation. Radiology 164:327–332

Rosen A, Korobkin M, Silverman PM, et al. (1984) Mesenteric vein thrombosis: CT identification. AJR 143:83–86

Rosenoff SH, DeVita VT, Hubbard S, et al. (1975) Peritoneoscopy in staging and follow-up of ovarian cancer. Semin Oncol 2:223–228

Roub LW, Drayer BP, Orr DP, et al. (1979) Computed tomographic positive contrast peritoneography. Radiology 131:699–704

Shetty MR (1990) Metastatic tumors of the umbilicus: a review 1830–1989. J Surg Oncol 45:212–215

Silverman PM, Baker ME, Cooper C, Kelvin FM (1987) Computed tomography of mesenteric disease. Radiographics 7:309–320

Solomon A, Rubinstein Z (1984) Importance of the falciform ligament, ligamentum teres, and splenic hilus in the spread of malignancy as demonstrated by computed tomography. Gastrointest Radiol 9:53–56

Sugarbaker PH (1996) Observations concerning cancer spread within the peritoneal cavity and concepts supporting an ordered pathophysiology. In: Sugarbaker PH (ed) Peritoneal carcinomatosis: principles of management. Kluwer, Boston, pp 79–100

Sugarbaker PH, Averbach AM (1996) Krukenberg syndrome as a natural manifestation of tumor cell entrapment. In: Sugarbaker PH (ed) Peritoneal carcinomatosis: principles of management. Kluwer, Boston, pp 163–191

Takano H, Sekiya T, Miyakawa K (1990) Analysis of mesenteric thickening on computed tomography. Nippon Acta Radiological 50:1519–1523

Takiff H, Calabria R, Yin L, et al. (1985) Mesenteric cysts and intra-abdominal cystic lymphangiomas. Arch Surg 120:1266–1269

Tyrrel RT, Montemayor KA, Bernardino ME (1990) CT density of mesenteric, retroperitoneal, and subcutaneous fat in cirrhotic patients: comparison with control subjects. AJR 155:73–75

Walensky RP, Venbrux AC, Prescott CA, Osterman FA Jr (1996) Pseudomyxoma peritonei. AJR 167:471–474

Walgore MP, Stephens DH, Soule EH, et al. (1981) Lipomatous tumors of the abdominal cavity: CT appearance and pathologic correlation. AJR 137:539–545

Walkey MM, Freidman AC, Sohotra P, et al. (1988) CT manifestations of peritoneal carcinomatosis. AJR 150:1035–1041

Weill FS, Perriguey G, Belloir A, et al. (1983) Ultrasonic anatomical study of the lesser omental sac: a pictorial essay. Eur J Radiol 3:142–147

Weill FS, Costaz R, Guetarni S, et al. (1990) Le diagnostic échographique des métastases péritonéales chez les malades ascitiques. J Radiol 71:365–368

Weiss SM, Wengert PA, Harkavy SE (1994) Incisional recurrence of gallbladder cancer after laparoscopic cholecystectomy. Gastrointest Endosc 40:244–246

Whitehead R (1995) Gastrointestinal and oesophageal pathology. Churchill Livingstone, New York

Young RC, Decker DG, Wharton JT, et al. (1983) Staging laparotomy in early ovarian cancer. JAMA 250:3072–3076

Section 3: Diseases

10 Inflammatory Disease

R.M. Gore, G.G. Ghahremani, and F.H. Miller

CONTENTS

10.1
Introduction

Ulcerative colitis and Crohn's disease, collectively known as idiopathic inflammatory bowel disease (IBD), remain a diagnostic and therapeutic challenge. While other inflammatory diseases of the gut are distinguished either by a specific etiologic agent or by the nature of the inflammatory activity, ulcer-

R.M. Gore, MD, Professor and Vice Chairman, Department of Diagnostic Radiology, Evanston Hospital-McGaw Medical Center of Northwestern University, 2650 Ridge Avenue, Evanston, IL 60201, USA
G.G. Ghahremani, MD, Professor and Chairman, Department of Diagnostic Radiology, Evanston Hospital-McGaw Medical Center of Northwestern University, 2650 Ridge Avenue, Evanston, IL 60201, USA
F.H. Miller, MD, Assistant Professor and Chief of Gastrointestinal Radiology, Northwestern Memorial Hospital, Northwestern University Medical School, 710 N. Fairbanks Ct., Chicago, IL 60611, USA

ative colitis and Crohn's disease are disorders of unknown etiology, with an uncertain and unpredictable course and a variable response to medical and surgical management (Debinski and Kamm 1997; Brzezinski and Lashner 1997).

Patients with IBD require prompt diagnosis and treatment both to relieve their symptoms and to minimize potential complications. Radiologic studies play a crucial role in determining the initial site and extent of intestinal involvement, therapeutic response, and detection and follow-up of complications. This chapter reviews the radiologic features of IBD useful for diagnosis and provides differential diagnostic guidelines.

10.2
Ulcerative Colitis

Ulcerative colitis is an inflammatory disease of unknown origin that primarily involves the colorectal mucosa but may later extend to other layers of the bowel wall (Debinski and Kamm 1997). The disease characteristically begins in the rectum and extends proximally to involve part or all of the colon.

10.2.1
Plain Film Features

In patients who present with a severe acute colitis, the following plain film findings can be used to assess the severity and extent of the disease: (a) the amount and location of fecal residue, (b) the appearance of the mucosal margins, (c) the width and number of visible haustra, (d) the colonic caliber, and (e) the thickness of the colorectal wall (Bartram 1976; Rice 1968).

The presence of fecal residue provides a clue to the extent of the colitis. If no fecal residue is seen, the patient probably has an active pancolitis. If the residue extends down into the sigmoid colon, a limited proctitis is more likely. As a general rule, fecal residue is noted only proximal to the inflamed segment of the colon (PRANTERA et al. 1991).

In active colitis, the colonic mucosal edge on plain films may be granular, indistinct, or disrupted rather than having its normal smooth appearance. Only edematous mucosal islands remain when there is extensive ulceration. Mottled-appearing intramural gas shadows indicate either extremely deep ulceration or transmural perforation with entrapped gas in pericolic soft tissues (BARTRAM 1977).

Widening of the haustral markings greater than 5–6 mm is an early manifestation of bowel wall edema in ulcerative colitis. It is often more obvious on plain films than the mucosal granularity or ulceration it accompanies. Haustral thickness should be assessed only where there is an adequate amount of air in the colon because the appearance of these markings may be misleading if the colon is collapsed or incompletely distended (BARTRAM and LAUFER 1992). Furthermore, the distal half of the colon may normally have decreased haustration, particularly in elderly patients with atonic or redundant colons (BARTRAM 1977).

The caliber of the air-filled colon, as seen on plain films, can provide a clue to the diagnosis of colitis. The diameter of the normal transverse colon is less than 5.5 cm. In chronic, *burned-out* ulcerative colitis, the colon becomes tubular and narrowed. In patients with fulminant colitis, a diameter greater than 6–7 cm suggests toxic megacolon with risk of perforation (BARTRAM 1983).

Mural thickness can also be assessed by measuring the distance between the pericolic fat line and gas-filled lumen. Normally, it is less than 3–5 mm but can increase to more than 10 mm in chronic ulcerative or granulomatous colitis (BARTRAM 1983).

10.2.1.1
Toxic Megacolon

Toxic megacolon occurs in up to 5% of patients with ulcerative colitis and represents a severe, life-threatening complication (HALPERT 1987). Pathologically, there is transmural inflammation with fissuring ulcers penetrating into the muscularis propria, often extending to the serosa. Exudates from diffusely inflamed mucosa seep deeply through the serosa and may lead to signs of peritonitis even without frank perforation (RIDDELL 1997). These changes are accompanied by vasculitis of the small arterioles, inflammation and destruction of ganglion cells of the myenteric and submucosal plexuses, and

myocytolysis in the muscularis propria (PRESENT 1993).

Colonic dilation is the hallmark of toxic megacolon on abdominal plain films, with the mean diameters of the most dilated segments ranging between 8.2 and 9.2 cm (Fig. 10.1). A lumen caliber greater than 5 cm indicates ulceration to the muscle layer and should be considered the threshold for dilation in fulminating colitis. Initially, only a short segment of colon may be involved.

The transverse colon has long been considered the focus of disease, but this is only a reflection of the fact that the transverse colon is the least dependent portion of the large intestine on supine view radiographs. Indeed, rolling the patient into the prone position has been advocated as a means of decreasing intraluminal pressures and transverse colon caliber. This measure may help prevent the development of toxic megacolon in patients with fulminant colitis.

Visualization of residual mucosal islands is a common finding in toxic megacolon and indicates severe disruption of the mucosa. Although the colon wall is thin pathologically, it appears thickened ra-

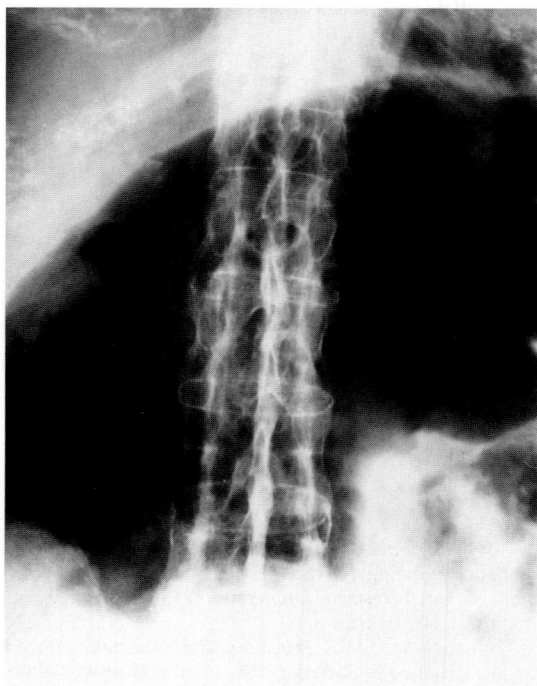

Fig. 10.1. Ulcerative colitis: toxic megacolon. Plain abdominal film shows marked dilation of the transverse colon associated with loss of the normal haustral pattern indicating profound inflammation and extensive ulceration. Note the ankylosing spondylitis

diologically, presumably as a result of subserosal or omental edema. A radiolucent stripe may be present running parallel to the colon, and this probably represents the pericolic fat line. The normal haustral pattern is always lost in toxic megacolon owing to the profound inflammation and extensive ulceration.

10.2.2
Barium Enema Features

In patients with known or suspected ulcerative colitis, the barium enema is performed to (a) confirm the clinical diagnosis, (b) assess the extent and severity of disease, (c) differentiate ulcerative colitis from Crohn's disease and other colitides, (d) follow the course of disease, and (e) detect complications.

10.2.2.1
Granular Pattern

The earliest pathologic changes of ulcerative colitis are hyperemia and the accumulation of inflammatory cells in the mucosa (GELLER 1994). These changes are manifested by a loss of normal mucosal translucency and obscuration of the submucosal pattern on endoscopy (LAUFER et al. 1976). Subtle thickening of the mucosa or haustral edema may be present radiographically, but these findings are often appreciated only in retrospect. With progressive edema and hyperemia, the mucosa develops a granular pattern (RIDDELL 1997). The smooth, sharp, and distinct appearance of the colonic margin seen on normal double-contrast studies is replaced by an amorphous, thickened, and indistinct mucosal line (Fig. 10.2a). There is a gradual transition between the normal and abnormal mucosa which extends over several centimeters. This granularity should be distinguished from the granular appearance of chronic ulcerative colitis. In the latter, the mucosal surface pattern is coarser and there are significant changes in colonic contour (Fig. 10.2b).

In acute disease, the granular pattern is primarily a result of abnormalities in the quality and quantity of mucus produced by the involved mucosa. Histologically, there is a reduction in the number of goblet cells, which contain less than the normal complement of mucin. Normal mucus is essential to normal barium coating of the gut (RIDDELL 1997). Any process, whether benign or malignant, infectious or inflammatory, which alters mucin production will

affect mucosal coating and visualization. In chronic, burned-out ulcerative colitis, the granular pattern is due to granulation tissue that reepithelializes the mucosa.

10.2.2.2
Mucosal Stippling

During the acute, granular phase of ulcerative colitis, inflammatory cells accumulate at the base of the

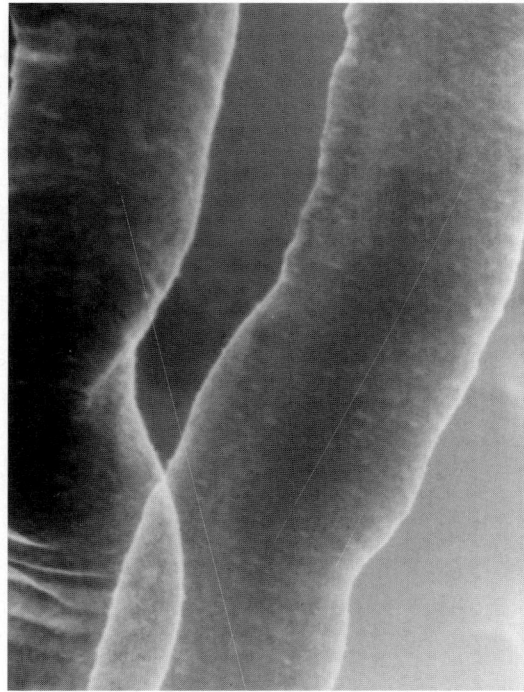

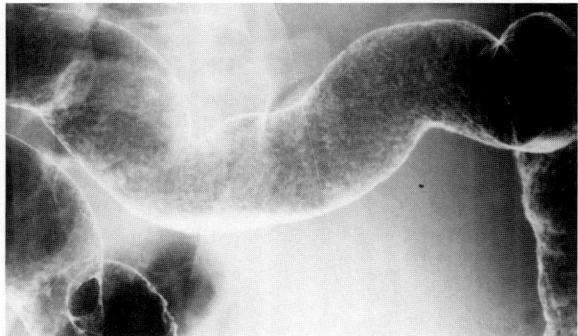

Fig. 10.2 a,b. Ulcerative colitis: mucosal granularity. **a** Fine mucosal granularity, characteristic of acute disease, is evident on this spot film of the proximal descending colon. Note the loss of haustra. Disease is continuous, circumferential, and symmetrical. **b** The mucosal granularity is much coarser in longstanding disease. Note the loss of haustration and colonic shortening. (From GORE and LAUFER 1994)

mucosal crypts. Cellular debris tends to block the crypts of Lieberkühn, leading to the formation of crypt abscesses (RIDDELL 1997). These microabscesses eventually erode into the lumen of the colon. The ulcers deepen and barium flecks become adherent to them, producing mucosal stippling (LAUFER 1975). This resembles white paint applied by dabbing a dark surface with the end of a fairly dry paintbrush (GORE 1991) (Fig. 10.3).

10.2.2.3
Collar Button Ulcers

With disease progression, the ulcers of the crypt abscess breach the lamina propria and muscularis mucosae and less resistant areolar tissue of the submucosa (RIDDELL 1997). The involved submucosa becomes necrotic and the ulcers extend laterally, causing further undermining (Fig. 10.4). This undermining is contained by the muscularis propria on the serosal side and by the muscularis mucosae on the lumen side of the colon. The ulcers are frequently related to the taeniae. The mucosal defect is small relative to the degree of undermining, producing a flask-like, "collar button" ulcer (LICHTENSTEIN et al. 1979).

As these ulcers enlarge and interconnect, the collar button ulcer configuration is lost, producing a network of residual islands of mucosa and inflammatory pseudopolyps (SUEKANE et al. 1990).

10.2.2.4
Polyps

A variety of different mucosal protrusions may be demonstrated in patients with ulcerative colitis on barium studies (LICHTENSTEIN 1987). Their appearance and significance depend on the stage of disease and pathologic origin.

10.2.2.4.1
INFLAMMATORY PSEUDOPOLYPS
In patients with severe ulcerative colitis, there is extensive mucosal and submucosal ulceration in which

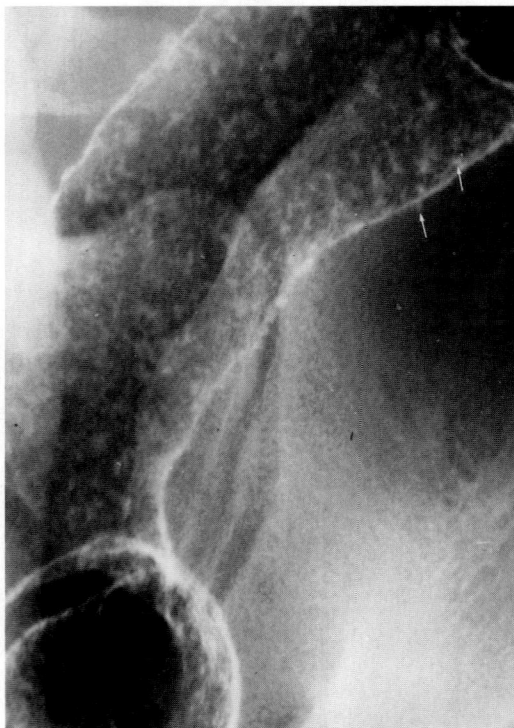

Fig. 10.3. Ulcerative colitis: mucosal stippling. When microabscesses at the base of the crypts of Lieberkühn erode into the lumen, they accumulate punctate collections of barium (*arrows*), producing mucosal stippling

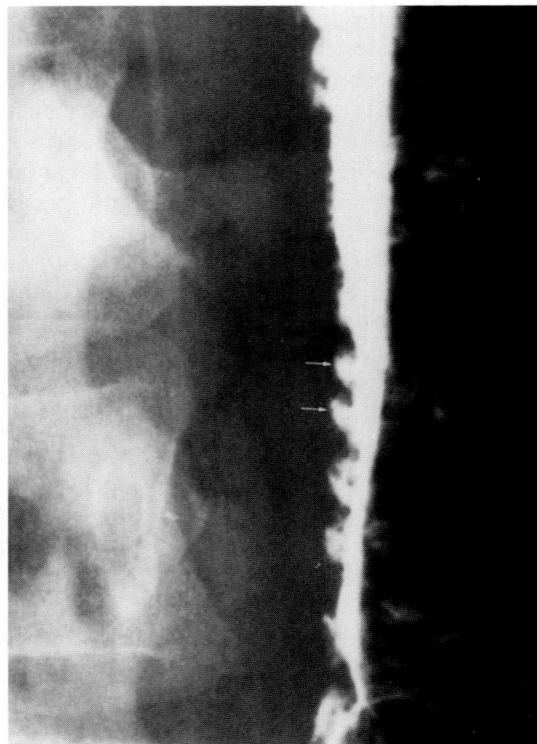

Fig. 10.4. Ulcerative colitis: collar button ulcers. Spot film of the descending colon discloses multiple flask-like ulcers (*arrows*) with a flat base. The ulceration is limited to the layers superficial to the muscularis propria

only small islands of mucosa and submucosa may survive. The inflamed edematous mucosa protrudes above the surrounding areas of ulceration, giving a polypoid appearance (Fig. 10.5) (PRICE and MORSON 1987). Since these "polyps" merely represent the remnants of preexisting mucosa and submucosa rather than new growths, they are called pseudopolyps. Inflammatory pseudopolyps are the natural progression of collar button ulcers: the ulcers extend and interconnect so that the pseudopolyp rather than the ulcers becomes the major radiologic finding (LICHTENSTEIN 1987). Inflammatory pseudopolyps usually occur in ulcerative colitis but may also be seen in Crohn's disease. The cobblestoning pattern seen in Crohn's disease is, in fact, a type of pseudopolyp in which larger islands of preserved mucosa are surrounded by linear and transverse ulcerations (GORE and LICHTENSTEIN 1994).

10.2.2.4.2
POSTINFLAMMATORY PSEUDOPOLYPS

When IBD goes into remission, the regenerated mucosa has a tendency to overgrow in some patients. This overgrowth often results in polypoid lesions that may be small and round, long and filiform (Fig. 10.6a), or proliferate into a bush-like structure (Fig. 10.6b) simulating a villous adenoma (KELLY et al. 1986). Since the regenerating mucosa is histologically normal, it is not a true neoplasm but a pseudopolyp (RIDDELL 1997). Because this occurs during mucosal healing, it is called a postinflammatory pseudopolyp. These polyps represent the aftermath of a severe attack of colitis and may be the only sign of previous disease.

Mucosal bridges are also postinflammatory pseudopolyps in which a bridge of mucosa survives between islands of mucosa surrounded by ulceration (HAMMERMAN et al. 1978). With remission, the underside of the mucosal bridge and the underlying ulcer reepithelialize (BROZNA et al. 1985).

Postinflammatory pseudopolyps can also be seen in ischemic and infectious colitis as well as in patients with Crohn's colitis (ZEGEL and LAUFER 1978). Filiform polyps have also been described in the esophagus, stomach, and small bowel in patients with Crohn's disease (BRAY 1983; WALKER et al. 1996).

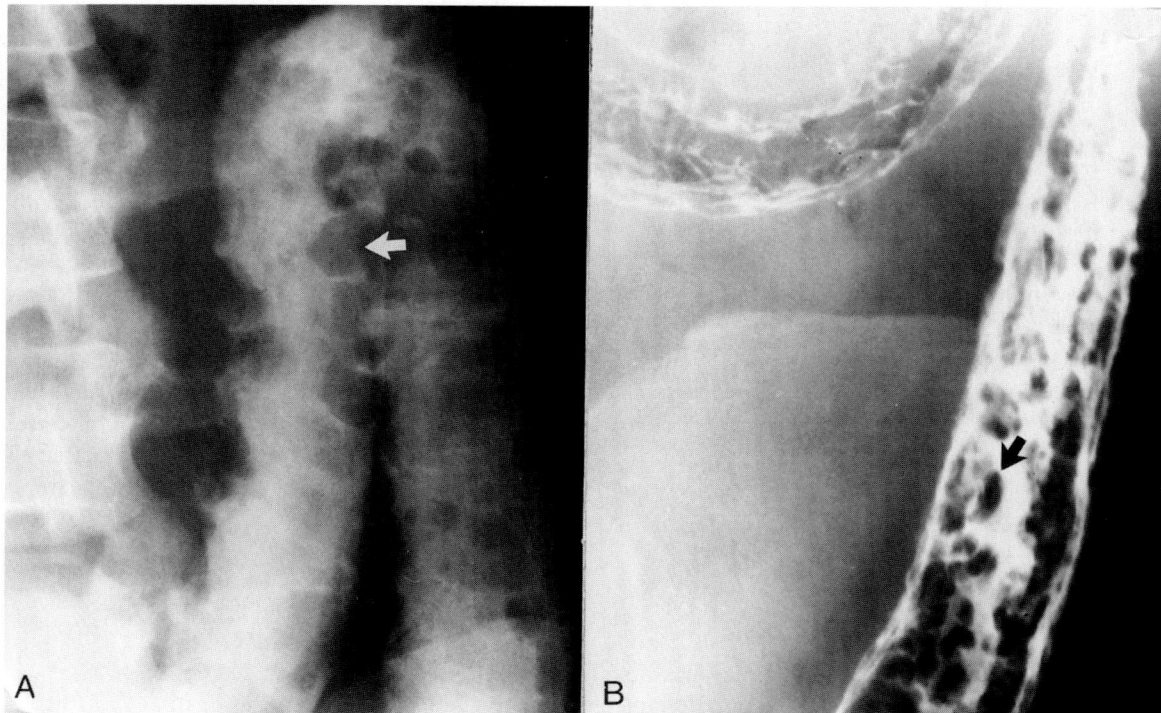

Fig. 10.5 a,b. Ulcerative colitis: inflammatory pseudopolyps. Sessile polypoid masses (*arrows*) are identified on single-contrast (**a**) and double-contrast (**b**) barium enema studies. They represent inflamed and swollen mucosal islands situated between areas of extensive ulceration. (From GORE and LAUFER 1994)

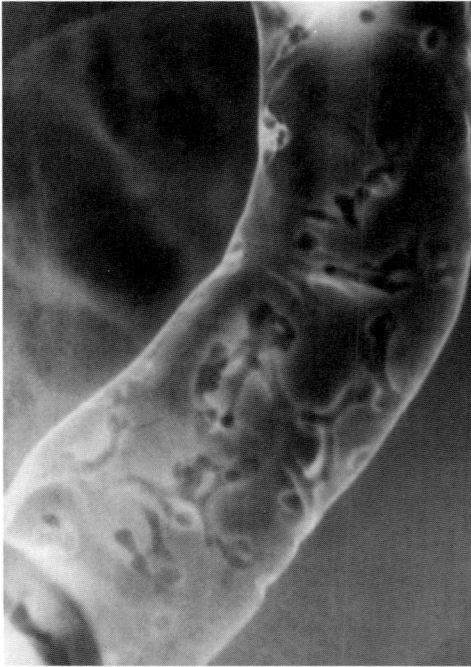

a

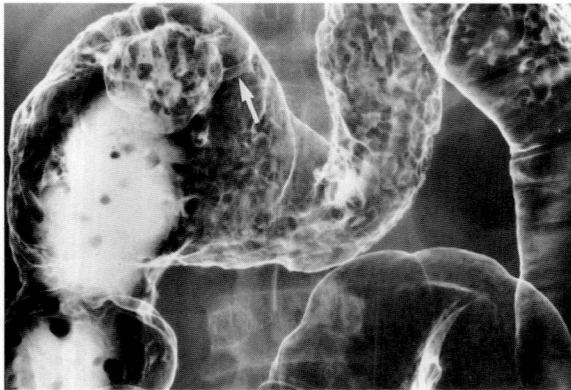

b

Fig. 10.6 a,b. Healed inflammatory bowel disease: postinflammatory pseudopolyps. **a** Filiform pseudopolyps are demonstrated in the distal descending colon in a patient with healed ulcerative colitis. Note the absence of active ulceration. (From GORE and LAUFER 1994). **b** Multiple postinflammatory pseudopolyps are seen in the ascending, transverse, and proximal descending colon in this patient with quiescent Crohn's disease. Note the giant pseudopolyp in the hepatic flexure and bridging pseudopolyp (*arrow*). (From GORE 1991)

10.2.2.5
Backwash Ileitis

In 10%–40% of patients with chronic ulcerative pancolitis, the distal 5–25 cm of ileum is inflamed (PRICE and MORSON 1987). This ileitis occurs only in the presence of pancolitis and usually resolves 1–2 weeks following colectomy. Although small ulcer-

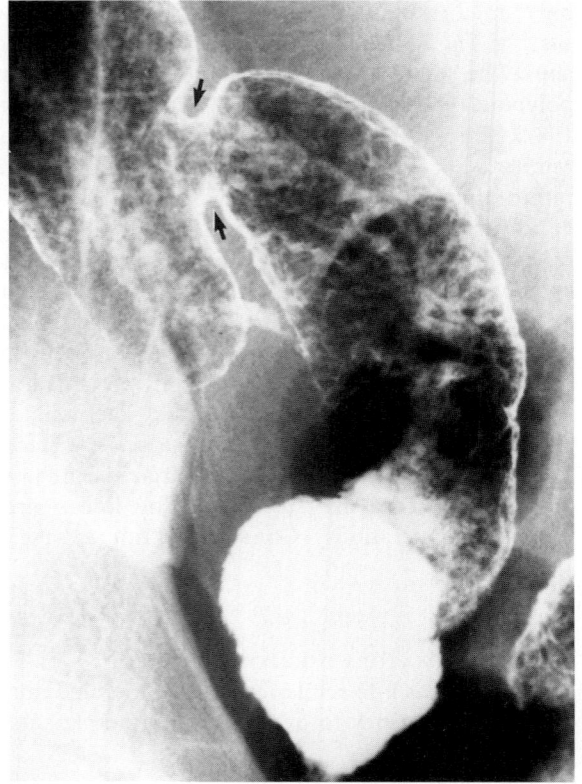

Fig. 10.7. Ulcerative colitis: backwash ileitis. The ileocecal value is patulous (*arrow*) and the dilated terminal ileum has a granular appearance in this patient with chronic ulcerative pancolitis. (From GORE and LAUFER 1994)

ations may be present, this is not a primary inflammation of the ileum. Indeed, the distal ileum can be used to form an ileostomy or pouch (COHEN and MCLEOD 1996). The pathogenesis of this disorder is uncertain but may relate to the reflux of colonic contents into the small bowel, hence the term "reflux" or "backwash" ileitis.

Barium studies reveal a chronic pancolitis associated with a patulous and fixed ileocecal valve that easily refluxes, and persistent dilatation of the terminal ileum (Fig. 10.7). The normal fold pattern is absent and the mucosa has a granular appearance (GARDINER 1977).

10.2.2.6
Blunting or Loss of Haustral Clefts

Haustra are formed by the taeniae coli which "shorten" the colon in an accordion-like fashion. They are fixed anatomic landmarks in the proximal colon because the circular muscle is fused to the

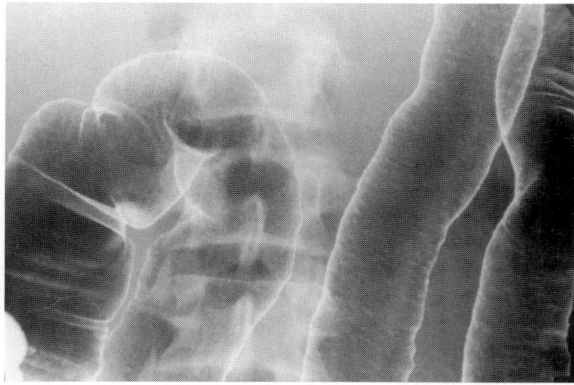

a

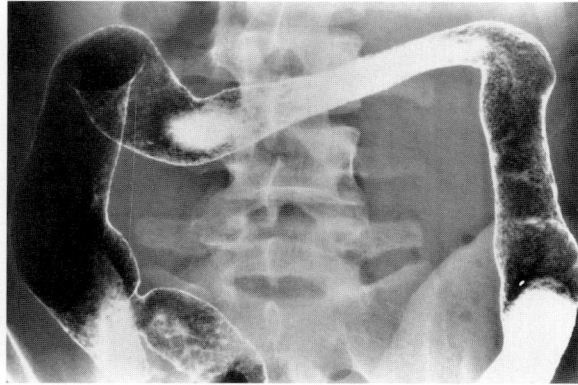

b

Fig. 10.8 a,b. Haustral alterations: acute and chronic ulcerative colitis. **a** In acute disease, the haustrations distal to the hepatic flexure are absent due to relaxation of the taeniae. The mucosa is granular and stippled, but the colon is not shortened because contraction and hypertrophy of the muscularis

mucosae have not yet developed at this early stage of disease. (From GORE and LAUFER 1994). **b** In chronic ulcerative colitis, the colon is ahaustral, shortened, tubular, and narrow. The muscularis mucosae is hypertrophied and chronically contracted. (From GORE and LAUFER 1994)

taeniae. In the distal colon, haustra are created by active contraction of the taeniae. Consequently, the colon can normally be devoid of haustra distal to the mid-transverse colon; loss of haustra in the proximal colon is always abnormal (GORE 1992).

In ulcerative colitis, the haustra are often lost for two reasons: alterations in the muscle tone of the taeniae in acute disease and colonic shortening in chronic disease (GORE 1992). In acute ulcerative colitis, the taeniae coli become relaxed and this is associated with abolition of the haustral pattern (Fig. 10.8a) in the involved segment (KOLODNY 1970). With healing, the haustra may reappear as the taeniae regain tone (GORE 1995). In chronic ulcerative colitis, the haustra are lost (Fig. 10.8b) as a result of fixed contraction and massive hypertrophy of the muscularis mucosae, often by a factor of 40-fold (GOULSTON and McGOVERN 1969). Forceful contraction of this hypertrophied longitudinal muscle may pull the mucosa away from the submucosa, producing diffuse or segmental narrowing of the lumen (GORE 1992). This contraction also causes shortening of the colon. As a result, the normal accordion-like array of colon on the taeniae is lost (GORE 1995).

10.2.3
CT Features

The subtle mucosal abnormalities that characterize the early stages of ulcerative colitis are beneath the spatial resolution of computed tomography (CT). With progressive disease, severe mucosal ulceration can denude certain portions of the colonic wall, lead-

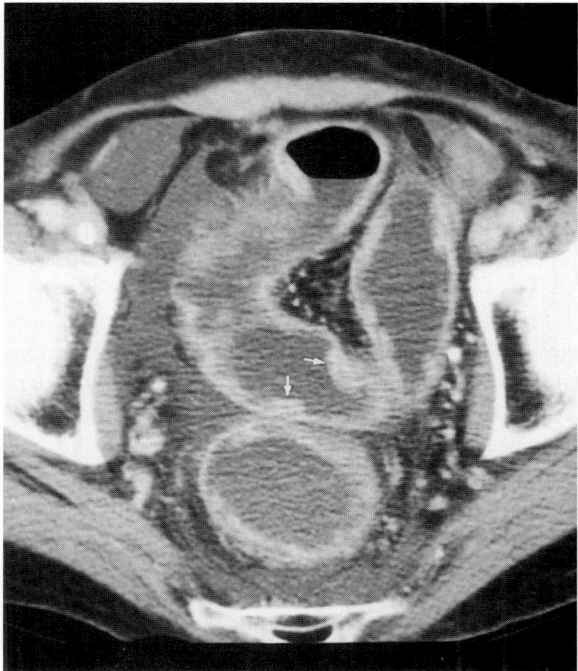

Fig. 10.9. Acute ulcerative colitis: inflammatory pseudopolyps. CT of the rectosigmoid colon shows residual islands of inflamed mucosa (*arrows*) protruding above the denuded colonic surface. Ascites is present as well

ing to inflammatory pseudopolyps (Fig. 10.9). When sufficiently large, these pseudopolyps can be visualized on CT. Mural thinning, unsuspected perforations (Fig. 10.10), and pneumatosis can be detected on CT in patients with toxic megacolon (SISKIND et al. 1985). In this regard, CT can be quite helpful in

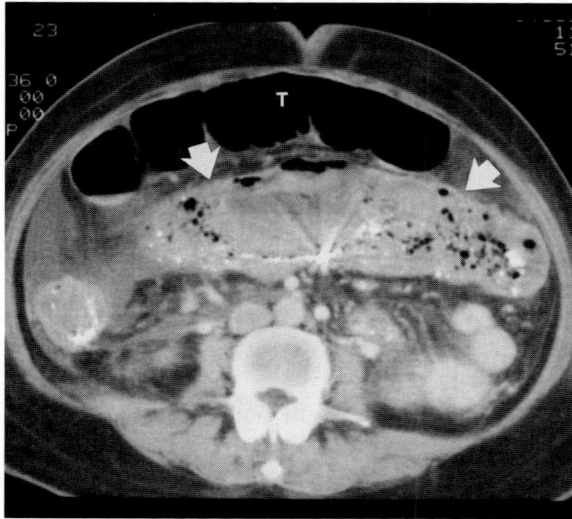

Fig. 10.10. CT scan revealing unsuspected perforation and abscess (*arrows*) in a patient with fulminant ulcerative colitis and toxic megacolon who was not improving clinically despite intensive medical management. This CT scan prompted colectomy and surgical abscess drainage. *T*, Transverse colon. (From GORE et al. 1996)

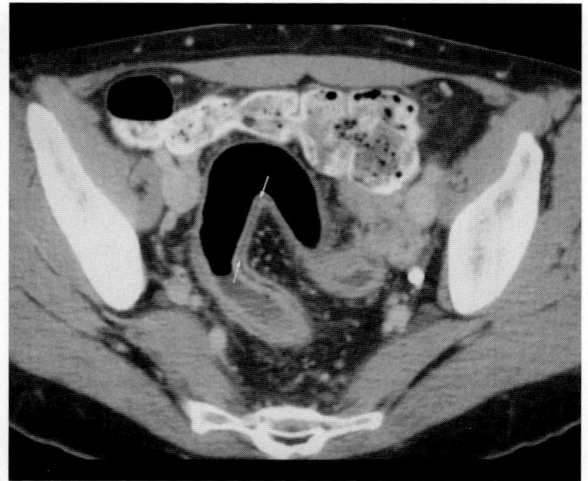

Fig. 10.11. Mural thickening in acute ulcerative colitis. CT section through rectosigmoid shows diffusely inflamed and thickened mucosa. Note that the edematous submucosal layer (*arrows*) of low attenuation is paralleled by the external layer of muscularis propria and internal layer of mucosa, both of which have higher attenuation. This mural stratification is typical of ulcerative colitis. (From GORE and LAUFER 1994)

determining the urgency of surgery in patients with stable plain abdominal films yet a deteriorating clinical course. Postinflammatory pseudopolyps can also be seen on CT (ARCHIBALD et al. 1988).

Mural thickening and lumen narrowing are common CT features of subacute and chronic ulcerative colitis. The mucosa becomes thickened due to hypertrophy of the muscularis mucosae in chronic ulcerative colitis. Additionally, the lamina propria is thickened due to round cell infiltration in both acute and chronic ulcerative colitis. The submucosa becomes thickened due to the deposition of fat, or, in acute and subacute cases, edema (Fig. 10.11). Submucosal thickening further contributes to luminal narrowing (KLEIN et al. 1995).

On CT, these mural changes produce a target or halo appearance when axially imaged (Fig. 10.11): the lumen is surrounded by a ring of soft tissue density (mucosa, lamina propria, hypertrophied muscularis mucosae), which is surrounded by a low-density ring (edema or fatty infiltration of the submucosa), which in turn is surrounded by a ring of soft tissue density (muscularis propria) (KLEIN et al. 1995). This mural stratification is not specific and can also be seen in Crohn's disease, infectious enterocolitis, pseudomembranous colitis, ischemic and radiation enterocolitis, mesenteric venous thrombosis, bowel edema and graft-versus-host dis-

ease (BALTHAZAR 1991, MULDOWNEY et al. 1995; PHILPOTTS et al. 1994).

Rectal narrowing and widening of the presacral space (Fig. 10.12a) are radiologic hallmarks of chronic ulcerative colitis (GORE and LAUFER 1994). High-resolution CT depicts the anatomic alterations that underlie these rather dramatic morphologic changes (Fig. 10.12b,c). The rectal lumen is narrowed due to the previously described mural thickening that attends chronic ulcerative colitis. As a result, the rectum has a target appearance on axial scans, which should not be mistaken for the external anal sphincter, mucosal prolapse, or the levator ani muscles. The increase in the presacral space is caused by proliferation of the perirectal fat. On CT this fat is characterized by an increased number of nodular and streaky soft tissue densities and an abnormal attenuation value 10–20 HU higher than the normal extraperitoneal or mesenteric fat (GORE et al. 1984). These fatty changes relate to a number of factors, including ex vacuo replacement by fat of the void produced by rectal lumen narrowing and lipodystrophy resulting from an influx of inflammatory cells and edema (GORE 1989). Edematous adipose tissue and enlarged lymph nodes are often observed in the perirectal region at the time of abdominoperineal resections in patients with chronic ulcerative colitis.

Normal   Chronic Ulcerative Colitis

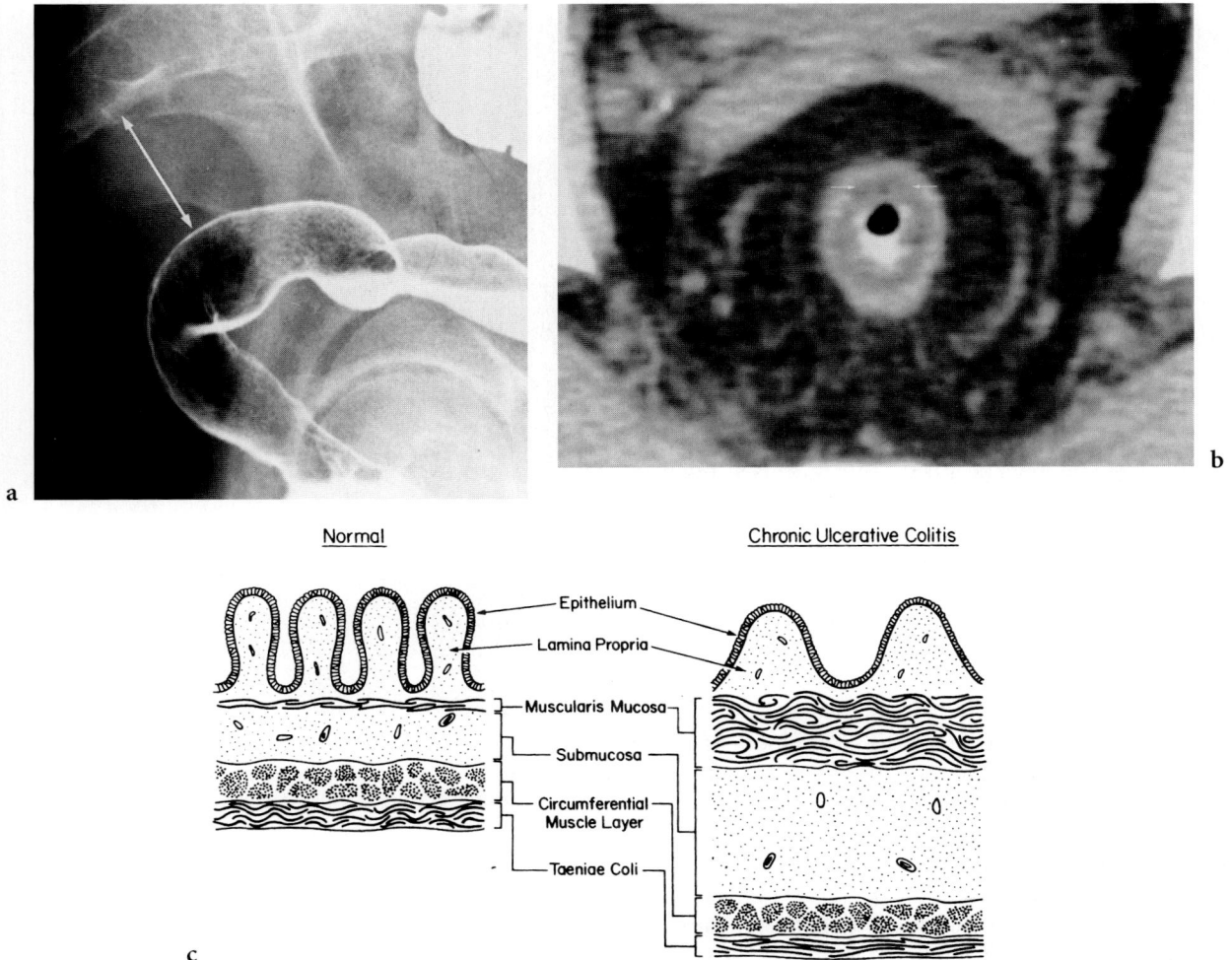

Fig. 10.12 a–c. Mural thickening in chronic ulcerative colitis. **a** Lateral view of the rectum on double-contrast barium enema shows narrowing of the lumen, granular appearance of the mucosa, loss of the valves of Houston, and significant widening of the presacral space (*arrows*). **b** Corresponding pelvic CT in a different patient reveals the target sign of the rectum. The middle, low-density ring (*arrows*), which is seen in chronic disease, is due to fatty infiltration. The widened presacral space is filled with abnormal fat with higher than normal attenuation and increased number of lymph nodes. **c** Diagram depicting the marked hypertrophy of the muscularis mucosae that attends chronic ulcerative colitis. This longitudinally oriented muscle is chronically contracted, which shortens and narrows the involved colon. The submucosa also widens and is infiltrated by fat, further narrowing the lumen. (From GORE 1992)

10.3
Crohn's Disease

Crohn's disease is a chronic granulomatous process that causes transmural inflammation of the bowel wall, often extending to the serosa and mesenteric lymph nodes (BRZEZINSKI and LASHNER 1997). Any portion of the alimentary tract may be involved, but the terminal ileum and proximal colon are most commonly affected (WILLS et al. 1997).

10.3.1
Plain Film Features

Radiographic findings of small bowel obstruction can be seen in patients with Crohn's disease. While it is uncommon to visualize the stenotic segment on plain film, the dilated loops proximal to or between stenotic areas can be seen. When confined to the colon, Crohn's disease has plain film features similar to ulcerative colitis. An extended gas-filled stricture of the colon is suggestive of granulomatous colitis, but it can also be present in carcinoma, healing ischemic colitis, and ulcerative colitis. Toxic megacolon can also develop in patients with Crohn's disease (SISKIND et al. 1985).

10.3.2
Barium Enema Features

10.3.2.1
Mucosal Granularity

The earliest radiologic manifestation of Crohn's disease of the small bowel is mucosal granularity (GLICK and TEPLIK 1985). This is caused by alteration in villous morphology: edema, hyperplasia, clubbing, fusion, and inflammatory cell infiltrate (GOLDBLUM and PETRAS 1997).

10.3.2.2
Lymphoid Hyperplasia

Lymphoid follicles are a normal component of gut-associated lymphatic tissue (KELVIN et al. 1979). They are aggregates of lymphocytes surrounding germinal centers that straddle the muscularis mucosae. Lymphoid follicles have an average macroscopic density of 3.8 per cm of adult human colon (LANGERMAN and ROWLAND 1986). They are seen in 50% of barium studies performed on children and 13% of air contrast barium enemas in adults (LAUFER and DESA 1978). Lymphoid follicles appear as 1- to 3-mm elevations in the mucosa without a ring shadow (LAUFER and COSTOPOULOS 1978).

Lymphoid follicles may enlarge (Fig. 10.13) in a wide variety of infectious, neoplastic, immunologic, and inflammatory diseases of the gut, including Crohn's disease (ERGERG and LINDSTROM 1979; KENNEDY et al. 1982). Prominent lymphoid follicles have also been observed in older patients with colonic adenomas and carcinomas (BRONEN et al. 1983).

10.3.2.3
Aphthous Lesions

As the lymphoid follicles enlarge, the overlying mucosa may ulcerate (Fig. 10.14), producing the aphthous lesion (FUJIMURA et al. 1996). These small superficial ulcers have erythematous margins and are seen on a background of normal or near-normal

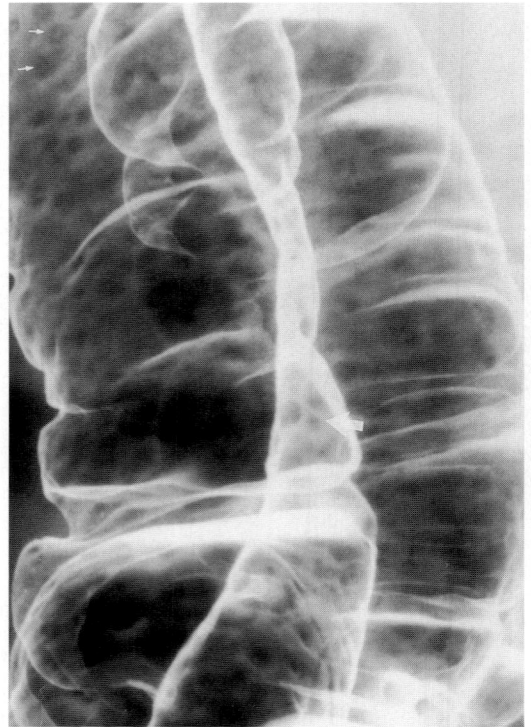

Fig. 10.13. Crohn's disease: lymphoid hyperplasia and aphthoid ulcers. Spot film of the splenic flexure shows large lymphoid follicles (*large arrow*), some of which have begun to ulcerate (*small arrows*)

mucosa (GOLDBLUM and PETRAS 1997). This is in direct contrast to ulcerative colitis, in which ulceration invariably occurs against a background of diffuse, continuous, and circumferential inflammation (SIMPKINS and GORE 1994). Radiologically, aphthae are recognized as punctate central collections of barium surrounded by a radiolucent halo about 1 mm in diameter, producing a "target" or "bull's eye" appearance. Aphthae may be isolated, found in clusters, or involve the entire colon (SIMPKINS 1977).

Aphthoid lesions are found in 44%–72% of patients with Crohn's disease and may be the only abnormality found in an otherwise normal colon (HIZAWA et al. 1994). These ulcers are nonspecific and also occur in amebiasis, salmonella, shigellosis, herpes, cytomegalovirus infection, Behçet's disease, ischemic colitis, and *Yersinia* enterocolitis (GORE and GHAHREMANI 1995).

10.3.2.4
Cobblestoning

Aphthous lesions may regress, remain stable, or, as is more common, enlargen and deepen (NI and

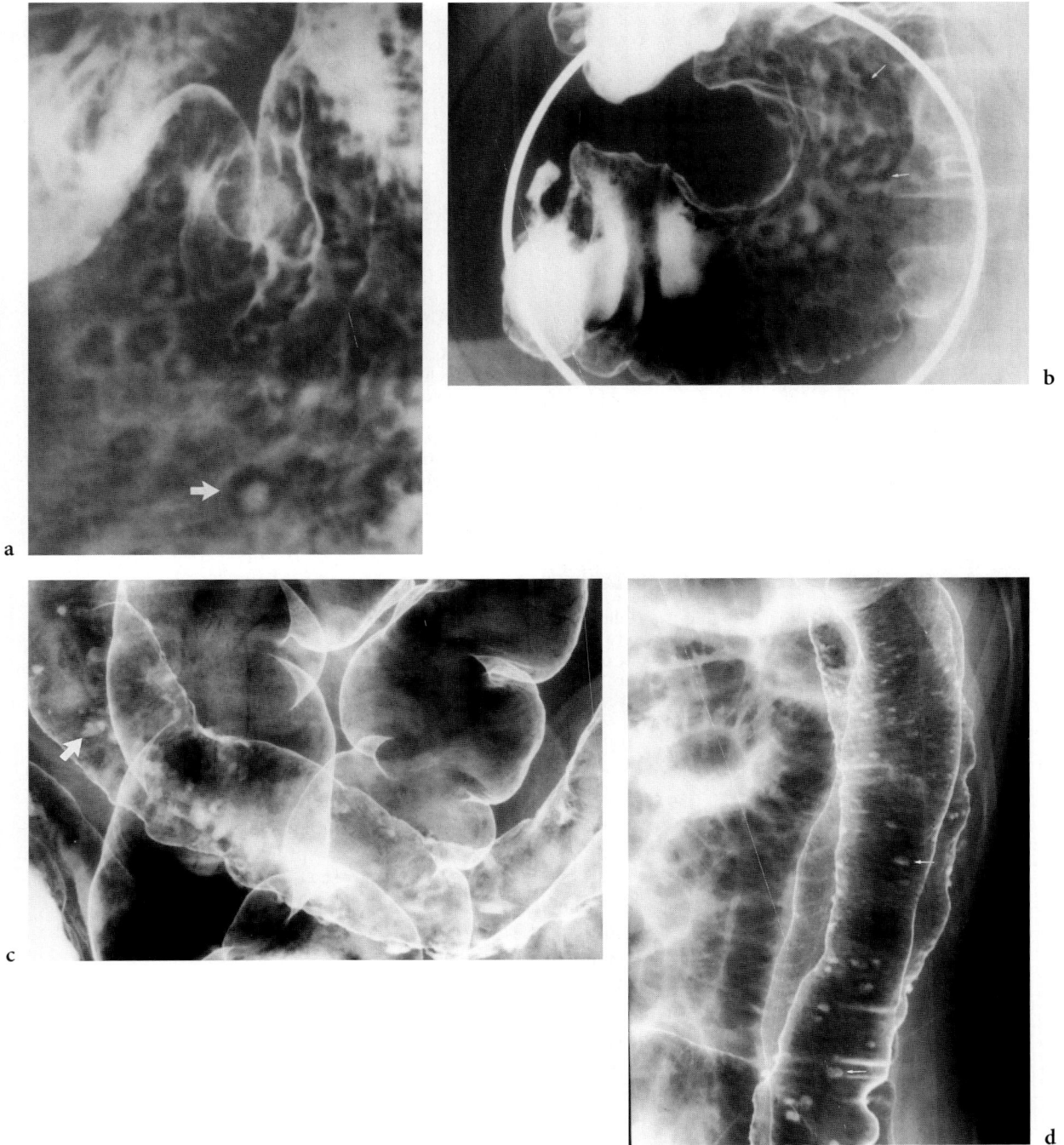

Fig. 10.14 a–d. Crohn's disease: aphthoid ulcerations. Double-contrast barium studies in different patients demonstrate aphthae (*arrows*) of varying size in the stomach (a), cecum (b), transverse colon (c), and splenic flexure (d). These aphthoid ulcers appear as central collections of barium surrounded by a thin radiolucent halo, producing a target or "bull's eye" appearance. (b From GORE and LAUFER 1994; c from GORE and LAUFER 1994)

GOLDBERG 1986). As the aphthae expand, they become irregular in outline and lose their surrounding lucent halo (TREMAINE 1996). Adjacent ulcers may coalesce, forming a network of longitudinal linear ulceration and transverse fissuring, with edematous intervening mucosa producing a raised, "cobbled" appearance (Fig. 10.15) (GOLDBLUM and PETRAS 1997). As mentioned earlier, this is actually one of many forms of inflammatory pseudopolyposis (LICHTENSTEIN 1987).

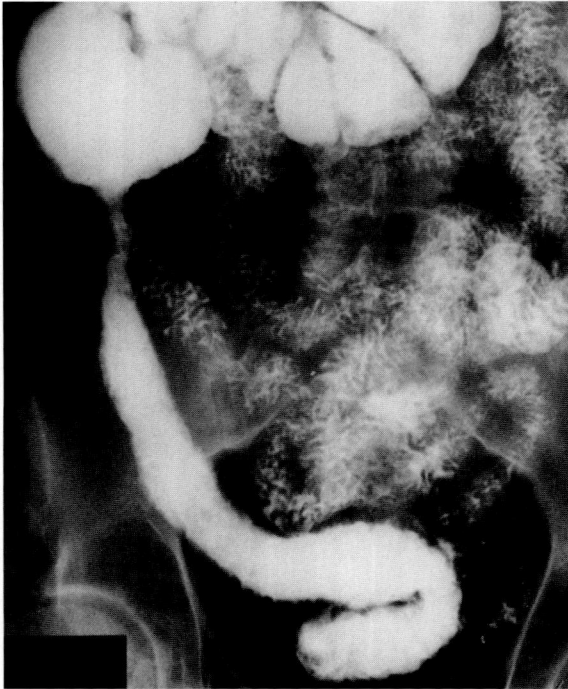

Fig. 10.15. Crohn's disease: cobblestoning. Spot film of the distal ileum demonstrates nodular mucosa caused by islands of preserved epithelium surrounded by a network of ulcerations. This is recurrent disease in a patient who has undergone resection of the terminal ileum and cecum and ileal-ascending colon anastomosis

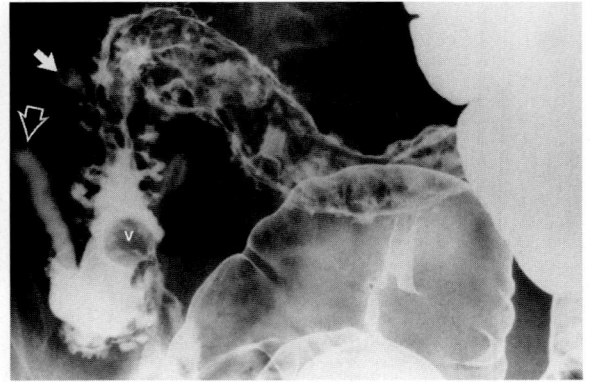

Fig. 10.16. Crohn's disease: deep, fissuring ulcers. Deep ulcers (*solid arrow*) that penetrate beyond the submucosa are seen in the right colon on this double-contrast barium enema. Note the thick ileocecal valve (*V*) and sparing of the left colon and rectosigmoid. Contrast these ulcers with the more superficial collar button ulcers of the ulcerative colitis in Fig. 10.4. *Open arrow*, suphepatic appendix. (From GORE and LAUFER 1994)

10.3.2.5
Deep Ulcerations

Fissuring ulcers are a distinctive feature of Crohn's disease. They typically penetrate beyond the submucosa (Fig. 10.16), resulting in knife-shaped or "rose thorn" fistulas (BUCKWELL et al. 1980). These fissures do not cause pneumoperitoneum because the surrounding serosa is inflamed and bowel loops become adherent to one another and to adjacent peritoneal surfaces (STRONG and FAZIO 1993).

10.3.2.6
Pericolic Sinus Tracking

Long interconnecting fistulas are common in Crohn's colitis and occur in the muscularis mucosae or subserosa paralleling (Fig. 10.17) the bowel lumen (GOLDBLUM and PETRAS 1997). When not associated with neoplasia or diverticula, paracolic sinus tracts are very suggestive of Crohn's disease.

10.3.2.7
Fistulae and Sinus Tracks

Fistulae and sinus tracks (Fig. 10.18) are hallmarks of Crohn's disease, affecting approximately 20%–40% of patients (GOLDBLUM and PETRAS 1997). The morphology and anatomic sites of fistulae are protean: enteroenteric, enterocolic, colo-colic, enterovesical, enterovaginal, enterocutaneous, enterovenous, anorectal, duodenopancreatic, gastrocolic, colobronchial, and enterospinal (FLUECKIGER et al. 1990; MICHELASSI et al. 1993; PICHNEY et al. 1992).

10.3.2.8
String Sign

When the lumen of the terminal ileum becomes markedly narrowed due to Crohn's disease, its radiologic appearance is referred to as the "string sign." This sign was originally reported in acute, prestenotic regional enteritis to describe a very narrowed ileum simulating a frayed string (GOLDBLUM and PETRAS 1997). It results from mucosal ulceration and spasms similar to the "Stierlin sign" observed in ileocecal tuberculosis. This spasm is reversible. The term "string sign" is now more commonly used to describe fixed, chronic narrowing due to fibrosis and thickening of the bowel wall (Fig. 10.19) that occurs in the cicatrizing phase of Crohn's disease (SIMPKINS 1988).

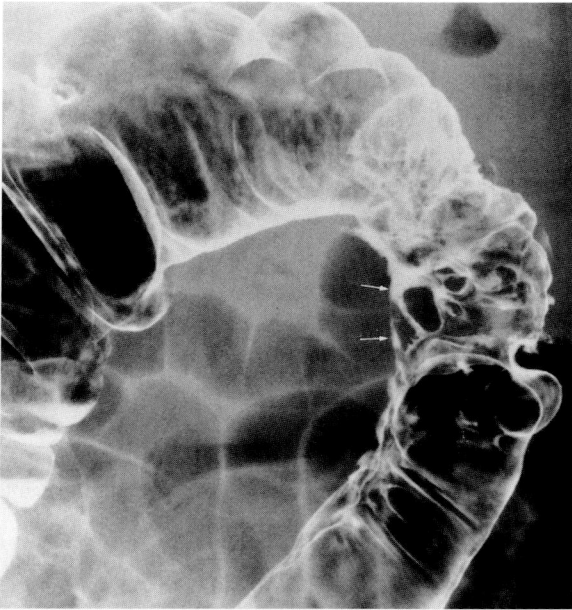

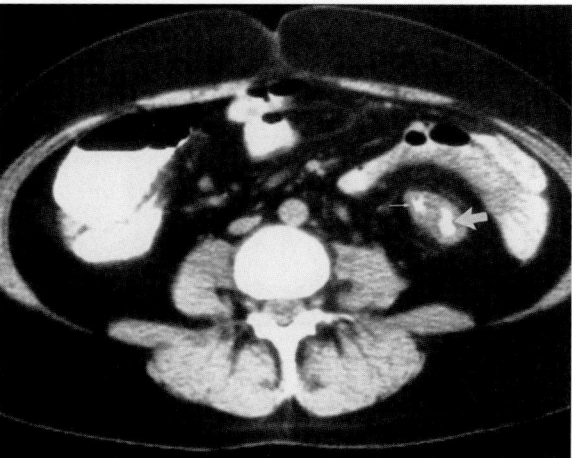

Fig. 10.17 a,b. Crohn's disease: pericolic sinus tracking. **a** Recurrent Crohn's disease characterized by ulcerations and pericolic sinus tracks (*arrows*) is shown at the anastomosis in this patient who had undergone resection of the transverse colon. **b** CT scan shows the lumen (*thick arrow*) and sinus track (*thin arrow*)

10.3.2.9
Lumen Narrowing and Strictures

Crohn's disease is a transmural inflammatory process which produces gut wall thickening and fibrosis leading to narrowing of the lumen (Fig. 10.20) and shortening of the gut as well (MARK et al. 1989). In ulcerative colitis, narrowing results from thickening and contraction of the muscularis mucosae rather than fibrosis. Strictures are asymmetric in Crohn's

disease and tend to be less smooth and circumferential than those seen in ulcerative colitis. Strictures occur in 21% of patients with small bowel disease and 8% of Crohn's colitis cases (GOLDBLUM and PETRAS 1997; RIDDELL 1997).

10.3.2.10
Sacculations

The transmural fibrosis of Crohn's disease is often asymmetric. It occurs predominantly on the mesenteric side of the gut, where it is often accompanied by "creeping fat" of the mesentery. The relatively unaffected side (usually antimesenteric) remains pliable and tends to bulge when intraluminal pressure increases due to peristalsis. Outpouchings (Fig. 10.21) may eventually develop (GOLDBLUM and PETRAS 1997). This is similar to the so-called sacculations or pseudodiverticula seen in scleroderma.

10.3.2.11
Anorectal Disease

Anorectal complications (Fig. 10.22) are common in patients with Crohn's disease and include anal fissures, ulcers, abscess, internal hemorrhoids, and stenosis with induration; skin lesions such as erosion, skin tags, ulceration, maceration, external hemorrhoids, and abscess; and fistulas – anal canal to skin, rectum to skin, and rectovaginal (GUILLAUMIN 1986). Anal disease develops in 36% of all patients with Crohn's disease, 25% of those with only small bowel involvement, 67% of patients with colonic disease, and nearly all patients with rectal disease (MCLEOD and COHEN 1997).

In approximately one-fourth of patients, the anal disease may antedate overt intestinal disease often by as many as 4 years (MCLEOD and COHEN 1997). Accordingly, development of these anorectal disorders warrants radiologic investigation of the entire gastrointestinal tract.

10.3.2.12
Distribution

Any portion of the gut from the mouth to the anus may be involved by Crohn's disease (YOUSEM et al. 1988). Twenty percent of cases are isolated to the colon, 20% are restricted to the small bowel, and 60% involve the colon and small bowel simultaneously. In

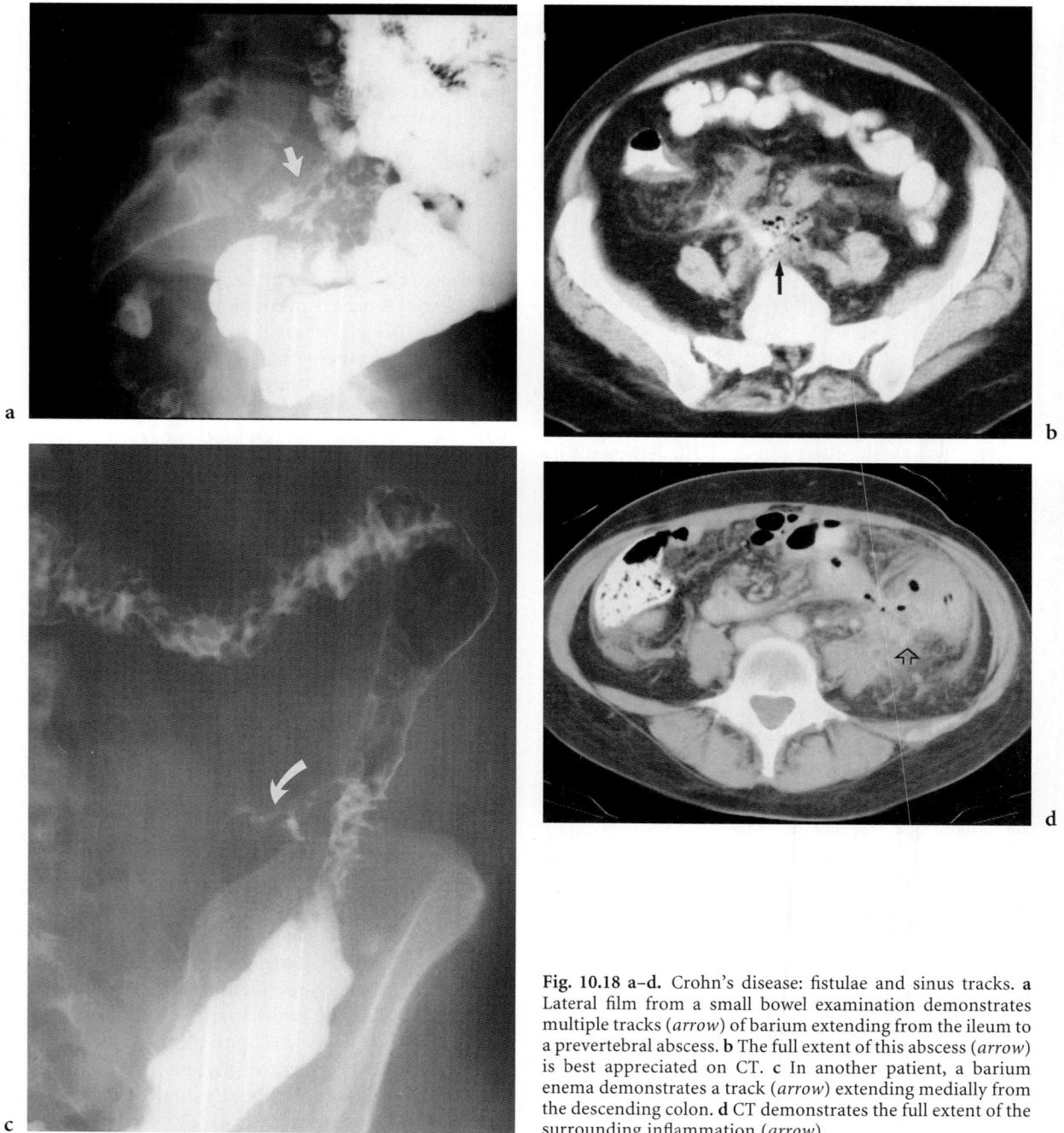

Fig. 10.18 a–d. Crohn's disease: fistulae and sinus tracks. a Lateral film from a small bowel examination demonstrates multiple tracks (*arrow*) of barium extending from the ileum to a prevertebral abscess. b The full extent of this abscess (*arrow*) is best appreciated on CT. c In another patient, a barium enema demonstrates a track (*arrow*) extending medially from the descending colon. d CT demonstrates the full extent of the surrounding inflammation (*arrow*)

5%–10% of these patients, upper gastrointestinal in-volvement is seen (GORE and GHAHREMANI 1986). It is unusual to see isolated esophageal or gastroduode-nal Crohn's disease, however. Regardless of loca-tion, similar radiographic-pathologic findings obtain: there is discontinuous, patchy, and asym-metric disease involvement (SIMPKINS and GORE 1994).

10.3.3
CT Features

Crohn's disease is manifested on CT by bowel wall thickening ranging between 1 and 2 cm (GOLDBERG et al. 1983; SCHOLTEN et al. 1995). This thickening, which occurs in up to 83% of patients, is most fre-quently observed in the terminal ileum, but other

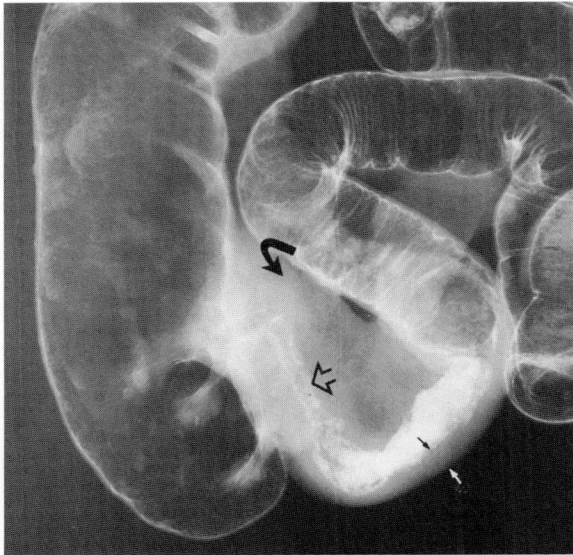

Fig. 10.19. Crohn's disease: string sign. Double-contrast examination of a resected specimen of the distal ileum and proximal colon shows narrowing of the lumen of the terminal ileum (*open arrow*) associated with mural thickening (*small arrows*) and creeping fat of the mesentery (*curved arrow*)

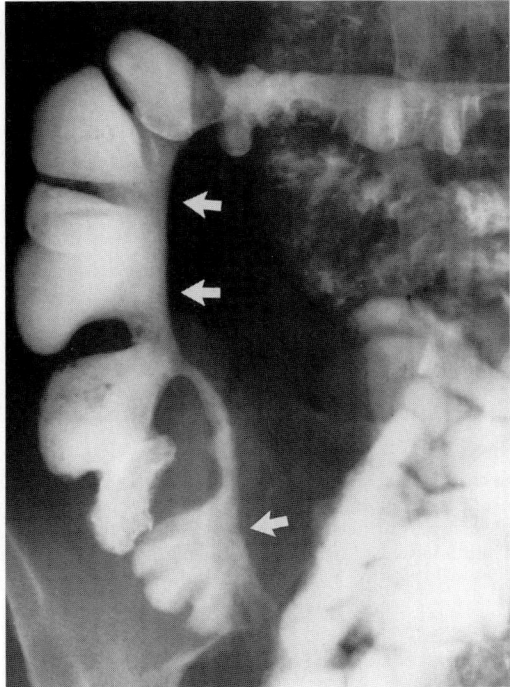

Fig. 10.21. Crohn's disease: sacculations. Sacculations of the terminal ileum are seen in this patient with ileocolitis. Notice the fibrosis on the mesenteric side of the gut (*arrows*) and "ballooning" of the antimesenteric border. (From GORE and LAUFER 1994)

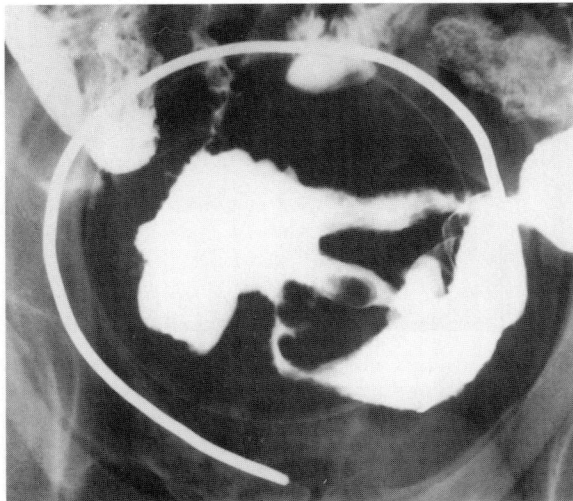

Fig. 10.20. Crohn's disease: stricture. Several regions of severe narrowing are identified on this spot film of the distal ileum

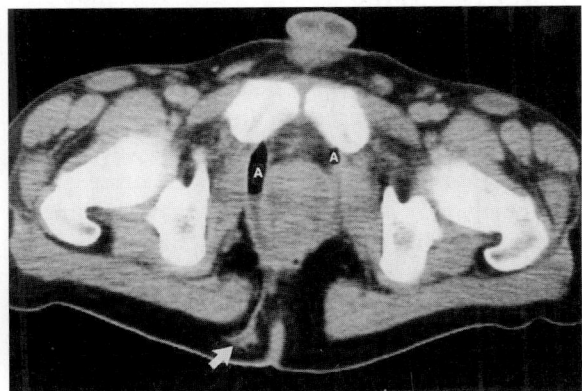

Fig. 10.22. Crohn's disease: anorectal disease. A perirectal sinus tract (*arrow*) extends through the fat of the right ischiorectal fossa into the right buttock. Perirectal abscesses (A) containing air are seen lateral to the rectum

portions of the small bowel, colon, duodenum, stomach, and esophagus may be similarly affected (PHILPOTTS et al. 1994; GORE and GHAHREMANI 1986).

During the acute, noncicatrizing phase of Crohn's disease, the small bowel and colon maintain mural stratification (Fig. 10.23a) and often have a target or double halo appearance (GORE et al. 1996a). As in

ulcerative colitis, there is a soft tissue density ring (corresponding to mucosa), which is surrounded by a low-density ring with an attenuation near water or fat (corresponding to submucosal edema or fat infiltration respectively), which in turn is surrounded by

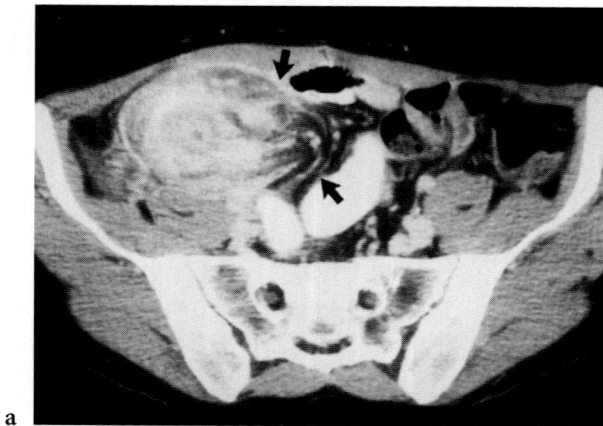

a

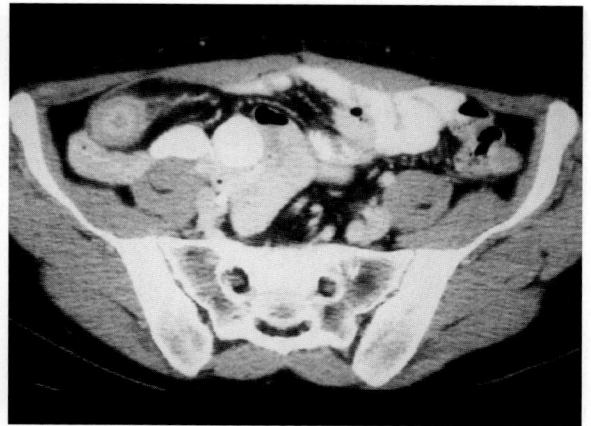

b

Fig. 10.23 a,b. Acute, noncicatrizing phase of Crohn's disease: target sign. **a** Contrast-enhanced CT of terminal ileum shows intense enhancement of mucosa and muscularis propria-serosa. Mural stratification is present as the edematous, thickened submucosa of low attenuation (*black arrows*) contrasts with the other bowel wall layers, producing the target sign.

The peri-intestinal fat also shows marked inflammatory change. The patient presented with low-grade obstruction of the small bowel and fever. (From GORE et al. 1996). **b** A scan of the same region obtained following intensive steroid and antibiotic therapy shows marked reduction in the inflammation. (From GORE et al. 1996a)

a higher density ring (muscularis propria) (GORE et al. 1994; JONES et al. 1986). Inflamed mucosa and serosa may show significant contrast enhancement following bolus intravenous contrast administration, and the intensity of enhancement correlates with the clinical activity of disease (JACOBS and BIRNBAUM 1995).

The CT demonstration of mural stratification, i.e., the ability to visualize distinct mucosal, submucosal, and muscularis propria layers, indicates that transmural fibrosis has not occurred and that medical therapy may be successful in ameliorating lumen compromise (GORE et al. 1996a). The edema and inflammation of the bowel wall which cause mural thickening and lumen obstruction are reversible to some extent (Fig. 10.23b). A modest decrease in wall thickness often produces a dramatic increase in lumen cross-sectional area and resolution of the patient's obstructive symptoms (Fig. 10.24). In patients with longstanding Crohn's disease and transmural fibrosis, mural stratification is lost so that the affected bowel wall typically has homogeneous attenuation on CT (GORE 1989). Homogeneous attenuation of the thickened bowel wall (Fig. 10.25) in the presence of good intravascular contrast medium levels and thin section scanning suggests irreversible fibrosis so that anti-inflammatory agents may not provide significant reduction in bowel wall thickness (GORE et al. 1996b). If these segments become sufficiently narrow, surgery or stricturoplasty may be necessary to relieve the patient's obstruction (ALEXANDER-WILLIAMS 1997).

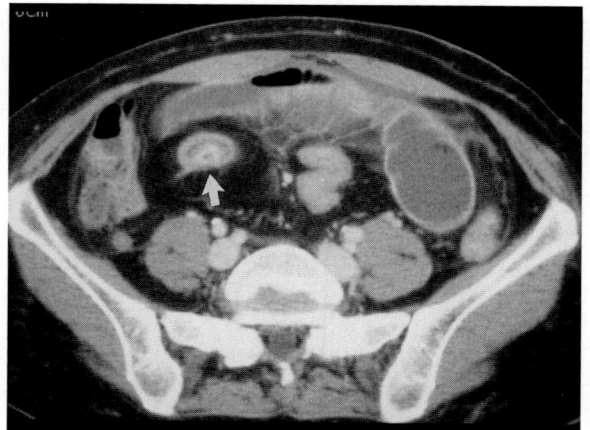

Fig. 10.24. Crohn's disease: bowel obstruction. Contrast-enhanced CT shows lumen narrowing, mural thickening, and a target sign (*arrow*) of the distal ileum causing small bowel obstruction. Mural stratification is maintained. The ability to visualize various layers of bowel wall suggests that the stenosis may be reversible with medical therapy

10.3.3.1
Mesenteric Involvement

The palpation of an abdominal mass or separation of bowel loops on a small bowel series in a patient with Crohn's disease evokes a large differential diagnosis: abscess, phlegmon, "creeping fat" or fibrofatty proliferation of the mesentery, bowel wall thickening, and enlarged mesenteric lymph nodes. Each of these disorders has significantly different prognostic and

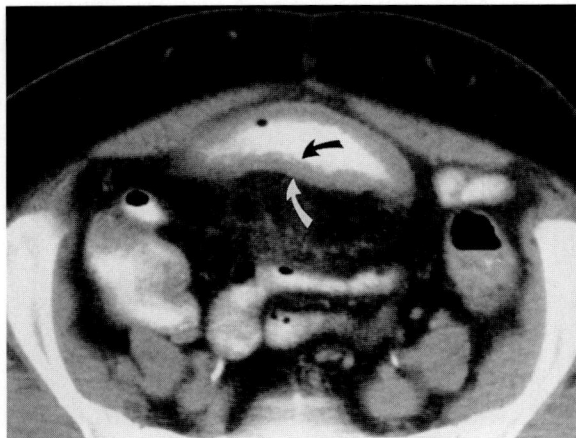

a

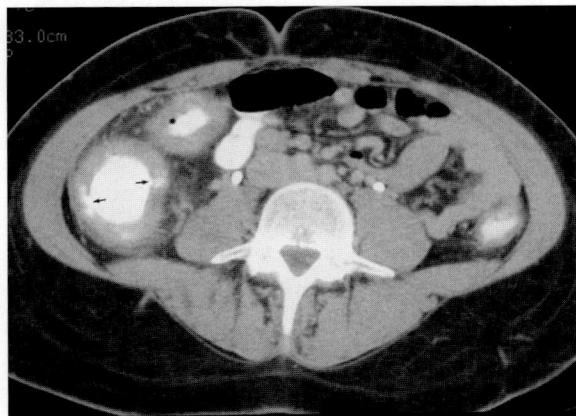

b

Fig. 10.25 a,b. Chronic cicatrizing Crohn's disease in which loss of mural stratification often indicates irreversible transmural fibrosis. **a** Pelvic CT scan reveals homogeneous mural thickening (*arrows*) of the distal ileum. **b** CT scan in another patient reveals deep ulcers (*black arrows*) penetrating the otherwise homogeneously thickened walls of the ascending colon. The terminal ileum (*black dot*) and descending colon are also involved. Note the increased linear and nodular densities in the mesenteric fat surrounding the inflamed intestinal segments. Prominent lymph nodes are present in the small bowel mesentery. (From GORE et al. 1996a)

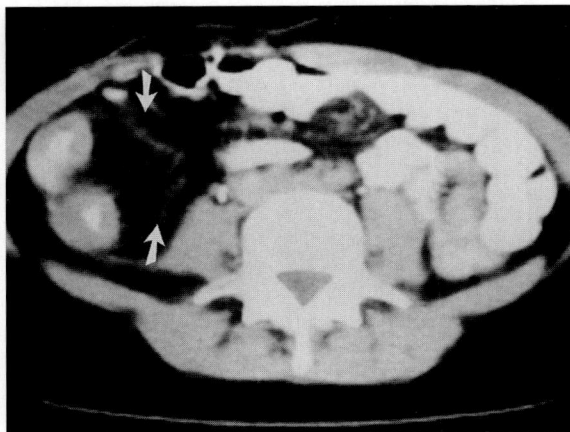

Fig. 10.26. Creeping mesenteric fat in Crohn's disease. CT shows homogeneously thickened walls of ileum and ascending colon. On their medial aspect, note the abnormal mesenteric fat with an increased number of strand-like densities (*arrows*). Note too the separation of normal small bowel loops from these diseased segments due to this abnormal mesenteric fat. (From GORE et al. 1996a)

therapeutic implications (FISHMAN et al. 1987). This diagnostic dilemma is further complicated by the fact that many patients are receiving immunosuppressive therapy that can mask signs and symptoms. CT can readily differentiate the extraluminal manifestations of Crohn's disease (OREL et al. 1987).

10.3.3.2
Fibrofatty Proliferation of the Mesentery

Fibrofatty proliferation, also known as "creeping fat" of the mesentery, is the most common cause of sepa-

ration of bowel loops seen on small bowel series in patients with Crohn's disease (JABRA et al. 1991). On CT (Fig. 10.26), the sharp interface between bowel and mesentery is lost and the attenuation value of the fat is elevated by 20–60 HU due to the influx of inflammatory cells and fluid (GORE and GOLDBERG 1982). Mesenteric adenopathy with lymph nodes ranging in size between 3 and 8 mm may also be present (GORE et al. 1984). If these lymph nodes are larger than 1 cm, the presence of lymphoma or carcinoma, both of which occur with greater frequency in Crohn's disease, must be excluded.

Contrast-enhanced CT scans often show hypervascularity of the involved mesentery manifesting as vascular dilatation, tortuosity, prominence, and wide spacing of the vasa recta (Fig. 10.27). These distinctive vascular changes have been called "vascular jejunization of the ileum" or the "comb sign" (MEYERS and McGUIRE 1995). Identification of this hypervascularity should suggest active disease and may be useful in differentiating Crohn's disease from lymphoma or metastases, which tend to be hypovascular lesions.

10.3.3.3
Abscess

Some 15%–20% of patients with Crohn's disease eventually develop an intra-abdominal abscess (KEIGHLEY et al. 1982). Abscesses (Fig. 10.28) are

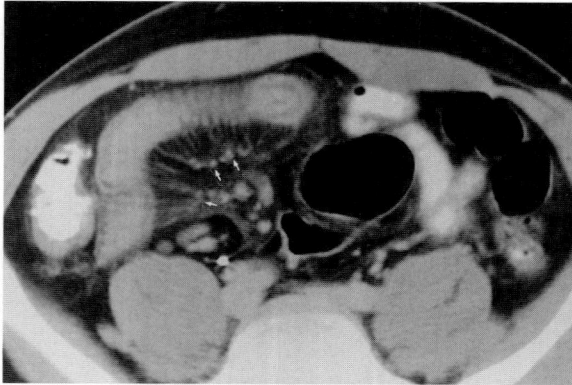

Fig. 10.27. Vascular engorgement of the ileal mesentery associated with active Crohn's disease. CT shows vascular dilation, tortuosity, and prominence of the vasa recta (*arrows*) on the mesenteric side of the ileum – the comb sign. The diseased ileal loop shows mural thickening and target appearance. Also note the prominent mesenteric lymph nodes. (From GORE et al. 1996a)

Fig. 10.28 a,b. Abscess formation complicating Crohn's disease. **a** CT reveals a midline abscess (*A*) posterior to the anterior peritoneal reflection. Note the thickened ileum (*arrows*) and the enlarged blood vessels supplying this abnormal segment. **b** Psoas abscess (*A*) in a different patient. Note the fistula to the small bowel (*open arrow*) and contrast-fluid-and-air level (*solid arrow*). (From GORE 1987)

most frequently associated with small bowel disease or ileocolitis (RIBEIRO et al. 1991). Once developed, an abscess can burrow through the adjacent tissue or break open and drain spontaneously into another part of the bowel and/or adjacent organs. Abscesses usually result from sinus tracts, fistulas, perforations, or surgical operations for Crohn's disease.

An intra-abdominal abscess may be difficult to diagnose on clinical grounds in patients with Crohn's disease because symptoms may be inconspicuous, masked by corticosteroids, or mistaken for an exacerbation of disease. Barium studies and endoscopy can only suggest the presence of an abscess indirectly by mass effect, spiculation of the mucosa, or identification of a fistula (HYDE and GERZOF 1994). Also these studies do not evaluate the ischiorectal fossa, psoas muscle, and solid abdominal organs, common locations of abscess formation. Cross-sectional imaging is required to confirm the diagnosis and reveal the full extent and location of the abscess cavity (LAMBIASE et al. 1988). CT is the prime imaging tool employed for percutaneous drainage (Fig. 10.29) of Crohn's related abscesses (CASOLA et al. 1987; DOEMENY et al. 1988).

10.3.3.4
Phlegmon

A phlegmon is an ill-defined, inflammatory mass in the mesentery or omentum that may resolve completely with antibiotics or progress to form an ab-

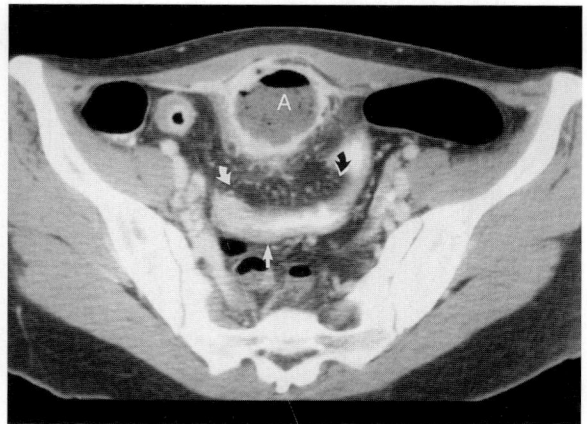

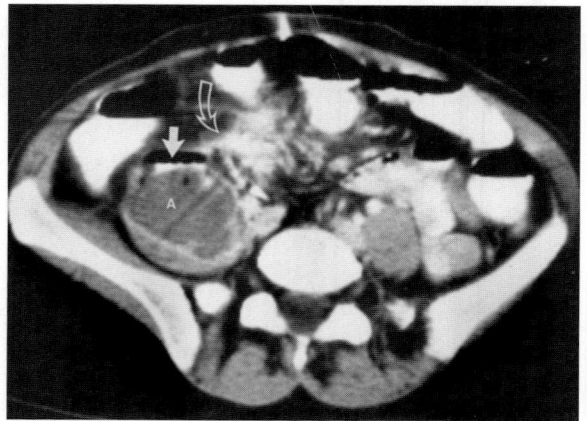

scess (GORE et al. 1985). Phlegmons are another common cause of mesenteric mass effect in patients with Crohn's disease. On CT (Fig. 10.30), a phlegmon produces loss of definition of surrounding organs and a "smudgy" or "streaky" appearance of the adjacent mesenteric or omental fat (GORE 1987).

10.3.4
Transrectal Ultrasound Features

Transrectal ultrasound can show the following abnormalities in patient's with Crohn's disease: (a) mural thickening; (b) perianal and perirectal abscesses (Fig. 10.31) and fistulas; (c) heterogeneity of the anal sphincter (VAN OUTRYVE et al. 1991). Rectal

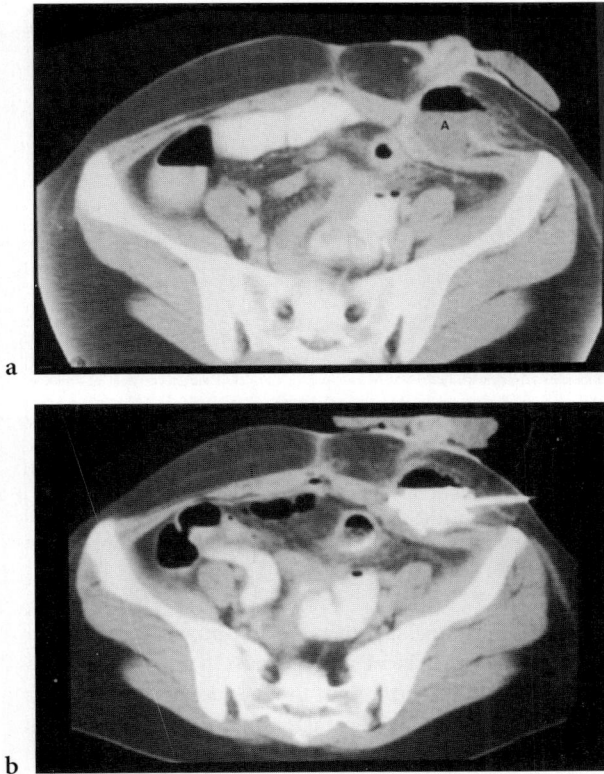

a

b

Fig. 10.29 a,b. Percutaneous abscess drainage. **a** A peristomal abscess (*A*) is demonstrated in this patient who had undergone a colectomy due to Crohn's disease. **b** A percutaneous catheter drains this collection

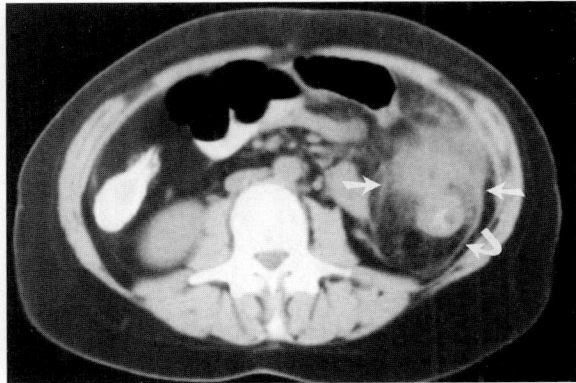

Fig. 10.30. Phlegmon associated with Crohn's colitis. Unenhanced CT scan shows homogeneous mural thickening of the descending colon, a pericolic phlegmon (*straight arrows*), and fascial thickening (*curved arrow*)

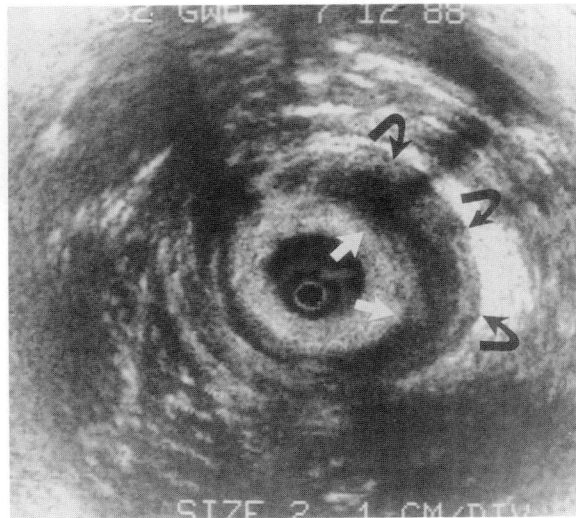

Fig. 10.31. Transrectal ultrasound image of perirectal abscess. A semilunar-shaped fluid collection with internal echoes (*arrows*) is identified at the level of anal sphincter, just below the supralevator ani muscle in this patient with Crohn's disease. (From HILL et al. 1992)

wall thickening (>4 mm) is often accompanied by loss of mural stratification in Crohn's disease.

The anal sphincter derives from the rectal muscular layer as a sharply delineated ellipsoid that is uniformly hypoechoic. When involved by Crohn's disease, the sphincter becomes heterogeneous with echogenic zones interspersed between the normal hypoechoic regions. Also in patients with active proctologic disease, the shortening and narrowing of the anal canal during squeezing and elongation with dilatation during straining are less pronounced (GORE 1995). Fistula and sinus tracts appear as a dotted column of echo-rich gas bubbles with reverberation on transrectal ultrasound. Abscesses are characterized sonographically as predominantly hypoechoic areas that contain echogenic elements corresponding to debris and gas bubbles. The wall of the abscess is usually thick and irregular and some posterior acoustic enhancement may be seen.

Some authors advocate routine screening transrectal ultrasound because this technique is capable of defining pararectal and para-anal abscesses and

fistula that develop extramurally without mucosal lesions (BUTANI and HAWES 1997).

10.3.5
Magnetic Resonance Imaging Features

Magnetic resonance imaging (MRI) provides a similar perspective (Fig. 10.32) to CT in that images demonstrate the overall topography of the abdomen. This imaging technique has several inherent advantages: lack of ionizing radiation, multiplanar imag-

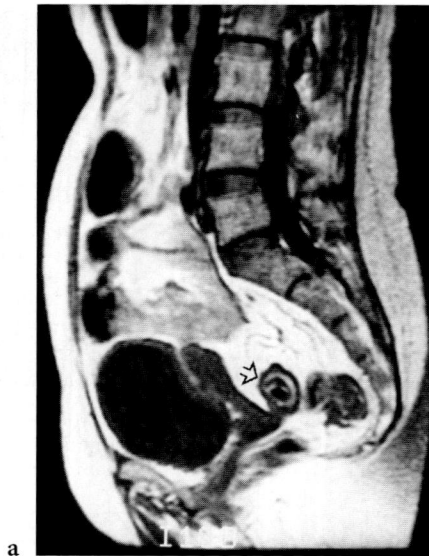

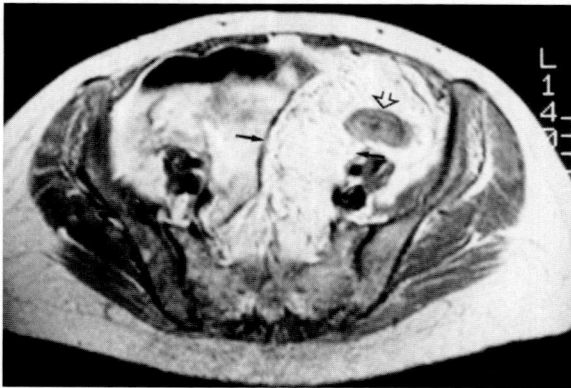

Fig. 10.32 a,b. Crohn's disease: MR findings. Sagittal (**a**) and axial (**b**) T1-weighted images through the sigmoid colon demonstrate mural thickening (*open arrows*). Notice also the creeping mesenteric fat, which has an increased number of blood vessels (*solid arrows*)

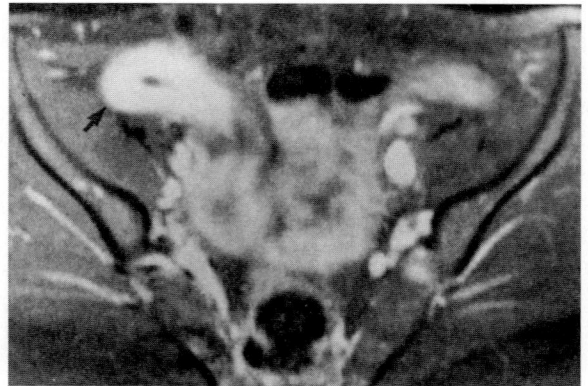

Fig. 10.33. Crohn's disease of the terminal ileum: contrast-enhanced MR findings. Axial scan of the pelvis obtained following the intravenous administration of Gd-DTPA shows severe inflammation with marked wall thickening and mural enhancement of the distal ileum (*arrow*). The degree of enhancement correlates with the degree of inflammation. (From SHOENUT et al. 1993)

ing capability, and superb soft tissue contrast (ANDERSON et al. 1994). Disadvantages which have generally precluded the routine use of MRI in the evaluation of IBD include respiratory and bowel motion artifact, lack of a satisfactory oral contrast agent, high signal intensity of intra-abdominal fat, and the long imaging times used in conventional spin-echo sequences.

Many of the limitations of MRI have been overcome by employing breath-holding imaging [fast low angle shot (FLASH)], fat suppression, and an intravenous contrast agent, gadopentate dimeglumine (Gd-DTPA) (SEMELKA et al. 1991). With these new techniques, MRI can show the extent and severity of inflammatory changes (Fig. 10.33) of

the gut that correlate with endoscopic and histologic findings from surgical specimens (GIOVAGNONI et al. 1993). Mural thickening of the gut can also be appreciated with MRI. When fast imaging sequences are combined with intravenous contrast (Gd-DTPA) administration and fat-suppressed imaging, a good correlation between bowel wall thickness, length of diseased bowel, and severity of inflammation has been reported (SHOENUT et al. 1993). Indeed, the percent contrast enhancement compares very well with severity of inflammation based on endoscopic and surgical findings. Gd-DTPA is a nonspecific extracellular space contrast agent that increases the T1 relaxation of surrounding water protons, thereby producing relative tissue brightening. This tissue brightening is transmural in Crohn's disease but not present in the submucosa in ulcerative colitis, an important differentiating feature of these two colitides (SHOENUT et al. 1993). The actively inflamed wall enhances because of increased delivery of the agent and increased capillary permeability. On T1-weighted MR sequences, the fat may have low signal intensity streaks and strands. These areas may enhance following Gd-DTPA administration on gradient echo images (SHOENUT et al. 1993).

10.3.6
Transabdominal Ultrasound Features

The thickness of the colonic and small bowel wall can be appreciated sonographically and the validity of employing mural thickening in establishing the diagnosis of IBD has a reported sensitivity of 67%–86% and specificity of 87%–100% (KIMMEY et al. 1990). Indeed, some authors suggest employing ultrasonography as a screen for IBD (WIJERS et al. 1993; BOZKURT et al. 1994). When suspicion of disease is low, normal ultrasonography may be sufficient to avoid barium examination. When abnormal gut is seen or clinical suspicion is high, despite a normal ultrasound study, barium examination should be performed (LIM et al. 1994).

In patients with active Crohn's disease, the colon wall can be up to 1.5 cm in thickness. Mural stratification is typically lost as well (LIMBERG 1989). Using criteria listed in Table 10.1, the sensitivity of ultrasound in detecting active Crohn's disease was 91% with a specificity of 100%; the figures for active ulcerative colitis were 89% and 97% respectively (LIM et al. 1994). Several sonographic caveats should be mentioned. In patients with only aphthoid ulcerations, typical wall stratification is maintained in patients with Crohn's disease, suggesting the disease is not yet transmural (PEDERSEN et al. 1986). In patients with ulcerative colitis who have large and extensive pseudopolyps, the thickness of the colon wall may approach 1.5 cm and mural stratification may be lost (LIMBERG and OSSWALD 1994).

Several authors, however, have questioned the utility of ultrasound in differentiating ulcerative colitis and Crohn's colitis on the basis of bowel wall changes alone (SCHWERK et al. 1992). Documentation of continuous or discontinuous involvement, combined with evidence of mesenteric disease, abscess, and/or fistulae can assist differentiation (LIMBERG 1988).

In a recent paper employing hydrocolonic ultrasonography, 93% of patients with Crohn's disease showed loss of mural stratification, and the wall appeared hypoechoic and clearly thickened. In contrast, mural stratification was maintained in ulcerative colitis (HATA et al. 1994). Indeed, hydrocolonic ultrasonography could differentiate Crohn's disease from ulcerative colitis in 93% of cases. Colonic Crohn's disease and ulcerative colitis were detectable by this technique with a sensitivity of 96% and 91% respectively (HATA et al. 1992).

The thickened bowel wall in Crohn's disease produces a "target," "bull's eye," or "cockade" appearance that must be differentiated from chronic ulcerative colitis, diverticulitis, lymphoma, ischemic colitis, and pseudomembranous colitis (LIMBERG 1990).

Ultrasonography has also been successful in diagnosing recurrent disease in patients who have had surgical resections (SHERIDAN et al. 1993; DiCANDIO et al. 1986).

Sonographically, creeping fat of the mesentery is hypoechoic, compared with normal fat due to edema (PERA et al. 1988).

10.4
Carcinoma

The risk of developing colorectal cancer is significantly higher in patients with ulcerative colitis and Crohn's colitis than in the general population, although the precise magnitude of this risk is uncertain (BANSAL and SONNENBERG 1996). Recent studies suggest an annual incidence of 10% after the first decade of ulcerative colitis. The risk of colorectal cancer also increases with increasing extent of disease; 75%–80% of patients who develop cancer have pancolitis (Fig. 10.34).

Carcinomas associated with ulcerative colitis are multiple in nearly 25% of cases and more often flat and scirrhous than in patients without colitis and thus harder to detect.

Cancer screening has become a popular and controversial issue in patients with IBD. Since the 1960s, mucosal dysplasia has been considered a precursor of colon cancer or at least a marker of colons at risk for developing cancer. Mucosal dysplasia is often detected near or remote from the neoplasm in ulcerative colitis patients with carcinoma. Dysplasia, however, is patchy, inconsistent, and unpredictably distributed in the colon. Accordingly, colonoscopy with multiple random biopsies as well as biopsies from masses or raised areas is recommended. Flow cytometry searching for aneuploidy has been advocated as a means of increasing the specificity and prognostic significance of the histologic results (JASS 1997).

Table 10.1. Crohn's disease versus ulcerative colitis: sonographic features (modified from LIMBERG 1989)

Active Crohn's disease
  Loss of mural stratification
  Clearly thickened, hypoechoic bowel wall
  Haustral loss
  Decreased compressibility
  Diminished peristalsis

Acute ulcerative colitis
  Mural stratification maintained
  Moderately thickened, hypoechoic bowel wall
  Haustral loss
  Decreased compressibility
  Diminished peristalsis

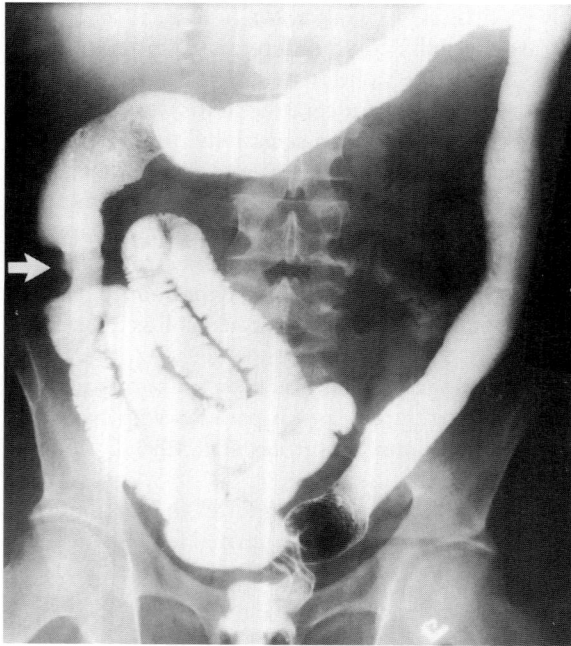

Fig. 10.34. Carcinoma complicating ulcerative colitis. A 3-cm mass (*arrow*) is present in the transverse colon in this patient with "burned out" pancolitis

Several studies have shown that certain dysplastic lesions are radiologically visible. When the dysplasia is elevated and plaque-like or multinodular, it manifests en face as irregular nodular areas with sharply angulated borders, having a "mosaic tile" appearance (FECZKO 1987). Tangentially, these lesions project only 1–2 mm above the adjacent normal mucosa (GORE and LAUFER 1994). When the dysplasia assumes a more polypoid form, it is indistinguishable from an adenomatous polyp. Unfortunately, most dysplasias occur in flat mucosa and therefore are not detectable on double-contrast barium studies.

The management of high-risk patients with panulcerative colitis requires regular radiologic and endoscopic surveillance for the detection of dysplasia. The role of the radiologist is to determine the extent of the colitis and the configuration of the colon to aid the endoscopist and to draw attention to any area suggestive of dysplasia or carcinoma.

10.5
Extraintestinal Complications

Extraintestinal manifestations develop in one-quarter to one-third of patients with IBD (LEVINE and LUKAWSKI-TRUBISH 1995). They can be divided into three categories: (a) those intimately related to disease activity or extent of disease and responsive to therapy directed at the bowel disease (i.e., arthritis, iritis); (b) those whose course is independent of underlying bowel disease (i.e., sclerosing cholangitis, ankylosing spondylitis); (c) those that are due to an inadequate or disordered intestinal function (i.e., cholelithiasis, nephrolithiasis) (LICHTMAN and SARTOR 1994; DANZI 1988).

10.5.1
Hepatobiliary Complications

The most frequent serious manifestations of extraintestinal IBD occur in the liver and the biliary tract (VIERLING 1994). As a rule, these complications do not correlate with disease activity, duration, or severity with the exception of fatty infiltration, which occurs in patients who tend to be more seriously ill, debilitated, and malnourished (BALAN and LA RUSSO 1995).

10.5.1.1
Hepatic Steatosis

Fatty liver is found on liver biopsy in 20%–25% of patients with IBD and may be caused by fat malabsorption, hyperalimentation, sepsis, protein-losing enteropathy, malnutrition, and corticosteroids (WEWER et al. 1991). The imaging features of fatty liver are variable and depend on the amount of fat deposited, its distribution within the liver, and the presence of associated hepatic disease. CT is the best noninvasive technique for the detection of hepatic steatosis because there is an excellent correlation between hepatic parenchymal CT attenuation and the amount of hepatic triglyceride found on liver biopsy specimens. Fatty deposition is usually diffuse; however, involvement can be focal, lobar, segmental, or scattered in a bizarre pattern that rapidly appears and disappears (HYAMS et al. 1995).

10.5.1.2
Cholelithiasis

Some 30%–50% of patients with Crohn's disease develop gallstones, especially those who have extensive terminal ileal disease or who have undergone ileal resection (WILLIAMS and HARNED 1987). These patients form lithogenic bile because of bile salt malabsorption or loss of the enterohepatic circulation. Ultrasound is the premier means of diagnosing gallstones.

10.5.1.3
Primary Sclerosing Cholangitis

Primary sclerosing cholangitis occurs in fewer than 2%–5% of patients with IBD; it is more commonly associated with ulcerative colitis (SCHRUMPF et al. 1988). Ultrasound and CT can directly visualize the fibrous mural thickening of the larger bile ducts that characterize this disease (ZEMAN 1995). The thickening may be concentric or asymmetric and usually measures 2–5 mm. Other signs suggesting the diagnosis include focal duct dilatation (Fig. 10.35), discrepancy between the size of the intrahepatic and extrahepatic bile ducts, focal clustering of intrahepatic ducts, and discontinuous areas of minimal intrahepatic biliary dilatation without associated hepatic, porta hepatis, or pancreatic masses. The cholangiographic signs of beading, pruning, and nodular mural thickening can also be seen on cross-sectional imaging, but usually with less detail and precision.

Computed tomography and ultrasound offer three major advantages in evaluating patients with known or suspected sclerosing cholangitis (ZEMAN 1995). First, they are noninvasive techniques that are quite safe in these patients who often need multiple serial examinations. Second, they can visualize the entire biliary tract in cases where strictures

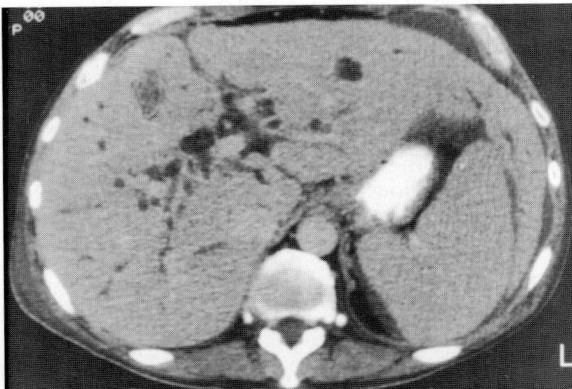

Fig. 10.35. Sclerosing cholangitis complicating ulcerative colitis. Note focal areas of bile duct "beading" and dilatation. (From GORE et al. 1996a)

obstruct the flow of contrast medium during cholangiography, occasionally leaving large portions of the intrahepatic ducts unexamined. Finally, CT and ultrasound can depict complications of sclerosing cholangitis such as cirrhosis and portal hypertension, as well as soft tissue masses associated with cholangiocarcinoma (MacCARTY 1994).

10.5.1.4
Liver Abscess

More than 30 cases of hepatic abscess complicating Crohn's disease have been reported. In one institution, they accounted for 8% of all liver abscesses (MIR-MADJLESS et al. 1986). They most commonly develop in patients with longstanding disease but may occur as the initial manifestation of Crohn's disease (VAKIL et al. 1994). Steroids and other immunosuppressive agents, perforation, intra-abdominal abscess, and anastomotic leaks are all predisposing factors to the development of a hepatic abscess (Fig. 10.36) in patients with Crohn's disease (DARNELL et al. 1995; FUKUYA et al. 1991).

10.5.2
Pancreatic Complications

Approximately 1%–2% of patients with Crohn's disease develop pancreatitis due to a variety of causes: (a) drugs such as steroids, azathiopine, or metronidazole; (b) choledocholithiasis; (c) fistula from the adjacent gut; (d) sclerosing cholangitis; (e) dysfunction of the sphincter of Oddi or stenosis of the descending duodenum leading to obstruction of the duct or reflux of duodenal contents into the duct; (f) autoantibodies against pancreatic acinar cells (WEBER et al. 1993; SPIESS et al. 1992; EISNER et al. 1993). Regardless of the cause, cross-sectional imaging is needed to help confirm the diagnosis of pancreatitis and more importantly its complications (MATSUMOTO et al. 1989).

10.5.3
Urinary Tract Complications

10.5.3.1
Nephrolithiasis

Between 2% and 10% of patients with Crohn's disease develop nephrolithiasis due to water and elec-

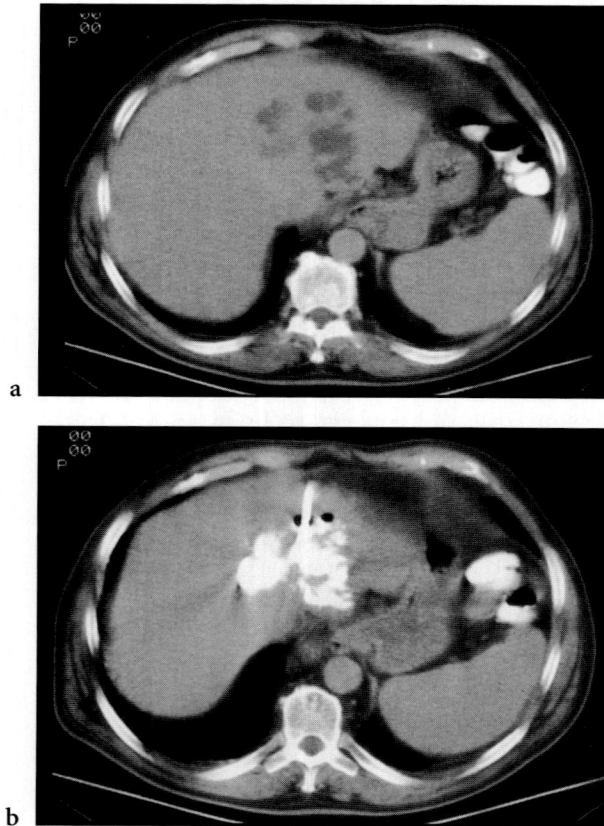

Fig. 10.36 a,b. Liver abscess associated with Crohn's disease. **a** Non-contrast CT scan shows a multilocated, low-density mass in the left lobe of the liver (*arrows*). **b** This abscess, in which all the locules communicated, was percutaneously drained

trolyte losses in diarrhea, malabsorption, and large ileostomy output. Oxalate stones are most common and because they are not calcified, may not be visible with conventional radiologic techniques (BANNER 1987). Noncontrast CT scans and, to a lesser degree, ultrasound detect these stones more readily.

10.5.3.2
Hydronephrosis

Hydronephrosis may develop in patients with Crohn's disease for a variety of reasons including: calculous disease or obstruction due to the inflammatory effect of an abscess or phlegmon or the mass effect of creeping fat of the mesentery (BANNER 1987). CT is useful in detecting both the hydronephrosis and the obstructing mass.

10.5.3.3
Fistulae

Fistulae may develop between diseased gut and the kidney in patients with Crohn's disease, leading to a renal or perinephric abscess (BANNER 1987). More commonly, enterovesical fistulae develop. While these fistulae should first be evaluated with conventional barium studies, excretory urography, and cystography, the origin of the fistula may be edematous and prevent contrast opacification and tiny fistulous tracts may not be seen. Indeed, conventional studies detect fewer than 50% of enterovesical fistulae; CT has a nearly 90% success rate (MERINE et al. 1989). CT scans are initially obtained with only oral and rectal contrast administration. The presence of gas and small amounts of contrast entering through the fistula may be obscured if the bladder is opacified following the intravenous injection of iodinated contrast medium.

10.5.4
Musculoskeletal Complications

10.5.4.1
Arthropathy

Arthritis is one of the most common extraintestinal manifestations of IBD and it is manifested as a peripheral arthritis and/or sacroiliitis-spondylitis (BJÖRKENGREN et al. 1987). The radiologic findings of peripheral enteropathic arthritis are usually minimal and best seen, if at all, with conventional radiographs (MÜNCH et al. 1986). The changes in the axial skeleton (see Fig. 10.1), affecting 3%–16% of patients with IBD, are similar to ankylosing spondylitis (McENIFF et al. 1995). CT and MRI can often detect the subtle changes of early sacroiliitis before they become apparent on plain films: bilateral, usually symmetric joint narrowing with osseous erosions followed by sclerosis, more pronounced on the iliac side of the articulation (SCOTT et al. 1990). Eventually bony ankylosis occurs (MEUWISSEN et al. 1997).

10.5.4.2
Avascular Necrosis

Osteonecrosis is a rare complication of IBD and usually occurs in the following clinical settings: during or after corticosteroid therapy; during total parenteral nutrition, especially with lipid emulsions; and most recently as a direct complication of the disease without other precipitating factors (SCHORR-LESNICK and BRANDT 1988; VAKIL and SPARBERG 1989).

Magnetic resonance imaging is the best imaging technique for establishing this diagnosis, with a reported sensitivity of 97% and specificity of 98%. On T1-weighted images, areas of low signal intensity may be seen beneath the articular surface. Alternatively, a band or bands of low signal intensity are seen surrounding a central area of higher signal intensity. On T2-weighted images, areas of low signal intensity can become bright, and regions of high signal intensity remain high.

Asymptomatic and radiologically normal hips may have early signs of avascular necrosis on CT studies (FREEMAN and KWAN 1993). These include subtle alterations in trabecular pattern, joint space integrity, and femoral head and acetabular contour which may be undetected or ill-defined on plain films.

10.5.4.3
Osteomyelitis–Septic Arthritis

Septic arthritis of the hip can complicate a psoas or retroperitoneal abscess tracking through the greater sciatic notch. MRI and CT show these changes prior to their recognition on plain films.

The iliac bone (Fig. 10.37) and sacrum are the most frequent sites of osteomyelitis in patients with

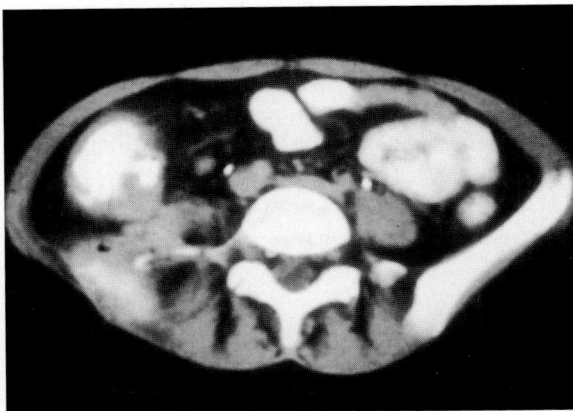

Fig. 10.37. Pelvic osteomyelitis complicating Crohn's disease. CT scan shows osteomyelitis involving the right iliac crest secondary to a fistula to the distal ileum. Notice the mural thickening of the cecum. (From GORE et al. 1996a)

Crohn's disease (SCHWARTZ et al. 1987). They are almost invariably the result of an adjacent pelvic abscess or enteric fistula (GHAHREMANI 1973). Accordingly, osteomyelitis is usually diagnosed on cross-sectional imaging when the abscess is identified. CT findings in osteomyelitis include cortical bone destruction, intraosseous gas, increased attenuation of the bone marrow, narrowing of the medullary cavity, serpentine drainage tracts, and the presence of an involucrum or sequestrum (MILLER and MILLER 1987). On MR, the marrow space of the involved bone demonstrates decreased signal on T1-weighted images and increased signal on T2-weighted images. Cortical destruction or thickening and edema or abscess formation in the soft tissues can also be demonstrated on MRI.

Spinal epidural abscess has been reported from fistulization of a presacral or psoas abscess in patients with Crohn's disease (PIONTEK et al. 1992). Indeed, prevertebral, intraforaminal, and epidural gas may be seen on CT and MRI studies (LAMPORT et al. 1994).

10.5.4.4
Psoas Abscess

Crohn's disease complications now accounts for 73% of all psoas abscesses (COHEN and McLEOD 1996). On the right, a psoas abscess (see Fig. 10.28b) may develop secondary to terminal ileal disease and on the left it can result from sigmoid or jejunal involvement. Most patients with psoas abscess have well-established Crohn's disease but the clinical manifestations may be very nonspecific (RICCI and MEYER 1985). Occasionally, psoas abscess may be seen at the initial presentation of disease. CT has emerged as the single best examination for its diagnosis. CT can also direct percutaneous abscess drainage in these patients (MILLWARD et al. 1986).

Primary rectus sheath abscesses have also been reported as a complication of Crohn's disease and may be visualized on CT, MRI, or ultrasound (SUNG et al. 1993).

10.6
Differential Diagnosis of Colitis

Ulcerative colitis and Crohn's disease are responsible for the majority of cases of enterocolitis in North America and Europe. Infectious enteritis and colitis, however, are occurring more frequently due to: increased global travel and immigration; the indiscriminate use of antibiotics; and more widespread immunosuppression resulting from the AIDS epidemic, chemotherapy, and bone marrow, stem cell, and organ transplantation (THOENI and MARGULIS 1980; GORE and GHAHREMANI 1995; SCHMITT and WEXNER 1993). Since the small bowel and colon only have a limited variety of response to a wide variety of insults, it is not surprising that the infectious enterocolitides often simulate the clinical (Table 10.2) and radiologic (Table 10.3) features of IBD (CHENEY and WONG 1993; LAVY et al. 1992). The definitive diagnosis of infectious or idiopathic inflammatory bowel disease ultimately rests on histologic and bacteriologic documentation.

The differentiation of Crohn's colitis and ulcerative colitis is important because each disease has different therapeutic and prognostic implications (SHANAHAN and TARGAW 1992). Patients with ulcerative colitis have a higher risk of developing cancer. They can also have a curative colectomy and are candidates for sphincter-preserving surgery (DEAN and DOZOIS 1997). Patients with Crohn's disease, however, are not candidates for ileal reservoirs because disease may recur in the ileum (STRONG 1997). The following double-contrast barium enema features (Tables 10.4, 10.5) enable the correct diagnosis to be made in most patients:

1. Ulcerative colitis is a contiguous, confluent, circumferential, and symmetric disease that begins in the rectum and extends proximally.
2. Crohn's disease is a patchy, discontinuous disease with asymmetric involvement that can lead to pseudodiverticula.
3. The following types of ulcerations are characteristic of Crohn's disease: aphthoid, discrete, deep (>3 mm), fissuring, and rose thorn.
4. Granular mucosa is typical in ulcerative colitis but not in Crohn's colitis.
5. Severe anal and perianal disease is characteristic of Crohn's disease but is exceptionally rare in ulcerative colitis.
6. Spontaneous fistula and sinus tracts are a hallmark of Crohn's disease.

There are certain CT findings that can help differentiate granulomatous and ulcerative colitis (Table 10.6). Mural stratification is seen in 61% of patients with chronic ulcerative colitis but only 8% of patients with chronic granulomatous colitis. Also mean colon wall thickness in chronic ulcerative colitis is 7.8 mm, significantly smaller than in Crohn's colitis (11 mm). Finally, the outer contour of the thickened colonic wall is smooth and regular in 95% of ulcerative colitis cases while serosal and outer mural irregularity is present in 80% of granulomatous colitis patients.

Differentiation between these two diseases can be made on radiologic grounds in 90%–95% of patients. This distinction is easier to make in the early stages of disease, because the early manifestations are particularly distinctive. When the disease is chronic or when there have been numerous exacerbations and remissions, the distinction may be more difficult. For example, ulcerative colitis in remission may become discontinuous, whereas granulomatous colitis may involve the entire colon.

Table 10.2. Inflammatory bowel disease: clinical differential diagnosis (from SHANAHAN and TARGAN 1992)

Ulcerative colitis	Crohn's disease
Pancolitis	Ileal and jejunal
Helicobacter infection	*Yersinia* enterocolitis
Shigellosis	Salmonellosis
Salmonellosis	Tuberculosis
Cytomegalovirus infection	*Strongyloides* infection
Escherichia coli infection	Lymphoma
Clostridium difficile infection	Radiation enteritis
Amebiasis	Carcinoid
Behçet's disease	Eosinophilic enteritis
Graft-versus-host disease	Carcinoma (rare)
Radiation colitis	Ileocecal
Diverticular disease	Tuberculosis
Ischemic colitis	Typhlitis
Proctosigmoiditis	Amebiasis
Herpes simplex infection	Graft-versus-host
Gonorrhea	disease
Chlamydia infection	Appendicitis
	Carcinoma
	Colonic
	Ischemia
	Diverticulitis
	Carcinoma
	Amebiasis
	Tuberculosis
	Ischemic colitis
	Radiation colitis
	Chlamydia infection

10.7
Conclusion

The radiologic diagnosis of ulcerative colitis and Crohn's disease is challenging. It embraces a variety of examination techniques that must be performed and interpreted with care if the radiologist is to make a significant contribution to patient management.

Table 10.3. Inflammatory bowel disease: radiologic differential diagnosis (from BARTRAM and LAUFER 1992)

Feature	Commonly found in:	May occur in:
Granular mucosa	Ulcerative colitis	Early Crohn's colitis (rare)
Ulceration		
Discrete	Crohn's colitis *Yersinia* infection Behçet's disease	Amebiasis Ischemia Tuberculosis
Confluent (shallow)	Ulcerative colitis	Crohn's disease Amebiasis
Confluent (deep)	Crohn's disease	Ischemia Amebiasis Tuberculosis *Strongyloides* infection
Stricture		
Symmetric	Ulcerative colitis *Chlamydia* infection	Tuberculosis
Asymmetric	Crohn's disease Ischemia Tuberculosis	
Fistula	Crohn's disease *Chlamydia* infection	Tuberculosis Actinomycosis
Inflammatory polyps	Ulcerative colitis Crohn's disease Schistosomiasis Colitis cystica profunda	Ischemia (rare)
Small bowel disease	Crohn's disease *Yersinia* infection Tuberculosis Pseudomembranous	Ulcerative colitis (backwash ileitis) Behçet's disease Ischemia
Skip lesions	Crohn's disease Tuberculosis Amebiasis	*Chlamydia* infection
Toxic megacolon	Ulcerative colitis	Crohn's disease Ischemia Amebiasis

Table 10.4. Ulcerative colitis: barium enema features

Acute changes	Chronic changes
Mucosal granularity	Lumen narrowing
Mucosal stippling	Haustral loss
Collar button ulcers	Loss of rectal valves
Haustral thickening or loss	Widened presacral space
Inflammatory polyps	Backwash ileitis
	Postinflammatory pseudopolyps

Table 10.5. Crohn's colitis: barium enema findings

Early changes	Late changes
Nodular lymphoid hyperplasia	Fissures
Aphthoid ulcerations	Fistula
Deep ulcerations	Haustral loss
Cobblestone appearance	Sacculations
Asymmetric involvement	Postinflammatory pseudopolyps
Inflammatory pseudopolyps	Inflammatory abscess
Segmental distribution	Strictures
Skip lesions	

Table 10.6. CT features of ulcerative colitis versus Crohn's disease (adapted from PHILPOTTS et al. 1994)

CT feature	Ulcerative colitis	Crohn's colitis	P
Mural thickness (in mm)	7.8 ± 1.9[a]	11.0 ± 5.1[a]	<0.0002
Submucosal fat (%)	61	8	0.0001
Isolated right colon involvement (%)	0	38	<0.0004
Fibrofatty mesenteric proliferation (%)	0	49	<0.0004
Abscess (%)	0	35	<0.0007

[a] Mean $\pm$ SD.

An understanding of the anatomic and pathophysiologic basis of the radiologic features of IBD is important to fully appreciate the natural history and differentiating features of these perplexing diseases.

References

Alexander-Williams J (1997) Surgical maneuvers in Crohn's disease. In: Allan RN, Rhodes JM, Hanauer SB (eds) Inflammatory bowel diseases. Churchill-Livingstone, New York, pp 707–712

Anderson CM, Brown JJ, Balfe DM, et al. (1994) MR imaging of Crohn disease: use of perflubron as a contrast agent. J Magn Reson Imaging 4:491–496

Archibald GR, Scholz FJ, Larsen CR (1988) Computed tomographic findings of giant intestinal pseudopolyposis. Gastrointest Radiol 13:155–159

Balan V, La Russo NF (1995) Hepatobiliary disease in inflammatory bowel disease. Gastroenterol Clin North Am 24:647–663

Balthazar EJ (1991) CT of the gastrointestinal tract: principles and interpretation. AJR 156:23–32

Banner MP (1987) Genitourinary complications of inflammatory bowel disease. Radiol Clin North Am 25:199–204

Bansal P, Sonnenberg A (1996) Risk factors for colorectal cancer in inflammatory bowel disease. Am J Gastroenterol 91:44–48

Bartram CI (1976) Plain abdominal x-ray in acute colitis. Proc R Soc Med 1:383–391

Bartram CI (1977) Radiology in the current assessment of ulcerative colitis. Gastrointest Radiol 1:383–391

Bartram CI (1983) Complications of ulcerative colitis. In: Bartram CI (ed) Radiology in inflammatory bowel disease. Marcel Dekker, New York, pp 63–118

Bartram CI, Laufer I (1992) Inflammatory bowel disease. In: Laufer I, Levine MS (eds) Double contrast gastrointestinal radiology, 2nd edn. Saunders, Philadelphia, pp 580–645

Björkengren AG, Resnick D, Sartoris DJ (1987) Enteropathic arthropathies. Radiol Clin North Am 25:189–198

Bozkurt T, Richter F, Lux G (1994) Ultrasonography as a primary diagnostic tool in patients with inflammatory disease and tumors of the small intestine and large bowel. J Clin Ultrasound 22:85–91

Bray JF (1983) Filiform polyposis of the small bowel in Crohn's disease. Gastrointest Radiol 8:155–156

Bronen RA, Glick SN, Teplick SH (1983) Diffuse lymphoid follicles of the colon associated with colonic carcinoma. AJR 142:105–109

Brozna JP, Fisher RL, Barwick KW (1985) Filiform polyposis: an unusual complication of inflammatory bowel disease. J Clin Gastroenterol 7:451–458

Brzezinski A, Lashner BA (1997) Natural history of Crohn's disease. In: Allan RNJ, Rhodes JM, Hanauer SB (eds) Inflammatory bowel diseases, 3rd edn. Churchill Livingstone, New York, pp 475–486

Buckwell NA, Williams GT, Bartram CI, et al. (1980) Depth of ulceration in acute colitis. Gastroenterology 79:19–25

Butani MS, Hawes RH (1997) Endoluminal ultrasound. In: Allan RNJ, Rhodes JM, Hanauer SB (eds) Inflammatory bowel diseases, 3rd edn. Churchill Livingstone, New York, pp 285–290

Casola G, van Sonnenberg E, Neff CC (1987) Abscess in Crohn's disease: percutaneous drainage. Radiology 163:19–22

Cheney CP, Wong RKH (1993) Acute infectious diarrhea. Med Clin North Am 77:1169–1192

Cohen Z, McLeod RS (1996) Inflammatory bowel disease. In: Zuidema GD (ed) Shackelford's surgery of the alimentary tract, vol 4, 4th edn. Saunders, Philadelphia, pp 53–71

Danzi JT (1988) Extraintestinal manifestations of idiopathic inflammatory bowel disease. Arch Intern Med 148:297–302

Darnell A, Brullet E, Campo R, Donoso L (1995) Liver abscesses as initial presentation of Crohn's disease. Am J Gastroenterol 90:1363–1364

Dean PA, Dozois SR (1997) Surgical options – ileoanal pouch. In: Allan RNJ, Rhodes JM, Hanauer SB (eds) Inflammatory bowel diseases, 3rd edn. Churchill Livingstone, New York, pp 761–772

Debinski H, Kamm MA (1997) Natural history of ulcerative colitis. In: Allen RN, Rhodes JM, Hanuer SB (eds) Inflammatory bowel diseases, 3rd edn. Churchill Livingstone, New York, pp 463–474

DiCandio G, Mosca F, Campatella A (1986) Sonographic detection of postsurgical recurrence of Crohn's disease. AJR 146:523–526

Doemeny JM, Burke DR, Meranze SG (1988) Percutaneous drainage of abscesses in patients with Crohn's disease. Gastrointest Radiol 13:327–341

Eisner TD, Goldman IS, McKinley MJ (1993) Crohn's disease and pancreatitis. Am J Gastroenterol 88:583–586

Ergerg O, Lindstrom C (1979) Superficial lesions in Crohn's disease of the small bowel. Gastrointest Radiol 4:389–392

Feczko PJ (1987) Malignancy complicating inflammatory bowel disease. Radiol Clin North Am 25:157–174

Fishman EK, Wolf EJ, Jones B, et al. (1987) CT evaluation of Crohn's disease: effect on patient management. AJR 148:537–541

Flueckiger F, Kullnig P, Melzer G, Posch E (1990) Colobronchial and gastrocolic fistulas: rare complication of Crohn's disease. Gastrointest Radiol 15:288–290

Freeman HJ, Kwan WCP (1993) Brief report: non-corticosteroid-associated osteonecrosis of the femoral heads in two patients with inflammatory bowel disease. N Engl J Med 1314–1316

Fujimura Y, Kamoi R, Iida M (1996) Pathogenesis of aphthoid ulcers in Crohn's disease: correlative findings by magnifying colonoscopy, electron microscopy, and immunochemistry. Gut 38:724–732

Fukuya T, Hawes DR, Lu CC, et al. (1991) CT of abdominal abscess with fistulous communication to the gastrointestinal tract. J Comput Assist Tomogr 15:445–449

Gardiner GA (1977) "Backwash ileitis" with pseudopolyposis. AJR 129:506–507

Geller SA (1994) Pathology of inflammatory bowel disease: a critical appraisal in diagnosis and management. In: Targan SR, Shanahan F (eds) Inflammatory bowel disease: from bench to bedside. Williams and Wilkins, Baltimore, pp 336–351

Ghahremani GG (1973) Osteomyelitis of the ilium in patients with Crohn's disease. AJR 118:364–370

Giovagnoni A, Misericordia M, Terilli F (1993) MR imaging of ulcerative colitis. Abdom Imaging 18:371–375

Glick SN, Teplik SK (1985) Crohn's disease of the small intestine: diffuse mucosal granularity. Radiology 154:313–316

Goldberg HI, Gore RM, Margulis AR, Moss AA, Baker E (1983) Computed tomography in the evaluation of Crohn disease. AJR 140:277–282

Goldblum JR, Petras RE (1997) Histopathology of Crohn's disease. In: Allan RN, Rhodes JM, Hanauer SB (eds) Inflammatory bowel disease, 3rd edn. Churchill-Livingstone, New York, pp 311–316

Gore RM (1987) Cross-sectional imaging of inflammatory bowel disease. Radiol Clin North Am 25:115

Gore RM (1989) CT of inflammatory bowel disease. Radiol Clin North Am 27:717–730

Gore RM (1991) Inflammatory bowel disease: anatomic-pathologic basis of radiographic findings. In: Gore RM (ed) Categorical course on gastrointestinal radiology. American College of Radiology, Reston, Va. pp 77–87

Gore RM (1992) Colonic contour changes in chronic ulcerative colitis: reappraisal of some old concepts. AJR 158:59–61

Gore RM (1995) Characteristic morphologic changes in chronic ulcerative colitis. Abdom Imaging 20:275–278

Gore RM, Ghahremani GG (1986) Upper gastrointestinal tract Crohn's disease. Crit Rev Contemp Radiol 25:305–331

Gore RM, Ghahremani GG (1995) Radiological investigation of acute inflammatory and infectious bowel disease. Gastroenterol Clin North Am 24:353–384

Gore RM, Goldberg HI (1982) Computed tomographic evaluation of the gastrointestinal tract in diseases other than primary adenocarcinoma. Radiol Clin North Am 781–798

Gore RM, Laufer I (1994) Ulcerative and granulomatous colitis: idiopathic inflammatory bowel disease. In: Gore RM, Levine MS, Laufer I (eds) Textbook of gastrointestinal radiology. Saunders, Philadelphia, pp 1098–1141

Gore RM, Lichtenstein JE (1994) The gastrointestinal tract: anatomic-pathologic basis of radiologic findings. In: Taveras JM, Ferrucci JT (eds) Radiology: diagnosis – imaging – intervention. Lippincott, Philadelphia, Chap 4, pp 1–42

Gore RM, Marn CS, Kirby DF, Vogelzang RL, Neiman HL (1984) CT findings in ulcerative, granulomatous, and indeterminate colitis. AJR 143:279–284

Gore RM, Cohen MI, Vogelzang RL, Neiman HL (1985) Value of computed tomography in the detection of complications of Crohn's disease. Dig Dis Sci 30:701–709

Gore RM, Balthazar EJ, Ghahremani GG, Miller FH (1996a) CT features of ulcerative colitis and Crohn's disease. AJR 167:3–15

Gore RM, Ghahremani GG, Miller FH (1996b) Cross-sectional imaging in the evaluation of Crohn's disease. In: Prantera C, Korelitz BI (eds) Crohn's disease. Marcel Dekker, New York, pp 145–185

Goulston SJM, McGovern VJ (1969) The nature of benign strictures in ulcerative colitis. N Engl J Med 281:290–295

Guillaumin E, Jeffrey RB, Shea WJ (1986) Perirectal inflammatory disease: CT findings. Radiology 161:153–157

Halpert RD (1987) Toxic dilatation of the colon. Radiol Clin North Am 25:147–158

Hammerman AM, Shatz BA, Susman N (1978) Radiographic characteristics of colonic "mucosal bridges": sequelae of inflammatory bowel disease. Radiology 127:611–614

Hata J, Haruma K, Yamanaka H, et al. (1994) Ultrasonographic evaluation of the bowel wall in inflammatory bowel disease: comparison of in vivo and in vitro studies. Abdom Imaging 19:395–399

Hata J, Haruma K, Suenaga K (1992) Ultrasonographic assessment of inflammatory bowel disease. Am J Gastroenterol 87:443–447

Hill MC, Smith LE, Huntington DK, et al. (1992) Endorectal sonography in the evaluation of the rectum. Ultrasound Q 10:29–56

Hizawa K, Iida M, Kohrogi N, et al. (1994) Crohn disease: early recognition and progress of aphthous lesions. Radiology 190:451–455

Hyams J, Markowitz J, Treem W, Davis P, Grancher K, Daum F (1995) Characterization of hepatic abnormalities in children with inflammatory bowel disease. Inflam Bowel Dis 1:27–33

Hyde C, Gerzof SG (1994) Abdominal abscess. In: Gore RM, Levine MS, Laufer I (eds) Textbook of gastrointestinal radiology. Saunders, Philadelphia, pp 1553–1569

Jabra AA, Fishman EK, Taylor GA (1991) Crohn disease in the pediatric patient: CT evaluation. Radiology 179:495–498

Jacobs JE, Birnbaum BA (1995) CT of the inflammatory disease of the colon. Semin Ultrasound CT MRI 16:91–101

Jass JR (1997) Histopathology – dysplasia and cancer. In: Allan RNJ, Rhodes JM, Hanauer SB (eds) Inflammatory bowel diseases, 3rd edn. Churchill Livingstone, New York, pp 317–328

Jones B, Fishman EK, Hamilton SR, et al. (1986) Submucosal accumulation of fat in inflammatory bowel disease: CT/pathologic correlation. J Comput Assist Tomogr 10:759–763

Keighley MRB, Eastwood D, Ambrose NS, et al. (1982) Incidence and microbiology of abdominal and pelvic abscess in Crohn's disease. Gastroenterology 83:1271–1275

Kelly JK, Langeuin JM, Price KM (1986) Giant and symptomatic inflammatory polyps of the colon and idiopathic inflammatory bowel disease. Am J Surg Pathol 10:420–428

Kelvin FM, May RJ, Norton GA (1979) Lymphoid follicular pattern of the colon in adults. AJR 133:831–835

Kennedy PJ, Koehler RE, Shackelford GD (1982) The clinical significance of large lymphoid follicles of the colon. Radiology 142:41–46

Kimmey MB, Wang KY, Haggitt RC (1990) Diagnosis of inflammatory bowel disease with ultrasound. Invest Radiol 25:1085–1090

Klein VHM, Wein B, Adam G, Ruppert D, Günther RW (1995) Computed tomography of Crohn's disease and ulcerative colitis. Fortschr Röntgenstr 163:9–15

Koelbel G, Schmiedl V, Major MC, et al. (1985) Diagnosis of fistulae and sinus tracts in patients with Crohn's disease: value of MR imaging. AJR 144:1229–1233

Kolodny M (1970) Reversible right colonic strictures in chronic ulcerative colitis. Radiology 97:83–84

Lambiase RE, Cronan JJ, Dorfman GS (1988) Percutaneous drainage of abscesses in patients with Crohn disease. AJR 150:1043–1045

Lamport RD, Cheskin LJ, Moscatello SA, Nikoomanesh P (1994) Sterile epidural and bilateral psoas abscesses in a patient with Crohn's disease. Am J Gastroenterol 89:1086–1087

Langerman JM, Rowland R (1986) The number and distribution of lymphoid follicles in the human large intestine. J Anat 194:189–194

Laufer I (1975) The radiologic demonstration of early changes in ulcerative colitis by double contrast techniques. J Can Assoc Radiol 26:116–121

Laufer I, Costopoulos L (1978) Early lesions of Crohn's disease. AJR 130:307–311

Laufer I, Desa D (1978) Lymphoid follicular pattern: a normal feature of the pediatric colon. AJR 130:51–55

Laufer I, Mullens JE, Hamilton J (1976) Correlation of endoscopy and double contrast radiography in the early stages of ulcerative colitis and granulomatous colitis. Radiology 118:1–5

Lavy A, Militianu D, Eidelman S (1992) Diseases of the intestine mimicking Crohn's disease. J Clin Gastroenterol 15: 17–23

Levine JB, Lukawski-Trubish D (1995) Extraintestinal considerations in inflammatory bowel disease. Gastroenterol Clin North Am 24:633–646

Lichtenstein JE (1987) Radiologic-pathologic correlation in inflammatory bowel disease. Radiol Clin North Am 25:3–24

Lichtenstein JE, Madewell JE, Feigen DS (1979) The collar button ulcer. Gastrointest Radiol 4:79–84

Lichtman SN, Sartor RB (1994) Extraintestinal manifestations of inflammatory bowel disease: clinical aspects and natural history. In: Targan SR, Shanahan F (eds) Inflammatory bowel disease: from bench to bedside. Williams and Wilkins, Baltimore, pp 317–335

Lim JH, Ko YT, Lee DH, et al. (1994) Sonography of inflammatory bowel disease: findings and value in differential diagnosis. AJR 163:343–347

Limberg B (1988) Diagnosis of inflammatory and neoplastic large bowel diseases by conventional abdominal and colonic sonography. Ultrasound Q 6:151–156

Limberg B (1989) Diagnosis of acute ulcerative colitis and colonic Crohn's disease by colonic sonography. J Clin Ultrasound 17:25–30

Limberg B (1990) Sonographic features of colonic Crohn's disease: comparison of in vivo and in vitro studies. J Clin Ultrasound 18:161–166

Limberg B, Osswald B (1994) Diagnosis and differential diagnosis of ulcerative colitis and Crohn's disease by hydrocolonic sonography. Am J Gastroenterol 89:1051–1057

MacCarty RL (1994) Noncalculous inflammatory disorders of the biliary tract. In: Gore RM, Levine MS, Laufer I (eds) Textbook of gastrointestinal radiology. Saunders, Philadelphia, pp 1727–1745

Mark MD, Foley MT, Banks PA (1989) Multiple strictures in Crohn's disease of the small bowel: a benign variant. Am J Gastroenterol 84:1047–1050

Matsumoto T, Matsui T, Iida TJ (1989) Acute pancreatitis as a complication of Crohn's disease. Am J Gastroenterol 84: 804–807

McEniff N, Eustace S, McCarthy C (1995) Asymptomatic sacroiliitis in inflammatory bowel disease: assessment by computed tomography. Clin Imaging 19:258–262

McLeod RS, Cohen Z (1997) Perianal Crohn's disease. In: Allan RNJ, Rhodes JM, Hanauer SB (eds) Inflammatory bowel diseases, 3rd edn. Churchill Livingstone, New York, pp 615–622

Merine D, Fishman EK, Kuhlman JE, Jones B, Bayless TM, Siegelman S (1989) Bladder involvement in Crohn disease: role of CT in detection and evaluation. J Comput Assist Tomogr 13:90–93

Meuwissen SGM, Crusius JBA, Peña AS, Dekker-Saeys AJ, Dijkmans BAC (1997) Spondyloarthropathy and idiopathic inflammatory bowel diseases. Inflamm Bowel Dis 3:25–37

Meyers MA, McGuire PV (1995) Spiral CT demonstration of hypervascularity in Crohn disease: "vascular jejunalization of the ileum" or the "comb sign." Abdom Imag 20:327–332

Michelassi F, Stella M, Balestracci T (1993) Incidence, diagnosis and treatment of enteric and colorectal fistulae in patients with Crohn's disease. Ann Surg 218:660–666

Miller LK, Miller JW (1987) Pelvic osteomyelitis complicating Crohn's disease: diagnosis by computed tomography. Am J Gastroenterol 82:371–372

Millward SF, Ramsewak W, Fitzsimons P (1986) Percutaneous drainage of iliopsoas abscess in Crohn's disease. Gastrointest Radiol 11:289–290

Mir-Madjless SD, McHenry MC, Farmer RG (1986) Liver abscess in Crohn's disease. Gastroenterology 91:987–993

Muldowney SM, Balfe DM, Hammerman A, Wick MR (1995) "Acute" fat deposition in bowel wall submucosa: CT appearance. J Comput Assist Tomogr 19:390–393

Münch H, Purrmann J, Reis HE (1986) Clinical features of inflammatory joint and spine manifestations in Crohn's disease. Hepatogastroenterology 33:123–127

Myhr GE, Myrvold HE, Nilsen G, et al. (1994) Perianal fistulas: use of MR imaging for diagnosis. Radiology 191:545–549

Ni X-Y, Goldberg HI (1986) Aphthoid ucers in Crohn's disease: radiographic course and relationship to bowel appearnce. Radiology 158:589–592

O'Donovan AN, Somers S, Farrow R, Mernagh JR, Sridhar S (1997) MR imaging of anorectal Crohn's disease: a pictorial essay. Radiographics 17:101–107

Orel SG, Rubesin SE, Jones BK, et al. (1987) Computed tomography vs barium studies in the acutely symptomatic patient with Crohn disease. J Comput Assist Tomogr 11: 1009–1016

Outwater E, Schiebler ML (1993) Pelvic fistulas: findings on MR images. AJR 160:327–330

Pedersen BH, Gronvall S, Dorph S, et al. (1986) The value of dynamic ultrasound scanning in Crohn's disease. Scand J Gastroenterol 21:969–974

Pera A, Cammarota T, Comino E, et al. (1988) Ultrasonography in the detection of Crohn's disease and in the differential diagnosis of inflammatory bowel disease. Digestion 4:180–189

Philpotts LE, Heiken JP, Westcott MA, Gore RM (1994) Colitis: use of CT findings in differential diagnosis. Radiology 190:445–449

Pichney LS, Fantry GT, Graham SM (1992) Gastrocolic and duodenocolic fistulas in Crohn's disease. J Clin Gastroenterol 15:205–211

Piontek M, Hengels K-J, Hefter H (1992) Spinal abscess and bacterial meningitis in Crohn's disease. Dig Dis Sci 37: 1131–1135

Prantera C, Lorenzetti R, Davoli M (1991) The plain abdominal film accurately estimates extent of active ulcerative colitis. J Clin Gastroenterol 13:231–236

Present DH (1993). Toxic megacolon. Med Clin North Am 77:1129–1142

Price AB, Morson BC (1987) Inflammatory bowel disease: the surgical pathology of Crohn's disease and ulcerative colitis. Hum Pathol 6:7–22

Ribeiro MB, Greenstein AJ, Yamazaki Y, Aufses ATL (1991) Intra-abdominal abscess in regional enteritis. Ann Surg 213:32–36

Ricci MA, Meyer KK (1985) Psoas abscess complicating Crohn's disease. Am J Gastroenterol 80:970–977

Rice RP (1968) Plain abdominal film roentgenographic diagnosis of ulcerative disease of the colon. Radiology 90:544–579

Riddell RH (1997) Histopathology of ulcerative colitis. In: Allan RN, Rhodes JM, Hanauer SB (eds) Inflammatory bowel diseases, 3rd edn. Churchill Livingstone, New York, pp 291–310

Rutgeerts R, Peeters M, Geboes K (1992) Infectious agents in inflammatory bowel disease. Endoscopy 26:565–569

Safrit HD, Mauro MA, Jaques PF (1987) Percutaneous abscess drainage in Crohn's disease. AJR 148:859–862

Schmitt SL, Wexner SD (1993) Bacterial, fungal, parasitic, and viral colitis. Surg Clin North Am 73:1055–1072

Scholten ET, des Plantes BGZ, Falke THM (1995) Computed tomography of the large bowel wall. Choice of slice thickness and intraluminal contrast medium. Invest Radiol 30: 275–284

Schorr-Lesnick B, Brandt LJ (1988) Selected rheumatologic and dermatologic manifestations of inflammatory bowel disease. Am J Gastroenterol 83:216–223

Schrumpf E, Fausa O, Elgjo K, Kolmannskog F (1988) Hepatobiliary complications of inflammatory bowel disease. Semin Liver Dis 8:201–209

Schwartz CM, Demos TC, Wehner JM (1987) Osteomyelitis of the sacrum as the initial manifestation of Crohn's disease. Clin Orthop 222:181–185

Schwerk WB, Beck HK, Raith M, et al. (1992) A prospective evaluation of high resolution sonography in the differential diagnosis of inflammatory bowel disease. Eur J Gastroenterol Hepatol 4:173–182

Scott WW Jr, Fishman EK, Kuhlman JE, Caskey CI (1990) Computed tomography evaluation of sacroiliac joints in Crohn's disease. Skeletal Radiol 19:207–210

Semelka RC, Shoenut JP, Silverman R (1991) Bowel disease: prospective comparison of CT and 1.5T pre- and post-contrast MRI imaging with T1-weighted fat-suppressed and breath-hold FLASH sequences. J Magn Reson Imaging 1:625–632

Shanahan F, Targan SR (1992) Inflammatory bowel disease. In: Kelley WN (ed) Textbook of internal medicine, 2nd edn. Lippincott, Philadelphia, pp 489–502

Sheridan MB, Nicholson DA, Martin DF (1993) Transabdominal ultrasonography as the primary investigation in patients with suspected Crohn's disease or recurrence: a prospective study. Clin Radiol 48:402–404

Shoenut JP, Semelka RC, Silverman R (1993) Magnetic resonance imaging in inflammatory bowel disease. J Clin Gastroenterol 17:73–78

Simpkins KC (1977) Aphthoid ulcers in Crohn's colitis. Clin Radiol 28:601–604

Simpkins KC (1988) Inflammatory bowel disease: ulcerative and Crohn's colitis. In: A textbook of radiologic diagnosis, vol 4. Lippincott, Philadelphia, pp 473–498

Simpkins KC, Gore RM (1994) Crohn's disease. In: Gore RM, Levine MS, Laufer I (eds) Textbook of gastrointestinal radiology. Saunders, Philadelphia, pp 2660–2681

Siskind BN, Burrell MI, Klein ML, Princenthal RA (1985) Toxic dilatation in Crohn disease with CT correlation. J Comput Assist Tomogr 9:193–195

Spencer JA, Ward J, Beckingham IJ, Adams C, Ambrose NS (1996) Dynamic contrast-enhanced MR imaging of perianal fistuals. AJR 167:735–741

Spiess SE, Braun M, Vogelzang RL, Craig RM (1992) Crohn's disease of the duodenum complicated by pancreatitis and common bile duct obstruction. Am J Gastroenterol 87: 1033–1036

Stoker J, Hussain SM, van Kempen D, Elevelt AJ, Lameris JS (1996) Endoanal coil in MR imaging of anal fistulas. AJR 166:360–362

Strong SA (1997) Crohn's disease of the colon-segmental resection. In: Allan RNJ, Rhodes JM, Hanauer SB (eds) Inflammatory bowel diseases, 3rd edn. Churchill Livingstone, New York, pp 615–622

Strong SA, Fazio VW (1993) Crohn's disease of the colon, rectum, and anus. Surg Clin North Am 73:933–963

Suekane H, Iida M, Matsui T (1990) Radiographic demonstration of longitudinal ulcers in patients with ulcerative colitis. Gastrointest Radiol 15:333–337

Sung W-C, McKinley MJ, Harvey LP (1993) Rectus sheath abscess in Crohn's disease. Am J Gastroenterol 88:793–794

Thoeni RF, Margulis AR (1980) Radiology in inflammatory disease of the colon: an area of increased interest for the modern clinician. Invest Radiol 15:281–296

Tremaine WJ (1996) Pathology and pathophysiology of symptoms. In: Prantera C, Korelitz BI (eds) Crohn's disease. Marcel Dekker, New York, pp 93–112

Vakil N, Sparberg M (1989) Steroid-related osteonecrosis in inflammatory bowel disease. Gastroenterology 96:62–67

Vakil N, Hayne G, Sharma A (1994) Liver abscess in Crohn's disease. Am J Gastroenterol 89:1090–1095

Van Outryve MJ, Pelckmans PA, Michielsen PP, Van Maercke YM (1991) Value of transrectal ultrasonography in Crohn's disease. Gastroenterology 101:1171–1177

Vierling JM (1994) Hepatobiliary diseases in patients with inflammatory bowel disease. In: Targan SR, Shanahan F (eds) Inflammatory bowel disease: from bench to bedside. Williams and Wilkins, Baltimore, pp 654–667

Walker RS, Breuer RI, Victor T, Gore RM (1996) Crohn's esophagitis: a unique cause of esophageal polyposis. Gastrointest Endosc 43:511–515

Weber P, Seibold F, Jenss H (1993) Acute pancreatitis in Crohn's disease. J Clin Gastroenterol 17:286–291

Wewer V, Gluud C, Schlichting P (1991) Prevalence of hepatobiliary dysfunction in a regional group of patients with chronic inflammatory bowel disease. Scand J Gastroenterol 26:97–102

Wijers OB, Tio TL, Tytgat GNJ (1993) Ultrasonography and endosonography in the diagnosis and management of inflammatory bowel disease. Endoscopy 24:559–567

Williams SM, Harned RK (1987) Hepatobiliary complications of inflammatory bowel disease. Radiol Clin North Am 25:175–188

Wills JS, Lobis IF, Denstman FJ (1997) Crohn's disease: State of the art. Radiology 202:597–610

Worlicek H, Lutz H, Heyder N, et al. (1987) Ultrasound findings in Crohn's disease and ulcerative colitis: a prospective study. J Clin Ultrasound 153:153–163

Yousem DM, Fishman EK, Jones B (1988) Crohn's disease: perirectal and perianal findings at CT. Radiology 167:331–334

Zegel H, Laufer I (1978) Filiform polyposis. Radiology 127: 615–619

Zeman RK (1995) The role of noninvasive screening in suspected sclerosing cholangitis. Abdom Imaging 20:113–114

11 Less Conventional Inflammatory Diseases

S.H. OMINSKY

CONTENTS

11.1
Helicobacter pylori Peptic Disease

11.1.1
History

Since its discovery little more than a decade ago, *Helicobacter pylori* bacterial infection has been recognized as the leading cause of peptic ulcer disease, playing a causal role in 95% of duodenal ulcers and 60%–70% of gastric ulcers (LEE 1994). Some types of gastric cancer and lymphoma may also be the result of chronic *H. pylori* infection (PARSONNET et al. 1991, 1994). This association of a bacterial infection with peptic disease and malignancy is a dramatic

S.H. OMINSKY, MD, Department of Radiology, University of California, San Francisco, 505 Parnassus Avenue, Box 0628, A344a, San Francisco, CA 94143-0628, USA

shift in thinking about the causation of a common and important group of diseases and is unparalleled in the late twentieth century, where medical advancements are usually measured in small incremental steps. The *H. pylori* peptic ulcer association also has many implications for radiologists and surgeons as well as gastroenterologists.

Since the time of BEAUMONT's description in 1833 of a young man with a gastric fisula who demonstrated increased hydrochloric acid (then called muriatic acid) and hyperemic gastric mucosa in response to anxiety and anger (BEAUMONT 1959, reprinted from 1833), acid and ulcer disease have been firmly linked. Treatment of peptic disease attempted to counteract the effect of acid on gastric mucosa with neutralizers such as dairy products. Surgery to decrease the vagal phase of acid secretion and partial gastrectomy to remove the parietal cell secreting portion of the stomach were mainstays in the treatment of recurrent ulcer up into the 1960s and were effective although not without side-effects, such as dumping syndrome and diarrhea. In the 1970s and 1980s newer antacid medications such as H_2 blockers and more recently proton pump inhibitors were developed which sharply reduced acid production. However, relapses occurred with cessation of medications, resulting in prolonged therapy of expensive medications, also not without side-effects.

The acid environment of the stomach was considered too hostile for bacterial growth although spiral bacteria were seen in the stomach in the late nineteenth century. In 1979, at the Royal Perth Hospital in Western Australia, J.R. WARREN observed what he termed "*Campylobacter*-like organisms" in biopsy specimens of antral mucosa which had infiltrates of lymphocytes, plasma cells, and neutrophils, components of "chronic active gastritis." MARSHALL and WARREN (1984) then showed in a prospective study of 100 patients undergoing endoscopy that *Campylobacter* bacteria could be isolated in more than 90% of patients with chronic active gastritis, including all 13 patients with duodenal ulcer and 14 of 18 patients with gastric ulcer. MARSHALL and

WARREN also demonstrated a decreased relapse rate in duodenal ulcer patients treated with bismuth for *H. pylori* eradication (MARSHALL et al. 1988). Many subsequent studies have silenced the skeptics by showing that eradication of *H. pylori* results in rapid peptic ulcer healing and lasting cure (GRAHAM et al. 1992; HENTSCHEL et al. 1993).

11.1.2
Detection

The *H. pylori* bacteria has had several name changes. The bacterium was described in initial publications as a *Campylobacter*-like organism; the name was subsequently changed to *Campylobacter pyloridis*, *Campylobacter pylori*, and then the current name, *Helicobacter pylori*. The organism is a motile, spiral microaerophilic bacterium that is difficult to culture although it grows well when incubated with carbon dioxide. Since culturing is difficult it is usually reserved for research studies to determine susceptibility to antibiotic drugs. The bacterium is seen on gastric biopsy specimens stained with hematoxylin and eosin, and also with Warthin-Starry staining. Diagnosis can be made by histologic examination of endoscopic biopsy specimens. A quick inexpensive diagnostic technique is the CLO test, which is a color test requiring an endoscopic biopsy. This test uses a pH-sensitive dye to detect any increases in pH caused by production of ammonia from urea. Urease is present in high concentrations in *H. pylori* infection and will hydrolyze urea to form ammonia and carbon dioxide. A breath urea test is also a sensitive, noninvasive test for the presence of *H. pylori* infection. This test also relies on the enzymatic hydrolysis of urea by urease in the stomach using ingested urea labeled with either carbon-13 or carbon-14. If urease is present, carbon dioxide will be produced and be detected in the breath. The advantage of the carbon-13 breath test is that the isotope is not radioactive, but expensive mass spectrometry instrumentation is required to detect carbon-13. Carbon-14 can be detected by a relatively inexpensive liquid scintillation counter but it is a beta emitter and there is a very small radiation dose estimated to be about one eight-hundredth of the radiation dose from natural sources during the course of a year (STUBBS and MARSHALL 1993).

Serologic testing using an enzyme-linked immunoabsorbent assay (ELISA) has been used widely in epidemiologic studies but only indicates that infection has occurred at some time in the past.

Breath tests indicate whether a patient is actively infected with *H. pylori* and whether treatment has been effective (PHILLIPS 1995). The noninvasive urea breath test is as accurate in predicting *H. pylori* status in untreated patients as the invasive CLO and histopathology tests. A saliva serology test which may be helpful in epidemiologic studies and in screening dyspeptic patients has also been developed (CHRISTIE et al. 1996).

11.1.3
Prevalence

Helicobacter pylori is a worldwide infection, with prevalence rates higher in underdeveloped countries. Infection at a younger age is also seen in these countries. Approximately 10% of Americans under the age of 30 years are infected and the number increases to 60% of Americans over the age of 60 years. The vast majority of infected people are asymptomatic. Data suggest that low socioeconomic status and a high population density enhance acquisition of *H. pylori* infection. The exact mechanism of transmission has not been determined but direct person-to-person contact from oropharyngeal secretions is suspected (DRUMM et al. 1990). Twin studies have also shown a genetic susceptibility to *H. pylori* infection (GRAHAM et al. 1994). Possible factors for infection would include the genetic susceptibility of the individual, the degree of contamination of the general environment, sanitation practices in the home, the degree of crowding and the presence of small children in the home.

With such a high prevalence of infection it is most important to determine why some people become symptomatic and others do not. One possible infectious model would be tuberculosis, which infects about one-third of the world's population but which is silent in more than 90% of cases. It is generally thought that individual immunologic differences play the primary role in who will or will not have clinical disease (BLASER 1994). Another infectious model is *Entamoeba histolytica*. Again, a large percentage of the world's population is infected but only a small percentage has clinical disease. The determinant in this infection is the particular strain of *Entamoeba* with one of the two strains being more virulent. A third model is group A streptococci infection. In the absence of antibiotic treatment, about 0.4% of cases of nonepidemic streptococcal pharyngitis lead to acute rheumatic fever whereas epidemic strains increase the rate almost tenfold to

3.0%. In this model the bacterial strain plus immunologic factors combine to determine disease occurrence. It seems likely that *H. pylori* infection will be found to be related to the group A streptococci model, with both immunologic factors and bacterial strains as determinants of disease (BLASER 1994). Current research is focusing on strain variations in lipopolysaccharide structure, the production of cagA-encoded protein, the production of vacuolating cytotoxin, and enhanced activation of neutrophils.

11.1.4
Pathophysiology

Helicobacter pylori infection in the gastric antrum stimulates inflammatory mediators such as interleukin-8, which is a potent activator of neutrophils. Interleukin-8, other interleukins, and tissue necrosis factor-α may also affect gastric acid secretion. In patients with duodenal ulcer disease, gastritis is primarily confined to the antrum and the acid-providing portion of the stomach is spared. Increased acid levels in the duodenum lead to gastric metaplasia – the appearance of patches of gastric type mucus cells interspersed between absorptive and goblet cells of the duodenal eptihelium. Gastric metaplasia is a consistent histologic finding in chronic duodenitis. Gastric metaplasia allows colonization of *H. pylori* in the duodenum. As a result of chronic inflammation in the bulb, mucosal resistance is impaired and persistent high acid load on the weakened mucosa leads to erosive duodenal and frank ulceration.

Gastric ulcer disease is associated with a more diffuse gastritis affecting both the antrum and the body of the stomach. An acute neutrophilic response and a more chronic lymphocyte-plasma cell response occurs. The plasma cells infiltrate the superficial mucosa and lymphoid nodules are found in the deeper mucosa as a result of chronic antibody stimulation. With chronic infection there may be atrophy of glands and intestinal metaplasia with replacement of normal glandular epithelium by goblet cells and cells containing acid mucin. Why only some patients infected by *H. pylori* develop duodenal and gastric ulcers is unknown. In addition to different virulence of *H. pylori* strains, other factors may include the patient's ability to produce differing levels of acid and individual host immune response variations. Over-stimulation of the immune response may result in increased production of antibodies. IgG in particular and activated neutrophils may produce epithelial damage and eventual ulceration (ERNST et al. 1994). Environmental factors such as stress, smoking, and diet are also likely co-factors in the development of ulceration.

11.1.5
Cancer

Chronic gastritis is considered an important risk factor for the development of the sequence of gastric mucosal atrophy, intestinal metaplasia, and finally gastric cancer. It has been demonstrated (KUIPERS et al. 1995) in cohort studies that atrophic gastritis and intestinal metaplasia are much more likely to occur in subjects infected with *H. pylori* than in uninfected control subjects. The aforementioned study also showed that atrophic gastritis is not a direct and inevitable consequence of aging, but the result of infection. In another large cohort study (PARSONNET et al. 1991) it was shown that *H. pylori* was associated with an increased risk for both diffuse and intestinal types of adenocarcinoma in the body and antrum but not in the cardia. Interestingly, this cohort study also showed a negative correlation of carcinoma and peptic ulcer disease.

Since the incidence of *H. pylori* infection is many times higher than the incidence of carcinoma, there must also be co-factors in the development of cancer. Long-term infection starting in childhood might increase the risk for the atrophic gastric-intestinal metaplasia. Long-standing chronic infection with repeated cell turnover may increase the risk of cell mutation and malignancy. Other possible co-factors are diet, strain virulence, and individual immune response levels. Young patients under the age of 45 years with gastric carcinoma are more likely to be infected by *H. pylori* (KOKKOLA et al. 1996). Patients with gastric lymphoma were found to be significantly more likely to be infected with *H. pylori* than controls (PARSONNET et al. 1994). The same study showed no association between non-gastric non-Hodgkin's lymphoma and *H. pylori* infection. Most gastric non-Hodgkin's lymphomas arise in areas of chronic gastric inflammation. One subgroup of gastric lymphomas are low-grade B-cell lymphomas that arise in mucosa-associated lymphoid tissue (malt tumors) rather than lymph nodes. One study showed a 100% association of gastric malt tumors with *H. pylori*-positive mucosal biopsy specimens (WOTHERSPOON et al. 1991). Another study has shown complete tumor regression in five of six malt

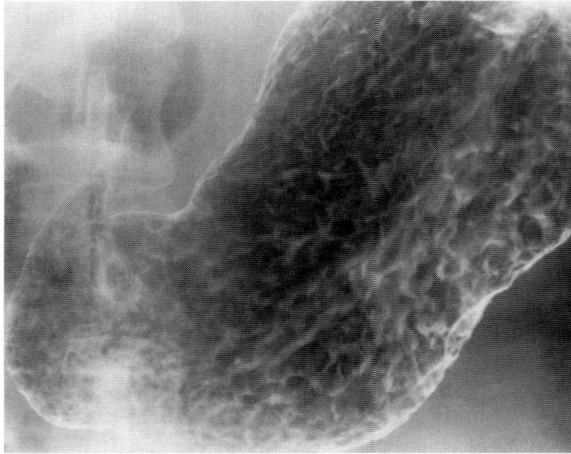

Fig. 11.1. Extensive nodular fold thickening with biopsy showing acute and chronic gastritis

tumors using antibiotic therapy for *H. pylori* (WOTHERSPOON et al. 1993).

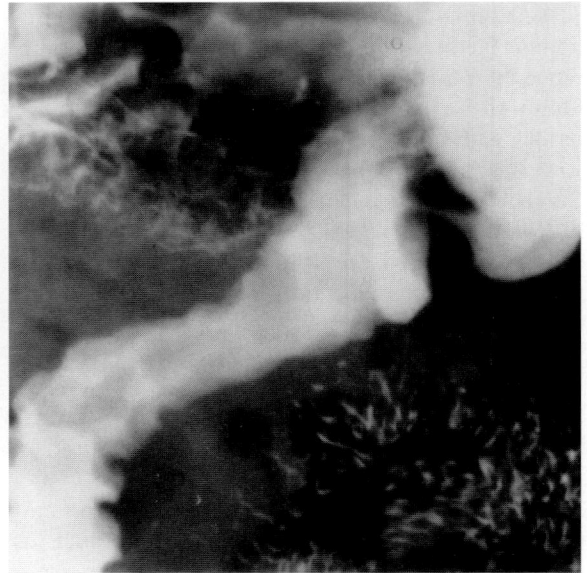

Fig. 11.2. Typical diffuse fold thickening of duodenitis in a young patient not taking NSAID medication

11.1.6
Radiologic Diagnosis

The primary finding in *H. pylori* gastritis is thickening of the folds of the antrum and body (Fig. 11.1). A study of 15 *H. pylori*-infected pediatric patients aged 9–16 years, using single- and double-contrast techniques, demonstrated enlarged folds in seven patients. Two patients had fold enlargement confined to the body of the stomach, three had body and antral fold thickening, and two had antral and duodenal fold enlargement (MORRISON et al. 1989). In a larger series (SOHN et al. 1995), adult patients with *H. pylori* diagnosed in endoscopy biopsy specimens were matched with a noninfected control group with a high percentage of gastritis on endoscopic biopsy. *H. pylori* patients had a significantly higher percentage of thick folds, thickened lobular folds, and enlarged areae gastricae. There was no statistical difference with other radiologic findings such as erosions, ulcers, or antral narrowing or polyps. The gastric ulcers in *H. pylori* patients were larger than ulcers in control patients and were associated with thickened antral folds while none of the control ulcer patients had thickened folds. Thickened antral folds on computed tomography (CT) simulating gastric carcinoma have also been described (URBAN et al. 1991). There are no studies in the literature evaluating the radiographic appearance of *H. pylori*-infected patients with duodenal ulcer and duodenitis. However, since it is clear that *H. pylori* is the main cause of duodenal ulcer and duodenitis [rare exceptions include Zollinger-Ellison syndrome and ulceration due to nonsteroidal anti-inflammatory drugs (NSAIDs)], the standard radiologic findings of these diseases should be seen (Fig. 11.2).

There is also little in the literature about the radiographic appearance of gastric carcinoma in *H. pylori*-infected patients. There is one report of gastric malt lymphoma in a *H. pylori* patient demonstrating innumerable less than 5 mm nodular elevations in the gastric body and fundus in addition to markedly thickened and scalloped antral folds (LEVINE et al. 1996). Gastric malt tumors have been described as being exophytic or relatively flat on endoscopy, with associated thick folds, erosions, or ulcers (SEIFERT et al. 1993), so that a variety of radiologic findings might be expected.

11.1.7
The Future

The medical and surgical management of gastric and duodenal ulcer disease has changed rapidly with the discovery of the role of *H. pylori* infection. Vagotomy and partial gastrectomy for acid control are no longer necessary for recurrent disease. Bleeding and perforation can be handled with a patch or oversewing. Acid control and eradication of *H. pylori* can be left for drug therapy (WITTE 1995). Current drug regimens include a triple therapy combination of bismuth, tetracycline, and metronidazole or a combination therapy of amoxicillin or similar broad-spectrum antibiotic such as clarithromycin combined with the ion pump inhibitor omeprazole (WALSH and PETERSON 1995). The decreased acid environment in the stomach caused by the ion pump inhibition seems to potentiate the effect of the antibiotic on *H. pylori*. Drug resistance is not now a problem, but there are treatment failures and alternative antibiotics may be necessary. Research is also underway in the development of an effective vaccine which, if found, could dramatically reduce morbidity and mortality from peptic ulcer and gastric malignancy.

The algorithm for treatment of peptic disease has changed. With a simple breath test diagnosis can be made by the internist and general practitioner and only patients with treatment failure need be referred to the gastroenterologist for endoscopy. Some patients may be treated empirically for *H. pylori* without confirmation of infection. Individuals who are seronegative for *H. pylori* and are not taking NSAIDs can be reassured that they do not have peptic ulcer disease (SOBALA et al. 1991). Endoscopy and radiographic evaluation will be reserved for treatment failure, evaluation of reflux and diagnosis of malignancy. pH monitoring can be expected to further reduce the need for radiologic evaluation in patients with reflux symptoms.

Since it has been demonstrated that gastroenterologists are 2–3 times more likely to be infected with *H. pylori*, possibly through contact with orogastric secretions during endoscopy (PETERSON 1986), radiology personnel should make sure to use standard precautions against infection when in possible contact with oral or orogastric patient secretions during procedures such as nasogastric tube placements, enteroclysis, and swallowing studies.

11.2
Gastrointestinal Tract Opportunistic Infections in the Immunocompromised Host

In addition to the increase in the number of patients with AIDS, there has also been an increase in the number of patients who are immune-suppressed as part of transplant therapy and tumor therapy. It is important to be aware of the many manifestations of opportunistic infections and graft-versus-host disease in the gastrointestinal tract.

11.2.1
Esophagitis

The commonest cause of esophagitis in immunocompromised patients is *Candida albicans*. Esophagitis and oropharyngeal candidiasis has a high predictive value (90%) for esophageal candidiasis (WILCOX et al. 1995). Candidiasis typically will present with diffuse mucosal irregularity and progress to a nodular, shaggy mucosal pattern with barium filling the interstices between *Candida* plaques (Fig. 11.3a). Rarely *Candida* can be localized (Fig. 11.4) or may simulate a tumor mass. Deep ulceration can also occur. Complications include stricture and microabscesses in the spleen, liver, and kidneys (WALL and JONES 1992).

Localized involvement of the esophagus is more typical of herpes, cytomegalovirus (CMV), human immunodeficiency virus (HIV), or idiopathic ulcer. There is ulceration usually with a normal background mucosa. CMV ulcers are often located near the esophagogastric junction. Tuberculosis and actinomycosis can cause ulcers and sinus tracts from adjacent infected mediastinal nodes. Specific diagnosis of viral esophagitis by endoscopic biopsy is critical since the treatments differ for CMV (ganciclovir), herpes (acyclovir), and idiopathic ulcer (corticosteroids).

11.2.2
Gastritis

Gastritis due to *Candida* and CMV produces variable patterns. The primary findings are ulcerations and thick folds. In CMV gastritis barium studies can show thickened folds, aphthous ulcers, superficial and deep ulceration, and fistula formation. CT can show a markedly thickened gastric wall and coarse thickened folds mimicking lymphoma and carcinoma (FARMEN et al. 1992).

11.2.3
Enteritis

The two main organisms causing enteritis in AIDS patients are *Cryptosporidium* and *Mycobacterium avium-intracellulare* (MAI). The protozoan *Cryptosporidium* usually involves the proximal small bowel, causing regular thick folds and increased bowel secretions (Fig. 11.5). Mesenteric lymphadenopathy is uncommon. MAI infection often involves the

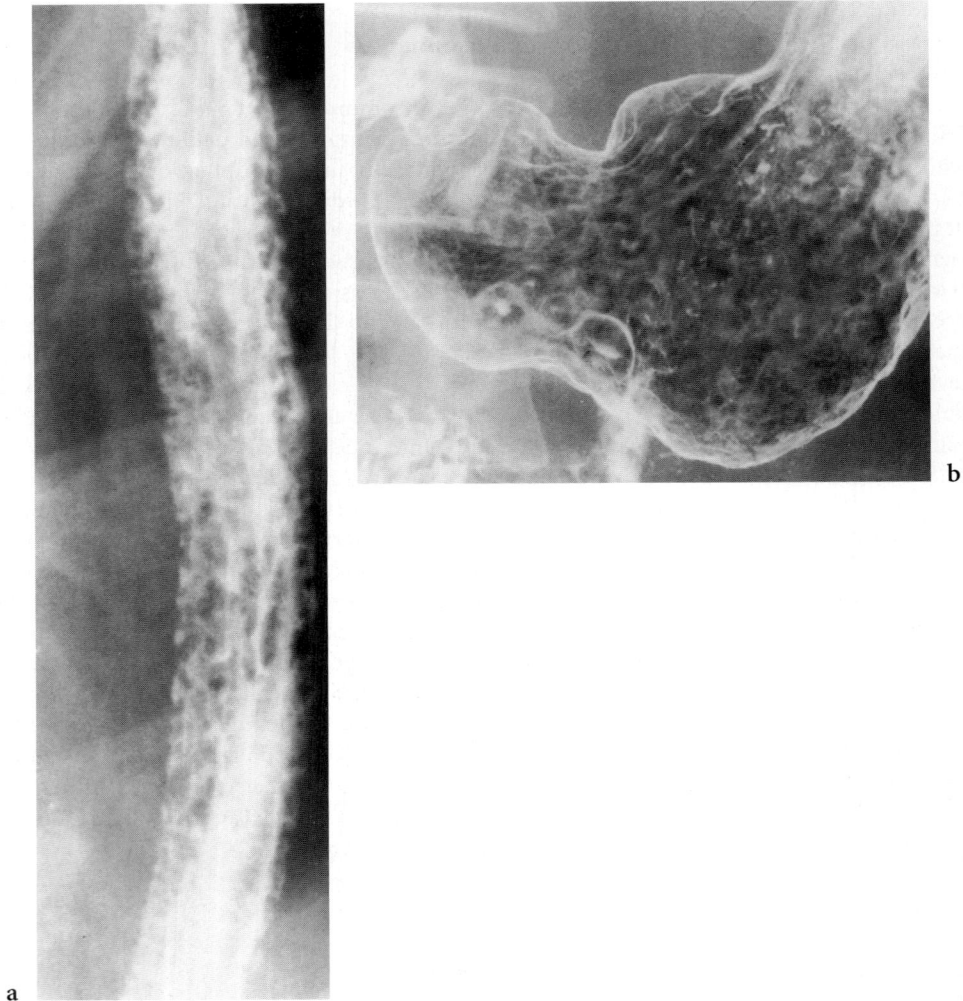

Fig. 11.3. a Coarse shaggy appearance of diffuse candidiasis of the esophagus in a patient with AIDS. **b** The same patient's stomach demonstrates numerous filling defects with central ulceration due to Kaposi sarcoma

middle and distal small bowel, producing irregular fold thickening and mild dilatation. Separation of bowel loops can be seen due to the frequent occurrence of extensive mesenteric lymphadenopathy. Like *Candida*, MAI can cause microabscesses in the solid organs of the abdomen. Rarely, enlarged lymphoid follicles in enteritis patients may act as lead points for intussusception (Fig. 11.6).

11.2.4
Colitis

Cytomegalovirus colitis has a wide range of findings. The pathology is similar to CMV gastritis. Early disease may show small nodules or aphthous ulcers

with a normal mucosal background. As disease progresses, thickened irregular mucosal and deep ulcerations can be seen. Distribution is often in a continuous manner without skip areas. Plain films may show thick mucosal, bowel dilatation, and occasionally pneumotosis and perforation (COLLINS et al. 1993). In one study of 24 patients with biopsy-proven CMV, CT showed circumferential wall thickening in 17 (cf. Fig. 11.7 for such a finding), deep mural ulceration in 15, mural edema in 15, and pericolonic stranding in 23. Lymphadenopathy was seen in only 4 patients (MURRAY et al. 1995). Diagnosis by biopsy is important since ganciclovir is effective therapy in 75% of patients. *Salmonella, Shigella* (Fig. 11.8), adenovirus, and coxsackie A and B also produce severe forms of colitis with watery diarrhea and hemor-

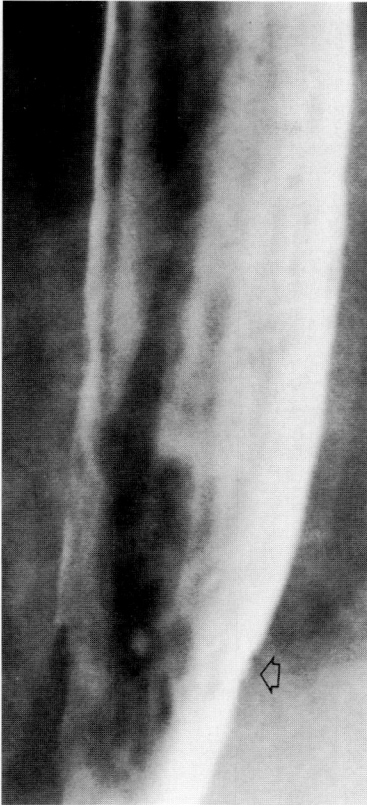

Fig. 11.4. Minimal fold thickening and several aphthous ulcerations including an ulcer in profile (*arrow*) in the lower esophagus secondary to candidiasis. This leukemic patient also had aphthoid ulcers in her mouth

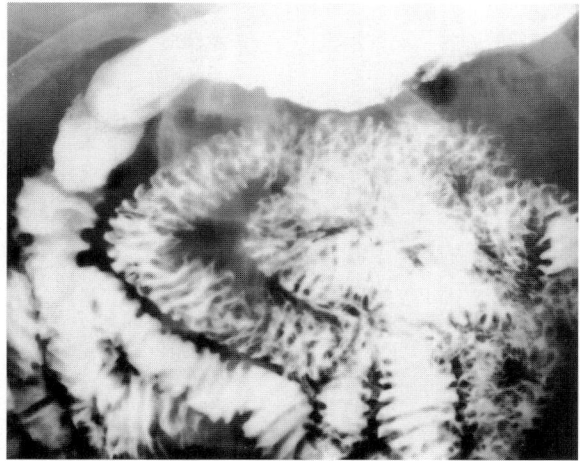

Fig. 11.5. Diffuse jejunal fold thickening with slight nodularity due to *Cryptosporidium* in an AIDS patient

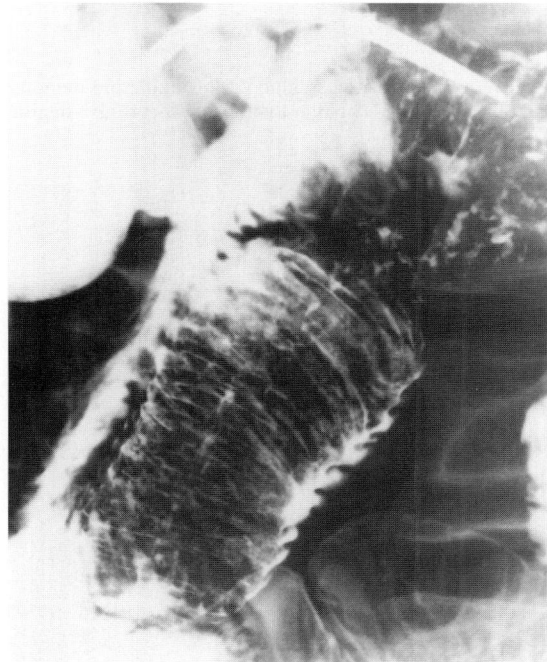

Fig. 11.6. Small bowel intussusception with a thin string of barium in the collapsed inner loop in a patient with AIDS and recurrent abdominal pain. At surgery the lead point was a focal area of thickened lymphoid tissue

rhage which can be fatal in immune-compromised patients. Tuberculosis most often involves the cecal region and ileum, and lymphadenopathy is usually confined to the right lower quadrant. Barium studies show thick folds, irregular contours, ulcerations, and strictures (Fig. 11.9). CT findings include thickening of the ileocecal valve and medial wall of the cecum with exophytic extension to the adjacent ileum and enlarged low-density nodes (BALTHAZAR et al. 1990).

11.2.5
Cholangitis

AIDS-related cholangitis may have one of four patterns: (a) isolated distal papillary stenosis, (b) diffuse intrahepatic strictures similar to sclerosing cholangitis, (c) a combination of diffuse intrahepatic and extrahepatic strictures (Fig. 11.10), and (d) long extrahepatic bile duct stricture (CELLO 1989). CMV and *Cryptosporidium* are the usual etiologic agents and the clinical picture includes fever, right upper quadrant pain, elevated white cell count, and abnormal liver function tests, especially alkaline phosphatase.

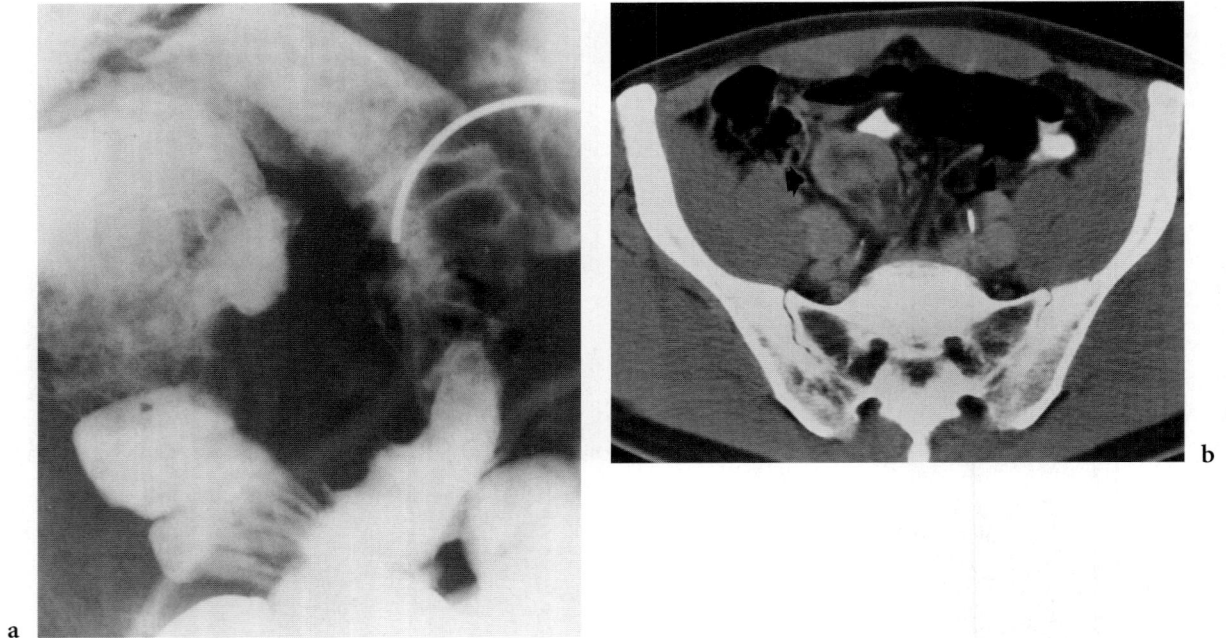

Fig. 11.7. a Close-up of a small bowel examination demonstrating enlarged terminal ileal folds and slight luminal narrowing. **b** CT of the same AIDS patient with CMV ileitis also demonstrates circumferential wall thickening (*arrow*)

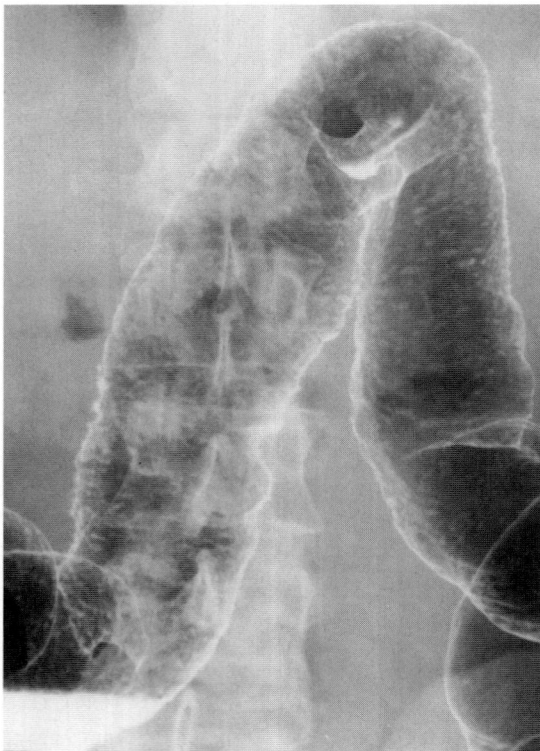

Fig. 11.8. An AIDS patient with recurrent diarrhea despite antibiotic therapy with innumerable tiny ulcerations in the transverse colon. Both *Salmonella* and *Shigella* were obtained from stool cultures. (Courtesy of R. Sollitto, MD)

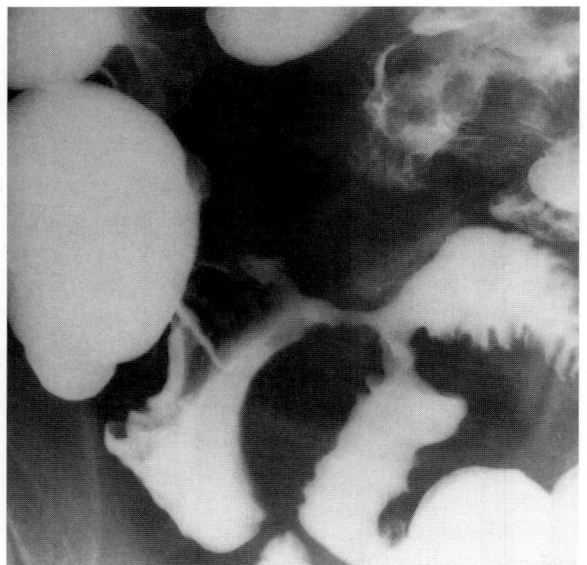

Fig. 11.9. An AIDS patient with tuberculosis of the terminal ileum and cecum with a fistula to adjacent ileum. (Courtesy of R. Sollitto, MD)

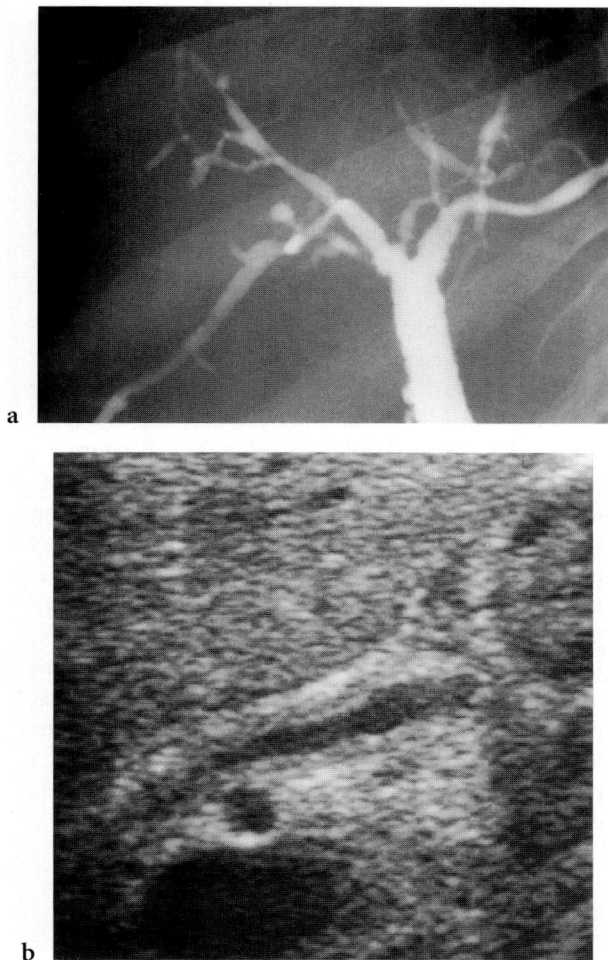

Fig. 11.10. a AIDS cholangitis secondary to *Cryptosporidium*. ERCP examination shows irregular wall contour of the common bile duct and main hepatic ducts. b Ultrasonography in the same patient demonstrates marked thickening of the wall of the common bile duct

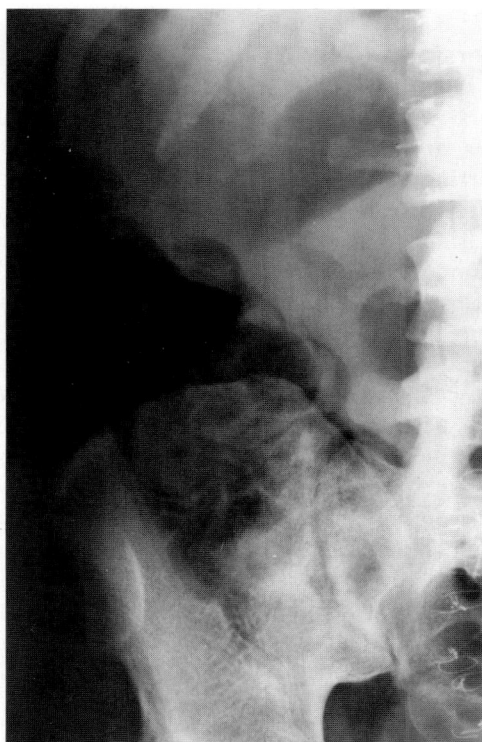

Fig. 11.11. Close-up of the right lower quadrant demonstrating extensive right colon intramural gas and dilatation in a leukemic patient with typhlitis

11.2.6
Graft Versus Host Disease

Graft versus host disease (GVHD) occurs when the immune-competent graft reacts to the immune-incompetent host. The major organ target in the acute form is the small bowel with severe mucosal inflammation and diarrhea. Radiographically there is diffuse fold thickening or fold effacement producing a featureless "ribbon bowel." Colonic involvement can also occur with spasm, ulceration, and thickened mucosa, simulating ulcerative colitis. The chronic form of GVHD affects the skin, producing a scleroderma-like pattern. The esophagus is also affected with desquamation followed by web and stricture formation (Wall and Jones 1992).

11.2.7
Typhlitis

Typhlitis is an acute inflammation of the cecum and appendix originally described in patients with leukemia and severe neutropenia. It can also be seen in patients with aplastic anemia, lymphoma, transplantation, and AIDS. It can be caused by leukemic or lymphomatous infiltrates, ischemia, focal pseudomembranous colitis, or other infection, frequently CMV. Plain film findings of typhlitis are small bowel obstruction, right lower quadrant mass, thickened bowel wall due to submucosal edema, and intramural gas (Fig. 11.11). CT findings demonstrate cecal and terminal ileal wall thickening with decreased attenuation suggesting edema and attenuation of adjacent fat (Merine et al. 1987). Prompt administration of fluids and antibiotics is necessary to avoid bowel necrosis and perforation. CT is helpful in the assessment of the effectiveness of therapy.

11.3
Diversion Colitis

Diversion colitis, also called bypass colitis, exclusion colitis, or disuse colitis, is an inflammatory process occurring in segments of the colon excluded from the fecal stream (GLOTZER et al. 1981). Hartmann's pouch and mucous fistula following ileostomy or colostomy are the common sites of diversion colitis. Most patients with temporary diversion of the fecal stream are asymptomatic. Symptoms occur 3–36 months after diversion and are manifested by mucoid or bloody discharge from the anus or mucous fistula. The discharge may be purulent. There may be abdominal or pelvic pain, low-grade fever, tenesmus, and anal fistula (GIARDIELLO et al. 1995). Endoscopically there may be erythema and friability in milder cases and spontaneous bleeding, exudation, superficial ulceration and nodularity, inflammatory polyp formation, and stricture in more severe disease following prolonged diversion. Radiologic changes of edema, nodularity, aphthous ulceration, and stricture can be seen.

The histologic changes are in the region of the crypts with foci of cryptitis and crypt abscesses but preservation of crypt architecture, in contrast to the crypt distortion typical of ulcerative colitis. The cause is related to an absence of short chain fatty acids normally produced as by-products of fecal stream bacterial metabolism of undigested carbohydrates and fecal stream fiber. These short chain fatty acids – acetate, proprionate, and butyrate – are an important energy source of colonocytes. The preferred treatment of diversion colitis is surgical reanastomosis; if this is not feasible, therapy comprises topical replacement of short chain fatty acids. This is accomplished by instilling solutions containing fatty acids several times per day through the anus or mucous fistula opening, and having the patient remain supine for 30 min.

11.4
Disinfectant Colitis

Radiologists should be aware of the colitis following a normal colonoscopy caused by colonoscopy disinfectants. The common endoscope disinfectant solutions hydrogen peroxide and glutaraldehyde are injurious to colonic mucosa and direct contact can result in colitis. There are some differences between hydrogen peroxide and glutaraldehyde. Glutaraldehyde causes direct injury to crypt epithelium while hydrogen peroxide compromises mucosal stroma (RYAN and POTTER 1995). Hydrogen peroxide causes an immediate formation of white mucosal plaques, originally called pseudolipomatosis, secondary to diffuse emphysema with minute gas cysts filling the lamina propria and separating crypts. Mucosal hemorrhage and ulceration may occur with tenesmus and bloody diarrhea (JONAS et al. 1988). Glutaraldehyde does not result in an immediate mucosal reaction that can be recognized by the endoscopist but mucosal contact during endoscopy will also produce symptoms of hematochezia, fever, and tenesmus within 48 h. Barium enema may show thickened colonic folds and CT can show circumferential thickening of the colonic wall in a left-sided distribution (BIRNBAUM et al. 1995). CT may be helpful in monitoring resolution of mural thickening following supportive therapy. Disinfectant solution contact is usually secondary to insufficient rinsing in automatic instrument-washing machines. These require proper machine maintenance, maintenance of satisfactory volumes of rinse water, and frequent changes of the rinse water. Preprocedure rinsing of channels and exterior endoscope components with tap water is also recommended. Another source of exposure is inadvertent channel flushing with glutaraldehyde included on the endoscopy tray instead of water.

11.5
Clostridium difficile Disease

Clostridium difficile is the primary cause of pseudomembranous colitis which is characterized by 1- to 3-mm raised plaques. The disease was originally described in 1893 and the plaques were thought to resemble the pseudomembranes seen in the pharynx in diphtheria, which was then a common disease. The organism was discovered in 1935 and was difficult to isolate and grow in pure culture, probably accounting for its name. The normal human colonic flora prevents colonization of *C. difficile*, but such colonization may occur following disturbance of the normal flora by antibiotics, especially broad-spectrum antibiotics such as ampicillin, clindamycin, cephalosporin, and aminoglycosides. *C. difficile* produces two toxins, toxin A, an enterotoxin which is responsible for the colitis, and toxin B, a cytotoxin which has little potency. Toxin A elicits an acute inflammatory response with activation of neutrophils, mast cells, and macrophages. There is destruction of mucosa, primarily at the tips of the villi. Histologically, the pseudomembranes are com-

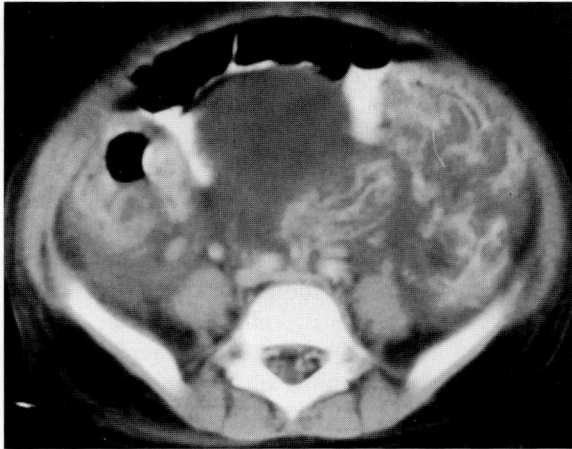

Fig. 11.12. CT examination of a 3-year-old with *C. difficile* colitis occurring after appendectomy and antibiotic therapy. There is diffuse fold thickening of left-sided colon loops

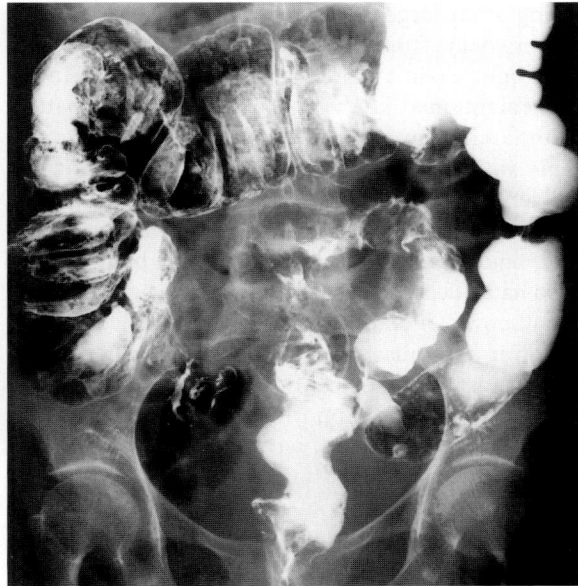

Fig. 11.13. Marked fold thickening of rectal and sigmoid folds in a patient with diarrhea. Rectal biopsy demonstrated extensive arteriolar amyloid deposition. Repeat barium enema 1 year later showed uniform narrowing of the rectum and sigmoid

posed of necrotic debris, mucus, and inflammatory cells (POTHOULAKIS and LA MONT 1993). Diagnosis is usually made by enzyme immunoassay for toxins A and B. Treatment using metronidazole or vancomycin is effective. There is a wide spectrum of disease presentations with mild, moderate, and fulminant forms of diarrhea and crampy pain. Morbidity from dehydration or perforation is more likely to occur in older or debilitated patients.

The radiologic findings also vary depending on the severity of the colitis. Plain film and barium enema examinations may show bowel dilatation and mucosal dedma with haustral thickening. Nodularity and plaques may also be seen (LOUGHRAN et al. 1982). Barium enema is not recommended in advanced disease because of the risk of perforation. CT shows diffuse wall thickening usually involving the more distal colon and rectum (Fig. 11.12), but disease can be limited to the right colon and transverse colon (BOLAND et al. 1994). The bowel wall thickening may be nodular with a shaggy mucosal contour. A sign thought to specific for *C. difficile* colitis is the accordian sign, which is the combination of broad transverse bands of closely spaced nodular haustra and thin columns of trapped contrast material (FISHMAN et al. 1991).

11.6
Amyloid Colitis

Amyloidosis may occur anywhere in the gastrointestinal tract but is most commonly found in the small intestine. The most common site of deposition is in and around the walls of arterioles in submucosal tissue. In addition to vascular infiltration, amyloid usually involves the mucosal and muscular layers of the bowel. Recent biochemical analysis has been able to demonstrate at least four different amyloid proteins. Patients with secondary or reactive systemic amyloidosis from chronic inflammatory diseases such as tuberculosis, rheumatoid arthritis, ankylosing spondylitis and ulcerative colitis have amyloid A protein. Patients with primary amyloidosis or multiple myeloma have light chain amyloid protein. Familial amyloidosis patients have prealbumin protein and patients undergoing long-term hemodialysis have B_2-microglobulin protein.

In a study correlating the different protein types with radiologic findings and biopsy specimens, TADA and his colleagues (1994) noted that patients with secondary amyloid were likely to demonstrate a fine granular elevation of bowel mucosa with double-contrast technique which correlated with amyloid type deposits in the lamina propria causing villi expansion. Patients with light chain protein from primary amyloidosis or multiple myeloma were more likely to have more massive amyloid deposits in the muscularis mucosa, resulting in more polypoid nodularity and diffuse wall thickening. Diffuse thickening of the large or small bowel wall may be due to either edema from acute ischemia (Fig. 11.13) or diffuse light chain amyloid protein infiltration. In the aforementioned study by TADA et al., one patient with familial amyloid had a marked delay in transit time which may have been due to preferential involvement of myenteric plexus by prealbumin protein. The one patient in the study with B$_2$-microglobulin protein from chronic hemodialysis also had a delay in barium transit time and large and small bowel dilatation with extensive amyloid deposition in the muscularis propria. When there is extensive arteriolar deposition of amyloid leading to ischemia, colonic abnormalities such as diffuse edema, loss of haustra, narrowing, and ulceration, the findings are indistinguishable from radiation colitis or other forms of ischemic colitis (SELIGER et al. 1971).

11.7
Cystic Fibrosis and Colonic Stricture

More than 90% of cystic fibrosis patients have pancreatic insufficiency and require enzymes to reduce steatorrhea. Colonic strictures have recently been reported in the ascending colon in young patients taking high doses of pancreatic enzymes (SMYTH et al. 1994). Predisposing factors include a young age group, previous intestinal surgery, and prolonged use of high-lipase products. Pathologically there is striking fibrosis and a lack of inflammatory change or granulomas to distinguish it from Crohn's disease, which has a high incidence in cystic fibrosis patients. The strictures are irreversible and require surgery. Early symptoms are abdominal pain, diarrhea, and hematochezia, and colonoscopy may show erythematous mucosa with friability and bleeding usually in the cecal region (LLOYD-STILL 1995). Ultrasound findings may show thickened colonic walls and decreased peristalsis. In early disease, the wall thickness on ultrasound examination may decrease when patients change to lower strength enzymes (MACSWEENEY et al. 1995). Radiologic findings in later stages of disease include loss of haustra, a lead pipe colon, and a focal stricture. The pathophysiology is unknown.

11.8
Collagenous and Lymphocytic Colitis

Two newer colitides that radiologists should be cognizant of, even though radiologic findings have not been described, are collagenous colitis (KINGHAM et al. 1986) and lymphocytic colitis (GIARDIELLO et al. 1989). Both colitides present with chronic watery diarrhea and crampy abdominal pain in middle-aged and older patients. Collagenous colitis has a 20:1 female to male predominance while lymphocytic colitis has close to a 1:1 female to male ratio. The pathology of both entities demonstrates an increase in intraepithelial lymphocytes. Collagenous colitis is distinguished by the additional finding of an increase in subepithelial collagen similar to the findings of increased small bowel subepithelial collagen seen in collagenous sprue, a variant of celiac disease. Lymphocytic colitis patients may have increased titers of antinuclear antibodies, antiparietal cell antibodies, antimicrosomal antibodies, and HLA A1 antigens. Endoscopy is normal in both diseases. Diagnosis is made by colonic biopsy and multiple biopsies may be necessary. Both colitides are treated with anti-inflammatory medications such as sulfasalazine or prednisone. Patients with collagenous colitis unresponsive to medical therapy have been successfully treated with surgical diversion of the fecal stream (JÄRNEROT et al. 1995). No malignant potential is known for either colitis.

References

Balthazar EJ, Gordon R, Hulnick D (1990) Tuberculosis: CT and radiologic evaluation. Am J Roentgenol 154:499–503

Beaumont W (1959) Experiments and observations on the gastric juice and the physiology of digestion (reprinted from 1833). Dover Publications, New York, pp 9–28

Birnbaum BA, Gordon RB, Jacobs JE (1995) Glutaraldehyde colitis: radiologic findings. Radiology 195:131–134

Blaser MJ (1994) *Helicobacter pylori* phenotypes associated with peptic ulceration. Scand J Gastroenterol 29 (Suppl 205):1–5

Boland GW, Lee MJ, Cats AM, et al. (1994) Antibiotic-induced diarrhea: specificity of abdominal CT for the diagnosis of *Clostridium difficile* disease. Radiology 191:103–106

Cello JP (1989) Acquired immunodeficiency syndrome cholangiopathy: spectrum of disease. Am J Med 86:539–546

Christie JML, McNulty CAM, shepherd NA, et al. (1996) Is saliva serology useful for the diagnosis of *Helicobacter pylori*? Gut 39:27–30

Collins CD, Blandshard C, Gleeson JA, et al. (1993) Cytomegalovirus colitis in AIDS: plain abdominal radiographic findings. Clin Radiol 48:127–130

Drumm B, Perez-Perez GI, Blaser MJ, et al. (1990) Interfamilial clustering of *Helicobacter pylori* infection. N Engl J Med 322:359–363

Ernst PB, Jin Y, Reyes VE, et al. (1994) The role of the local immune response in the pathogenesis of peptic ulcer formation. Scand J Gastroenterol 29 (Suppl 205):22–28

Farmen J, Lerner ME, Ng C, et al. (1992) Cytomegalovirus gastritis: protean radiologic features. Gastrointest Radiol 17:202–206

Fishman EK, Kavuru MK, Jones BJ, et al. (1991) Pseudomembranous colitis: CT evaluation of 26 cases. Radiology 180:57–60

Giardiello FM, Lazenby AJ, Bayless TM, et al. (1989) Lymphocytic (microscopic colitis) – clinicopathologic study of 18 patients and comparison to collagenous colitis. Dig Dis Sci 35:33–40

Giardiello FM, Lazenby AJ, Bayless TM (1995) The new colidites collagenous, lymphocytic and diversion colitis. Gastroenterol Clin North Am 24:717–729

Glotzer DJ, Glick ME, Golman H (1981) Proctitis and colitis following diversion of the fecal stream. Gastroenterology 35:428–430

Graham DY, Lew GM, Klein PD, et al. (1992) Effect of treatment of Helicobacter pylori infection on the long-term recurrence of gastric and duodenal ulcer. Ann Intern Med 116:705–708

Graham DY, Malaty HM, Go MF (1994) Are there susceptible hosts to Helicobacter pylori infection? Scand J Gastroenterol 29 (Suppl 205):6–10

Hentschel E, Brandstatter G, Dragosics B, et al. (1993) Effect of ranitidine and amoxicillin plus metronidazole on the eradication of Helicobacter pylori and the recurrence of duodenal ulcer. N Engl J Med 328:308–312

Järnerot G, Tysk C, Bohr J, et al. (1995) Collagenous colitis and fecal stream diversion. Gastroenterology 109:449–455

Jonas C, Mahoney A, Murray J, et al. (1988) Chemical colitis due to endoscope cleaning solutions: a mimic of pseudomembranous colitis. Gastroenterology 35:428–430

Kingham JGC, Levison DA, Morson BC, et al. (1986) Collagenous colitis. Gut 27:570–577

Kokkola A, Valle J, Haapiainen R, et al. (1996) Helicobacter pylori infection in young patients with gastric carcinoma. Scand J Gastroenterol 31:643–647

Kuipers EJ, Uyterlinde AM, Pena AS, et al. (1995) Long-term sequelae of Helicobacter pylori gastritis. Lancet 345:1525–1528

Lee A (1994) Future research in peptic ulcer disease. Scand J Gastroenterol 29 (Suppl):51–58

Levine MS, Elmas N, Furth E, et al. (1996) Helicobacter pylori and gastric malt lymphoma. Am J Roentgenol 166:85–86

Lloyd-Still JD (1995) Cystic fibrosis and colonic stricture. J Clin Gastroenterol 21:2–5

Loughran CF, Tappin JA, Whitehouse GH (1982) The plain radiograph in pseudomembranous colitis due to Clostridium difficile disease. Radiology 191:103–106

Macsweeney E, Oades PJ, Buchdahl RM, et al. (1995) Relation of thickening of colon wall to pancreatic enzyme treatment in cystic fibrosis. Lancet 345:752–756

Marshall BJ (1986) Campylobacter pyloridis and gastritis. J Infect Dis 153:650–657

Marshall BJ, Warren JR (1984) Unidentified curved bacilli in the stomach of patients with gastritis and peptic ulceration. Lancet 1:1311–1315

Marshall BJ, Goodwin CS, Warren JR, et al. (1988) Prospective double-blind trial of duodenal ulcer relapse after eradication of Campylobacter pylori. Lancet ii:1437–1442

Merine D, Fishman EK, Jones B, et al. (1987) Right lower quadrant pain in the immunocompromised patient: CT findings in 10 cases. Am J Roentgenol 149:1172–1179

Morrison S, Dahms BB, Hoffenberg E, et al. (1989) Enlarged gastric folds in association with Campylobacter pylori gastritis. Radiology 171:819–821

Murray JG, Evans SJ, Jeffrey PB, et al. (1995) Cytomegalovirus colitis in AIDS. Am J Roentgenol 165:67–71

Parsonnet J, Friedman GD, Vardersteen MS, et al. (1991) Helicobacter pylori infection and the risk of gastric carcinoma. N Engl J Med 325:1127–1131

Parsonnet J, Hansen S, Rodriquez L, et al. (1994) Helicobacter pylori infection and gastric lymphoma. N Engl J Med 330:1267–1271

Peterson WL (1986) Helicobacter pylori and peptic ulcer disease. N Engl J Med 524:1043–1048

Phillips M (1995) Breathtaking technology for the detection of Helicobacter pylori. Am J Gastroenterol 90:2089–2090

Pothoulakis C, La Mont JT (1993) Clostridium difficile colitis and diarrhea. Gastroenterol Clin North Am 22:623–637

Ryan CK, Potter GD (1995) Disinfectant colitis rinse as well as you wash (editorial). J Clin Gastroenterol 21:6–9

Seifert E, Schulte F, Weismuller J, et al. (1993) Endoscopic and bioptic diagnosis of malignant non-Hodgkin's lymphoma of the stomach. Endoscopy 25:497–501

Seliger G, Krassner RL, Beranbaum ER, et al. (1971) The spectrum of roentgen appearance in amyloidosis of the small and large bowel: radiologic pathologic correlation. Am J Roentgenol 100:63–70

Smyth RL, Van Velzen D, Smith AR, et al. (1994) Strictures of ascending colon in cystic fibrosis and high-strength pancreatic enzymes. Lancet 343:85–86

Sobala GM, Crabtree JE, Pentith JA, et al. (1991) Screening dyspepsia by serology to Helicobacter pylori. Lancet 338:94–94

Sohn J, Levine MS, Furth E, et al. (1995) Helicobacter pylori gastritis: radiographic findings. Radiology 195:763–767

Stubbs JB, Marshall BJ (1993) Radiation dose estimates for carbon-14 labeled urea breath test. J Nucl Med 34:821–825

Tada S, Iida M, Yao M, et al. (1994) Gastrointestinal amyloidosis: radiologic features by chemical types. Radiology 190:37–42

Urban BA, Fishman EK, Hruban RH (1991) Helicobacter pylori gastritis mimicking gastric carcinoma at CT evaluation. Radiology 179:689–691

Wall SD, Jones B (1992) Gastrointestinal tract in the immunocompromised host: opportunistic infections and other complications. Radiology 185:327–335

Walsh JH, Peterson WL (1995) The treatment of Helicobacter pylori infection in the management of peptic ulcer disease. N Engl J Med 333:984–991

Wilcox CM, Straub RF, Clark WS (1995) Prospective evaluation of oropharyngeal findings in human immunodeficiency virus-infected patients with esophageal ulceration. Am J Gastroenterol 90:1938–1941

Witte CL (1995) Vagotomy and gastrectomy for duodenal ulcer. J Clin Gastroenterol 20:2–3

Wotherspoon AC, Ortiz-Hidalgo C, Falzon MR, et al. (1991) Helicobacter pylori-associated gastritis and primary B-cell gastric lymphoma. Lancet 338:1175–1176

Wotherspoon AC, Doglioni C, Diss TC, et al. (1993) Regression of primary low-grade B-cell gastric lymphoma of mucosa-associated lymphoid tissue type after eradication of Helicobacter pylori. Lancet 342:575–577

Wotherspoon AC, Doglioni C, Diss TC, et al. (1994) Regression of primary low grade B-cell lymphoma of mucosa-associated lymphoid tissue type after eradication of Helicobacter pylori. Gastroenterology 107:1835–1838

12 Neoplastic Disease

M. Maruyama, Y. Baba, N. Takemoto, S. Kaku, K. Koizumi, S. Kai, and T. Sakai

CONTENTS

12.1
Introduction

The use of classic barium radiology for investigation of the gastrointestinal tract has been declining worldwide. Against this background, the information provided by the technique has become less reliable: the less the need for it, the smaller the number of skilled radiologists. The better diagnostic yield of endoscopy, and especially video endoscopy, has been recognized, with the consequence that much more reliance has been placed on endoscopy.

Nevertheless, it is certain that classic barium radiology still has advantages over other diagnostic modalities such as computed tomography (CT), ultrasonography (US), and magnetic resonance imaging (MRI) for the diagnosis of many abnormalities of the gastrointestinal tract. In this chapter we attempt to illustrate the value of classic barium radiology in the diagnosis of neoplastic diseases of the alimentary tube.

12.2
Early and Superficial Esophageal Carcinoma

12.2.1
General Considerations

12.2.1.1
Definition and Classification

The term "early esophageal carcinoma" (EEC) refers to squamous cell carcinoma (SCC), and has been defined as a carcinoma which is limited to the mucosal membrane and submucosa without lymph node and distant metastases (Japanese Society for Esophageal Diseases 1992). The term "superficial esophageal carcinoma" (SEC) is used for a carcinoma which is limited to the mucosal membrane and submucosa, without regard to the presence or absence of metastases (Japanese Society for Esophageal Diseases 1992). However, because of the increased incidence of metastases and the poorer survival rates in cases with submucosal involvement, many clinical researchers consider that the term EEC, too, should be restricted to a carcinoma which is limited to the mucosal membrane (Shirakabe et al. 1990).

12.2.1.2
Prognosis

Lymph node metastases are rarely encountered in cases of mucosal cancer and the 5-year survival rate is quite favorable; by contrast, as mentioned above,

M. Maruyama, MD, Y. Baba, MD, N. Takemoto, MD, S. Kaku, MD, K. Koizumi, S. Kai, MD, T. Sakai, MD, Division of Internal Medicine, Cancer Institute Hospital, 1-37-1 Kami-Ikebukuro Toshima-ku, Tokyo 170, Japan

ep

lpm

mm

Invasive
depth

m1

ep

lpm

mm

m2

ep

lpm

mm

m3

ep: epithelium
lpm: lamina propria mucosae
mm: muscularis mucosae

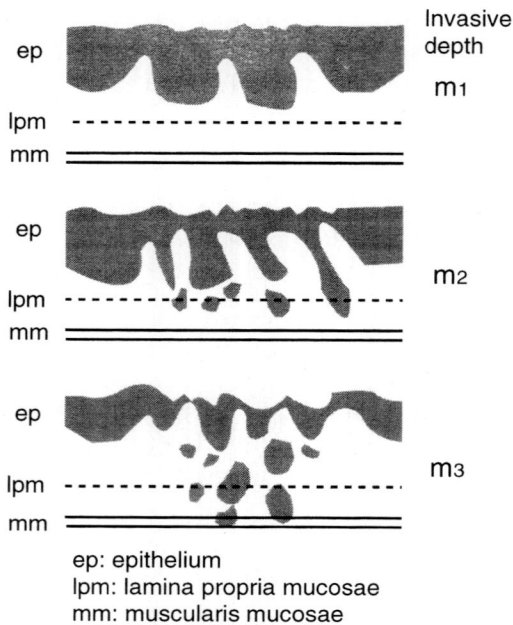

Fig. 12.1. Subclassification of invasive depth in SEC. *ep*, epithelium; *lpm*, lamina propria mucosae; *mm*, muscularis mucosae

lymph node metastases are frequently present when cancer involves the submucosa, and the 5-year survival rate is consequently comparable to that in patients with gastric cancer involving the propria muscle (MARUYAMA 1992).

12.2.1.3
Subclassification

Against this background, in 1992 the Committee for the Clinical Classification of Cancer proposed a subclassification of SEC that was expected to facilitate treatment decision-making (Japanese Society for Esophageal Diseases 1992). In this subclassification, mucosal carcinoma and carcinoma with submucosal involvement were each divided into three subgroups [m1, m2, and m3 (Fig. 12.1) and sm1, sm2, and sm3]. This new subclassification has proved of practical value in deciding upon the appropriateness of endoscopic mucosal resection (EMR), and is now widely used in Japan (MAKUUCHI et al. 1994).

Many reports have addressed the relation between the invasive depth of superficial carcinoma and lymph node metastasis, and it is accepted that no lymph node metastases are present in m1 and m2 cancers (MONMA et al. 1994); accordingly, EMR is indicated in such cases, though consideration must always be given to its impact on the quality of life of patients, who are usually males of advanced age.

Table 12.1. Macroscopic classification of type 0 superficial lesions

0-I	Superficial and protruding type
0-II	Superficial and flat type
0-IIa	Slightly elevated type
0-IIb	Flat type
0-IIc	Slightly depressed type
0-III	Superficial and distinctly depressed type

N.B. When a lesion reveals different morphologic patterns, two or more types are described together, with the predominant pattern preceding the others, e.g., type 0-IIc + IIa or 0-IIc + IIb.

12.2.2
Gross Pathology

12.2.2.1
Size of Mucosal Cancer

The maximum diameter of mucosal cancer typically ranges from 10 to 30 mm, exceptions being m1 cases comprising a microfocus measuring 5 mm or less (OHKURA et al. 1994). In addition, a superficial spreading type is encountered, in which the focus measures 5 cm or more. In our institution the superficial spreading type has accounted for 23.0% of mucosal carcinomas and 15% of all SECs (KAKU et al. 1995).

12.2.2.2
Macroscopic Classification

All mucosal carcinomas (m1–3) are of a macroscopic type designated 0-II (Table 12.1). Type 0-IIc accounts for 74% of cases, including both mixed and pure types. The mixed type (0-IIc + IIb and 0-IIc + IIa) is more frequent, accounting for 91% of type 0-IIc cases. The pure 0-IIc type is most often present in m1 and m2 cancer, while the mixed type is found in m3 and submucosal cancers (OHKURA et al. 1994). The presence of multiple foci is also characteristic of mucosal carcinoma (YAMAKI et al. 1994).

12.2.2.3
Gross Features of Mucosal Carcinoma

Elevated lesions (types 0-I and 0-IIa) are characterized by granularity or by a reticular pattern on their surface. Depressed Lesions (type 0-IIc) present gross finding of two types: (a) coalescent grooves (MARUYAMA 1992) or (b) irregular surface depression. A lesion consisting of coalescent grooves is very characteristic of mucosal carcinoma, and is not encountered in submucosal disease. Some lesions display transition from one type to the other; this is observed most prominently on Lugol-sprayed surgical and EMR specimens after fixation.

12.2.2.4
Location

The midthoracic esophagus is the most frequent site of superficial carcinoma, accounting for 64.4% of cases. The lower intrathoracic esophagus is the second most frequent site, accounting for 20.5% of cases, and the upper intrathoracic esophagus is the third most frequent (6.8% of cases) (NAKAGAWA and WATANABE 1994).

12.2.3
Diagnostic Imaging

In classic barium radiology, an effort is made to detect EEC on the initial radiographic examination while making reference to the abnormalities observed with endoscopy. and a detailed radiographic study is also performed following endoscopy. Initial radiographic examination using the double-contrast method has progressed so far as to enable the detection of m2 and m3 cancer, although recognition of the former is still rather difficult (NAGANO et al. 1995).

Endoscopic ultrasonography (EUS) is commonly used for assessment of the invasive depth of esophageal carcinoma, but it does tend to be used in different ways in different parts of the world: While in Western countries it is typically used for the assessment of T2 and T3 tumors and periesophageal lymph nodes, in Japan it is mainly employed to distinguish m1 and m2 from m3 cancer, and thus establish whether EMR is indicated.

It has been reported that EUS can make the differential diagnosis between m1 or 2 cancer and m3 cancer in 95% of cases (KONO et al. 1995). However, difficulty remains in the differentiation of minimal invasion from lymphatic proliferation, and the overall accuracy in the assessment of the invasive depth of SEC (m1–3 and sm1–3) was reported to be 79% by KONO et al.

12.2.3.1
Initial Radiographic Study

In the standard procedure for upper gastrointestinal

series, imaging is performed in the right anterior oblique and left anterior oblique projections. In each case two divided exposures are used, usually focusing on the upper esophagus in the first frame and on the lower esophagus in the second frame.

Double-contrast studies are the only tool for the detection of mucosal carcinoma. It is important for the patient to swallow as much air as possible together with a mouthful of contrast medium. Presence of air in the esophagus may be ensured by use of a tube with holes.

YAMAKI and co-workers (1994) reported that eight (80%) of the m1–2 carcinomas of the polypoid type (0-IIa) could be detected on the initial radiographic examination, whereas this was true for only two of six m3 cancers of the depressed type. NAGANO and co-workers (1995) reported on two mucosal carcinomas detected during mass screening for gastric cancer: one was observed at fluoroscopy and the other was picked up in the film reading. They also reported that three out of seven cases of submucosal cancer were detected by mass screening.

On the basis of their own experience, MAKUUCHI and associates (1995) emphasized the superiority of endoscopy over radiographic examination for the detection of mucosal carcinoma: indeed, they found that radiographic examination could detect only 4.7% (5/107) of mucosal carcinomas. It may be generally true that where there is a skilled endoscopist there is no skilled radiologist and vice versa!

In cases of mucosal carcinoma it is rare for an entire lesion to be visualized on the initial radiographic images. Usually only a part of the lesion is depicted as an abnormality of the esophageal mucosa in a frontal image, and slight marginal stiffness or rigidity may be present. The extent to which double-contrast images approximate to the gross characteristics of each type of mucosal carcinoma depends on the image quality.

An elevated lesion (0-IIa) is visualized as small coalescent nodules or a small area of granularity with a surface pattern of small plaque-like mucosal elevations (MARUYAMA 1992). A depressed lesion is visualized as a small faint pool of barium in a depression (Figs. 12.2a, 12.3) or one or two linear grooves. A lesion consisting of coalescent grooves is often delineated as a small depression (MARUYAMA 1992).

It is rare for wall stiffness or irregularity to be recognized in cases of m1 cancer; in m2 cancers, too, such stiffness or irregularity is either not observed or very faint (Fig. 12.3a) whereas in m3 cancers it is quite clearly seen. Visualization of these minimal wall abnormalities depends on the presence of a slight to moderate degree of lumen distension.

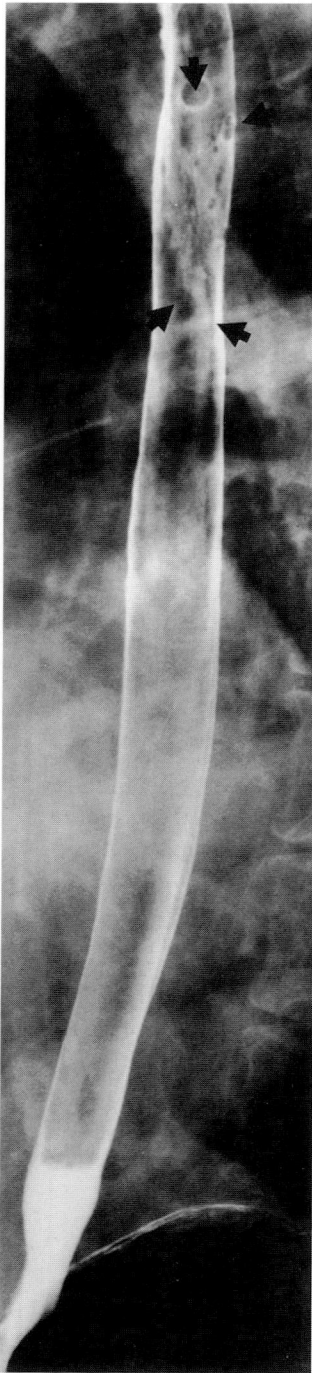

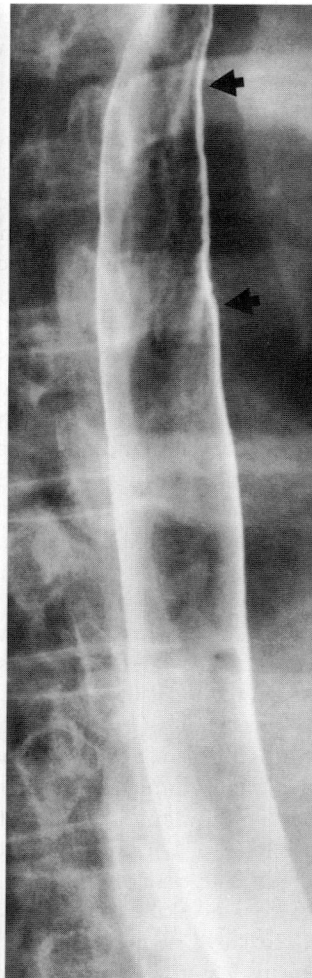

a,b

a,b

Fig. 12.3 a,b. Early carcinoma (type 0-IIa + IIc + IIb) of the middle intrathoracic esophagus with an invasive depth of m2 and measuring 90 × 50 mm. This case was detected on the initial radiographic examination (**a**). The lesion consists of a IIa part visualized as fine granularity and a IIc + IIb part faintly recognized as some pools of contrast medium extending to the distal side. The IIa part was noted on the initial study. In the detailed study the thickly coated margin corresponds quite closely to the extent of the entire lesion

Fig. 12.2 a,b. Early carcinoma (type 0-IIc) of the upper intrathoracic esophagus with an invasive depth of m3 and measuring 28 × 26 mm. This case (42-year-old female) was detected on the initial radiographic examination (*arrows*, **a**). The initial radiographic image seems of better quality than the detailed one (**b**)

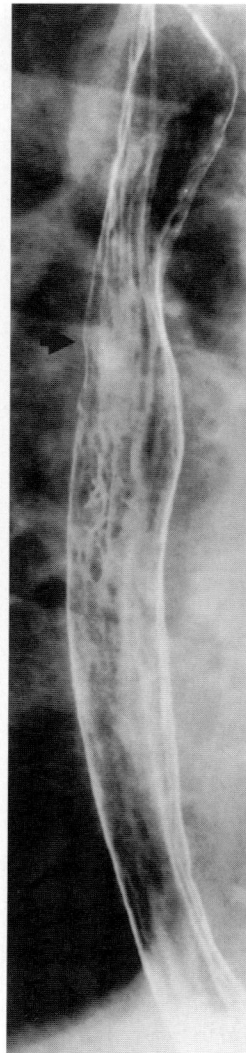

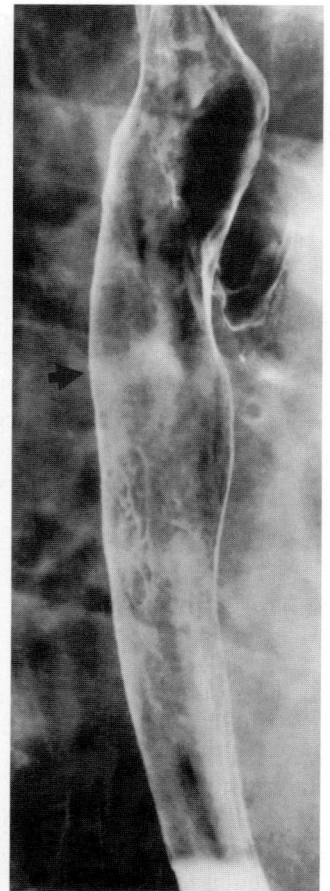

12.2.3.2
Detailed Radiographic Study

12.2.3.2.1

TECHNIQUE

Various devices have been proposed in order to obtain optimal lumen distension and barium coating of the esophageal mucosa. Effervescent granules are suitable when double-contrast images of the hy-

Fig. 12.4 a–d. Superficial carcinoma (type 0-IIc) of the lower intrathoracic esophagus with an invasive depth of m2 and measuring 15 × 13 mm. This case was detected with endoscopy and endoscopically resected. **a** The detailed radiographic study with slight lumen distension revealed a part of this IIc lesion and right wall stiffness (*arrows*). The fold defining the lesion is thickened. In **b** the lesion is visualized as a localized thickening of the mucosal fold with slightly less lumen distension than in **a** (*arrows*). **c** With moderate lumen distension the lesion is recognized as a faint pool of contrast medium (*arrows*). **d** An EUS image obtained with a 20-MHz probe reveals thickening of the second layer and thinning of the third layer, indicating the m2 level of cancerous invasion

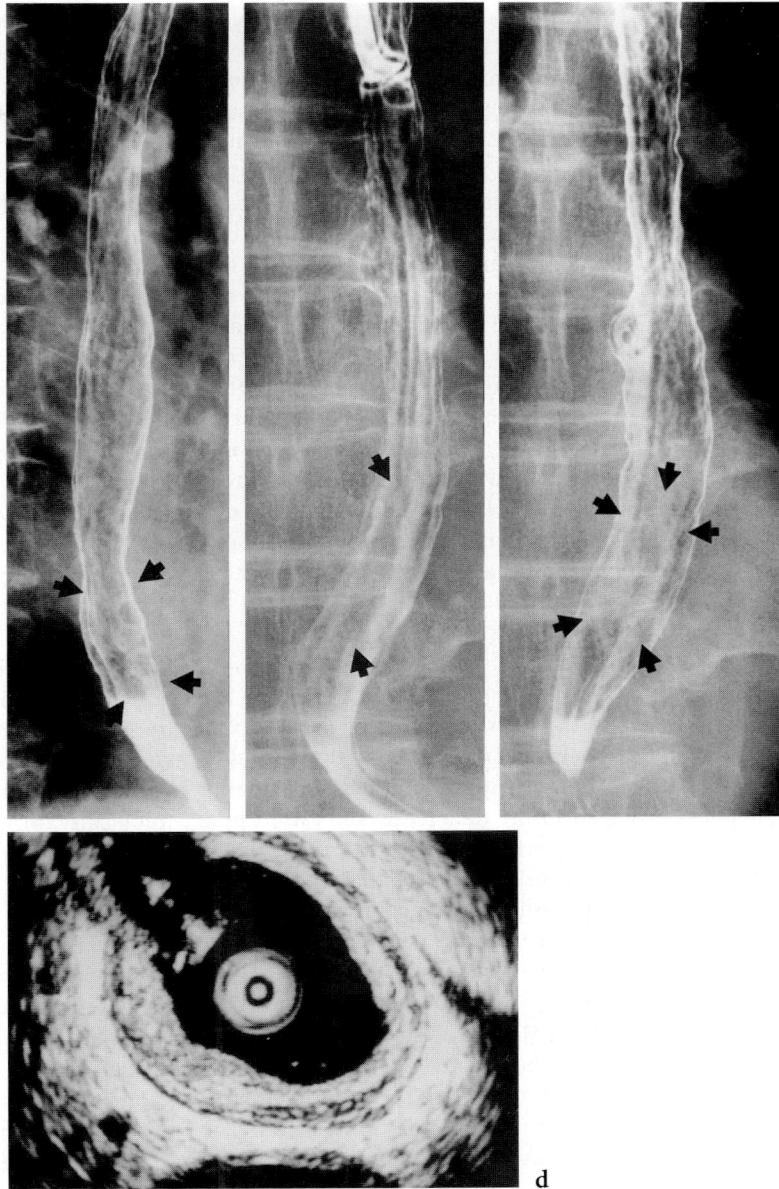

a–c

d

popharynx and cervical esophagus are to be obtained. The patient is asked to swallow a large volume of the barium, and filming is done immediately after the barium passes into this region.

A nasal or oral tube is preferred for acquisition of double-contrast images of a lesion located in the midthoracic esophagus. Between 30 and 50 ml of the barium is injected through the tube with the patient supine or prone, depending upon the location of the lesion. The fluoroscopic table is then tilted upright, and halted just before the barium passes the lesion. Air is injected with a syringe after confirming that a thin layer of barium is covering the lesion. In most cases optimal barium coating is achieved with a moderate degree of lumen distension (YAMAKI et al. 1994; SHIRAKABE et al. 1987), which is also best for the assessment of wall abnormalities. Nevertheless, the detailed study often results in unsatisfactory visualization (Fig. 12.4). In Fig. 12.4a a depressed lesion is faintly recognized in one phase of double-contrast radiography. It is visualized as thickening of a mucosal fold in another phase (Fig. 12.4b) and is nearly effaced with moderate lumen distension (Fig. 12.4c).

12.2.3.2.2

AIM

Repeat radiographic examinations may seem redundant to Western radiologists. However, there is a necessity for detailed examination to be performed prior to surgery or EMR. There is no doubt that the initial or screening radiographic examination can be improved by the information provided by the detailed radiographic examination. We consider the latter to be indispensable for assessment of the invasive depth of mucosal carcinoma, and especially for the distinction of m1 and m2 cancer from m3 cancer. The presence of m1 or m2 cancer is highly likely if a wall abnormality is not recognized or is very faint (MARUYAMA 1992). The deepest invasion front usually involves only a very small portion of the lesion which EUS often fails to detect. The detailed radiographic study is also useful for excluding the presence of multiple cancers which may be missed with endoscopy.

12.2.3.2.3

LIMITATIONS

Radiographically the gross features of m2 and m3 cancer can be delineated fairly well under favourable circumstances, though without the degree of completeness achieved in the detailed examination of a gastric cancer. Most m1 cancers are not recognized. Shadows from the ribs and chest interfere with the clear visualization of the esophageal mucosa.

As mentioned above, lesions consisting of coalescent grooves are often visualized as a surface depression even in the detailed radiographic study (SHIRAKABE et al. 1987). In addition, a depressed lesion (0-IIc) cannot be defined as sharply as a depressed early gastric cancer (Fig. 12.4). In the majority of cases this may be ascribed not only to the fact that a depression of the mucosal carcinoma of the esophagus is a wide erosion with blending edges but also to the erosion being much less deep than that of an early depressed carcinoma of the stomach (ARAKI et al. 1986).

12.2.4
Summary

In the initial radiographic study m1 and m2 cancers of the polypoid type are fairly easily detected. However, the detection of m1 cancer of the depressed type is nearly impossible, and the detection of m2 and m3 cancers of this type, though not impossible, is very difficult. The detailed radiographic study permits the visualization of m1 cancer of the depressed type, though often not with adequate clarity; the depiction of m2 and m3 cancers is frequently satisfactory.

12.3
MALT Lymphoma of the Stomach

12.3.1
General Considerations

The concept of mucosa-associated lymphoid tissue (MALT) was proposed by ISAACSON and WRIGHT in 1983, and malignant lymphoma developing from MALT has come to be called MALT lymphoma. In the last 10 years MALT lymphoma has been accepted as a type of extranodular B cell lymphoma of low-grade malignancy that shows different clinicopathologic features from ordinary lymphomas. Recently, the definition of MALT lymphoma has been expanded to include lesions of high-grade malignancy (CHAN and ISAACSON 1990).

The gross features of MALT lymphoma as defined by Isaacson are characterized by a superficial mucosal depression accompanied by nodularity and granularity that simulates IIc type early cancer. Histologically, MALT lymphoma displays densely proliferated centrocyte-like cells and lymphoepithelial lesions.

In Japan the concept of reactive lymphoreticular hyperplasia (RLH) of the stomach (NAKAMURA et al. 1966) was in the past commonly used for a lesion which consisted of non-neoplastic proliferation of lymphoid tissue. Recent progress in immunohistochemical and molecular biological analysis has shown that most cases of RLH are MALT lymphomas of low-grade malignancy. However, on the basis of detailed histological and immunohistochemical study, TAKANO and co-workers (1992) have reported that RHL can be divided into benign lymphoid hyperplasia (BLH) and atypical lymphoid hyperplasia (ALH). They have emphasized that BLH is an inflammatory change which mainly consists of secondary proliferation of the lymphoid apparatus associated with peptic ulcer, and that ALH should tentatively be regarded as a borderline lesion despite the fact that monoclonality of the B cells is seen in approximately 20% of cases.

There have been many reports dealing with the disappearance and regression of MALT lymphoma with the eradication of Helicobacter pylori (HP) (WOTHERSPOON et al. 1993; STOLTE and EIDT 1993). However, a lesion which disappears with eradication of HP in response to antibiotics cannot be considered a malignancy (SUEKANE et al. 1996). Although the monoclonality may be proved in biopsy specimens by the polymerase chain reaction (PCR) method, it does not represent substantial evidence of MALT lymphoma. Monoclonality may be seen in cases of reactive hyperplasia of lymph nodes because of the high sensitivity of the PCR method (WOTHERSPOON et al. 1993; HUSSELL et al. 1993). It should also be noted that there have been many reports on the spontaneous disappearance of malignant lymphoma of the stomach (TAKEUCHI et al. 1971; NAKANO et al. 1972; MATSUMOTO et al. 1993).

12.3.2
Gross Features

In our institution MALT lymphoma of low-grade malignancy accounted for 38.4% (5/13) of malignant lymphomas of the superficial spreading type and for 6.3% of all malignant lymphomas (5/79) which were surgically resected between 1961 and 1993. Their size ranged from 60 mm to 190 mm in maximum diameter, the mean being 98 mm. The invasive depth was limited to the mucosal membrane in one lesion, and reached the submucosal layer in four lesions. In other words, all MALT lymphomas were grossly classified as being of the superficial spreading type. On the other hand, the majority of tumor-forming types were histologically diagnosed as malignant lymphoma of high-grade malignancy. It should also be noted that the incidence of MALT lymphoma varies between institutions, depending on the diagnostic criteria employed (HISHIMA et al. 1996).

The mucosal depression of MALT lymphoma is not circumscribed as sharply as type IIc early cancer. It is vaguely demarcated by the presence of granules of various sizes which characterizes the surface of the mucosal depression in most cases. The granularity sometimes shows a cobblestone appearance when densely distributed. Ulceration is an associated finding in 60% of cases of MALT lymphomal (BABA et al. 1996). Small erosions and ulcers are seen scattered among the granules.

12.3.3
Radiographic Findings

Double-contrast images delineate best the gross findings of MALT lymphoma. Basically, MALT lymphoma shows an ill-defined mucosal depression that consists of granules of varioussizes (Figs. 12.5, 12.6).

Consequently, the overall impression is dissimilar to that of a type IIc early cancer, where the mucosal depression is usually well defined. The mucosal depression of type IIc early cancer is generally well circumscribed from the normal surrounding mucosa, and the surface granularity is not seen as dense as with MALT lymphoma even in cases of poorly differentiated carcinoma. In MALT lymphoma, slight mucosal convergence is visualized when ulceration is present. The lesion of MALT lymphoma is usually pliable as the lumen distension increases.

When the granularity is densely distributed in the depression it has a cobblestone appearance and produces irregular reticular shadows (Fig. 12.6). When the granularity in the depression is sparse, small irregular barium pools become prominent (Figs. 12.5b, 12.7). An earlobe-shaped mucosal elevation is also characteristic of MALT lymphoma (Fig. 12.7), and is often observed in the superficial type of malignant lymphoma.

12.3.4
Differential Diagnosis

Radiographically, the differential diagnosis of MALT lymphoma is difficult as its gross features are similar to those of high-grade malignant lymphomas of the superficial spreading type and certain other mimicking lesions (borderline lesions, ALH, BLH).

BABA and associates (1996) reported that the granules of various sizes were visualized both in MALT lymphoma and in the lesions that simulate it. They were densely distributed in all MALT lymphomas, in 57% of cases of ALH, and in 50% of high-grade malignant lymphomas of the superficial spreading type. The irregular reticular shadow was seen in many MALT lymphomas and borderline lesions while it was sparse in malignant lymphoma of the superficial spreading type, ALH, and BLH. Small irregular barium pools were observed in all MALT lymphomas and borderline lesions, in 71% of cases of ALH, in 63% of malignant lymphomas of the superficial spreading type, and in 50% of cases of BHL. BABA and associates concluded that the differences in the histologic findings in MALT lymphoma and simulating lesions did not reflect the differences in the radiographic findings.

Endoscopic ultrasonography does not allow the differential diagnosis between MALT lymphoma and simulating lesions, but it does reveal the depth of invasion beyond the submucosal layer (SUEKANE et al. 1996).

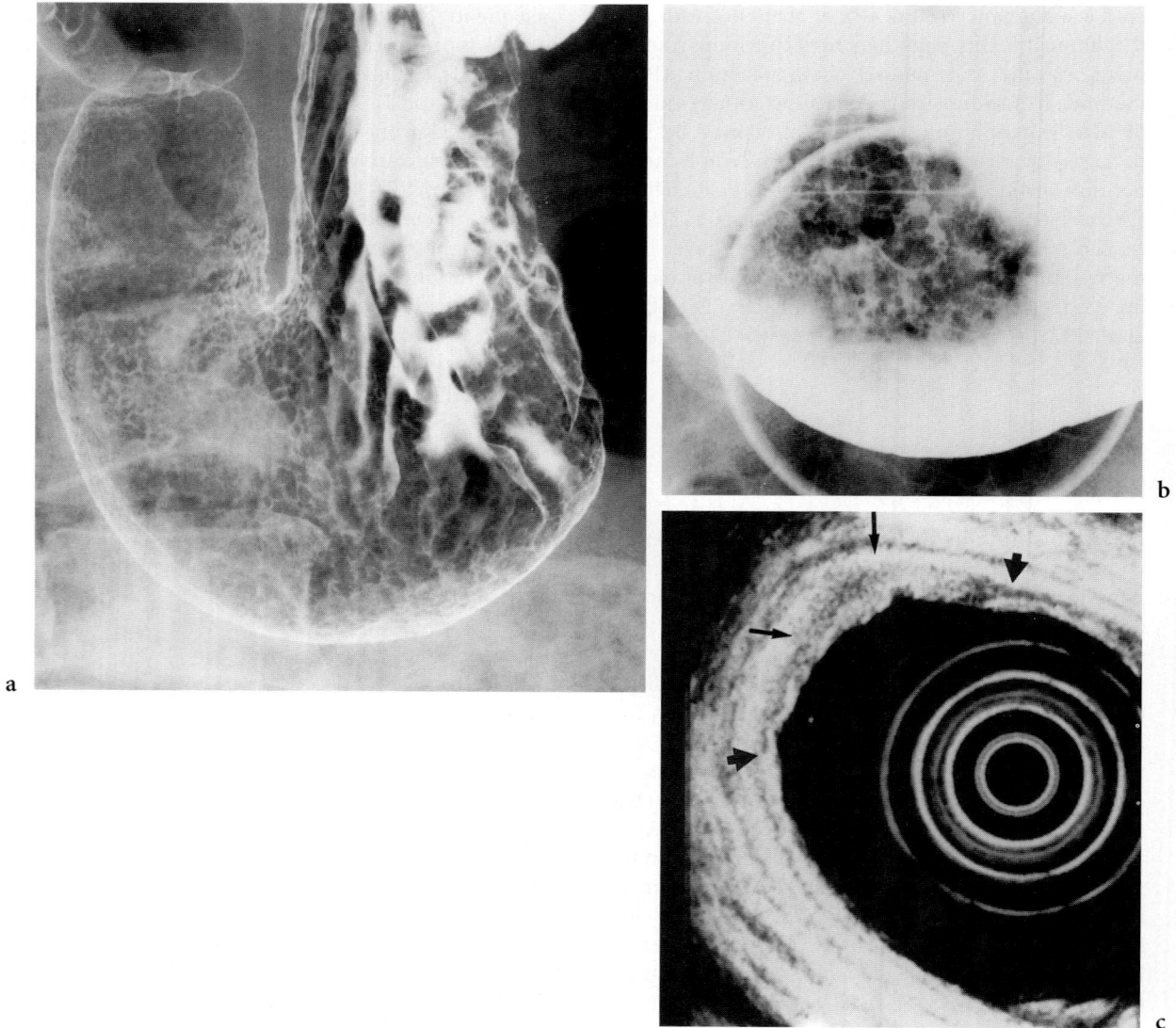

Fig. 12.5 a–c. MALT lymphoma in the incisura region with an invasive depth of sm and measuring 98 × 58 mm. **a** A lesion consisting of granules of various sizes is seen in the posterior wall but is not sharply defined. **b** A compression image delineates the granularity and irregular pools of contrast medium showing mucosal depressions. **c** On EUS, thickening of the second layer (*large arrows*) and thinning of the third layer (*small arrows*) indicate submucosal involvement by MALT lymphoma

12.3.5
Summary

In the radiographic diagnosis, MALT lymphoma and simulating lesions, including the borderline lesions, ALH, and BLH, should be treated as low-grade malignant lymphoma. The granules of various sizes, irregular reticular shadows, and small irregular barium pools are regarded as the characteristic radiographic findings.

12.4
Small Depressed Neoplasms of the Large Bowel

12.4.1
General Considerations

It has long been believed that depressed neoplasms (adenomas and carcinomas) are never encountered in the colon and rectum. Recently, however, a con-

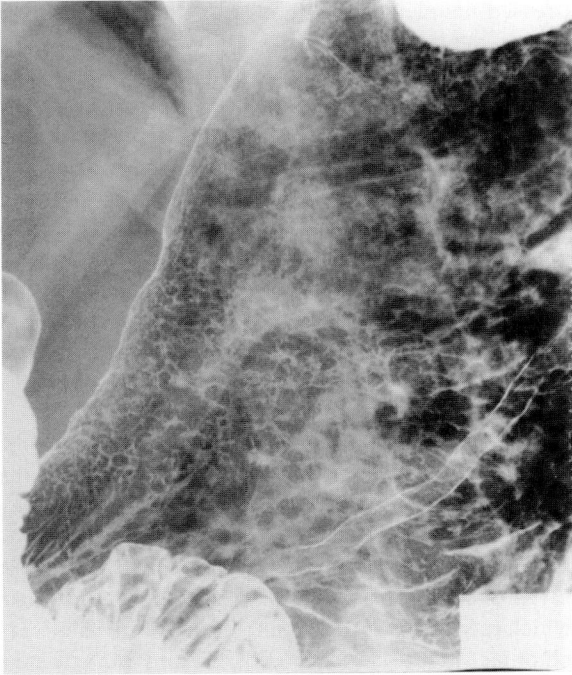

a

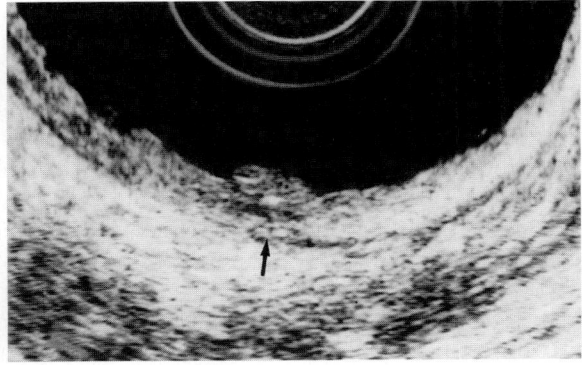

b

Fig. 12.6 a,b. MALT lymphoma in the posterior wall of the middle and lower gastric body with an invasive depth of sm and measuring 73 × 47 mm. The lesion consists of granules of various sizes and reticular shadows. The granularity shows a cobblestone appearance in the posterior wall of the greater curvature (**a**), and wall stiffness is noted. **b** EUS image showing thinning of the third layer, indicating submucosal involvement (*arrow*)

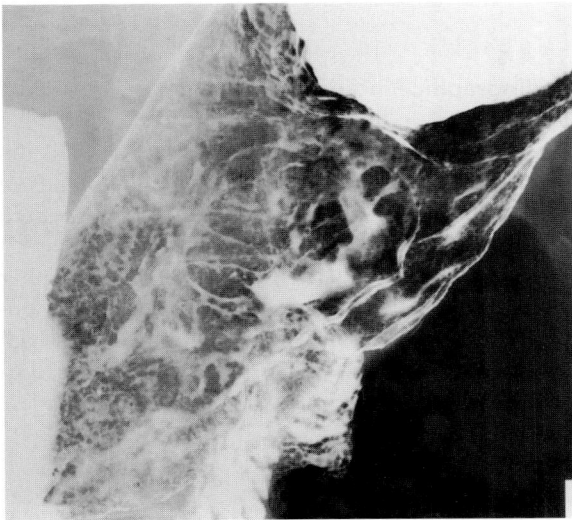

a

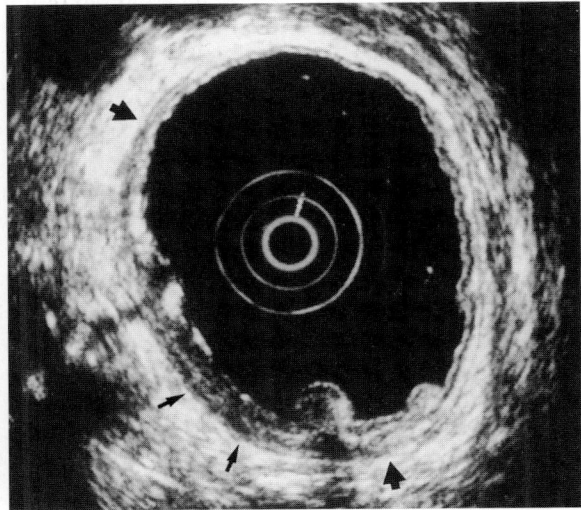

b

Fig. 12.7 a,b. MALT lymphoma in the posterior wall of the gastric body with an invasive depth of se (the serosa is involved) and measuring 80 × 65 mm. The lesion consists primarily of irregular mucosal depression and elevation simulating an earlobe. **b** On EUS the second layer is thickened and the third layer is extensively interrupted (*large arrows*). In addition, the outer line of the fifth layer is irregular and obscured by thickening of the fourth layer (*small arrows*). These findings indicate that the invasion reaches the subserosa

siderable number of flat and depressed colorectal neoplasms have been reported in Japan (KUDO 1993). The majority of them have been detected with colonoscopy, and have been smaller than 5 mm in maximum diameter. Histologically, such neoplasms are either adenomas or carcinomas, and show a high grade of dysplasia (in spite of their small size) when compared to ordinary adenomas (NAKAMURA 1994; WOLBER and OWEN 1991). Submucosal invasion is reported to be present in approximately 25% of the carcinomas even when their size is 5 mm or less (KUDO 1993).

In this section we consider not only depressed neoplasms (adenoma and carcinoma) measuring 5 mm and less but also those measuring 6–10 mm in maximum diameter because the destiny of those neoplasms measuring 5 mm or less can inevitably be discussed in terms of the morphogenesis of adenoma and carcinoma.

Early submucosal invasion is characteristic of this type of carcinoma (KUDO 1993), and may lead to rapid-growing carcinoma which may arise de novo (NAKAMURA 1994). In addition, it has been reported that expression of the K-ras codon 12-point mutation is less frequently observed in flat and depressed adenomas than in polypoid adenomas (YAMAGATA et al. 1994).

Radiographically, the visualization of depressed lesions has been nearly impossible until recently, when control of lumen distension in double-contrast radiography was found to be the key which enables the delineation of such a subtle mucosal alteration (FUJIYA and MARUYAMA 1997).

12.4.2
Definition

A small depressed neoplasm of the colon and rectum may be defined as an adenoma or carcinoma measuring 10 mm or less in maximum diameter in which there is a central depression on a flat mucosal elevation (type IIa + IIc), or a nearly pure depression (type IIc), or a depression surrounded by slightly raised mucosa (IIc + IIa) (Japanese Research Society for Cancer of the Colon and Rectum 1994).

It has been postulated that morphologically, lesions of type IIc and IIc + IIa are essentially different from lesions of type IIa + IIc (Kudo et al. 1995). On radiographs, however, lesions with a prominent depression cannot be distinguished from those with a less prominent depression, and in this section de-

pressed neoplasms are defined as flat lesions with a central depression regardless of its type.

Depressed neoplasms are commonly referred to as flat adenomas or flat neoplasms regardless of the presence or absence of the central depression. Depressed adenomas and carcinomas are included in the series of flat neoplasms described by WOLBER and OWEN (1991) although they did not mention in detail the presence of the depression.

12.4.3
Incidence

Depressed neoplasms account for a very low percentage of the total number of colorectal neoplasms detected. In Kudo's series (KUDO et al. 1995) they accounted for 2.7% (105/3824) of all colorectal neoplasms which were 5 mm or less, including eight invasive carcinomas, and for 1.5% (22/1475) of those which measured 6–10 mm, including 11 invasive carcinomas. In the series of FUJIYA and MARUYAMA (1997) they accounted for 5.7% (54/951) of lesions measuring 5 mm or less, and 1.3% (12/930) of those measuring 6–10 mm. In the latter series there were two invasive carcinomas measuring 5 mm or less and four invasive carcinomas measuring 6–10 mm. In our institution depressed neoplasms have accounted for 0.2% (13/4367) of all neoplasms measuring 5 mm or less, and 0.9% (17/1840) of those measuring 6–10 mm.

12.4.4
Radiographic Findings

There is no doubt that the detection of small depressed neoplasms of the large bowel by means of radiographic examination is not easy. In the Western literature there are very few reports of radiographic visualization (MATSUMOTO et al. 1993). On the other hand, radiographic images of small depressed neoplasms often appear in Japanese literature, although most such neoplasms have been visualized radiographically in the presence of colonoscopic images.

12.4.4.1
Contour and Central Depression

When radiography was performed prior to colonoscopy, FUJIYA and MARUYAMA (1997) found that

a

b

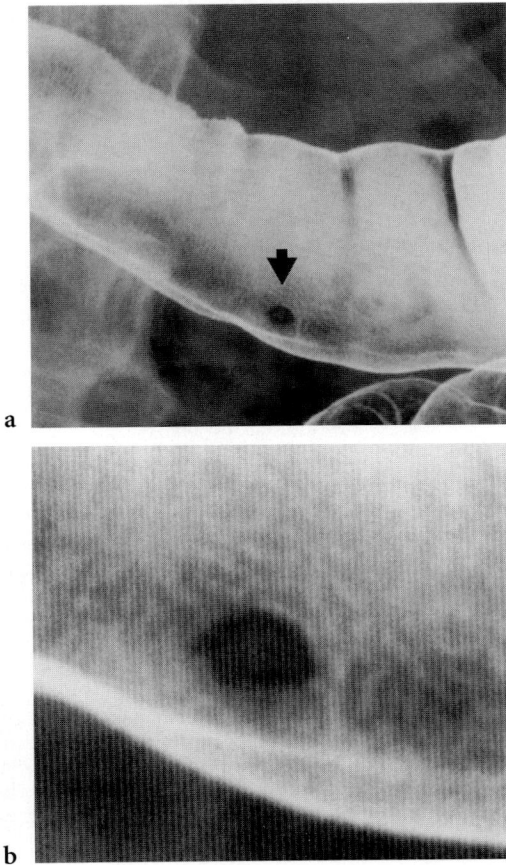

Fig. 12.8. a Depressed adenoma (flat adenoma with central depression, type IIa + IIc; *arrow*) measuring 4 mm in the transverse colon. **b** Enlarged (×3) image of **a**

Fig. 12.9. Depressed adenoma (type IIc + IIa) measuring 9 mm in the descending colon

the contour of 61.2% (23/37) of depressed neoplasms measuring 5 mm or less was visualized (Fig. 12.8), while the figure was 80% for those measuring 6–10 mm (Fig. 12.9). There is no other report on the radiographic delineation of small depressed neoplasms when the radiographic examination has been initially carried out in the absence of information from colonoscopy.

The results reported by FUJIYA and MARUYAMA (1997) are expected to be a landmark, helping to dispel any pessimism regarding the radiographic visualization of such neoplasms (cf. HAMILTON 1993). They also reported that the contour of all lesions measuring 5 mm or less could be visualized with the radiographic examination which followed colonoscopy when the lesions whose contour was only faintly visualized on radiographic examination were included. Their results suggest that it is much less difficult to delineate a small depressed lesion if

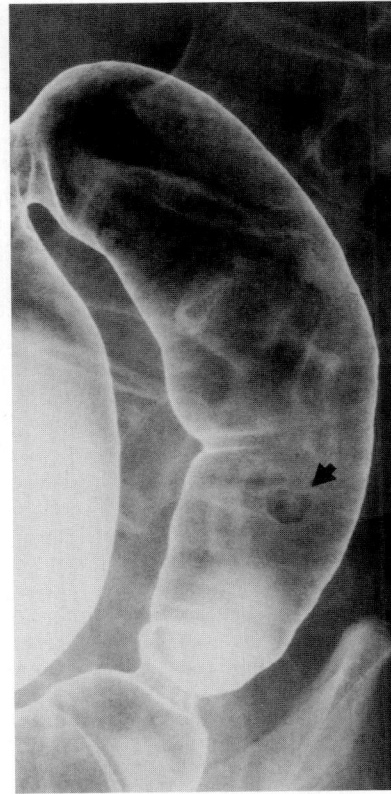

one is already aware of its presence, and that controlling the lumen distension may be the key to visualization of not only the contour but also the central depression (Figs. 12.8, 12.9).

In contrast, MATSUMOTO and co-workers (1995) reported that only 11 of 21 adenomas measuring 5 mm or less which were initially detected with colonoscopy were detected with radiographic examination, and that the central barium fleck (= central depression) was seen in seven of the 11 lesions detected radiographically.

The central depression is not delineated in most lesions whose contour is not visualized (FUJIYA and MARUYAMA 1997). Radiographically, however, we have not been able to distinguish between IIc or IIc + IIa lesions and IIa + IIc lesions (see Sect. 12.3.2 for definitions). MATSUMOTO and co-workers (1995), dealing with the same kind of morphology, classified their series into flat-topped elevations with either shallow or deep depression. In their classification the former are comparable to type IIa + IIc lesions, and the latter to type IIc or IIc + IIa lesions.

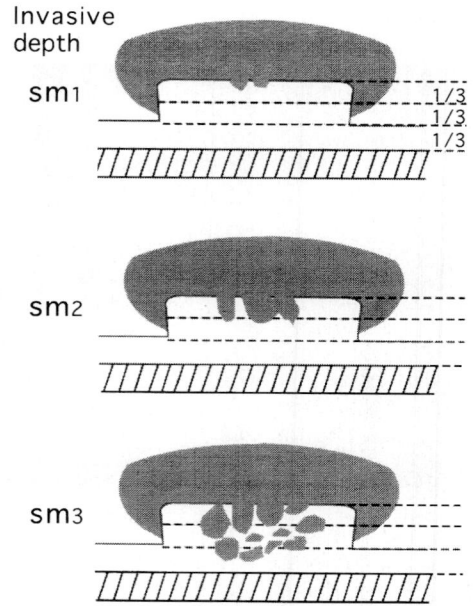

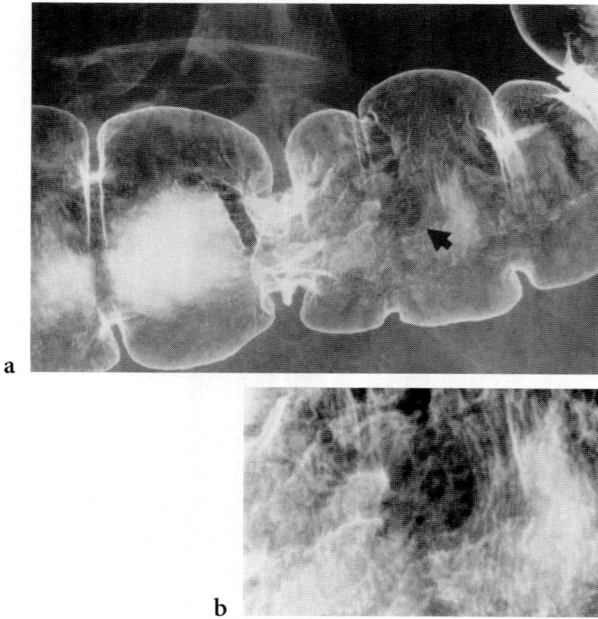

Fig. 12.10. a Minimally invasive carcinoma of the depressed type (type IIc), measuring 8 mm in the transverse colon (*arrow*). b Enlarged image (×2) of a. In this case only one cancerous gland invaded the submucosa (minimal invasion with positive p 53 staining)

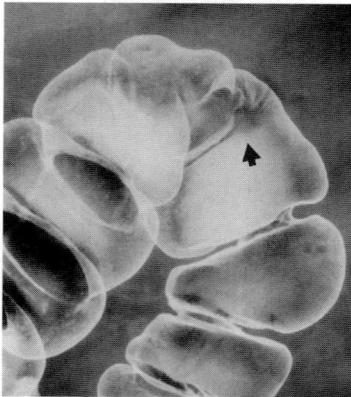

Fig. 12.11. Schematic representation of depth of submucosal invasion by colorectal cancer

Fig. 12.12 a,b. Depressed invasive carcinoma (sm2) of the left flexure, measuring 9 mm. A faint barium pool with mucosal fold convergence is noted in a (*arrow*), and the in-drawn sign in b (*arrow*) is suggestive of submucosal invasion. c The lesion is seen to be depressed on the resected specimen (*arrows*)

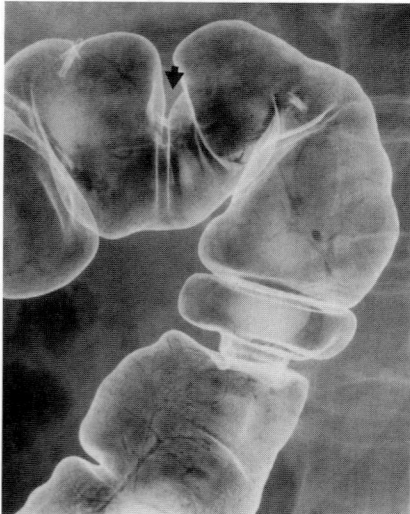

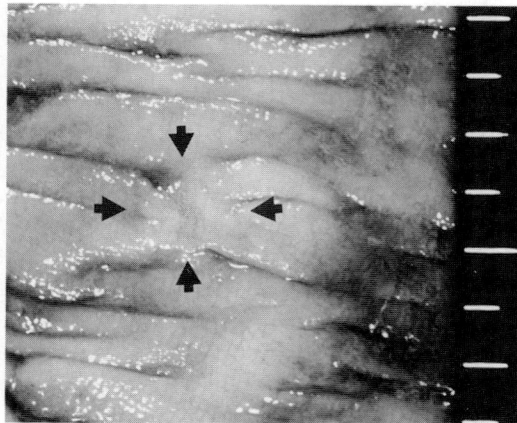

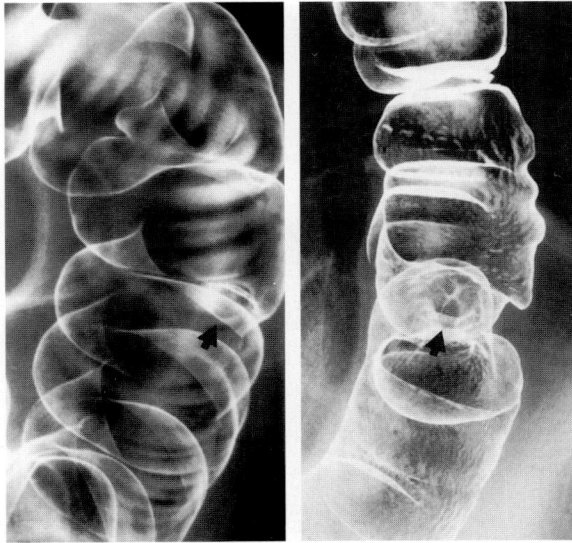

Fig. 12.13 a,b. Rapidly growing carcinoma. **a** There is a flat elevation measuring 9 mm in the descending colon (*arrow*). The presence of central depression may be suspected. This lesion was missed. **b** Within 1 year and 4 months the lesion had developed into a cancer with irregular depression (*arrow*), measuring approximately 17 mm (localized ulcerating type). Histologic examination after surgery disclosed the lesion to be an advanced carcinoma involving the subserosa. (From KOIZUMI et al. 1993)

12.4.4.2
Control of Lumen Distension

The macroscopic appearance of flat and depressed neoplasms on colonoscopy varies according to the degree of lumen distension. The more distended the lumen, the flatter a lesion becomes. Accordingly, a depression basically looks more shallow as the lumen is more distended. In our experience small depressed lesions may be classified into two groups: those with an obvious depression and those with a faint depression.

In this classification a lesion with a faint central depression does not always represent a type IIa + IIc lesion. A radiographic image of the depressed lesion depends on lumen distension, which by chance may have produced a faint depression. In our experience control of lumen distension seems the most important factor enabling the visualization of small depressed lesions (Fig. 12.10). The presence of the central depression does not necessarily indicate malignancy, especially when lesions measure 5 mm or less: it is much more frequently an indicator of malignancy when the depression measures 6–10 mm (cf. Fig. 12.12) (MARUYAMA 1992). The presence of an

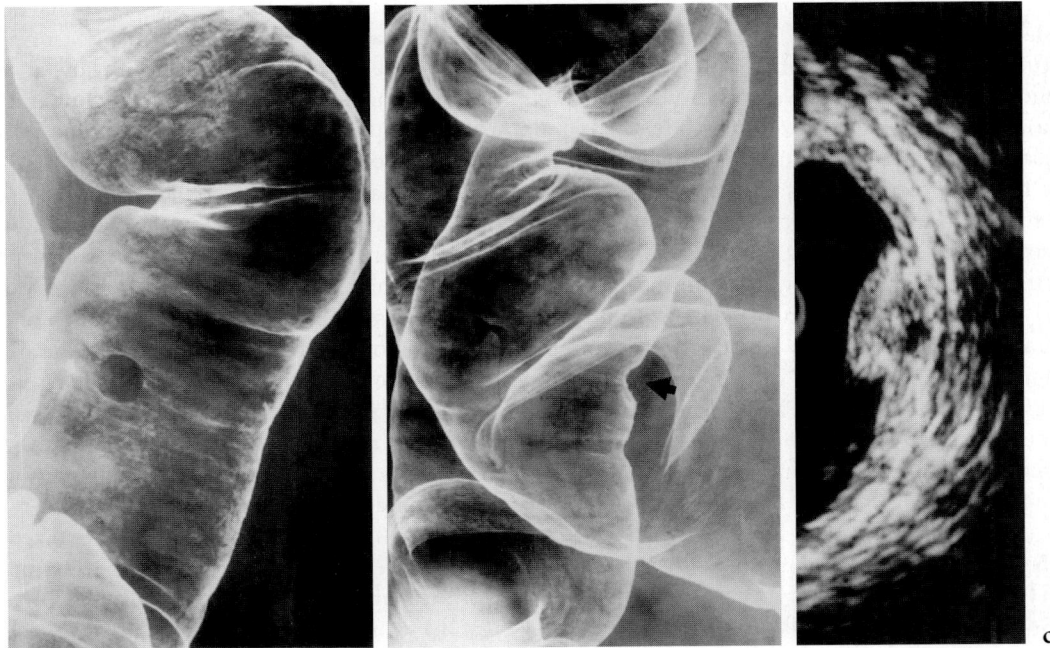

Fig. 12.14 a–c. Invasive carcinoma (sm2) of the elevated type in the descending colon, measuring 9 mm. No depression is noted on a frontal view (**a**). A profile image (**b**) reveals a definite in-drawn sign suggesting submucosal invasion (*arrow*). **c** EUS image showing thickening and interruption of the third layer. Cyst formation is also noted in the third layer. Histologically submucosal invasion was proved above the cyst formation, which was noncancerous.

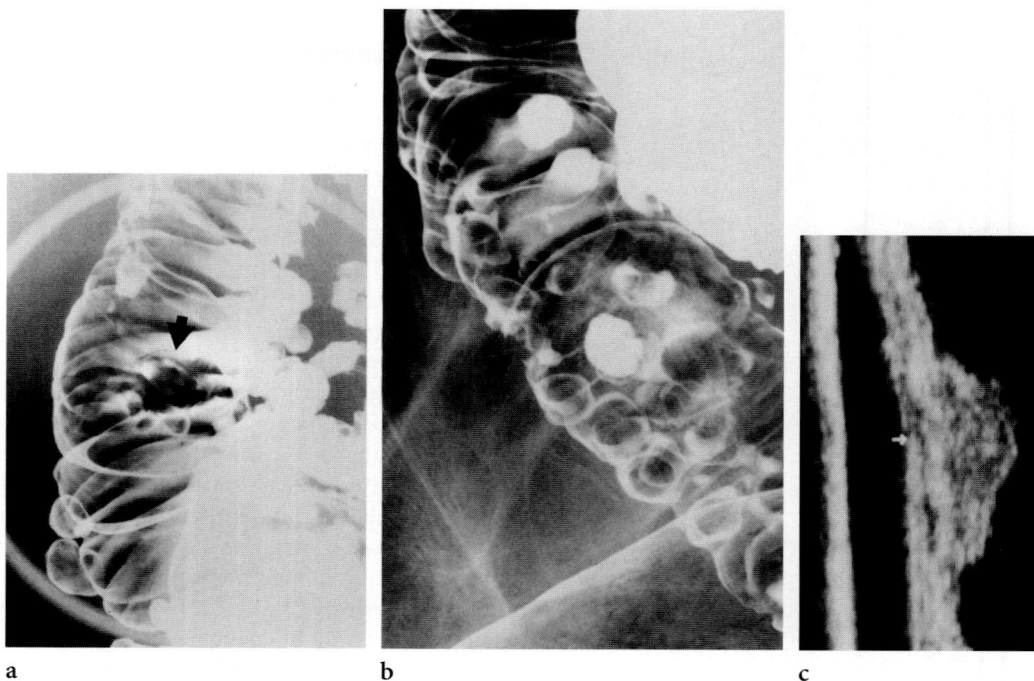

a   b   c

Fig. 12.15 a–c. Invasive carcinoma (sm2) of the elevated type in the ascending colon, measuring 10 mm. Some folds are retracted (*arrow*, **a**), and a definite in-drawn sign is noted (**b**). **c** A sonogram of the specimen reveals irregular thinning of the third layer (*arrow*) which corresponds to submucosal invasion (sm2).

"in-drawn" sign is also an indicator of malignancy when a lesion is delineated on a complete or nearly complete profile image (Figs. 12.12b, 12.14b, 12.15b) (MARUYAMA 1992). Sometimes mucosal fold convergence is seen in an invasive carcinoma (Fig. 12.12a), and it may even be present in adenomas and mucosal carcinomas, though it is slight in these lesions. Invasive carcinoma is usually classified into three subgroups (sm1, 2, 3) according to the grade of invasion (Fig. 12.11). KODAIRA et al. (1994) reported that lymph node metastasis was found in only 3.2% of sm1 cancers but in 11% and 12% of sm2 and sm3 cancers, respectively. Usually sm1 cancers cannot be distinguished from mucosal cancers and adenomas with EUS or radiography. This subclassification is considered useful for defining the indication for endoscopic mucosal resection.

12.4.5
Small Invasive Carcinoma
and Rapidly Growing Carcinoma

There is no doubt that a considerable number of small invasive and advanced carcinomas have recently been encountered in Japan. They are consid-

ered to have developed from depressed neoplasms (Case presentation 1993). However, this does not mean that all depressed neoplasms measuring 5 mm or less develop into invasive and advanced carcinomas, leaving aside the question of whether a cancer arises through the "adenoma-carcinoma sequence" or "de novo."

SASAKI and associates (1993) reported a case of invasive carcinoma which had been followed for about 5 years. In this case the initial radiographic and colonoscopic images revealed a depressed lesion (IIc + IIa) measuring 5 mm, and the initial colonoscopic biopsy showed adenoma with moderate atypia. Within about 5 years the lesion developed into a carcinoma with extensive submucosal invasion (IIc + IIa) and measuring 7 mm in maximum diameter. This case is an example of how a small invasive carcinoma can develop from a depressed lesion.

KOIZUMI and co-workers (1993) reported a case of advanced carcinoma invading the subserosa and measuring 16 mm in maximum diameter (Fig. 12.13b) which was considered to have developed from a flat lesion of 9 mm in size which had been demonstrated on a radiograph obtained 1 year and 4 months previously (Fig. 12.13a). In this case, however, the presence of the central depression was suggested on the original image by virtue of a faint barium pool (Fig. 12.13a). This case illustrates the possibility of a rapidly growing carcinoma (BURNETT and GREENBAUM 1981).

12.4.6
Clinical Significance

In Western countries there is a general consensus that small flat adenomas are of little clinical importance, although this was disputed by JARAMILLO and co-workers (1995) on the basis of their experience of colonoscopy in patients with flat colorectal neoplasms at Karolinska Hospital, Sweden.

BOND (1995) emphasized that the small flat adenoma (= small depressed neoplasm) represents an early stage of typical adenoma development.

The data reported in Japan to some extent support the statement of BOND (1995). In our institution depressed neoplasms measuring 6–10mm were much less frequently detected than such neoplasms measuring 5mm or less in spite of a general tendency for larger lesions (Figs. 12.9, 12.10) to be more easily detectable than small ones (Fig. 12.8). Similarly, in Kudo's series (KUDO 1993) there were 105 depressed neoplasms measuring 5mm or less but only 22 measuring 6–10mm.

Theoretically, in both Kudo's series and our own, there should have been many more depressed lesions larger than 6mm if depressed lesions measuring 5mm or less enlarge while retaining the same morphology. One therefore needs to consider the possibility that a depressed neoplasm may be transformed into a flat elevation without a central depression during the course of its development. Indeed, colonoscopically we have observed a number of small depressed neoplasms that have changed into flat mucosal elevations. Moreover, in our experience invasive carcinomas smaller than 10mm in maximum diameter do not always take the form of a depressed lesion (Figs. 12.14, 12.15); histologically there was no definite evidence that such cases had developed from a depressed lesion.

12.4.7
Summary

Small depressed neoplasms are clinically significant because there is a risk of rapidly growing carcinoma with early invasion although the possibility that most small depressed neoplasms are merely a precursor of ordinary adenoma cannot be excluded.

References

Araki K, Yamazaki S, Kumonn M (1986) A histological study on the typical Type IIb early gastric carcinoma (in Japanese). I-to-Cho 21:389–394

Baba Y, Kaku S, Sakata H, et al. (1994) Roentgenologic diagnosis of intramucosal carcinoma of the esophagus (in Japanese). I-to-Cho 29:301–317

Baba Y, Morita S, Masumoto H, et al. (1996) Image diagnosis of gastric malignant lymphoma and its mimicking lesions – focused on the low-grade malignant lymphoma (MALT lymphoma) (in Japanese). I-to-Cho 31:41–58

Bond JH (1995) Small flat adenomas appear to have little clinical importance in Western countries. Gastrointest Endosc 42:184–186

Burnett K, Greenbaum EI (1981) Rapidly growing carcinoma of the colon. Dis Colon Rectum 24:282–286

Case presentation (1993) Advanced colorectal carcinoma less than 10mm (in Japanese). I-to-Cho 28:1224–1245

Chan JC, Isaacson PG (1990) Relationship between high-grade lymphoma and low-grade B-cell mucosa-associated lymphoid tissue lymphoma (MALToma) of the stomach. Am J Pathol 136:1153–1164

Fujiya M, Maruyama M (1997) Small depressed neoplasm of the large bowel; its radiographic visualization and clinical significance. Abdominal Imaging 22:325–331

Hamilton SR (1993) flat adenomas: what you can't see can hurt you. Radiology 187:309–310

Hishima T, Koike M, Hayashi Y, et al. (1996) Histologic diagnosis of primary gastric lymphoma of mucosa-associated lymphoid tissue type through endoscopic biopsy specimen (in Japanese). I-to-Cho 31:33–40

Hussell T, Isaacson PG, Crabtree JE, et al. (1993) The response of cells from low grade B-cell gastric lymphoma of mucosa-associated lymphoid tissue type after eradication of Helicobacter pylori. Lancet 342:571–574

Isaacson PG, Wright DH (1983) Malignant lymphoma of mucosa-associated lymphoid tissue. Cancer 52:1410–1416

Japanese Research Society for Cancer of the Colon and Rectum (1994) General rules for clinical and pathological studies on cancer of the colon, rectum and anus, 5th edn. Kanehara-Shuppan, Tokyo

Japanese Society for Esophageal Diseases (1992) Guidelines for the clinical and pathologic studies on carcinoma of the esophagus, 8th edn (in Japanese). Kanehara-Shuppan, Tokyo

Jaramillo E, Watanabe M, Slezak P, et al. (1995) Flat neoplastic lesions of the colon and rectum detected by high-resolution video colonoscopy and chromoscopy. Gastrointest Endosc 42:114–122

Kaku S, Baba Y, Takemoto N, et al. (1995) Radiological diagnosis of the extensive superficial type esophageal cancer (in Japanese). I-to-Cho 30:985–999

Kodaira S, Yao T, Nakamura K, et al. (1994) Lymph node and distant metastases of 1806 cases of sm-cancer based on its subclassification (in Japanese). I-to-Cho 29:1137–1142

Koizumi K, Sakatani S, Kai S, et al. (1993) Surveillance of colorectal remnant after surgery for carcinoma (in Japanese). I-to-Cho 28:541–551

Kono T, Ohsima M, Endo M (1995) Diagnosis of early esophageal carcinoma with endoscopic ultrasound (in Japanese). I-to-Cho 30:365–373

Kudo S (1993) Endoscopic mucosal resection of flat and depressed types of early colorectal cancer. Endoscopy 25:455–461

Kudo S, Tamura S, Nakajima T, et al. (1995) Depressed type of colorectal cancer. Endoscopy 27:54–57

Makuuchi H, Mitomi T, Tajima T, et al. (1994) Endoscopic diagnosis of esophageal mucosal carcinoma (in Japanese). I-to-Cho 29:319–326

Makuuchi H, Ohmori Y, Yokoyama K, et al. (1995) Screening for early esophageal carcinoma with endoscopy (in Japanese). I-to-Cho 30:283–294

Maruyama M (1992) Early diagnosis of gastrointestinal cancer. In: Laufer I, Levin MS (eds) Double contrast gastrointestinal radiology, 2nd edn. Saunders, Philadelphia, P 496–532

Matsumoto T, Iida M, Kohrogi N, et al. (1993) Minute nonpolypoid adenomas of the colon depicted with barium enema examination. Radiology 87:377–380

Matsumoto T, Iida M, Kuwano Y, et al. (1995) Small nonpolypoid neoplastic lesions of the colon: endoscopic features with emphasis on their progression. Gastrointest Endosc 41:135–140

Monma K, Yoshida M, Yamada Y, et al. (1994) Endoscopic estimation of depth of invasion in cases with esophageal mucosal cancer (in Japanese). I-to-Cho 29:327–340

Nagano M, Mochizuki F, Chonan A, et al. (1995) Screening for early esophageal carcinoma with the initial radiographic examination (in Japanese). I-to-Cho 30:271–282

Nakagawa S, Watanabe H (1994) Mucosal carcinomas of the esophagus – their subclassification of depth of invasion, histologic risk factors and macroscopic features (in Japanese). I-to-Cho 29:273–288

Nakamura K (1994) Carcinoma de novo and diagnostic criteria of colorectal carcinoma (in Japanese). I-to-Cho 29 (Suppl):151–159

Nakamura K, Aoki M, Sugano H, et al. (1966) Reactive lymphoreticular hyperplasia of the stomach – report of 6 surgical cases (in Japanese). Ganno-Rinsho 12:691–696

Nakano H, Nakazawa S, Ito J, et al. (1972) A case of reticulum cell sarcoma of the stomach (in Japanese). I-to-Cho 7:375–382

Ohashi Y, Kumakura K, Sugiyama N, et al. (1973) Early reticulum cell sarcoma of the stomach; report of a case showing remarkable changes within a short time (in Japanese). I-to-Cho 8:195–203

Ohkura Y, Nishizawa M, Hosoi T (1994) Esophageal mucosal carcinoma: classification and the depth of invasion from the pathological point of view (in Japanese). I-to-Cho 29:263–271

Sasaki S, Maenou K, Fujiya M, et al. (1993) A five year follow up case of Type IIa + IIc colonic cancer (in Japanese). I-to-Cho 28:215–223

Shirakabe H, Yamaki G, Maruyama M (1987) A new proposal of macroscopic classification of superficial esophageal carcinoma (in Japanese). I-to-Cho 22:1349–1368

Shirakabe H, Yamaki H, Fukuchi S, et al. (1990) Some problems on macroscopic classification of early esophageal cancer from the standpoint of clinical diagnosis and treatment (in Japanese). I-to-Cho 25:1087–1103

Stolte M, Eidt S (1993) Healing gastric MALT lymphomas by eradicating H. pylori? Lancet 342:568

Suekane H, Iida M, Nakamura S, et al. (1996) Differential diagnosis between so-called reactive lymphoid hyperplasia (RLH) and mucosa-associated lymphoid tissue (MALT) lymphomas in the stomach – studies on radiographic, endoscopic, and endosonographic findings (in Japanese). I-to-Cho 31:59–72

Takano Y, Kato Y, Sugano H (1992) Histopathological and immunohistochemical study of atypical lymphoid hyperplasia and benign lymphoid hyperplasia of the stomach. Jpn J Cancer Res 83:288–293

Takeuchi T, Ito M, Murate H, et al. (1971) A case of early gastric reticulum-cell sarcoma; follow-up study with x-ray and gastroscope during the early stage (in Japanese). I-to-Cho 6:211–219

Wolber RA, Owen DA (1991) Flat adenomas of the colon. Hum Pathol 22:70–74

Wotherspoon AC, Doglioni C, Diss TC, et al. (1993) Regression of primary low-grade B-cell lymphoma of mucosa-associated lymphoid tissue type after eradication of Helicobacter pylori. Lancet 342:575–577

Yamagata S, Muto T, Uchida Y, et al. (1994) Lower incidence of K-ras codon 12 mutation in flat colorectal adenomas than in polypoid adenomas. Jpn J Cancer Res 85:147–151

Yamaki G, Unagami M, Tsurumaru M, et al. (1994) Newly proposed classification of esophageal mucosal carcinoma and its roentgenologic diagnosis (in Japanese). I-to-Cho 29:289–300

13 Infections of the Alimentary Tract in AIDS

J. YEE and S.D. WALL

CONTENTS

13.1
Introduction

With continued growth of the HIV epidemic, it is becoming increasingly important that radiologists are aware of the gastrointestinal manifestations of this illness. Most patients with AIDS will exhibit gastrointestinal symptoms at some time during the course of their disease, and clinical AIDS is often determined by identifying an opportunistic infection or neoplasm of the gastrointestinal tract. Hence, radiology often plays a key role in helping to determine the diagnosis as well as in directing the management.

13.2
Candidiasis

Oral thrush is one of the earliest and most common infections among HIV-positive individuals. *Candida albicans* is the most frequent cause of esophageal infection in AIDS patients. Indeed, *Candida* esophagitis occurring in an HIV-positive patient defines clinical AIDS in that individual. Patients with AIDS and esophageal candidiasis typically present with dysphagia or even sometimes odynophagia. Chest pain can develop and it may be severe. Although endoscopic findings are characteristic if creamy, white plaques covering an erythematous mucosa are seen, therapy often is instituted based on clinical symptoms alone. This is especially true if typical findings are present on esophagram. Radiographic findings include mucosal plaques that cause small filling defects generally oriented along the long axis of the esophagus in the early stages of disease. Fold thickening and abnormal motility are notable as well. A typical "cobblestone" appearance develops with progression of the infection, and this represents edema of the submucosa and adjacent tissues (Fig. 13.1). Advanced cases demonstrate the classic "shaggy" esophageal contour that is due to the trapping of barium within the interstices of confluent plaques and pseudomembranes (Fig. 13.2) (LEVINE et al. 1985). Deep ulcers in addition to sloughed mucosa contribute to the irregular appearance (LEVINE et al. 1987). AIDS patients tend to present in the more advanced stages of infection than do nonimmunosuppressed patients. Systemic candidiasis is a potentially fatal complication. Hematogenous dissemination of the infection can lead to the development of microabscesses in the liver, spleen, and kidneys. Contrast-enhanced CT scan demonstrates multiple tiny (less than 5 mm) hypodense lesions in these organs.

J. YEE, MD, Assistant Professor of Radiology, University of California, San Francisco; Chief, Computed Tomography and Gastrointestinal Radiology, Department of Radiology, Veterans Affairs Medical Center, 4150 Clement Street, San Francisco, CA 94121, USA
S.D. WALL, MD, Professor of Radiology, University of California, San Francisco; Chief, Angiography and Interventional Radiology, Assistant Chief of Radiology, Department of Radiology, Veterans Affairs Medical Center, 4150 Clement Street, San Francisco, CA 94121, USA

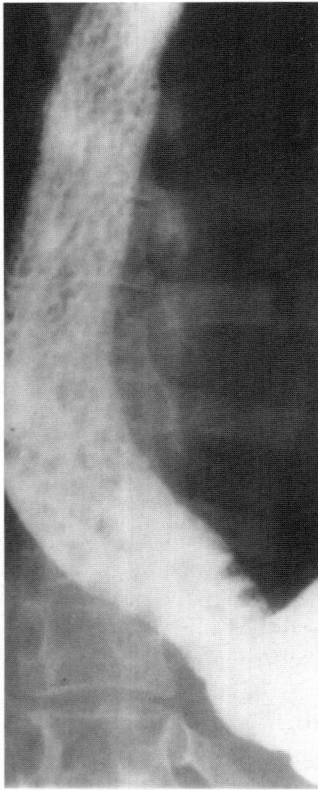

Fig. 13.1. Single-contrast esophagram demonstrating diffuse involvement of the esophagus with a cobblestone appearance representing edema of the submucosa and surrounding tissues due to *Candida* esophagitis

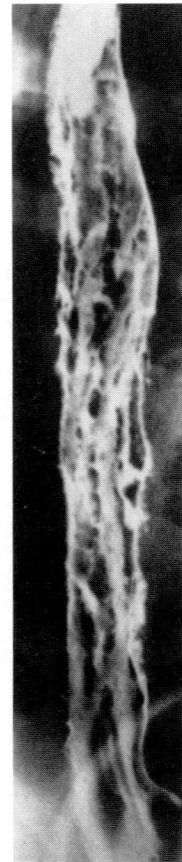

Fig. 13.2. Advanced *Candida* esophagitis with fold thickening, large filling defects, and an irregular "shaggy" esophageal contour

13.3
Herpes

Odynophagia is the most common presenting sympton in patients with herpes simplex virus (HSV) esophagitis. The causative organism can be either HSV 1 or HSV 2. Herpetic lesions in the mouth may provide a clue to the diagnosis although this does not exclude concomitant esophageal candidiasis. In the early stage of disease, endoscopy may reveal small vesicles although these are not always seen. Progression of disease leads to shallow ulcerations which then enlarge and coalesce. In the late stage of herpes esophagitis, diffuse ulcerations and an inflammatory exudate may produce an appearance that is indistinguishable from *Candida* esophagitis. The radiographic features of herpes esophagitis are best demonstrated on double-contrast esophagram, and these consist of mulitiple scattered superficial ulcers which are separated by normal appearing mucosa. Often these ulcers are diamond shaped, and a lucent

rim of edema is usually present (Fig. 13.3). Advanced cases of herpes esophagitis will demonstrate diffuse nodularity with cobblestoning and a markedly irregular esophageal contour that is identical to the findings of *Candida* esophagitis. When these findings are present on barium swallow, biopsy and histologic analysis are necessary for definitive diagnosis (LEVINE et al. 1987). The characteristic histologic findings include multinucleated giant cells and Cowdry type-A intranuclear inclusion bodies which typically are found along ulcer margins.

13.4
Cytomegalovirus

Cytomegalovirus (CMV) is the most common pathogen identified by culture in AIDS patients. Almost one-third of AIDS patients develop CMV infections of the gastrointestinal tract. CMV may cause disease

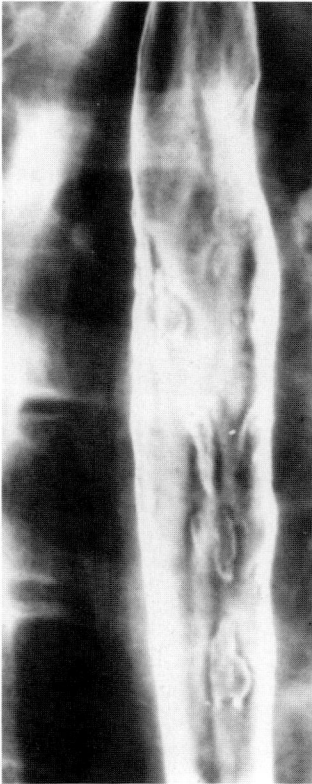

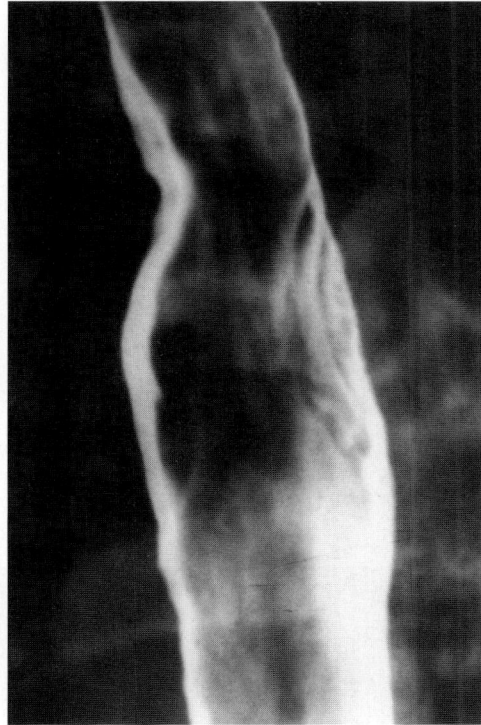

Fig. 13.4. A giant superficial esophageal ulceration is present against normal background esophageal mucosa. This is the typical appearance of cytomegalovirus esophagitis. However, radiographically this appearance is indistinguishable from the idiopathic ulceration of HIV infection, and biopsy with histopathologic examination is necessary for diagnosis

Fig. 13.3. Multiple discrete diamond-shaped ulcers are present with surrounding halos of edema. Note the normal appearance of the intervening background esophageal mucosa

in any segment of the luminal gastrointestinal tract (KOTLER 1991). However, the proximal colon and distal small bowel are more commonly infected than are the esophagus and stomach. Biopsy provides histologic diagnosis when the typical cytoplasmic and intranuclear inclusion bodies are found. Mucosal necrosis leading to ulceration is caused by a viral-induced vasculitis as evidenced by the presence of CMV inclusion bodies in the endothelial cells of blood vessel walls in areas of focal ulceration.

The typical radiographic appearance of CMV esophagitis is that of a discrete, giant (>2 cm) ulceration of the distal esophagus with a normal appearing surrounding mucosa (Fig. 13.4). This is very unlike the findings (noted above) in esophageal candidiasis (BALTHAZAR et al. 1987). This ulceration is evident on both endoscopy and barium esophagram, and a lucent halo of edema surrounding the ulcer is generally present. This appearance is similar to the large flat idiopathic esophageal ulceration which may be seen with early HIV infection

and seroconversion illness. The definitive diagnosis of CMV esophagitis is made by endoscopic biopsy and histopathologic examination. In patients with HIV disease, CMV ulcers of the distal esophagus have been found to extend into the esophagogastric junction, and they may cause fold thickening of the proximal stomach. However, CMV gastritis frequently involves the gastric antrum, and the appearance on barium examination is that of nodular wall thickening and circumferential antral narrowing with limited distensibility (BALTHAZAR et al. 1985b).

Colitis is the most commonly encountered site of gastrointestinal CMV infection. Radiographic features of CMV colitis include mucosal ulcerations that initially are shallow but become deeper (Fig. 13.5) (BALTHAZAR et al. 1985a). Giant ulcerations of the colon and terminal ileum due to CMV similar to the large CMV ulcerations seen in the esophagus have been reported (BALTHAZAR and MARTINO 1996). With progression of disease, edema and thickening of the colonic wall become evident. These findings can be observed on both barium examina-

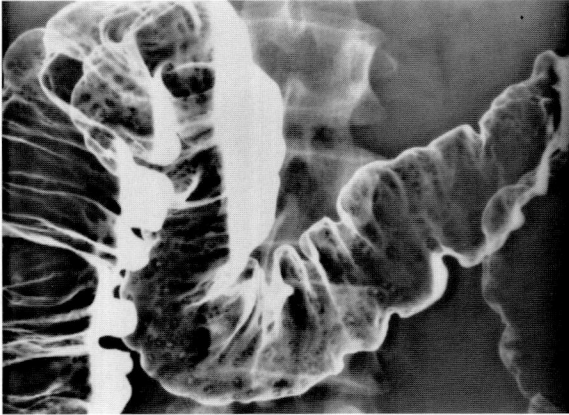

Fig. 13.5. Multiple small ulcerations due to cytomegalovirus are present throughout the colon. They are easily identified due to the surrounding lucent edematous rims

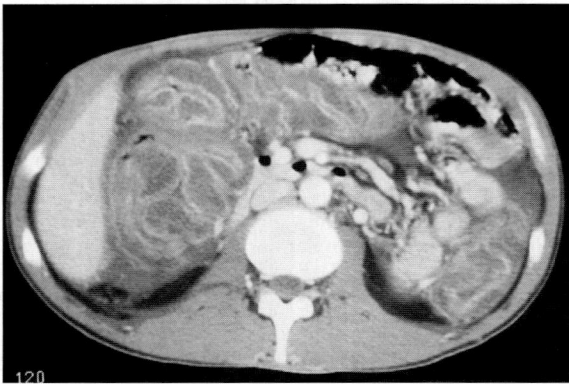

Fig. 13.7. Patient with CMV colitis demonstrating nodular high-density thickened wall of the ascending colon due to hemorrhage. The ascending colon is also dilated and fluid filled

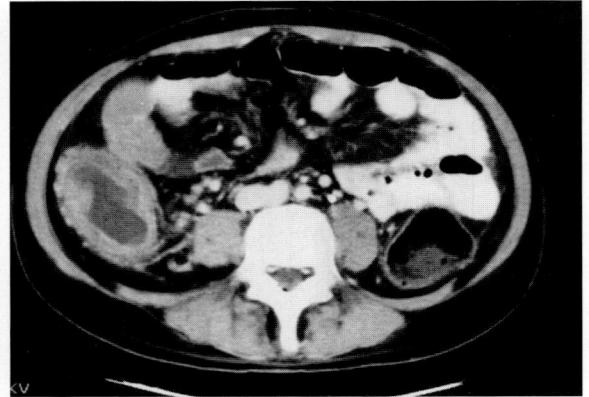

Fig. 13.6. Contrast-enhanced CT scan of a patient with cytomegalovirus colitis demonstrating marked low-density colonic wall thickening. There is enhancement of the mucosal and serosal bowel wall layers

tion and computed tomography. CMV colitis typically involves the cecum and ascending colon with involvement of the terminal ileum as well. The transverse colon is less commonly involved although a pancolitis may occur. Computed tomography (CT) with intravenous contrast demonstrates low-density edematous bowel wall with marked enhancement of the mucosal and serosal layers (Fig. 13.6). In advanced cases, hemorrhage into the bowel wall will cause areas of both increased and decreased nodular density (Fig. 13.7). Pneumatosis, toxic megacolon, and colonic perforation are findings associated with impending death. Lympadenopathy is usually not found in association with CMV colitis. CMV hepatitis has been reported in association with multiple

small hyperechoic liver lesions on ultrasound, and focal low-density liver lesions that are seen on CT. These have been noted histologically to represent focal areas of fatty infiltration.

13.5
Tuberculosis

Mycobacterium tuberculosis can involve the esophagus and the colon in patients with HIV disease. Esophageal tuberculosis in these patients is due to regional extension of infection from mediastinal lymph nodes (DE SILVA 1990). Barium radiography and CT demonstrate transmural inflammation of the esophagus with ulceration, and sinus tracts from the esophagus to the mediastinum may be demonstrated. Additionally, esophagoesophageal and esophagobronchial fistulas occur, as well as sinus tracts extending from the lumen of the esophagus to adjacent necrotic lymph nodes. Hence, esophageal tuberculosis generally is focal in the upper esophagus at the level of mediastinal adenopathy (Fig. 13.8).

Mycobacterium tuberculosis colitis generally is focal in the ileocecal area (BALTHAZAR et al. 1990). Radiographic findings include thickening of the ileocecal valve as well as the adjacent medial wall of the cecum. Frequently, the terminal ileum is also abnormal, with luminal narrowing and wall thickening. More extensive disease is demonstrated by diffuse, circumferential mural thickening of the cecum and the ascending colon. Regional

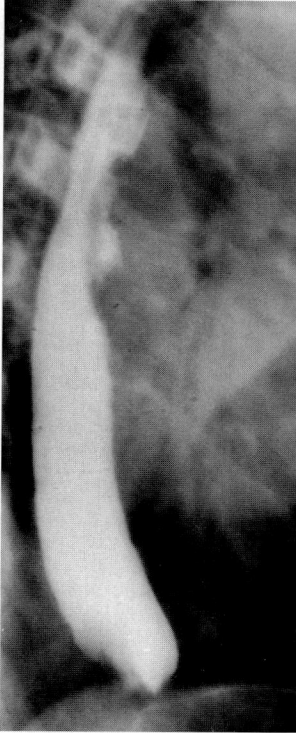

Fig. 13.8. A large penetrating ulcer is present in the proximal esophagus in this patient who had mediastinal adenopathy due to tuberculosis

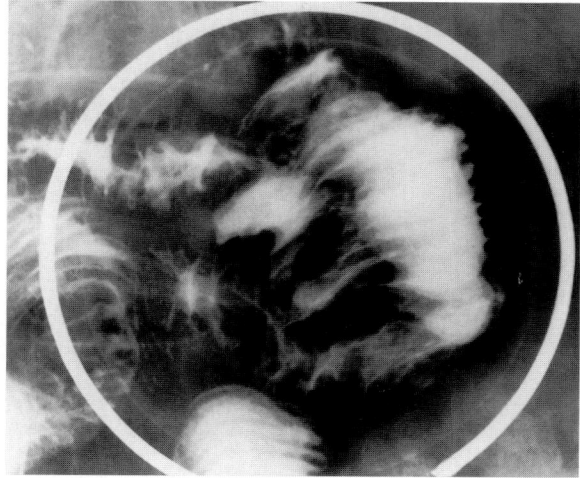

Fig. 13.9. Spot film from a small bowel study shows jejunal fold thickening which is irregular in appearance with areas of luminal narrowing due to MAI enteritis

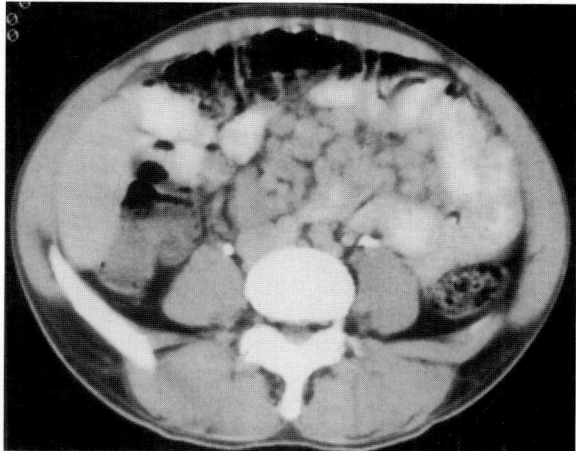

Fig. 13.10. CT scan of a patient with abundant mesenteric adenopathy due to MAI infection

lymphadenopathy is notable on computed tomography in most patients. The typical pattern of *Mycobacterium tuberculosis* colitis in patients with HIV disease is that of a cluster of low-density lumph nodes in the right lower quadrant adjacent to an abnormal terminal ileum and cecum (JEFFREY 1992).

13.6
Atypical *Mycobacterium*

Mycobacterium avium-intracellulare (MAI) infection of the gastrointestinal tract occurs most commonly in the small bowel. Clinical presentation of this enteritis is characterized by diarrhea, fever, and weight loss. Because the pathophysiology and radiographic findings of MAI enteritis are similar to those of Whipple's disease, it is often described as "pseudo-Whipple's disease" (MALIHA et al. 1991; VINCENT and ROBBINS 1985). Barium examination demonstrates mild small bowel dilatation as well as diffuse, irregular fold thickening (Fig. 13.9). The abnormal small bowel loops are often separated, and

this is well explained on CT by the presence of bulky mesenteric lymphadenopathy (Fig. 13.10). Additional large retroperitoneal adenopathy also occurs. Focal areas of central low attenuation may be present in the enlarged lymph nodes due to central necrosis (Fig. 13.11). Some researchers have found this pattern of low-density lymphadenopathy to be more common in tuberculosis than with MAI (RADIN 1991, 1995). Focal low-density microabscesses in the liver and/or spleen due to hematogenous dissemination of MAI are uncommon findings. Discrete low-density lesions in the liver or spleen are more commonly seen with disseminated tuberculosis.

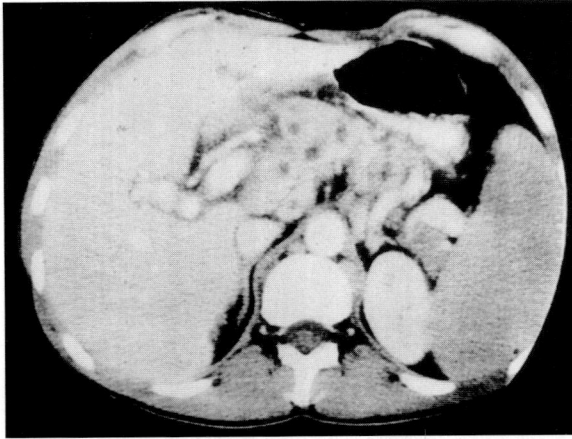

Fig. 13.11. Adenopathy due to MAI infection may have a typical appearance of enlarged lymph nodes with low-density centers

13.7
Cryptosporidiosis

Cryptosporidium is a small opportunistic protozoan that causes a severe chronic enteritis in patients with AIDS. This is manifested clinically by abdominal pain and voluminous watery diarrhea (GROSS et al. 1986). Dehydration and electrolyte abnormalities contribute to morbidity as well as mortality in these patients. Some patients are incapacitated with this secretory enteritis, passing as much as 7–10 l of fluid per day. Fecal-oral contamination and sexual contact are the most common routes of spread of *Cryptosporidium* in AIDS patients. Histologically, the mucosal damage is evident with partial villous atrophy, crypt hyperplasia, and cellular infiltrates (ANGUS 1990). The diagnosis of intestinal cryptosporidiosis is usually made by stool examination, although the organism can be identified on small bowel biopsy specimens. The most prominent radiographic finding on barium evaluation of the small bowel in patients with cryptosporidiosis is that of regular fold thickening of the duodenum and jejunum (Fig. 13.12) (BERK et al. 1984). However, the entire small bowel may be involved when disease has been longstanding. Mild small bowel dilatation and barium dilution due to hypersecretion often occur. *Isospora belli* is another protozoan that is often found histologically in association with *Cryptosporidium*, but generally does not cause disease in isolation. CT in patients with cryptosporidiosis demonstrates fluid-filled dilated segments of small bowel (Fig. 13.13).

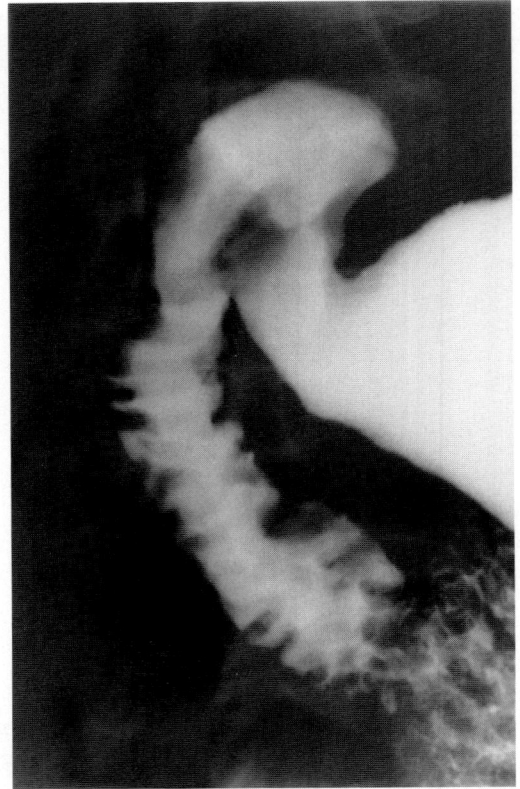

Fig. 13.12. Deformity of the postbulbar duodenum with fold thickening involving the second portion of the duodenum due to *Cryptosporidium* duodenitis

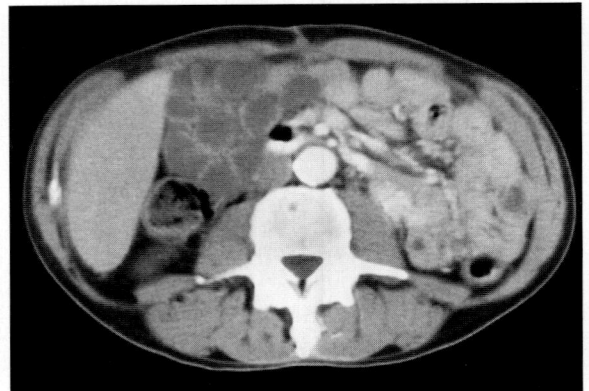

Fig. 13.13. CT scan in a patient with *Cryptosporidium* enteritis demonstrating several mildly dilated fluid-filled small bowel loops in the right abdomen

Lymphadenopathy is minimal or nonexistent, whereas it is typical (as described above) for MAI. Cryptosporidiosis is difficult to treat, showing only a mild response to octreotide, spiramycin, and other antibiotics (MEYERS et al. 1990).

13.8
Histoplasmosis

Fungal infection due to *Histoplasma capsulatum* is acquired via a respiratory route and is typically encountered in endemic areas such as eastern and central United States. Following inhalation of infectious spores, pneumonitis and adenopathy may develop. These typically resolve without significant sequelae. Person-to-person spread of histoplasmosis does not occur. Dissemination of disease occurs in children and in patients with compromised immune systems.

The gastrointestinal tract is involved in up to 75% of patients with the disseminated form of histoplasmosis (BALTHAZAR et al. 1993). Similar to CMV and tuberculosis, histoplasmosis tends to involve the cecum, ascending colon, and terminal ileum. Early barium findings consist of multiple mucosal ulcerations and edema. As the infection progresses, a large inflammatory mass may develop which can be difficult to distinguish from colon carcinoma. Colonic perforation has been reported as a complication of histoplasmosis. CT reveals the additional finding of associated abdominal adenopathy which may demonstrate central low density. Even with therapy, disseminated histoplasmosis infection has a poor prognosis and is associated with a high mortality.

13.9
Pneumocystis carinii

Pneumocystis carinii causes pneumonia in patients with AIDS, but sometimes dissemination results in abscesses of the abdominal organs and intestinal tract. Patients typically have a history of treatment with aerosolized pentamidine as prophylaxis to prevent the initial or recurrent episodes of *Pneumocystis carinii* pneumonia. This therapy is effective in treating the lungs, but aerosolized delivery of pentamidine results in an insufficient blood level to prevent dissemination (LUBAT et al. 1990). Hence, pneumonia may be prevented, but abscesses of other organs occur (SPOUGE et al. 1990).

Radiographically, focal areas of low attenuation are seen on contrast-enhanced CT scan (SACHS et al. 1991). Often these are associated with discrete, small foci of calcifications which are found histologically as well as radiographically (RADIN et al. 1990). Diagnosis may be made by percutaneous fine-needle aspiration with CT guidance (TOWERS et al. 1991). This is important as treatment with intravenous

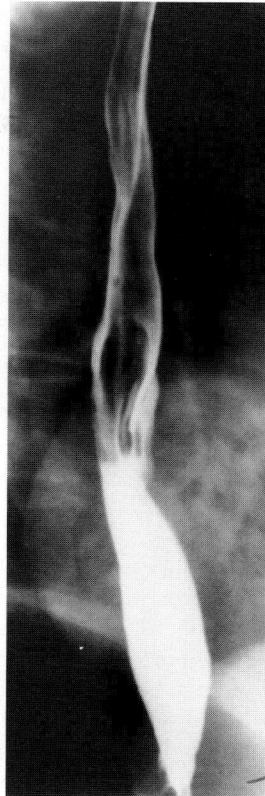

Fig. 13.14. Large shallow ulcer of the mid-esophagus due to HIV infection is seen in profile. Biopsy and histopathologic evaluation were negative for cytomegalovirus

pentamidine can be effective. Following successful eradication of the organism, the involved solid organ frequently becomes diffusely calcified.

13.10
HIV Infection

Gastrointestinal disease is common among individuals infected with HIV even prior to their progression to clinical AIDS. In fact, gastrointestinal signs and symptoms may be the first manifestation of HIV disease. This is common at the time of HIV seroconversion as many patients develop an acute infectious mononucleosis-like illness at that time. This is manifested clinically with gastrointestinal symptoms including nausea, vomiting, diarrhea, and odynophagia. The odynophagia is related to HIV ulceration of the esophagus (RABENECK et al. 1990). Endoscopy or barium swallow typically demonstrates a large (>2 cm) discrete, shallow ulceration of the distal esophagus against a normal background

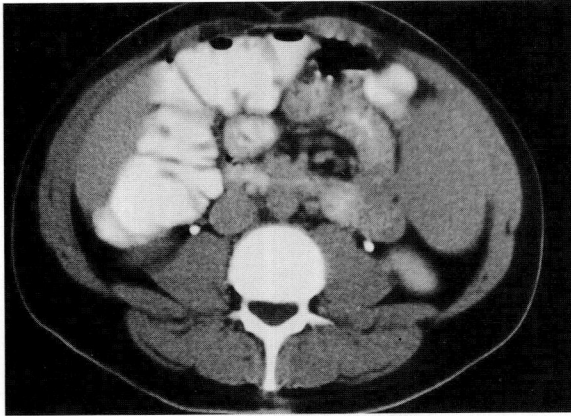

Fig. 13.15. CT scan in a patient with HIV-related enteritis demonstrating nonspecific mild small bowel wall thickening

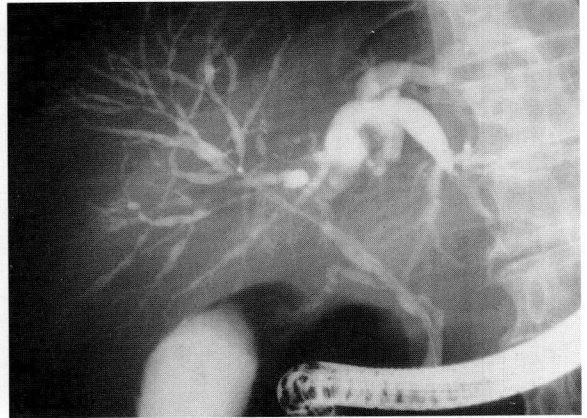

Fig. 13.16. Cholangiogram demonstrating multifocal intra-hepatic biliary ductal strictures causing a "beaded" appearance in a patient with AIDS cholangitis. The left intrahepatic bile ducts are more markedly dilated and a long stricture of the extrahepatic duct is present

mucosa (Fig. 13.14) (LEVINE et al. 1991). This appearance is like that seen with CMV ulceration of the esophagus in clinically ill AIDS patients. However, biopsy reveals no opportunistic organism, and the ulceration is thought to be caused by HIV itself (SOR et al. 1995). Signs and symptoms of HIV esophagitis are relieved with steroid treatment, although spontaneous resolution occurs as well. Furthermore, HIV has been isolated from the gut in patients with HIV disease who have not progressed to clinical AIDS. These patients often suffer from unremitting diarrhea, and this is thought to be due to an HIV enteropathy as no opportunistic organism is detectable. CT scan findings of HIV enteropathy are nonspecific, usually demonstrating mild small bowel wall thickening (Fig. 13.15) (PANTALEO et al. 1993).

After resolution of the influenza-like syndrome associated with early HIV seroconversion, there is generally a long interval until clinical AIDS is diagnosed. Indeed, the mean time between seroconversion to the diagnosis of clinical AIDS has lengthened to more than 10 years. It is during this interval that many patients suffer from a wasting-like syndrome that is often associated with diarrhea and HIV enteropathy. HIV has been isolated from the small bowel in many of these patients. Histologically focal crypt epithelial necrosis is thought to be related to HIV infection directly.

13.11
AIDS Cholangitis

Hepatobiliary disease can occur in patients with AIDS. Most often this is due to an acalculous inflam-

mation caused by opportunistic infection with *Cryptosporidium* or CMV (TEXIDOR et al. 1991). Both organisms are implicated by their presence in bile, gallbladder, and ductal mucosa as well as in the duodenal aspirates of symptomatic AIDS patients. *Microsporidia* infection has also been implicated as a cause of AIDS cholangitis (POL et al. 1993). Clinical presentation includes right upper quadrant pain, nausea, and vomiting. Liver enzyme abnormalities are present with a marked elevation of the alkaline phosphatase, but frequently normal serum bilirubin. The clinical and radiographic findings of AIDS-related cholangitis simulate those of primary sclerosing cholangitis (CAPPELL 1991). Cholangiography demonstrates alternating areas of stricture and focal dilatation involving the intra- and/or extrahepatic bile ducts (Fig. 13.16). Mural irregularities and intraluminal filling defects occur. Pruning with attenuation and decreased arborization of the intrahepatic bile ducts is frequently seen as well (FARMAN et al. 1994). It is notable that the radiographic feature that distinguishes AIDS-related cholangitis from that of primary sclerosing cholangitis is the presence of papillary stenosis in patients with AIDS (SCHNEIDERMAN et al. 1987). Indeed, some patients present with isolated papillary stenosis and only later develop intra- and extrahepatic bile duct irregularities as described above. Patients with papillary stenosis can be palliated with regard to signs and symptoms of AIDS cholangitis when sphincterotomy is performed via endoscopic retrograde cholangiopancreatography. Occasionally patients present with an isolated acalculus cholecystitis, and only later in the course of disease are associated biliary abnormalities noted.

13.12
Conclusion

HIV patients with gastrointestinal diseases often have multiple coexisting infections. Conventional infections often do not behave as they would in patients with intact immune systems. The clinical course of infections in HIV-positive individuals may show a slow response to treatment or may fail to respond entirely to therapy. Also clinical relapses of infections are common.

References

Angus KW (1990) Cryptosporidiosis and AIDS. Ballieres Clin Gastroenterol 4:425–441

Balthazar EJ, Martino JM (1996) Giant ulcers in the ileum and colon caused by cytomegalovirus in patients with AIDS. AJR 166:1275–1276

Balthazar EJ, Megibow AJ, Fazzini E (1985a) Cytomegalovirus colitis in AIDS: radiographic findings in 11 patients. Radiology 155:585–589

Balthazar EJ, Megibow AJ, Hulnick DH (1985b) Cytomegalovirus esophagitis and gastritis in AIDS. AJR 144:1201–1204

Balthazar EJ, Megibow AJ, Hulnick D, et al. (1987) Cytomegalovirus esophagitis in AIDS: radiographic features in 16 patients. AJR 149:919–923

Balthazar EJ, Gordon R, Hulnick D (1990) Ileocecal tuberculosis: CT and radiologic evaluation. AJR 154:499–503

Balthazar EJ, Megibow AJ, Barry M, Opulencia JF (1993) Histoplasmosis of the colon in patients with AIDS: imaging findings in four cases. AJR 161:585–587

Berk RN, Wall SD, McArdle CT, et al. (1984) Cryptosporidiosis of the stomach and small intestine in patients with AIDS. AJR 143:549–554

Cappell MS (1991) Hepatobiliary manifestations of acquired immunodeficiency syndrome, Am J Gastroenterol 86:1–15

de Silva R, Stoopack PM, Raufman JP (1990) Esophageal fistulas associated with mycobacterial infection in patients at risk for AIDS. Radiology 175:449–453

Farman J, Brunetti J, Baer JW, et al. (1994) AIDS-related cholangiopancreatographic changes. Abdom Imaging 19:417–422

Gross TL, Wheat J, Bartlett M, et al. (1986) AIDS and multiple system involvement with Cryptosporidium. Am J Gastroenterol 81:456–458

Jeffrey RB (1992) Abdominal imaging in the immune-compromised patient. Radiol Clin North Am 30:579–596

Kotler DP (1991) Gastrointestinal complications of the acquired immunodeficiency syndrome. In: Yamada T (ed) Textbook of gastroenterology. Lippincott, Philadelphia, pp 2086–2103

Levine MS, Macones PJ, Laufer I (1985) Candida esophagitis: accuracy of radiographic diagnosis. Radiology 154:581–587

Levine MS, Woldenberg R, Herlinger H, et al. (1987) Opportunistic esophagitis in AIDS: radiographic diagnosis. Radiology 165:815–820

Levine MS, Loercher G, Katzka DA, et al. (1991) Giant human immunodeficiency virus-related ulcers of the esophagus. Radiology 180:323–326

Lubat E, Megibow AJ, Balthazar EJ, et al. (1990) Extrapulmonary Pneumocystis carinii infection in AIDS: CT findings. Radiology 174:157–160

Maliha GM, Hepps KS, Maia DM, et al. (1991) Whipple's disease can mimic chronic AIDS enteropathy. Am J Gastroenterol 86:79–81

Meyers SA, Kuhlman JE, Fishman EK (1990) Enterovesical fistula in a patient with cryptosporidiosis and AIDS. Clin Imaging 14:143–145

Pantaleo G, Graziosi C, Fauci AS (1993) The immunopathogenesis of human immunodeficiency virus infection. N Engl J Med 328:327–335

Pol S, Romana CA, Richard S, et al. (1993) Microsporidia infection in patients with human immunodeficiency virus and unexplained cholangitis. N Engl J Med 328:95–99

Rabeneck L, Popovic M, Gartner S, et al. (1990) Acute HIV infection presenting with painful swallowing and esophageal ulcers. JAMA 263:2318–2322

Radin DR (1991) Intraabdominal Mycobacterium tuberculosis vs Mycobacterium avium-intracellulare infections in patients with AIDS: distinction based on CT findings, AJR 156:487–491

Radin DR (1995) HIV infection: analysis in 259 consecutive patients with abnormal abdominal CT findings. Radiology 197:712–722

Radin DR, Balcer LE, Katt EC, et al. (1990) Visceral and nodal calcifications in patients with AIDS-related Pneumocystis carinii infection. AJR 154:27–31

Sachs JR, Greenfield SM, Sohn M, et al. (1991) Disseminated Pneumocystis carinii infection with hepatic involvement in a patient with the acquired immune deficiency syndrome. Am J Gastroenterol 86:82–85

Schneiderman DJ, Cello JP, Laing FC (1987) Papillary stenosis and sclerosing cholangitis in the acquired immunodeficiency syndrome. Ann Intern Med 10:546–549

Sor S, Levine MS, Kowalski TE, Laufer I, Rubesin SE, Herlinger H (1995) Giant ulcers of the esophagus in patients with human immunodeficiency virus: clinical, radiographic, and pathologic findings. Radiology 194:447–451

Spouge AR, Wilson SR, Gopinath N, et al. (1990) Extrapulmonary Pneumocystis carinii in a patient with AIDS: sonographic findings, AJR 155:76–78

Texidor HS, Godwin TA, Ramirez EA (1991) Cryptosporidiosis of the biliary tract. Radiology 180:51–56

Towers MJ, Withers CE, Hamilton PA, et al. (1991) Visceral calcification in patients with AIDS may not always be due to Pneumocystis carinii. AJR 156:745–747

Vincent ME, Robbins AH (1985) Mycobacterium avium-intracellulare complex enteritis: pseudo-Whipple's disease in AIDS. AJR 144:921–922

14 Ischemic Disease

Z.C. TRAILL and D.J. NOLAN

CONTENTS

14.1
Introduction

Ischemia of the intestine has three causes: arterial occlusion, venous occlusion and nonocclusive or "low-flow" states. The commonest cause of arterial occlusive disease is arteriosclerosis affecting one or more of the major arteries supplying the intestine: the celiac axis and the superior and inferior mesenteric arteries (HILDEBRAND and ZIERLER 1980). The visceral arteries may also be narrowed or occluded by embolus, thrombus, blunt or penetrating trauma (MARKS et al. 1979), compression, or malignant infiltration. Emboli are usually cardiac in origin, in association with recent myocardial infarction or cardiac arrhythmia. Paradoxical embolus can occur in patients with a patent foramen ovale. Occlusion of tiny

Z.C. TRAILL, MD, Department of Radiology, John Radcliffe Hospital, Oxford, OX3 9DU, UK
D.J. NOLAN, MD, Consultant Radiologist, John Radcliffe Hospital, Oxford, OX3 9DU, UK

peripheral visceral arteries may occur in the vasculitides such as rheumatoid arthritis (KUEHNE et al. 1992) and systemic lupus erythematosus (GORE et al. 1983), and as a complication of radiation treatment (JOHNSON and CARRINGTON 1992).

Mesenteric venous occlusion is usually due to thrombosis (HILDEBRAND and ZIERLER 1980). However, mesenteric venous thrombosis accounts for only 5%–15% of cases of intestinal ischemia (GRENDELL and OCKNER 1982). Primary mesenteric venous thrombosis refers to cases of spontaneous occlusion of the mesenteric veins in the absence of a predisposing cause. Most cases of mesenteric venous thrombosis are secondary and are described in association with portal hypertension, cardiac disease, renal disease, intra-abdominal infection and inflammation, "hypercoagulable" states, and trauma (JOHNSON and BAGGENSTOSS 1949). Patients with cirrhosis may develop portal vein thrombosis which propagates back into the mesenteric veins. Impaired venous drainage may also result from mechanical compression of mesenteric veins by metastatic mesenteric tumor, particularly carcinoid tumor (GOLDSTONE et al. 1970), from small intestinal hernias, and from volvulus of the small intestine. Frequently multiple etiologic factors are present.

Nonocclusive mesenteric ischemia occurs in low-flow states such as severe hypovolemic shock and cardiac failure. Nonocclusive ischemia may also be produced by drugs which cause mesenteric arterial vasoconstriction such as cocaine (NALBANDIAN et al. 1985; FREUDENBERGER et al. 1990), ergot preparations, and digitalis.

14.2
Clinical Presentation

14.2.1
Acute and Subacute Intestinal Ischemia

The commonest cause of acute intestinal ischemia is sudden occlusion of the superior mesenteric artery.

Embolic occlusion is most common, with emboli characteristically lodging distal to the origin of the artery (CLARK and GALLANT 1984). Thrombotic occlusion is usually associated with arteriosclerotic disease and therefore occurs preferentially at the origin of the superior mesenteric artery. Characteristically the patient with mesenteric artery occlusion presents with sudden onset of abdominal pain, nausea, and vomiting (WILSON et al. 1987; CORDER and TAYLOR 1993). Initially the abdominal pain may be out of proportion to the physical findings. With the development of infarction, signs of peritonitis supervene. Laboratory findings are of limited value, although an elevated white cell count and plasma amylase are usual (CORDER and TAYLOR 1993). Prompt diagnosis is essential because of the rapidity with which the small intestine undergoes irreversible ischemic damage. Unfortunately the nonspecific nature of the clinical symptoms and signs means that delays in diagnosis are common, and the mortality remains high, up to 80%–90% (WILSON et al. 1987; HEYS et al. 1993).

Mesenteric venous occlusion is the cause of acute intestinal ischemia in a much smaller percentage of cases. A more insidious onset of symptoms is usual. Abdominal pain is often intermittent and may predate the patient's presentation by days or weeks (GRENDELL and OCKNER 1982). Nausea, vomiting, diarrhea, and melena may also occur. The white cell count is generally elevated (CLEMETT and CHANG 1975; ABDU et al. 1987). The prognosis is better than

with mesenteric arterial occlusion, with reported mortality rates of between 15% and 40% (CLAVIEN et al. 1988; RHEE et al. 1994). Spontaneous recovery may also occur (ABDU et al. 1987). However, there is a significant postoperative recurrence rate, up to 50% in some series, occasionally attributable to inadequate resection of intestine at operation (JONA et al. 1974; CLAVIEN et al. 1988).

Ischemia or infarction resulting from low-flow states typically produces a sudden onset of severe gastrointestinal symptoms. The clinical state of the patient, who will usually have an underlying cause such as cardiac disease or an episode of profound hypovolemia, may suggest the diagnosis.

14.2.2
Chronic Intestinal Ischemia

The clinical corollary of chronic intestinal ischemia resulting from arteriosclerotic narrowing or occlusion of the major visceral arteries is "intestinal angina." Most studies suggest that involvement of at least two of the three major visceral arteries is necessary to produce the characteristic symptoms of pain associated with eating and weight loss (MORRIS et al. 1962), although the same clinical syndrome is described in patients with involvement of the celiac axis alone (MORRIS et al. 1966; KENNEDY-WATT et al. 1967). An autopsy study of the major visceral arteries found no correlation between degrees of stenosis

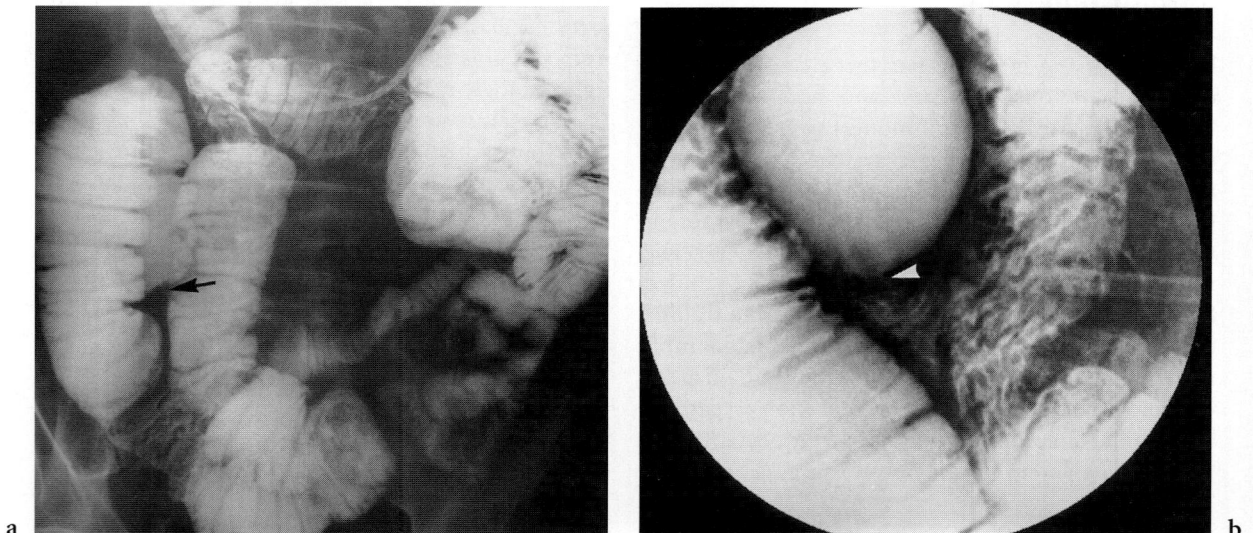

a

b

Fig. 14.1 a,b. Ischemic stricture causing intestinal obstruction. a Most of the small intestine is outlined with contrast medium during enteroclysis and a dilated segment of ileum is seen with an abrupt termination in the barium column (*arrow*). b A spot compression view shows a tight stricture in the ileum with proximal dilatation (*arrowhead*)

and previous gastrointestinal symptoms (CROFT et al. 1981). It seems that in most patients the slowly progressive nature of arteriosclerotic narrowing allows the development of a collateral circulation so that symptomatic narrowing is rare. In a few patients the collateral circulation is inadequate and these patients may benefit from a revascularization procedure (CALDERON et al. 1992).

Occasionally the ischemic process is localized, so-called focal segmental ischemia. The initial ischemic event may be subclinical, the patient presenting at a later stage with obstructive symptoms due to development of a fibrotic stricture (Fig. 14.1). Causes for this include distal vessel occlusion by embolus or thrombosis (GINAI et al. 1994), trauma causing either direct damage to the intestinal wall or a short mesenteric tear (MARKS et al. 1979), vasculitis, and radiation. The small vessel occlusive disease associated with the vasculitides and previous radiation treatment may produce a wide range of effects from asymptomatic alteration of intestinal peristaltic activity (QUELOZ and WOLOSHIN 1972) to obstructive symptoms (KUEHNE et al. 1992).

14.3 Pathophysiology

Early changes occur predominantly in the mucosa and submucosa with mucosal necrosis and the formation of a surface membrane and submucosal edema and hemorrhage (MORSON et al. 1990). At this early stage there is spasm of the intestinal smooth muscle. Continuing ischemia results in paralysis of the intestinal muscle so that the ischemic intestine becomes atonic. The intestinal wall and valvulae conniventes are thickened by edema and hemorrhage. Necrotic mucosa may slough into the intestinal lumen. Finally, with persisting ischemia, transmural necrosis and perforation may develop.

Alternatively the ischemic process may undergo resolution and repair, especially if localized. The common end result of this is an ischemic stricture.

14.4 Imaging of Ischemia and Infarction

14.4.1 Plain Radiographs

Most patients with suspected intestinal ischemia will have a plain radiograph of the abdomen. Unfortu-

nately, findings in the early stages of intestinal ischemia are notoriously nonspecific. Abnormal abdominal radiographs have been reported in between approximately 50% and 75% of patients with mesenteric vascular occlusion in several studies (NELSON and EGGLESTON 1960; TOMCHIK et al. 1970; RHEE et al. 1994). Smooth muscle spasm may empty the intestine of gas and liquid content, producing a "gasless" abdomen on early radiographs. As smooth muscle paralysis supervenes the intestine becomes atonic so that gas-distended intestinal loops are a frequent but nonspecific finding (CLEMETT and CHANG 1975). Fixity of intestinal loops as shown by an unchanging appearance on serial radiographs is also described (WANG and REEVES 1960). Dilatation of intestinal loops proximal to the atonic segment gives the radiographic appearance of obstruction. Thickening of the intestinal wall due to edema in combination with mucosal irregularity is highly suggestive of ischemia (Fig. 14.2) (TOMCHIK et al. 1970). "Thumb printing" along the mesenteric border of an intestinal loop is caused by focal hemorrhage (SCOTT et al. 1971). Air within the intestinal wall is a late finding indicating infarction. Transmural infarction may lead to intestinal perforation and free intraperitoneal air. Air within the portal or mesenteric veins

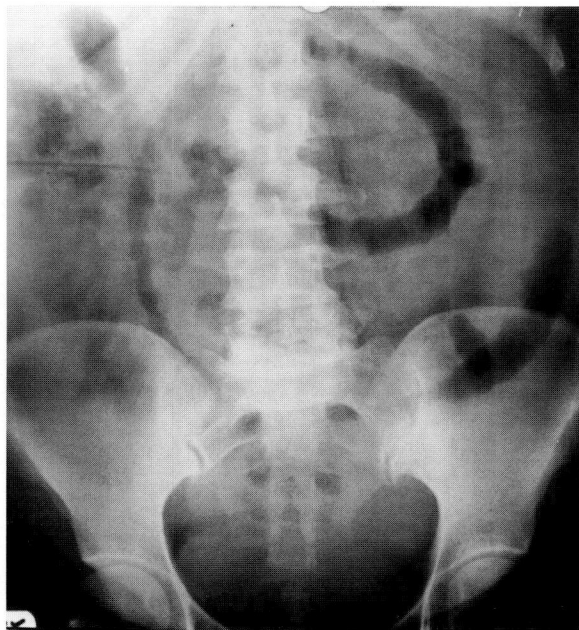

Fig. 14.2. Acute intestinal ischemia. Gas outlines a long atonic segment of narrowed small intestine with thickening, and in some areas effacement of the mucosal folds. Ischemic small intestine caused by mesenteric venous thrombosis was found at operation

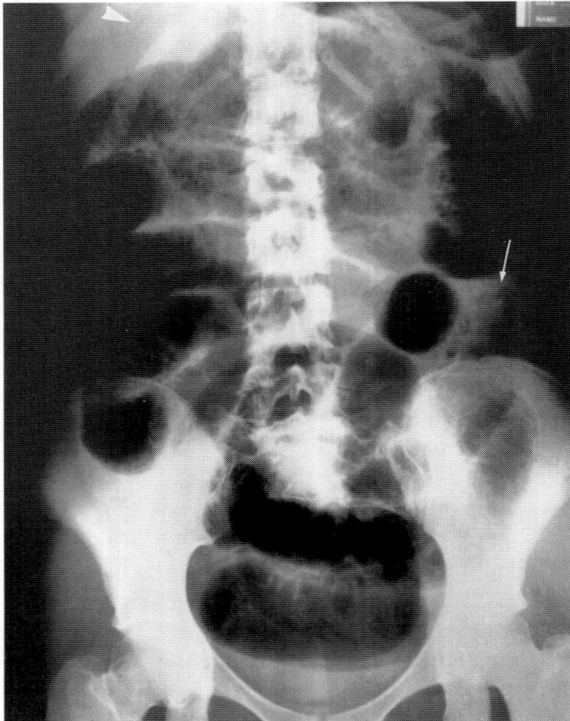

Fig. 14.3. Intestinal infarction. A plain abdominal radiograph shows intramural gas throughout the intestine, mostly seen as round discrete radiolucencies. The characteristic appearances of intramural gas seen in profile can also be identified (*arrow*). Gas is seen in the portal venous system (*arrowhead*)

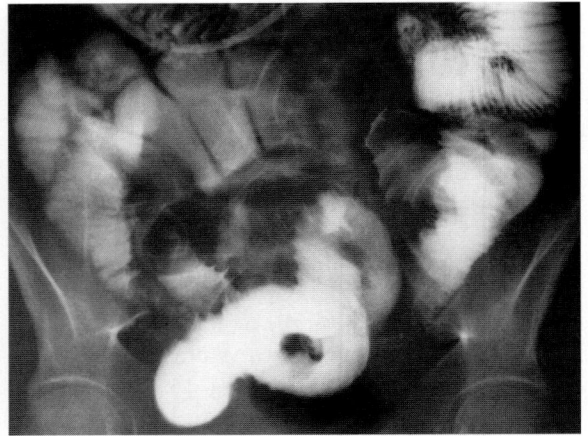

Fig. 14.4. Acute ischemia. Enteroclysis view showing marked thickening of the mucosal folds in the ileum of a 39-year-old woman who presented with acute abdominal pain 6 months after a right hemicolectomy for a cecal volvulus. Her symptoms resolved rapidly and a repeat examination 6 weeks later showed that the small intestine had returned to normal. (Reproduced from NOLAN 1983)

almost invariably indicates an extremely poor prognosis (Fig. 14.3).

14.4.2
Contrast Examinations

Barium studies are not indicated in suspected acute mesenteric ischemia but may be performed in patients with an atypical or subacute presentation. Barium studies reveal characteristic findings in intestinal ischemia (CLEMETT and CHANG 1975). Marked thickening of the intestinal wall and valvulae conniventes is the main finding (Fig. 14.4). This, in combination with mesenteric thickening, results in separation of adjacent barium-filled intestinal loops. Thumb printing may be apparent. Extensive submucosal hemorrhage and edema may give rise to the "stack of coins" or "picket-fence" appearance indistinguishable from that seen in some cases of hemophilia or intramural hemorrhage caused by anticoagulant therapy.

Ischemic strictures occurring as a consequence of healing of a localized ischemic lesion with fibrosis can be well demonstrated by barium examination (MARKS et al. 1979; GINAI et al. 1994). These strictures usually appear as short narrowed segments, sometimes with dilatation of proximal intestine. They are characteristically smoothly tapering but occasionally, particularly in the colon, they may be eccentric, producing "pseudodiverticula" or sacculation of the spared intestinal wall (IIDA et al. 1986).

14.4.3
Angiography

The role for emergency angiography in patients with suspected acute mesenteric ischemia has not been clearly defined. It has no place in patients with obvious infarction. If angiographic facilities are readily available, it has the advantages of possibly permitting the definitive diagnosis of mesenteric artery embolus or thrombosis, mesenteric vein thrombosis, and nonocclusive ischemia. It may effectively exclude these diagnoses. Finally it may allow endovascular therapy. Disadvantages include a high rate of negative examinations (CLARK and GALLANT 1984), the risks of the procedure, and the possibility of falsely attributing the patient's acute symptoms and signs to a long-standing, silent vascular lesion.

Mesenteric arterial embolus may be difficult to distinguish from mesenteric arterial thrombus at angiography. Thrombosis usually occurs in the first 3 cm of the artery while emboli usually lodge distal to this (CLARK and GALLANT 1984). Thrombotic occlusion usually appears as an abrupt vessel cut-off in contrast to embolic occlusion, which appears as a rounded filling defect in the artery with high-grade obstruction of distal flow of contrast (BAKAL et al. 1992) Mesenteric venous occlusion may be demonstrated as an intraluminal venous filling defect or as nonopacification of the mesenteric veins with evidence of a collateral venous circulation. The angiographic findings in nonocclusive mesenteric ischemia include patent mesenteric arteries and veins, increased mesenteric-aortic reflux of contrast material, and mesenteric arterial vasoconstriction with decreased arterial flow. These findings may be reversed by intra-arterial infusion of a vasodilator.

Angiography is the definitive investigation in patients with "intestinal angina." The lateral aortogram with early, rapid, serial filming demonstrates the origins of the major visceral arteries (Fig. 14.5) and the anteroposterior aortogram can assess the collateral

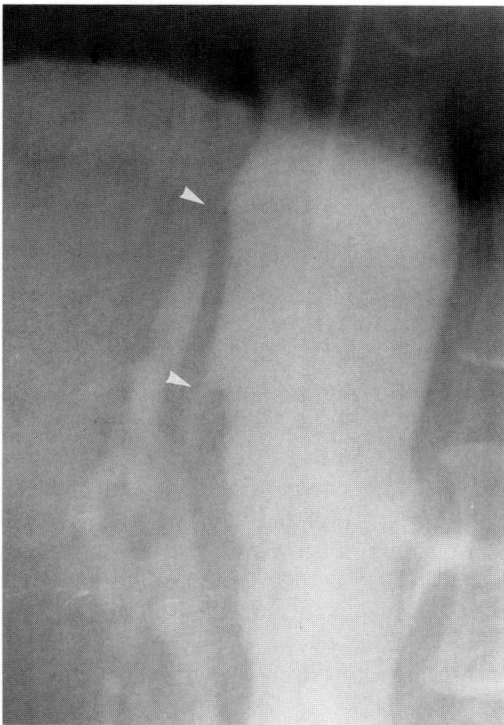

Fig. 14.5. Chronic mesenteric ischemia. Lateral aortogram showing stenosis of the celiac axis and superior mesenteric artery (*arrowheads*) in a patient with "intestinal angina." (Courtesy of Dr. E.W.L. Fletcher)

vessels. Doppler ultrasonography and magnetic resonance imaging are playing an increasing role in the investigation of this condition.

In 1963 HARJOLA first reported the syndrome of ligamentous compression of the celiac artery. Compression of the celiac trunk by the median arcuate ligament of the diaphragm is now a well recognized finding at angiography and surgery. Angiographic findings include stenosis of the proximal celiac trunk, poststenotic dilatation, and the presence of collateral vessels (DUNBAR et al. 1965). A recent study suggests that similar findings can be identified at computed tomography (CT) (PATTEN et al. 1991). Correlation of imaging findings with symptoms of intestinal angina and the efficacy of surgical resection of the ligamentous band remain controversial (BRANDT and BOLEY 1978).

14.4.4
Computed Tomography

In clinical practice the patient with acute mesenteric ischemia may present with nonspecific symptoms and signs and referral for emergency angiography may be inappropriate. In these circumstances contrast-enhanced CT is proving increasingly helpful.

Contrast-enhanced CT demonstrates mesenteric venous thrombus as a low attenuation filling defect within the vein (Fig. 14.6) (ROSEN et al. 1984; VOGELZANG et al. 1988). CT may also demonstrate the predisposing factor in cases of secondary mesenteric venous thrombosis. Thrombus or embolus may be shown in the proximal trunk of the mesenteric artery on CT, although not in the more distal branches (TAOUREL et al. 1996).

Several CT findings, including portal or mesenteric venous gas, focal thickening of the intestinal wall, and intramural gas, have been found to be highly suggestive of intestinal ischemia or infarction (FEDERLE et al. 1984; SMERUD et al. 1990). However, in one study, none of these features were present on the CT scans or plain abdominal radiographs of 8 out of 23 patients with mesenteric infarction proven at surgery or autopsy (SMERUD et al. 1990). TAOUREL et al. (1996) retrospectively compared the CT scans of 39 patients with surgically proven acute ischemia with those of 24 control patients with suspected acute mesenteric ischemia that was disproved at surgery. The CT scans were all performed with dynamic intravenous contrast-material enhancement. CT findings with a specificity of greater than 95% for the

a

b

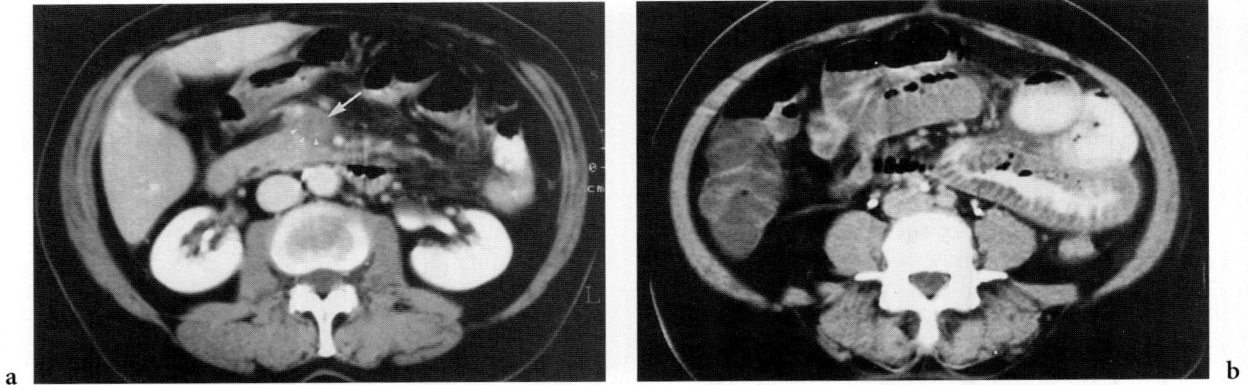

Fig. 14.6 a,b. Mesenteric vein thrombosis. **a** Contrast-enhanced CT scan showing thrombus within the superior mesenteric vein (*arrow*). Enhancement of the vessel wall is due to contrast medium in the vasa vasorum (*arrowheads*). **b** CT scan demonstrating marked thickening of the wall of the small intestine

diagnosis of acute mesenteric ischemia included superior mesenteric artery or superior mesenteric vein occlusion, intramural gas, portal venous gas, lack of enhancement of the bowel wall, and liver or splenic infarcts. The sensitivity of each of these findings was less than 30%. If the presence of at least one of these signs was used as the criterion for the diagnosis of mesenteric ischemia, CT had a sensitivity of 64%, a specificity of 92%, and an accuracy of 75%. Interestingly a very high proportion of patients (33%) had evidence of arterial or venous occlusion at CT compared with previous studies. This is likely to be due to the consistent use of a dynamic contrast-enhanced CT technique. CT was also valuable for assessing prognosis, with superior mesenteric artery thrombosis having a 100% negative predictive value for survival and superior mesenteric vein thrombosis having a 100% positive predictive value for survival.

Several recent studies have evaluated the role of CT in intestinal ischemia associated with closed-loop or incarcerated intestinal obstruction, so-called strangulating obstruction (BALTHAZAR et al. 1992; TAOUREL et al. 1995; FRAGER et al. 1996). Findings suggestive of intestinal ischemia or infarction in patients with small bowel obstruction included thickening and enhancement of the intestinal wall occasionally producing concentric rings of different densities, the "target" or "halo" sign, and pneumatosis. Strangulation was also associated with abnormalities in the attached mesentery, blurring or obliteration of mesenteric vessels, mesenteric fluid, or hemorrhage. CT signs of strangulation may be absent in proven cases: 6 out of 16 patients with proven strangulation reported by BALTHAZAR et al. (1992) had no CT signs of strangulation. In contrast, in a large series reported by FRAGER et al. (1996), CT correctly identified all 29 patients with intestinal ischemia as assessed at surgery out of a total of 60 patients with complete or high-grade small bowel obstruction. There were 12 CT diagnoses that were false-positive for intestinal ischemia. These findings would suggest that CT may be of value in patients with clinical or radiographic signs of high-grade intestinal obstruction in whom a trial of conservative management is planned. CT signs of strangulation would preclude such management.

14.4.5
Ultrasonography

Ultrasonography is often the initial investigation performed in patients with abdominal pain. Although a nonspecific finding, small bowel thickening detected sonographically should suggest the diagnosis of mesenteric ischemia in the appropriate clinical context. Duplex Doppler ultrasonography is helpful in evaluating the proximal visceral arteries in patients with "intestinal angina" (HARTNELL and GIBSON 1987). However, visualization of these vessels may be inadequate in a significant percentage of patients (ROOBOTTOM and DUBBINS 1993). The role of ultrasonography in the investigation of suspected acute mesenteric ischemia is limited by its inability to detect distal emboli and mesenteric vasoconstriction.

Ultrasonography is a useful imaging modality in the diagnosis of portal vein thrombosis (VAN GANSBEKE et al. 1985) and duplex Doppler ultrasonography is reliable for demonstrating the periportal collateral vessels in "cavernous transformation" of the portal vein due to chronic portal vein obstruction (WELTIN et al. 1985). However, it is less reliable in the diagnosis of mesenteric vein occlusion and CT is the preferred investigation if this disorder is suspected.

14.4.6
Magnetic Resonance Imaging

Magnetic resonance (MR) imaging allows non-invasive assessment of the mesenteric arteries and veins. Breath-hold gadolinium-enhanced MR angiography provides good depiction of the origins of the visceral arteries (PRINCE et al. 1995; HOLLAND et al. 1996). A recent paper suggests that MR imaging may have a role as a screening test for chronic mesenteric ischemia (BURKART et al. 1995). Phase-contrast cine MR imaging was used to measure flow in the mesenteric venous system in ten healthy volunteers and in ten patients with a clinical suspicion of chronic mesenteric ischemia. A postprandial augmentation of peak superior mesenteric vein flow was found in the volunteers and in patients without mesenteric ischemia. The percentage of flow augmentation was significantly lower in patients with chronic mesenteric ischemia.

Magnetic resonance imaging is also valuable in the diagnosis of portal and mesenteric venous thrombosis (Fig. 14.7). Fresh thrombus appears as a high signal abnormality within the vein or in the expected position of the vein on T1- and T2-weighted spin-echo images (ZIRINSKY et al. 1988). Older thrombus loses its T1 hyperintensity but remains high-signal on T2-weighted images. Gradient-

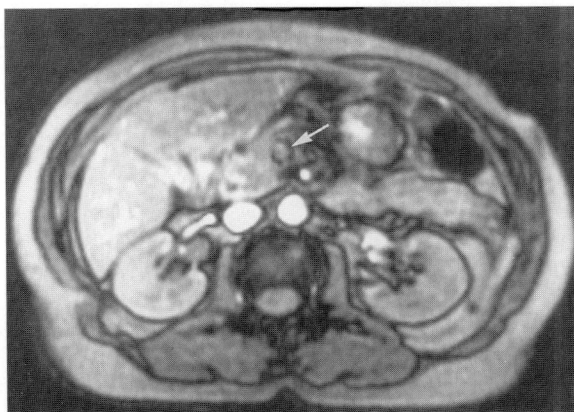

Fig. 14.7. Mesenteric vein thrombosis. Gradient-echo MR image showing absence of high signal in the superior mesenteric vein (*arrow*) indicating thrombosis. High signal from the aorta, inferior vena cava, and superior mesenteric artery indicates blood flow

echo sequences are useful in the differentiation of true thrombi from flow-related artifacts (HADDAD et al. 1992).

14.5
Radiation Enteritis

Chronic radiation enteritis is a form of chronic intestinal ischemia resulting from damage to vascular endothelial cells leading ultimately to endarteritis obliterans (MASON et al. 1970; HASLETON et al. 1985). The time interval between the radiation therapy course and the development of symptoms is highly variable, with latent periods as long as 25 years (MENDELSON and NOLAN 1985). Several factors increase the susceptibility of the intestine to radiation damage, including hypertension, atherosclerosis, and diabetes mellitus, presumably due to preexisting vascular damage (MARUYAMA et al. 1974). Previous pelvic inflammatory disease and infection (STROCKBINE et al. 1970) and previous laparotomy also increase the risk of radiation damage by adhesive immobilization of small intestinal loops within the treatment field (MASON et al. 1970; POTISH et al. 1979). Combination treatment with chemotherapy reduces the patient's radiation tolerance (JOHNSON and CARRINGTON 1992).

The small intestine, distal colon and rectum are the usual sites of radiation damage after abdominopelvic radiation. The distal ileum is the commonest site of small intestinal damage (MENDELSON and NOLAN 1985; YUHASZ et al. 1985). Patients with chronic radiation enteritis affecting the small intestine characteristically present with intermittent small intestinal obstruction, colicky abdominal pain, diarrhea, or malabsorption (MENDELSON and NOLAN 1985; TAYLOR et al. 1990). Chronic radiation enteritis of the rectum and sigmoid colon usually manifests itself as abdominal pain, diarrhea, or rectal bleeding (TAYLOR et al. 1990).

Patients with suspected chronic radiation enteritis of the small intestine require a barium examination. Enteroclysis (small bowel enema) is superior to the barium follow-through examination in the diagnosis of low-grade small intestinal obstruction due to its ability to distend maximally the intestine (MENDELSON and NOLAN 1985). Enteroclysis is therefore well suited to the investigation of chronic radiation enteritis, where stenoses and adhesions are common.

Barium studies reveal typical small intestinal changes in this condition which include mural thickening, thickening of the valvulae conniventes, fixity and angulation of small intestinal loops, absence of the mucosal fold pattern, nodular mucosal filling defects, single or multiple strictures, and evidence of intestinal obstruction (Figs. 14.8, 14.9) (Mason et al. 1970; Mendelson and Nolan 1985; Taylor et al. 1990). The "pool of barium" appearance due to featureless, matted loops of closely adherent small intestine is characteristic but rare. Ulceration, although often evident microscopically, is rarely detected during barium examination. Sinuses and fistulae are an uncommon finding. "Mucosal tacking," i.e. spiking and distortion of the mucosal folds on the antimesenteric border of the intestine due to adhesions to the mesentery, is often a feature (Mason et al. 1970). Barium examination underestimates the extent of radiation damage as determined at surgery (Mendelson and Nolan 1985). The diagnosis of radiation ileitis can also be made at CT, where matted loops of thick-walled intestine with increased density of the adjacent mesenteric fat are characteristic (Fishman et al. 1984).

Investigation of suspected chronic radiation damage in the rectum and sigmoid colon is usually by double-contrast barium enema although the single-contrast technique is preferred for demonstrating

fistulae. Typical findings include spasm, mucosal effacement producing a featureless mucosa or ulceration, strictures, widening of the presacral space, sinuses, and fistulae (Mason et al. 1970; Taylor et al. 1990). Strictures may be single or multiple and although usually smoothly tapering, they may occasionally be short with overhanging edges resembling a carcinoma (Mason et al. 1970). Perforation and abscess formation are very unusual.

14.6 Vasculitis

14.6.1 Systemic Lupus Erythematosus

Systemic lupus erythematosus is characterized histologically by "fibrinoid necrosis" of the small arteries, arterioles, and capillaries. Ischemia or infarction of both small intestine and colon are recognized complications (Shapeero et al. 1974; Gore et al. 1983). Some ischemic lesions may be reversible with steroid therapy (Shapeero et al. 1974). However, necrosis and perforation may also occur.

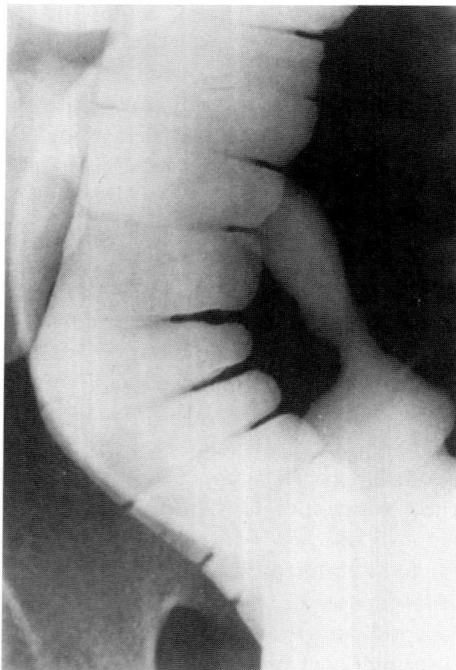

Fig. 14.8. Radiation stricture. A spot compression view taken at enteroclysis shows a short segment of narrowing in the distal ileum with slight dilatation of the more proximal ileum

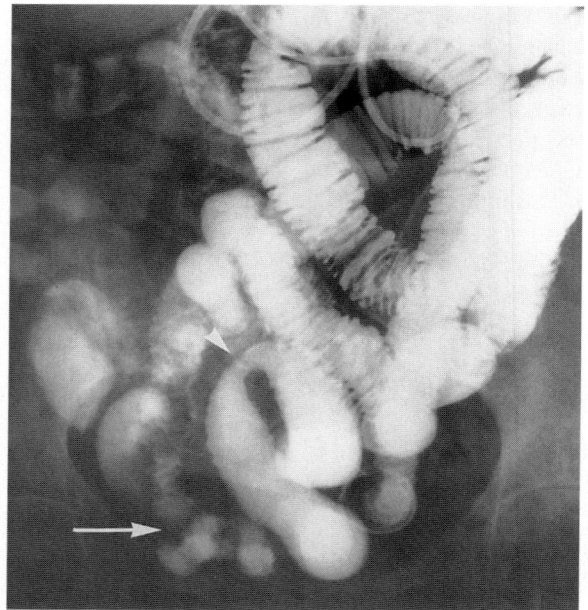

Fig. 14.9. Radiation enteritis. There are fairly extensive changes of radiation enteritis involving the ileum. Thickening of the valvulae is seen in a number of loops. In one loop there is a short segment of narrowing (*arrowhead*), thickening of the valvulae, and considerable effacement of the mucosal pattern. The more distal ileal loops (*arrow*) are contracted and distorted with thickening of the valvulae

14.6.2
Rheumatoid Vasculitis

Although vasculitis is common in rheumatoid arthritis, intestinal ischemia is rare. Nonetheless, it is an extremely serious complication with a mortality of 75% in one review of intestinal rheumatoid vasculitis (DE BRUM-FERNANDES et al. 1988). An ischemic small bowel stricture has recently been reported by KUEHNE et al. (1992).

14.6.3
Behçet's Disease

Involvement of the gastrointestinal tract occurs in 10%–15% of patients with Behçet's disease (ROSENBERGER et al. 1982). Ulceration and fissure formation are common and may result in hemorrhage or perforation. There is predominant involvement of the ileocecal region and the changes may be difficult to differentiate from those of Crohn's disease (Fig. 14.10).

14.6.4
Henoch-Schönlein Purpura

Gastrointestinal manifestations are a prominent feature of the syndrome of Henoch-Schönlein purpura due to a small vessel vasculitis (HANDEL and SCHWARTZ 1957). Mucosal edema and hemor-

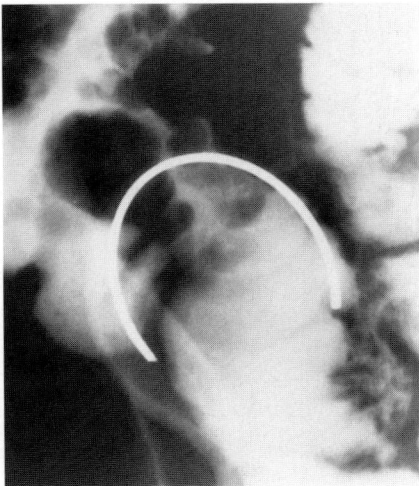

Fig. 14.10. Behçet's disease. Spot view at enteroclysis showing narrowing and irregularity of the terminal ileum with enlargement of the ileocecal valve. (Courtesy of Professor D.J. Allison and reproduced from NOLAN 1994)

rhage are common and ulceration may occur. However, these findings usually resolve and full-thickness necrosis and perforation are rare.

14.6.5
Polyarteritis Nodosa

Polyarteritis nodosa is characterized histologically by an inflammatory process involving all three layers of the small and medium-sized arteries leading to aneurysm formation, thrombosis, and infarction. In the intestine both ischemia and infarction with perforation may occur (CRAIG 1963).

14.6.6
Systemic Sclerosis

Systemic sclerosis (scleroderma) is a multisystem disorder in which abnormalities of the gastrointestinal tract are a prominent feature. The etiology is unknown but replacement of smooth muscle by fibrous tissue is responsible for many of the gastrointestinal manifestations. Deposition of collagen also occurs in the small vessels of the skin, suggesting that disease of small vessels may be central to the widespread pathology seen in this disorder (HUGHES 1987). Motility disturbances are common with decreased peristalsis in the esophagus and delayed transit in the small intestine and colon. Dilatation of intestine occurs particularly in the duodenal loop (ANDERSON 1974). Prominent pseudodiverticula are found in the small intestine (QUELOZ and WOLOSHIN 1972) and colon. Occasionally the "hide-bound" appearance is seen in the small intestine, where the valvulae conniventes appear thin and crowded together (HOROWITZ and MEYERS 1973).

14.7
Ischemic Colitis

The pathogenesis of ischemic colitis is poorly understood and, in many cases, multiple etiologic factors are probably present. Most cases occur spontaneously in the absence of a major vessel occlusion or an episode of profound hypotension (GANDHI et al. 1996). Patients are usually elderly and present with an acute onset of abdominal pain and bloody diarrhea.

Colonic ischemia is usually segmental, affecting the "watershed" areas of the splenic flexure and sigmoid colon between the territories of the superior and inferior mesenteric arteries and the inferior mesenteric artery and hemorrhoidal arteries respectively. Elsewhere an extensive collateral circulation protects the colon from ischemia. Unusual sites of ischemia may result from specific predisposing factors or a combination of risk factors. Acute ischemic proctitis has been reported as a complication of vascular surgical procedures and also of tumor encasement of the rectum (NELSON et al. 1992). WELCH et al. (1986) describe three patients with total colonic ischemia in whom more than one risk factor for ischemia was identified. Colonic distension, for example due to a distal obstructing carcinoma, may cause colonic ischemia as a result of impairment of venous drainage. In these circumstances the cecum is usually the most severely affected and the region that may perforate.

Spasm, submucosal edema, and hemorrhage are prominent in the early stages of colonic ischemia. More prolonged ischemia results in mucosal necrosis with ulceration. Depending on the severity of the ischemic insult, ischemic colitis may follow three courses: complete healing with no sequelae, healing with fibrosis resulting in stricture formation, and transmural necrosis and gangrene. Fibrotic healing may involve only a portion of the circumference of the bowel so that the spared areas balloon out to form pseudodiverticula.

Plain abdominal radiographs are often normal or nonspecifically abnormal but findings suggestive of ischemic colitis include narrowing of the affected colon with wall thickening and thumb printing (Fig. 14.11a). There may be dilatation of the proximal colon. Rarely toxic megacolon may occur. Barium studies are the most useful radiologic investigation in nongangrenous ischemic colitis. The instant single-contrast barium enema is valuable in the diagnosis of acute ischemic colitis, demonstrating the characteristic findings of thumb printing and narrowing of the involved segment (Fig. 14.11b). Double-contrast barium studies characteristically show thumb-printing and longitudinal ulcers (IIDA et al. 1986). Loss of thumb printing may occur with air insufflation on the double-contrast barium examination but this finding will usually be evident at some stage during the examination, often during the filling stage (BARTRAM 1979). Rarely the mucosal abnormality will be extensive and resemble an inflammatory or infectious colitis (SCHOLZ 1993). Strictures may occur in the healing phase and may be single or multiple. Eccentric involvement of the

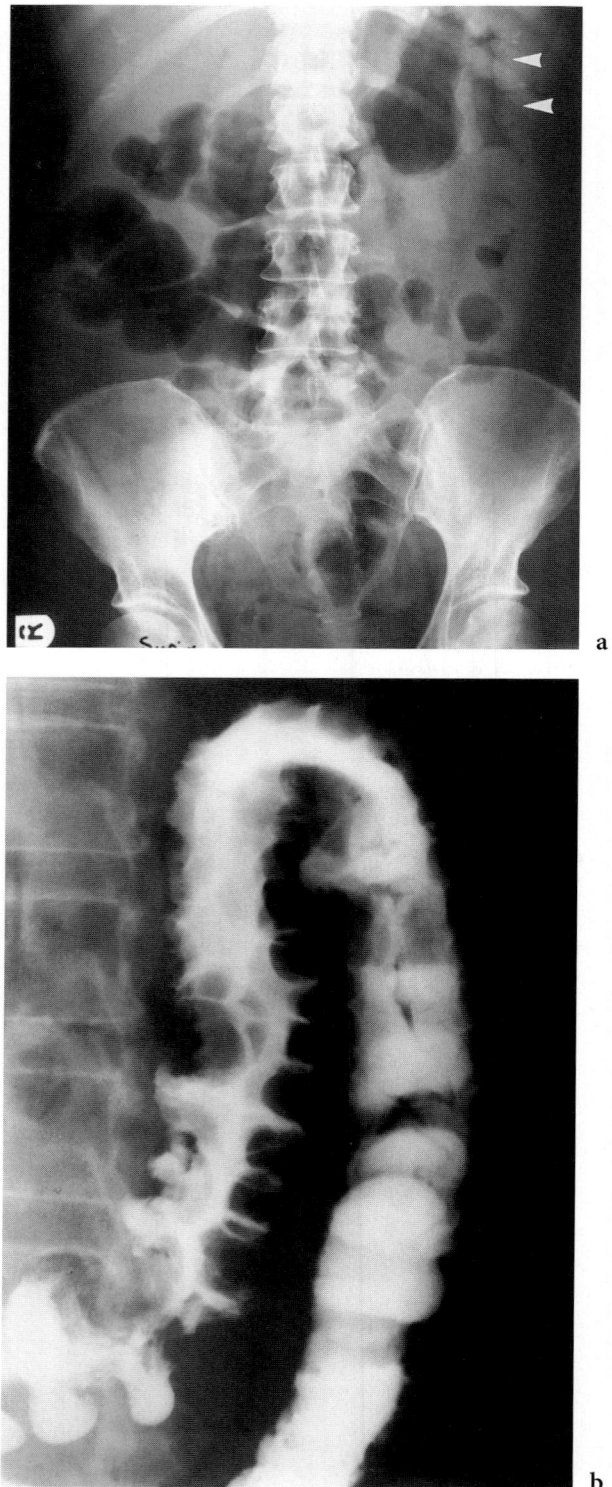

Fig. 14.11 a,b. Ischemic colitis. **a** Plain abdominal radiograph showing edema of the splenic flexure with a small amount of air in the lumen outlining a thumb printing appearance (*arrowheads*). **b** Spot view from a single-contrast barium examination also showing the characteristic thumb printing appearance

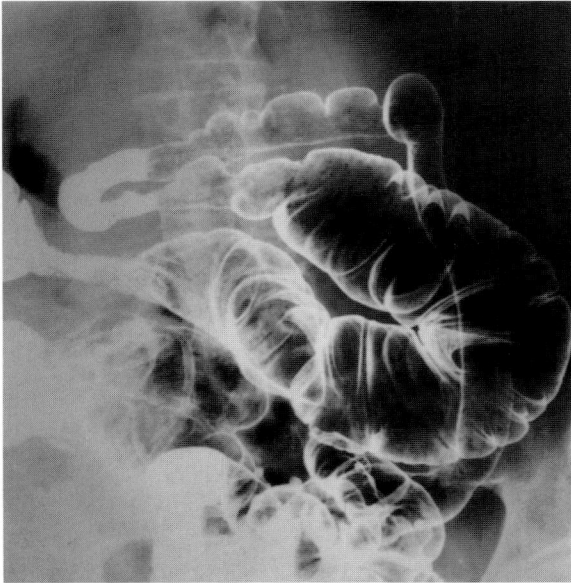

Fig. 14.12. Ischemic stricture. Barium enema shows a long stricture of the splenic flexure with pseudodiverticula

bowel wall by the ischemic process may result in pseudodiverticula (Fig. 14.12).

The CT findings in ischemic colitis are usually nonspecific, consisting in colonic wall thickening and, less commonly, ascites (JONES et al. 1982; PHILPOTTS et al. 1994). Rarely, intramural air will be present, which, although not pathognomonic for ischemia, should suggest the diagnosis in the appropriate clinical context.

References

Abdu RA, Zakhour BJ, Dallis DJ (1987) Mesenteric venous thrombosis – 1911 to 1984. Surgery 101:383–388

Anderson F (1974) Megaduodenum. Am J Gastroenterol 62:509

Bakal CW, Sprayregen S, Wolf EL (1992) Radiology in intestinal ischemia. Angiographic diagnosis and management. Surg Clin North Am 72:125–141

Balthazar EJ, Birnbaum BA, Megibow AJ, Gordon RB, Whelan CA, Hulnick DH (1992) Closed-loop and strangulating intestinal obstruction: CT signs. Radiology 185:769–775

Bartram CI (1979) Obliteration of thumbprinting with double-contrast enemas in acute ischemic colitis. Gastrointest Radiol 4:85–88

Brandt LJ, Boley SJ (1978) Celiac axis compression syndrome. A critical review. Am J Dig Dis 23:633–640

Burkart D, Johnson CD, Reading CC, Ehman RL (1995) MR measurements of mesenteric venous flow: prospective evaluation in healthy volunteers and patients with suspected chronic mesenteric ischemia. Radiology 194:801–806

Calderon M, Reul GJ, Gregoric ID, et al. (1992) Long-term results of the surgical management of symptomatic chronic intestinal ischemia. J Cardiovasc Surg 33:723–728

Clark RA, Gallant TE (1984) Acute mesenteric ischemia: angiographic spectrum. AJR 142:555–562

Clavien PA, Dürig M, Harder F (1988) Venous mesenteric infarction: a particular entity. Br J Surg 75:252–255

Clemett AR, Chang J (1975) The radiologic diagnosis of spontaneous mesenteric venous thrombosis. Am J Gastroenterol 63:209–215

Corder AP, Taylor I (1993) Acute mesenteric ischaemia. Postgrad Med J 69:1–3

Craig RDP (1963) Multiple perforations of the small intestine in polyarteritis nodosa. Gastroenterology 44:355

Croft RJ, Menon GP, Marston A (1981) Does "intestinal angina" exist? A critical study of obstructed visceral arteries. Br J Surg 68:316–318

de Brum-Fernandes AJ, Lucena-Fernandes M, Calvo I, Rodrigues CJ, de Souza AEL (1988) Small bowel necrosis: a rare, life-threatening complication of rheumatoid arthritis (letter). J Rheumatol 15:1313–1315

Dunbar JD, Molnar W, Beman FF, Marable SA (1965) Compression of the celiac trunk and abdominal angina. AJR 95:731–744

Federle MP, Chun G, Jeffrey RB, Rayor R (1984) Computed tomographic findings in bowel infarction. AJR 142:91–95

Fishman EK, Zinreich ES, Jones B, Siegleman SS (1984) Computed tomographic diagnosis of radiation ileitis. Gastrointest Radiol 9:149–152

Frager D, Baer JW, Medwid SW, Rothpearl A, Bossart P (1996) Detection of intestinal ischemia in patients with acute small-bowel obstruction due to adhesions or hernia: efficacy of CT. AJR 166:67–71

Freudenberger RS, Cappell MS, Hutt DA (1990) Intestinal infarction after intravenous cocaine administration. Ann Intern Med 113:715–716

Gandhi SK, Hanson MM, Vernava AM, Kaminski DL, Longo WE (1996) Ischemic colitis. Dis Colon Rectum 39:88–100

Ginai AZ, Hussain SM, Hordijk ML, den Hollander JC (1994) Case report: solitary ischaemic small bowel stenosis. Br J Radiol 67:405–407

Goldstone J, Moore WS, Hall AD (1970) Chronic occlusion of the superior and inferior mesenteric veins: report of a case. Am Surg 36:235–237

Gore RM, Marn CS, Ujiki GT, Craig RM, Marquardt J (1983) Ischemic colitis associated with systemic lupus erythematosus. Dis Colon Rectum 26:449–451

Grendell JH, Ockner RK (1982) Mesenteric venous thrombosis. Gastroenterology 82:358–372

Haddad MC, Clark DC, Sharif HS, Al Shahed MA, Aideyan O, Sammak BM (1992) MR, CT and ultrasonography of splanchnic venous thrombosis. Gastrointest Radiol 17:34–40

Handel J, Schwartz S (1957) Gastrointestinal manifestations of the Schönlein-Henoch syndrome. AJR 78:643–652

Harjola PT (1963) A rare obstruction of the coeliac artery. Ann Chir Gynaecol 52:547–550

Hartnell GG, Gibson RN (1987) Doppler ultrasound in the diagnosis of intestinal ischemia. Gastrointest Radiol 12:285–288

Hasleton PS, Carr N, Schofield PF (1985) Vascular changes in radiation bowel disease. Histopathology 9:517–534

Heys SD, Brittenden J, Crofts TJ (1993) Acute mesenteric ischaemia: the continuing difficulty in early diagnosis. Postgrad Med J 69:48–51

Hildebrand HD, Zierler RE (1980) Mesenteric vascular disease. Am J Surg 139:188–192

Holland GA, Dougherty L, Carpenter JP, et al. (1996) Breath-hold ultrafast three-dimensional gadolinium-enhanced MR angiography of the aorta and the renal and other visceral abdominal arteries. Radiology 166:971–981

Horowitz AL, Meyers MA (1973) The "hide-bound" small bowel of scleroderma: characteristic mucosal fold pattern. AJR 119:332–334

Hughes GRV (1987) Connective tissue diseases, 3rd edn. Blackwell, Oxford

Iida M, Matsui T, Fuchigami T, Iwashita A, Yao T, Fujishima M (1986) Ischemic colitis: serial changes in double-contrast barium enema examination. Radiology 159:337–341

Johnson CC, Baggenstoss AH (1949) Mesenteric vascular occlusion 1. Study of 99 cases of occlusion of veins. Mayo Clin Proc 24:628–636

Johnson RJ, Carrington BM (1992) Pelvic radiation disease. Clin Radiol 45:4–12

Jona J, Cummins GM, Head HB, Govostis MC (1974) Recurrent primary mesenteric venous thrombosis. JAMA 227:1033–1035

Jones B, Fishman EK, Siegelman SS (1982) Ischemic colitis demonstrated by computed tomography. J Comput Assist Tomogr 6:1120–1123

Kennedy-Watt J, Watson WC, Haase S (1967) Chronic intestinal ischaemia. BMJ 3:199–202

Kuehne SE, Gauvin GP, Shortsleeve M (1992) Small bowel stricture caused by rheumatoid vasculitis. Radiology 184:215–216

Marks CG, Nolan DJ, Piris J, Webster CU (1979) Small bowel strictures after blunt abdominal trauma. Br J Surg 66:663–664

Maruyama Y, Van Nagell JR, Utley J, Vider ML, Parker JC (1974) Radiation and small bowel complications in cervical carcinoma therapy. Radiology 112:699–703

Mason GR, Dietrich P, Friedland GW, Hanks GE (1970) The radiological findings in radiation-induced enteritis and colitis. A review of 30 cases. Clin Radiol 21:232–247

Mendelson RM, Nolan DJ (1985) The radiological features of chronic radiation enteritis. Clin Radiol 36:141–148

Morris GC, Crawford ES, Cooley DA, De Bakey ME (1962) Revascularization of the celiac and superior mesenteric arteries. Arch Surg 84:95–107

Morris GC, De Bakey ME, Bernhard V (1966) Abdominal angina. Surg Clin North Am 46:919–930

Morson BC, Dawson IMP, Day DW, Jass JR, Price AB, Williams GT (1990) Morson and Dawson's gastrointestinal pathology, 3rd edn. Blackwell, Oxford

Nalbandian H, Sheth N, Dietrich R, Georgiou J (1985) Intestinal ischemia caused by cocaine ingestion: report of two cases. Surgery 97:374–376

Nelson RL, Briley S, Schuler JJ, Abcarian H (1992) Acute ischemic proctitis. Dis Colon Rectum 35:375–380

Nelson SW, Eggleston W (1960) Findings on plain roentgenograms of the abdomen associated with mesenteric vascular occlusion with a possible new sign of mesenteric venous thrombosis. AJR 83:886–894

Nolan DJ (1983) Radiological atlas of gastrointestinal disease. John Wiley, New York

Nolan DJ (1994) Vascular disorders of the small intestine. In: Freeny PC, Stevenson GW (eds) Margulis and Burhenne's alimentary tract radiology, 5th edn. Mosby, St. Louis, pp 649–658

Patten RM, Coldwell DM, Ben Menachem Y (1991) Ligamentous compression of the celiac axis: CT findings in five patients. AJR 156:1101–1103

Philpotts LE, Heiken JP, Westcott MA, Gore RM (1994) Colitis: use of CT findings in differential diagnosis. Radiology 190:445–449

Potish RA, Jones TK, Levitt SH (1979) Factors predisposing to radiation-related small-bowel damage. Radiology 132:479–482

Prince MR, Narasimham DL, Stanley JC, Chenevert TL, Williams DM, Marx MV, Cho KJ (1995) Breath-hold gadolinium-enhanced MR angiography of the abdominal aorta and its major branches. Radiology 197:785–792

Queloz JM, Woloshin HJ (1972) Sacculation of the small intestine in scleroderma. Radiology 105:513–515

Rhee RY, Gloviczki P, Mendonca CT, et al. (1994) Mesenteric venous thrombosis: still a lethal disease in the 1990s. J Vasc Surg 20:688–697

Roobottom CA, Dubbins PA (1993) Significant disease of the celiac and superior mesenteric arteries in asymptomatic patients: predictive value of Doppler sonography. AJR 161:985–988

Rosen A, Korobkin M, Silverman PM, Dunnick NR, Kelvin FM (1984) Mesenteric vein thrombosis: CT identification. AJR 143:83–86

Rosenberger A, Adler OB, Haim S (1982) Radiological aspects of Behçet disease. Radiology 144:261–264

Scholz FJ (1993) Ischemic bowel disease. Radiol Clin North Am 31:1197–1218

Scott JR, Miller WT, Urso M, Stadalnik RC (1971) Acute mesenteric infarction. AJR 113:269–279

Shapeero LG, Myers A, Oberkircher PE, Miller WT (1974) Acute reversible lupus vasculitis of the gastrointestinal tract. Radiology 112:569–574

Smerud MJ, Johnson CD, Stephens DH (1990) Diagnosis of bowel infarction: a comparison of plain films and CT scans in 23 cases. AJR 154:99–103

Strockbine MF, Hancock JE, Fletcher GH (1970) Complications in 831 patients with squamous cell carcinoma of the intact uterine cervix treated with 3000 rads or more whole pelvis irradiation. AJR 108:293–304

Taourel PG, Fabre JM, Pradel JA, Seneterre EJ, Megibow AJ, Bruel JM (1995) Value of CT in the diagnosis and management of patients with suspected acute small-bowel obstruction. AJR 165:1187–1192

Taourel PG, Deneuville M, Pradel JA, Régent D, Bruel JM (1996) Acute mesenteric ischemia: diagnosis with contrast-enhanced CT. Radiology 199:632–636

Taylor PM, Johnson RJ, Eddleston B, Hunter RD (1990) Radiological changes in the gastrointestinal and genitourinary tract following radiotherapy for carcinoma of the cervix. Clin Radiol 41:165–169

Tomchik FS, Wittenberg J, Ottinger LW (1970) The roentgenographic spectrum of bowel infarction. Radiology 96:249–260

Van Gansbeke D, Avni EF, Delcour C, Engelholm L, Struyven J (1985) Sonographic features of portal vein thrombosis. AJR 144:749–752

Vogelzang RL, Gore RM, Anschuetz SL, Blei AT (1988) Thrombosis of the splanchnic veins: CT diagnosis. AJR 150:93–96

Wang CC, Reeves JD (1960) Mesenteric vascular disease. AJR 83:895–908

Welch GH, Shearer MG, Imrie CW, Anderson JR, Gilmour DG (1986) Total colonic ischemia. Dis Colon Rectum 29:410–412

Weltin G, Taylor KJW, Carter AR, Taylor CR (1985) Duplex doppler: identification of cavernous transformation of the portal vein. AJR 144:999–1001

Wilson C, Gupta R, Gilmour DG, Imrie CW (1987) Acute superior mesenteric ischaemia. Br J Surg 74:279–281

Yuhasz M, Laufer I, Sutton G, Herlinger H, Caroline DF (1985) Radiography of the small bowel in patients with gynecologic malignancies. AJR 144:303–307

Zirinsky K, Markisz JA, Rubenstein WA, et al. (1988) MR imaging of portal venous thrombosis: correlation with CT and sonography. AJR 150:283–288

15 Traumatic Injury to the Bowel and Mesentery

M.P. Federle

CONTENTS

15.1 Etiology and Epidemiology

Traumatic injury to the bowel and mesentery is relatively uncommon but can be life-threatening if diagnosis and repair are delayed. Penetrating injuries of the peritoneal cavity from stab wounds or high-velocity gunshot are usually not a diagnostic problem for radiologists as these patients almost invariably have open surgical exploration. Low-velocity shotgun wounds may not penetrate the abdominal wall, and computed tomography (CT) may be requested to confirm evidence of penetration into the peritoneal cavity or retroperitoneal organs. Stab wounds of the back or flank place the colon at risk and will be discussed below. Penetrating injuries of the rectosigmoid colon result from foreign body insertion. Water-soluble contrast enema examination can provide evidence of transmural laceration and/or intraperitoneal colonic involvement that requires surgical repair.

Bowel and mesenteric injuries are found in 5% of patients who have surgical exploration following blunt abdominal trauma (Buck et al. 1986; Cox 1984). Most injuries result from motor vehicle accidents, although direct blows and falls are common etiologies as well. Mesenteric injuries are about 3 times more frequent than bowel injuries and associ-

ated extra-gastrointestinal injuries are present in at least half of all cases.

Clinical or radiographic evidence of a horizontal (Chance) fracture of the spine or a lap-type seat belt hematoma of the abdominal wall is convincing evidence of substantial trauma to the bowel and mesentery (Asbun et al. 1990). Such injuries coexist so frequently that some trauma surgeons recommend surgical exploration of all such accident victims. Lacerations of the pancreas or left lobe of liver are also associated with bowel and mesenteric injuries. Mesenteric injuries are frequently mild and may consist of minor hemorrhage from torn veins. Such lesions, along with superficial liver lacerations, are the most common reason for nontherapeutic laparotomy, especially when the main criterion for surgery is a "positive" diagnostic peritoneal lavage (Buck et al. 1986; Fabian et al. 1986; Fischer et al. 1978). Other mesenteric injuries, however, are more important and torn mesenteric vessels can lead to life-threatening hemorrhage or bowel ischemia and necrosis.

Blunt trauma may result in injuries to the gut ranging from minor intramural hematoma to complete transection. Children more frequently develop hematoma rather than laceration, in large part because they are usually the victims of rather low-velocity trauma (falls, sports injuries, etc.) rather than motor vehicle accidents. Adult victims of car accidents more commonly have transmural laceration of bowel or substantial mesenteric hemorrhage.

15.2 Clinical Evaluation and Diagnostic Testing

Diagnosis of bowel injuries and differentiation of those requiring surgery from those than can be left to heal on their own are notoriously difficult. The classic clinical triad of absent bowel sounds, tenderness, and rigidity are absent in two-thirds of patients (Asbun et al. 1990; Burney et al. 1983). The signs of

M.P. Federle, MD, Department of Radiology, University of Pittsburgh Medical Center, DeSota at O'Hara Street, Pittsburgh, PA 15213, USA bowel injury may be masked by other abdominal or extra-abdominal injuries. Even patients with an intact sensorium may have no clear indications of peritonitis even with complete bowel transection, because the normal small bowel contents have a neutral pH and a low bacteria count. Morbidity and mortality rise rapidly, however, with delays in diagnosis as peritonitis develops; more than 50% of patients with duodenal or jejunal laceration will die if surgical repair is delayed for more than 2 days (Roman et al. 1971; Lucas and Ledgerwood 1975).

Diagnostic peritoneal lavage (DPL) consists of the sterile catheterization of the peritoneal cavity with infusion of 1 l of saline. The fluid is then recovered and examined for blood, and possibly bowel contents, amylase, and other contaminants. The reported accuracy of DPL for diagnosis of bowel injury varies considerably. Injuries to retroperitoneal segments of the duodenum and colon are not detected, and some cases of small bowel injury have normal or equivocal findings when DPL is performed soon after the trauma. DPL becomes more accurate with inter-

vals of time following the injury (Burney et al. 1983; Fabian et al. 1986; Fischer et al. 1978; Ryan et al. 1986).

Hematologic and biochemical tests such as serum amylase levels and differential blood count are of little value in the evaluation of acute injuries.

Plain radiographic studies also play a relatively minor role in acute setting of blunt abdominal trauma. Plain films are neither sensitive nor specific, and contrast studies of the gastrointestinal tract are usually contraindicated. Patients who must be evaluated for bowel trauma are also at risk for other visceral injuries. The presence of dense contrast media in the gut may preclude accurate subsequent evaluation by CT or angiography (Fig. 15.1).

15.3
Computed Tomography

Computed tomography is of proven value in diagnosing abdominal visceral injuries. The presence,

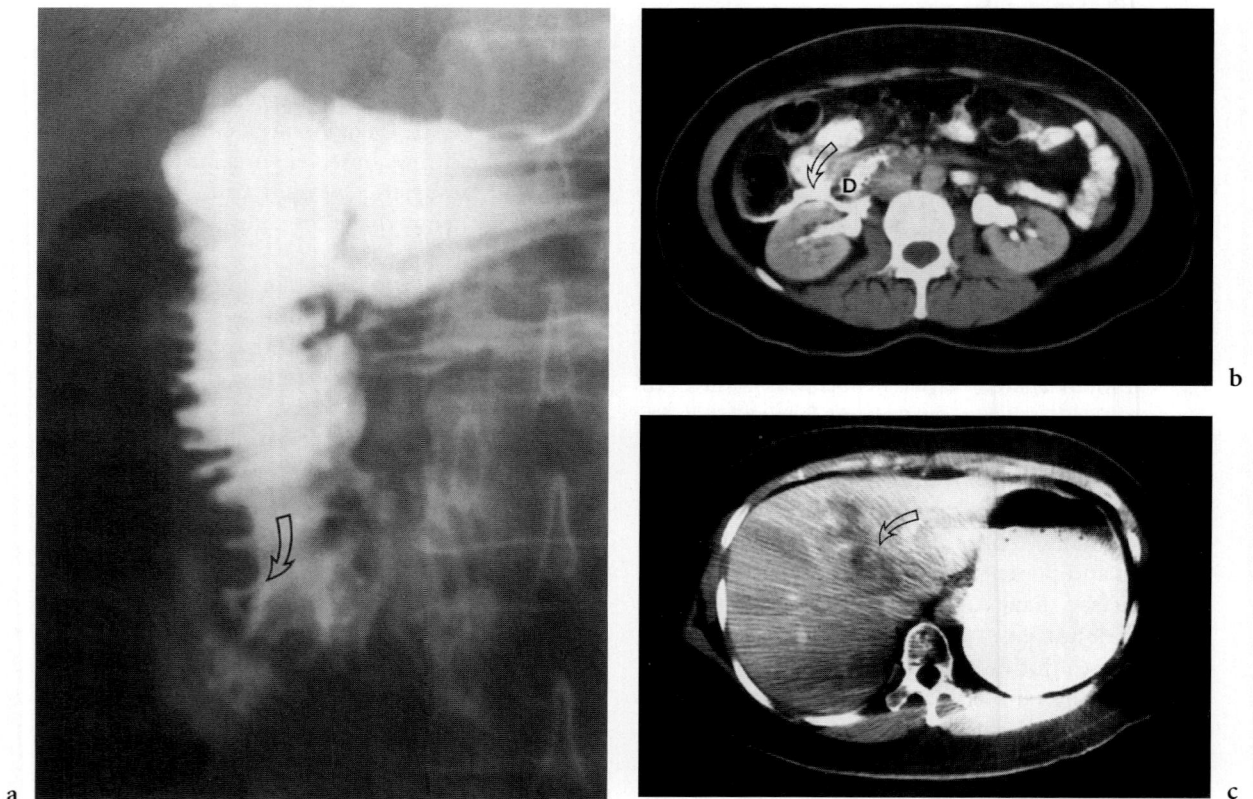

Fig. 15.1 a–c. Duodenal and hepatic laceration. **a** An upper gastrointestinal (UGI) series was requested first and demonstrates intramural hematoma and extravasation of oral contrast medium (*arrow*). **b** Subsequent CT also shows extra-luminal contrast medium (*arrow*) in the retroperitoneum. *D*, Duodenal lumen. **c** The excessively dense contrast medium within the stomach from the UGI series causes artifacts that nearly obscure the hepatic laceration (*arrow*)

amount, and even the source of hemorrhage are usually evident. The accuracy of CT in the diagnosis of bowel and mesenteric injuries remains controversial (COOK et al. 1986; DONAHUE et al. 1987), but excellent results have been reported from several trauma centers, all of which stress the need for optimal CT technique and expert interpretation. Several investigators have reported direct or indirect CT signs of bowel trauma in 85%–95% of initial CT evaluations, and in up to 100% of scans delayed up to 4 h after trauma (BULAS et al. 1989; DONAHUE et al. 1987; MIRVIS et al. 1992; MIYAKAWA et al. 1992; NGHIEM et al. 1993; RIZZO et al. 1989).

15.3.1
CT Techniques

All CT scans for evaluation of abdominal trauma are performed in a similar fashion, with all patients receiving 100–150 ml of intravenous contrast medium (2 ml/kg) as a sustained 2 ml/s bolus. Nonionic contrast is preferable to minimize adverse effects, including nausea. Scanning should be initiated after a 60-s delay to allow adequate and uniform enhancement of abdominal organs. Delays of 70–100 s can be used if a helical CT scanner is to be used.

Artifacts must be minimized, with removal or repositioning of ECG leads and various tubes and catheters from the upper abdomen whenever possible. If the arms cannot be positioned over the head or chest, they should be immobilized against the torso rather than allowing them to lie close to the CT detectors.

The use of oral contrast medium makes recognition of bowel wall thickening easier and is almost essential for identification of extravasation of bowel contents. While some physicians have expressed concern over possible dangers of aspiration of such contrast media, we have recently completed a review of more than 500 consecutive abdominal trauma CT scans and found no instances of aspiration or other adverse effects related to the performance of the CT scan (FEDERLE et al. 1995). Obtunded or uncooperative patients have 450 ml of a 2.5% solution of iodinated contrast medium (diatrizoate meglumine and sodium) administered through a nasogastric tube following endotracheal intubation. Alert, cooperative patients drink the same volume and concentration of contrast.

The CT images are reviewed at standard abdominal window width and level (350–400 HU and 45 HU, respectively). In addition, images should be reviewed at bone windows (for fractures) and lung windows for the purpose of detecting pneumothorax and pneumoperitoneum.

15.3.2
CT Findings

15.3.2.1
Extraluminal Gas

Free air in either the peritoneal cavity or the retroperitoneum after blunt trauma is highly suggestive of bowel perforation. Potential pitfalls include mistaking pneumothorax or gas in the abdominal wall for pneumoperitoneum. The intraperitoneal air may result from urinary bladder rupture, or the female genital tract. Performance of diagnostic peritoneal lavage prior to CT is a major potential pitfall, as patients usually have retained fluid and gas.

The presence of extraluminal gas may be subtle or even absent in cases of small bowel perforation. Viewing scans at a window width of more than 500 HU is essential. Free intraperitoneal gas is most frequently recognized in the subphrenic spaces, especially ventral to the dome of the liver (Fig. 15.2). The air may be trapped in the leaves of the mesentery and can often be found in a focal collection near the site of laceration (Fig. 15.3). Because the small bowel in the ambulatory patient is largely gasless, some cases of transmural laceration may have no extraluminal gas, even in the presence of extravasated oral contrast medium. CT evidence of free air is seen in less than 60% of cases with proved bowel laceration (DONAHUE et al. 1987; MIRVIS et al. 1992).

15.3.2.2
Extraluminal Fluid

Free intraperitoneal fluid in the absence of an apparent solid visceral injury is an important clue to possible bowel or mesenteric trauma, although small amounts of fluid in the pouch of Douglas or Morison may be found, particularly in young women, as a physiologic or clinically benign condition (LEVINE et al. 1995). In our original series of 28 patients with surgically proven bowel injuries, we found abdominal fluid collections in 27 (96%) (RIZZO et al. 1989). The fluid may be of low attenuation (<20 HU), possibly representing extravasated bowel contents; of intermediate density (25–50 HU) from hemo-

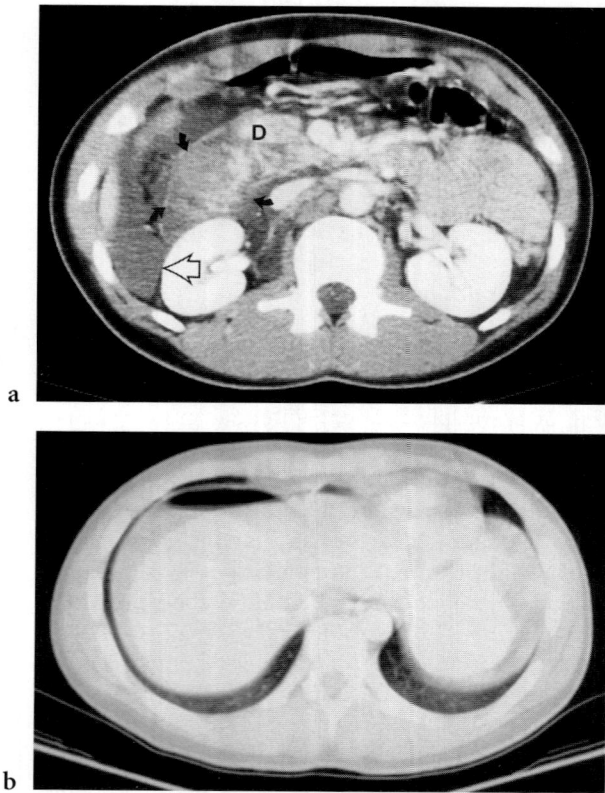

a

b

Fig. 15.2 a,b. Duodenal laceration. a Standard soft tissue window levels demonstrate disruption of the wall of the duodenum (*D*), extravasated contrast medium and blood in the retroperitoneum (*arrows*), and free intraperitoneal fluid (*open arrow*). b Lung window levels demonstrate free air and fluid under the right hemidiaphragm

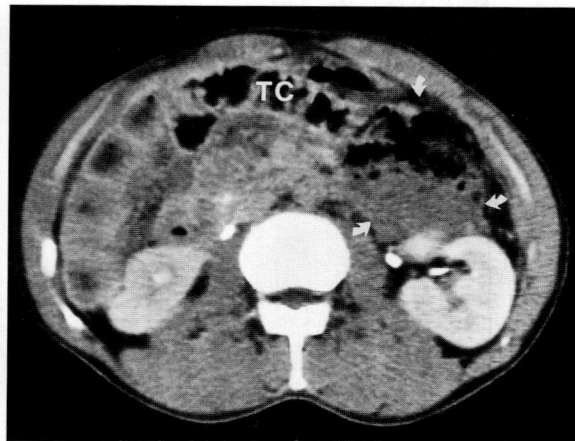

Fig. 15.3. Transverse colon transection. A focal collection of gas and mottled fluid (*arrows*) is present in the omentum and mesentery adjacent to the transected transverse colon (*TC*)

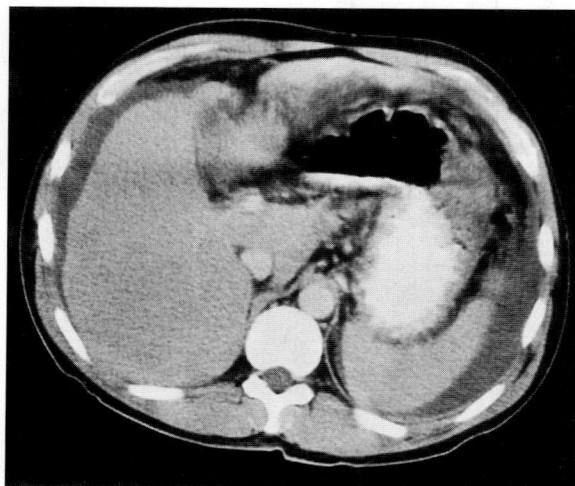

Fig. 15.4. Gastric hematoma and hemoperitoneum. The wall of the greater curvature of the stomach is focally thickened. Free intraperitoneal blood (40 HU) is present but the liver and spleen are normal. Bleeding mesenteric vessels were found at surgery

peritoneum (Fig. 15.4); or of very high density (>150 HU), representing extravasated oral contrast medium (FEDERLE and JEFFREY 1983).

Other causes of low-density fluid include preexisting ascites, ruptured gallbladder or urinary bladder, and transudation of fluid following severe hypotension and subsequent volume reexpansion.

Blood or other fluid lying between loops of bowel is an important and specific finding indicating injury of the bowel or mesentery. Bleeding from hepatic or splenic laceration accumulates in the subphrenic spaces and extends to the pelvis via the paracolic gutters, rarely extending into the mesentery (FEDERLE and JEFFREY 1983). Mesenteric blood often appears as triangular fluid collections in the immediate vicinity of the bleeding source (Fig. 15.5) (NGHIEM et al. 1993).

High-density clotted blood, the "sentinel clot" sign, is a reliable indicator of a focal source of bleeding and is often the most evident CT finding in subtle

gastrointestinal or mesenteric injuries (Fig. 15.5) (ORWIG and FEDERLE 1989).

The presence of very high density fluid presents an interesting diagnostic challenge but a specific diagnosis is usually possible (KWAUK et al. 1995). Laceration of large mesenteric veins or arteries results in diffuse intraperitoneal fluid that is isodense with contrast-opacified blood vessels if the scan is obtained while the bolus of IV contrast continues (Figs. 15.6, 15.7). (Scans completed after the bolus has been injected usually demonstrate extravasated blood that

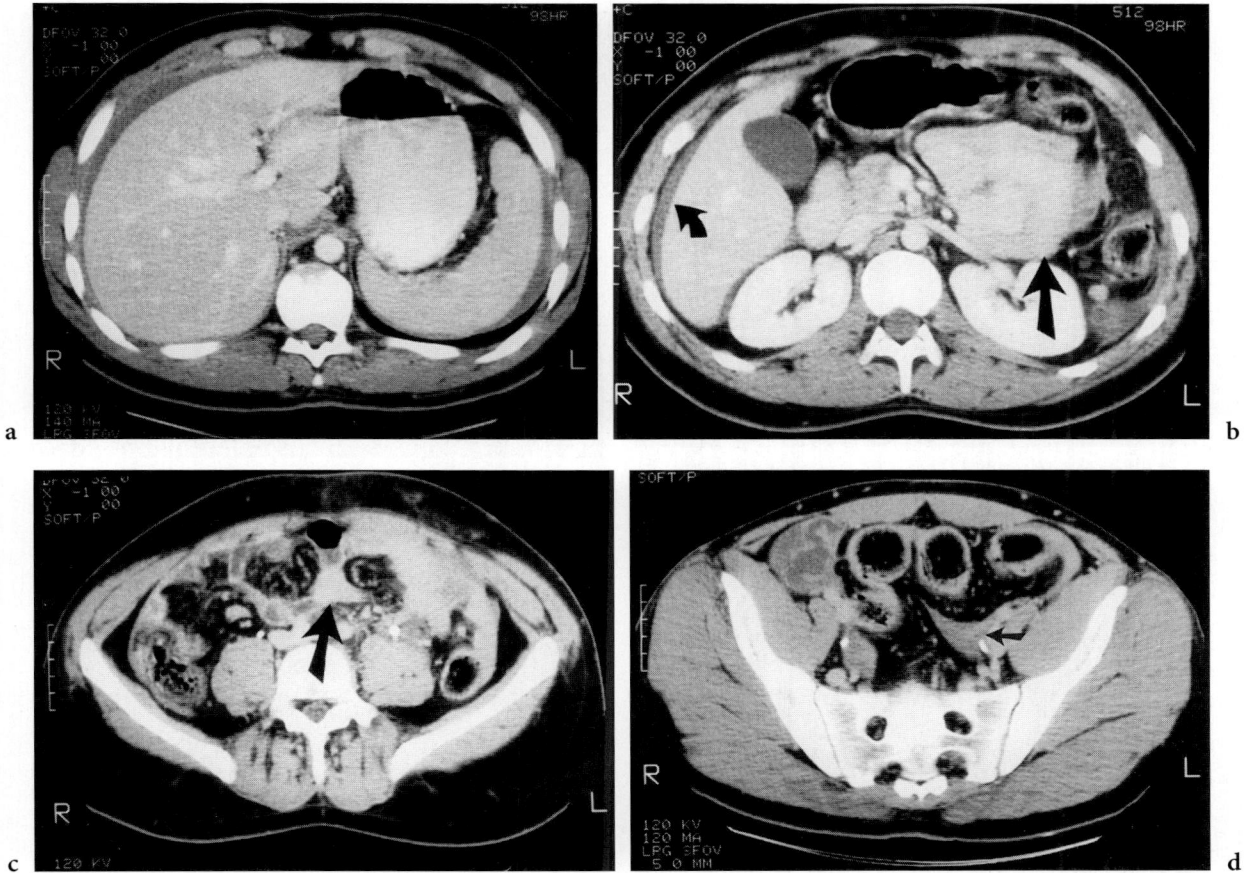

a

b

c

d

Fig. 15.5 a–d. Hemoperitoneum and mesenteric blood with "sentinel clot." a The liver and spleen are normal but blood is present in the subphrenic spaces. b The blood in the right subphrenic space (*curved arrow*) has an attenuation of 45 HU, while the blood surrounding proximal jejunal loops (*straight arrow*) is much more dense. This sentinel clot indicates a focal source of hemorrhage. c, d Lower sections show an additional sentinel clot in the mesentery, and characteristic triangular mesenteric collections of blood (*arrows*). Multiple mesenteric bleeding vessels were found at surgery

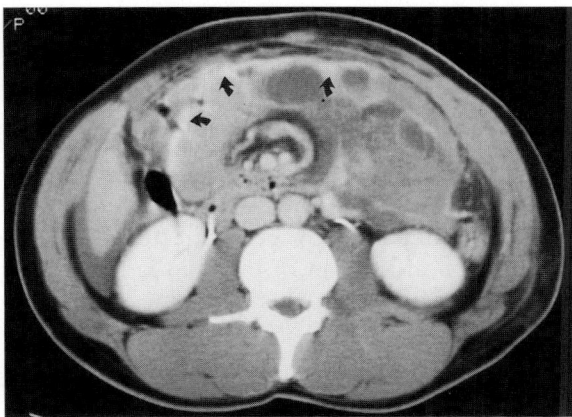

Fig. 15.6. Active extravasation of vascular contrast medium. High-attenuation fluid (*arrows*) that is isodense to blood vessels surrounds small bowel segments. Less dense hemoperitoneum is present in Morison's pouch. Torn large mesenteric veins were found at surgery

is hyperdensse to blood vessels.) In two published reports, actively bleeding arterial hemorrhage was easily recognized as focal or diffuse fluid having a mean attenuation of about 130 HU (range, 100–130 HU depending on the amount, rate, concentration, and timing of the IV contrast bolus) (Fig. 15.6) (JEFFREY et al. 1991; SHANMUGANATHAN et al. 1993).

Extravasated oral contrast medium should be isodense with intraluminal contrast in the affected or contiguous bowel segment. Bowel rupture is usually accompanied by pneumoperitoneum, focal bowel wall thickening, and focal hemorrhage (Figs. 15.7, 15, 8) (BULAS et al. 1989; DONAHUE et al. 1987; MIRVIS et al. 1992; RIZZO et al. 1989).

Rupture of the urinary bladder results in retroperitoneal collections of fluid that may be extremely dense (>200 HU) if a retrograde cystogram has pre-

Fig. 15.8 a,b. Jejunal laceration. Intramural hematoma causes thickening of the duodenum and jejunum. Extravasated oral contrast (*arrow*) indicates laceration of the wall

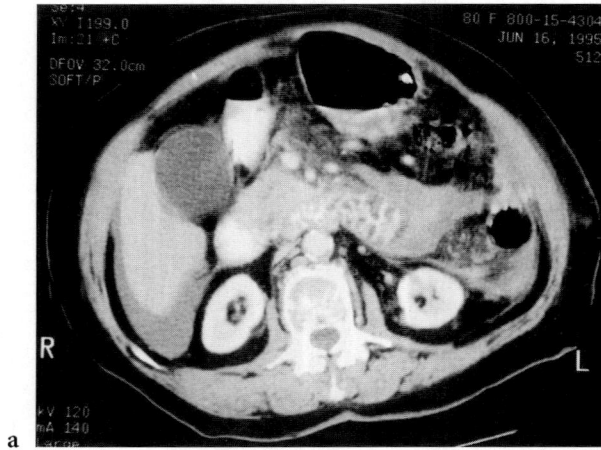

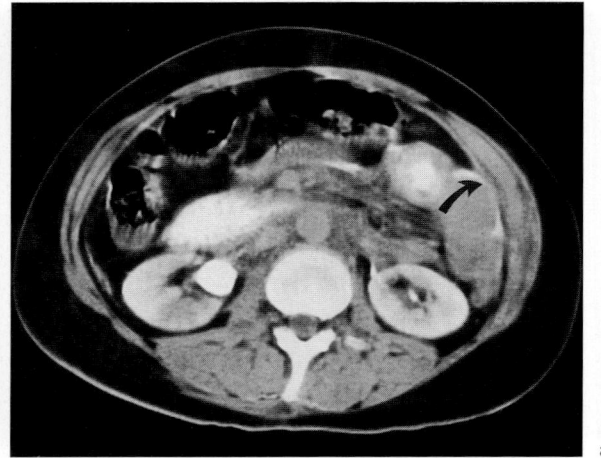

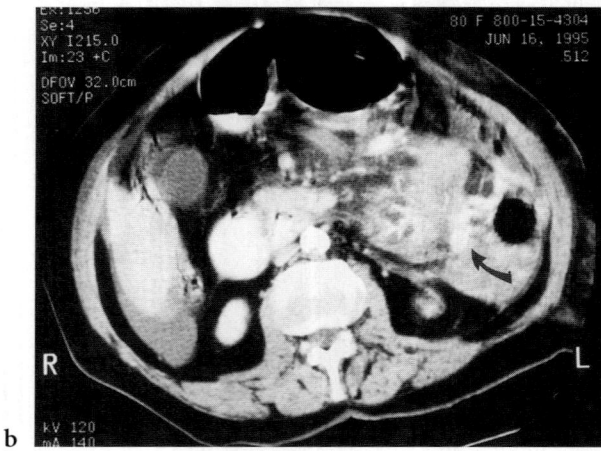

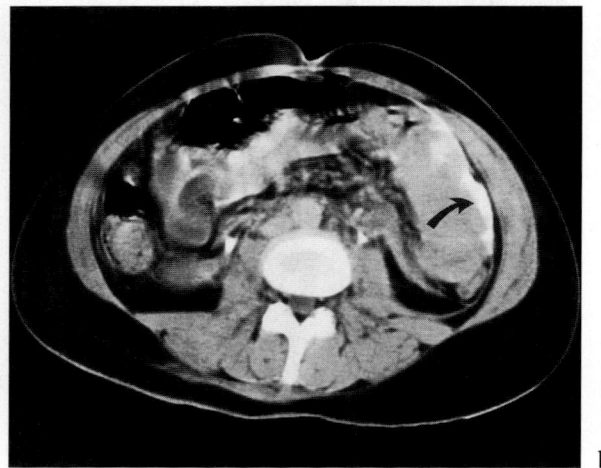

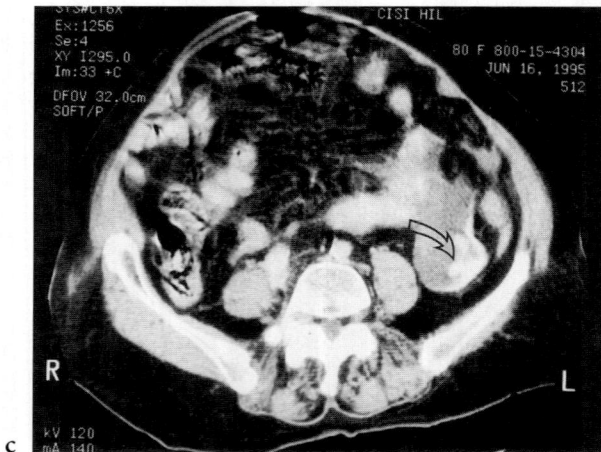

Fig. 15.7 a–c. Jejunal and mesenteric laceration; active extravasation. **a** Intramural hematoma in the transverse duodenum with adjacent sentinel clot. Hemoperitoeneum in Morison's pouch. **b** Near the ligament of Treitz a heterogeneous high attenuation collection includes fluid isodense with bowel contents (*curved arrow*). **c** A more caudal CT section shows mesenteric collection of fluid (*open arrow*) isodense with blood vessels, representing active arterial hemorrhage

ceded the CT scan. If no retrograde contrast has been administered, intraperitoneal bladder rupture usually results in large amounts of near water density ascitic fluid collecting within the dependent peritoneal recesses. Extraperitoneal bladder rupture is usually accompanied by pelvic fractures and the extraperitoneal location of the fluid is not usually mistaken for bowel contents (MEE et al. 1987).

15.3.2.3
Bowel Wall Thickening

Computed tomography can depict bowel wall hematomas as eccentric or circumferential thickening of the wall. Large focal hematomas may have

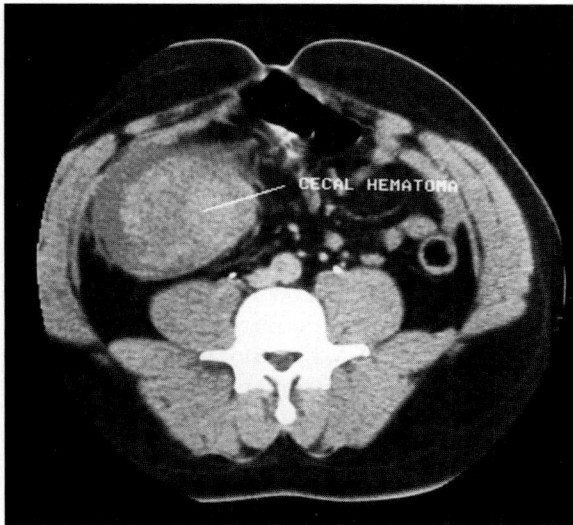

Fig. 15.9. Cecal hematoma. A high-attenuation mass obliterates the lumen of the cecum and ascending colon

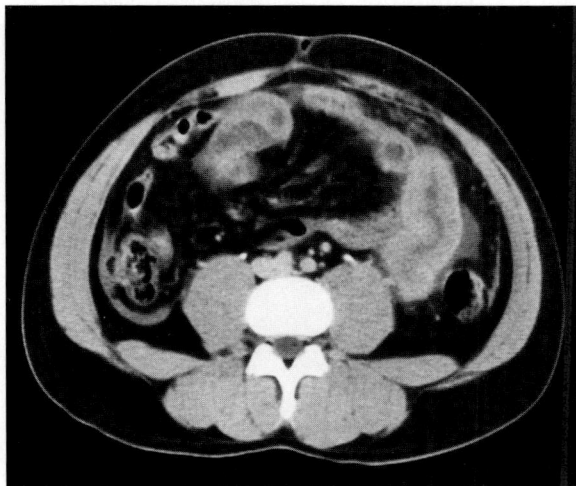

Fig. 15.10. Jejunal laceration. Wall thickening and serosal enhancement with an adjacent focal fluid collection indicate bowel perforation and focal peritonitis

Fig. 15.11 a,b. Diffuse bowel wall thickening due to shock. The wall of the small intestine is diffusely thickened and intensely enhanced. Transudated fluid is present in the mesentery and peritoneal recesses. Note also the "collapsed cava" sign, a flattened inferior vena cava and renal veins due to hypovolemia

characteristically high density (>60 HU) (Fig. 15.9), while more diffuse intramural hemorrhage precludes accurate determination of attenuation values. We have identified focal bowel wall thickening in about 75% of cases with surgically proven bowel injuries (DONAHUE et al. 1987). Intense enhancement of the bowel wall accompanied by bowel wall thickening and free intraperitoneal fluid correlates well with bowel preformation and peritonitis (Fig. 15.10) (HARA et al. 1992; MIRVIS et al. 1992).

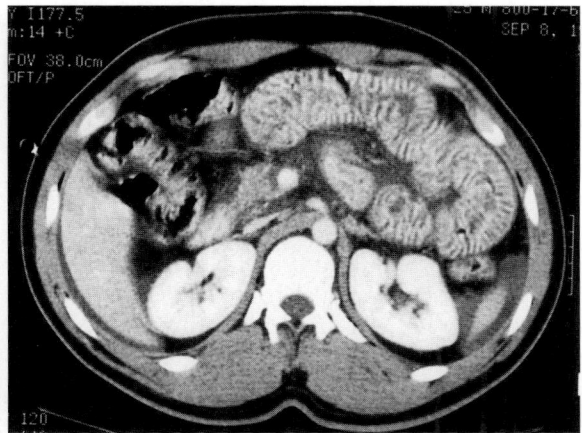

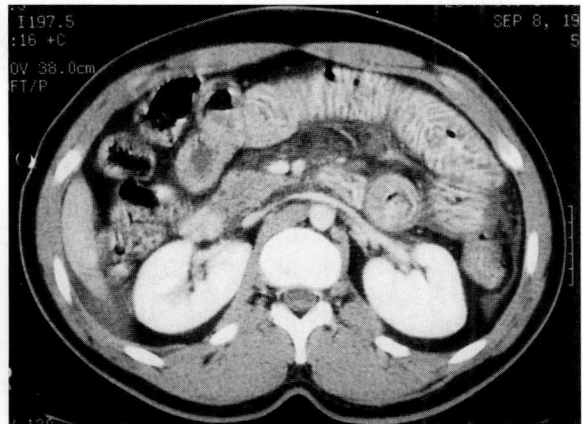

Bowel wall thickening itself is a nonspecific finding, and will be seen in many trauma patients who have preexisting bowel pathology (e.g., inflammatory bowel disease), ascites, or hypoproteinemia, among many potential causes. Diffuse bowel wall thickening is also found in response to hemodynamic instability (MIRVIS and SHANMUGANATHAN 1994) (Fig. 15.11). Other associated signs of hypotension or shock are poor perfusion and function of the spleen and kidneys, the "collapsed cava" sign (a slit-like appearance of the inferior vena cava and renal veins due to hypovolemia), and transmural exudation of low-density fluid into the peritoneal cavity (JEFFREY and FEDERLE 1988; TAYLOR et al. 1987).

15.3.3
CT Features of Specific Injuries

15.3.3.1
Stomach

Gastric rupture from blunt trauma is rare. It occurs more commonly in children but may affect adults, particularly if trauma occurs with a distended stomach (BRUNSTING and MORTON 1987; COURCY et al. 1984). Release of large amounts cf irritative gastric contents into the peritoneal cavity usually results in early diagnosis and intervention. Intramural hematoma has the CT apperance of focal wall thickening of high attenuation (Fig. 15.4).

15.3.3.2
Duodenum

The duodenum is one of the two most commonly injuries segments of the alimentary tract due to its fixed retroperitoneal location and its vulnerability to direct compression against the spine. In children intramural hematoma predominates, while adults usually have transmural laceration. Duodenal hematoma results in wall thickening, often of impressive degree and of characteristically high attenuation (>60 HU), with narrowing of the lumen (Fig. 15.12). Small amounts of fluid or infiltrated fat are often found in the right anterior pararenal space, even if the duodenal wall is intact. CT can reliably distinguish between duodenal hematoma and duodenal perforation. Perforation results in extraluminal gas or contrast material in the retroperitoneum (anterior pararenal space), with gas also present intraperitoneally in many cases due to tearing of fascial planes and peritoneum (BULAS et al. 1989; HOFER and COHEN 1989; KUNIN et al. 1993) (Figs. 15.13, 15.14).

Duodenal and pancreatic trauma often occur together and distinction between them on clinical or CT criteria can be difficult, especially in the absence of extravasation of duodenal contents. Clinical con-

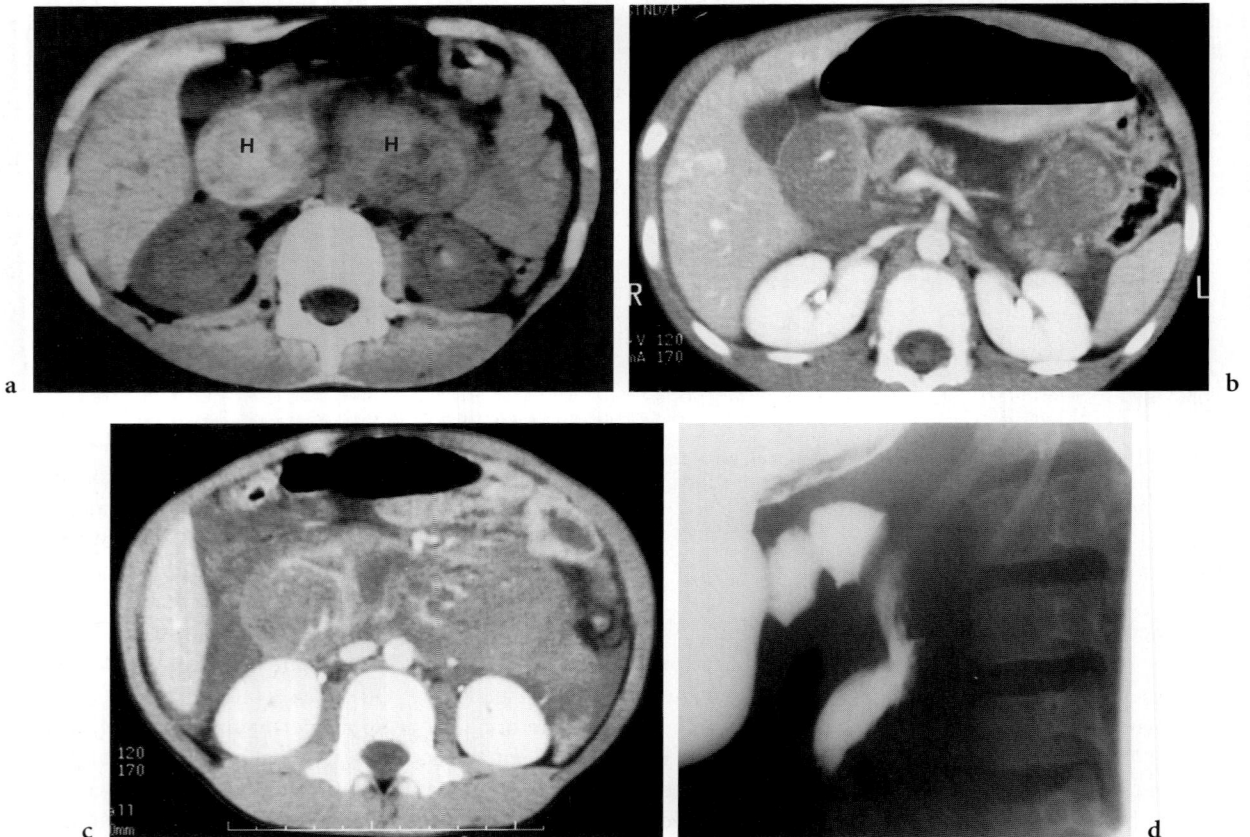

Fig. 15.12 a–d. Duodenal hematoma in a 7-year-old boy. **a** Noncontrast CT demonstrates a high attenuation mass (*H*) that follows the course of the duodenum. **b, c** The lumen of the duodenum is markedly narrowed throughou: its length. Intra-peritoneal and periduodenal retroperitoneal fluid is present, but no extravasation. **d** UGI series confirms intramural hematoma without laceration

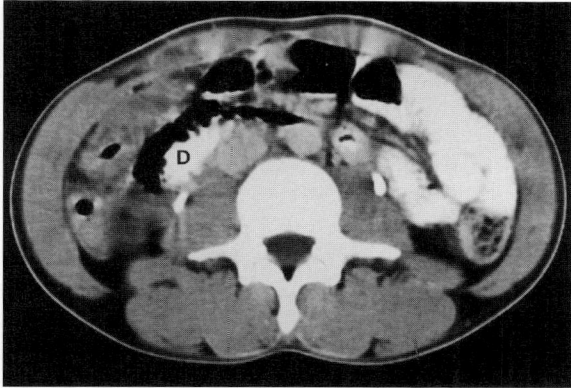

Fig. 15.13. Duodenal laceration. Extraluminal gas follows the course of the duodenum (*D*)

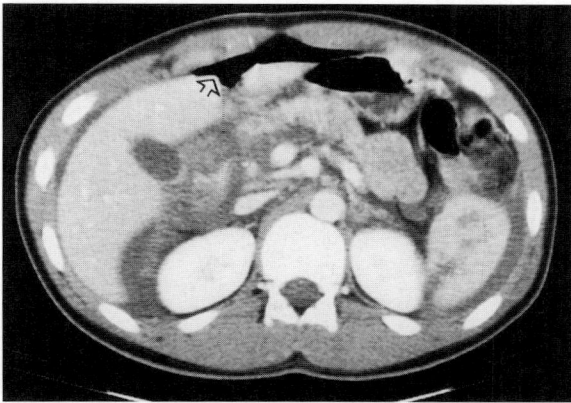

a

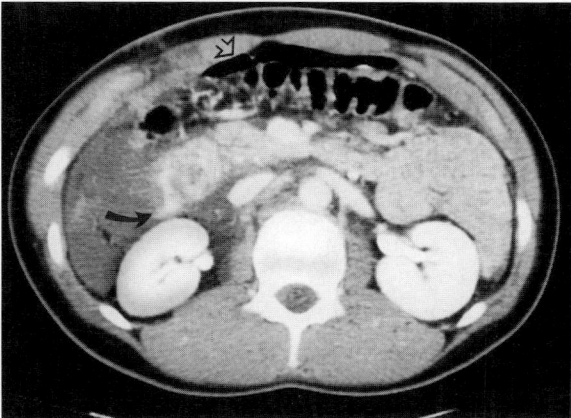

b

Fig. 15.14 a,b. Duodenal laceration. Hemoperitoneum and free intraperitoneal air (*open arrows*) are present. Extraluminal oral contrast (*curved arrow*) is adjacent to the intramural hematoma

cern over pancreatic or duodenal injury may require repeated CT evaluation, endoscopic evaluation with pancreatography, or surgical exploration. Delayed diagnosis and repair of duodenal laceration has a high morbidity and mortality.

15.3.3.3
Small Intestine

The most commonly injured segment of bowel is the proximal jejunum, because its fixation by the ligament of Treitz makes it vulnerable to shearing forces as well as direct compression. Less commonly, the distal ileum is injured near its fixation at the ileocecal valve. While intramural hematoma occurs in children, adults usually suffer transmural rupture of the jejunum along the antimesenteric surface. Because of the nonirritative composition and low bacterial count of intestinal chyme, abdominal pain and signs of peritonitis are slow to develop, leading to potential delays in clinical diagnosis (SCHERK et al. 1983).

The CT findings of intestinal trauma may be subtle but are almost invariably present and multiple. Intraperitoneal fluid is present in more than 90% of cases and the presence of adjacent clotted blood (the sentinel clot) is both common and specific for the site of bleeding (Figs. 15.5–15.8, 15.15). Recently, the Stanford group emphasized recognition of fluid collections between loops of bowel or within mesenteric leaves (NGHIEM et al. 1993). These collections are usually triangular or irregular in shape and are a specific sign of injury to the adjacent bowel or mesentery (Figs. 15.5, 15.10). Extravasation of oral contrast medium or air is a specific sign of perforation, but is seen in less than half of jejunal or ileal lacerations (Fig. 15.16). Intramural hematoma and intense mural enhancement are additional signs of focal trauma and inflammation (BULAS et al. 1989; DONAHUE et al. 1987; HARA et al. 1992; MIRVIS et al. 1992; MIRVIS and SHANMUGANATHAN 1994).

15.3.3.4
Colon

Compression of the upper abdomen caused by a steering wheel or lap-type seat belt predisposes patients to colonic injuries. Injuries of the transverse colon are usually intramural hematoma (Fig. 15.9) or serosal tears without fecal spillage, but any segment of the colon may be perforated, transected, or devascularized (Fig. 15.3). Colonic injuries are usually accompanied by injuries of other bowel or solid viscera (STRATE and GREICO 1983) (Fig. 15.17).

GUR and colleagues (1995) reported several young patients with inflammatory bowel disease who suffered isolated injuries of the colon and terminal ileum including complete transection following relatively minor trauma. They postulate that the stiff diseased bowel wall and mesentery, characteristic of

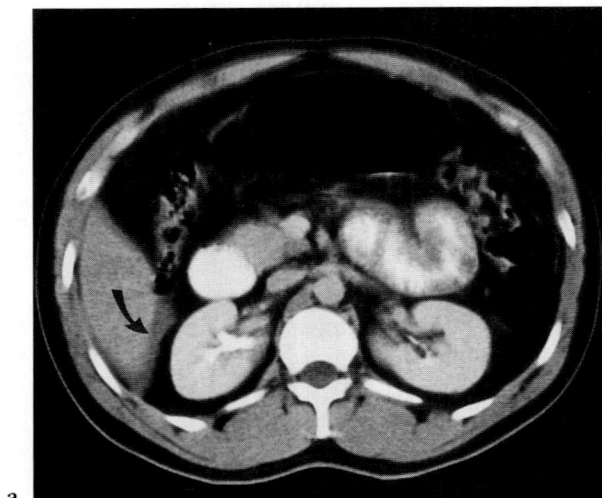

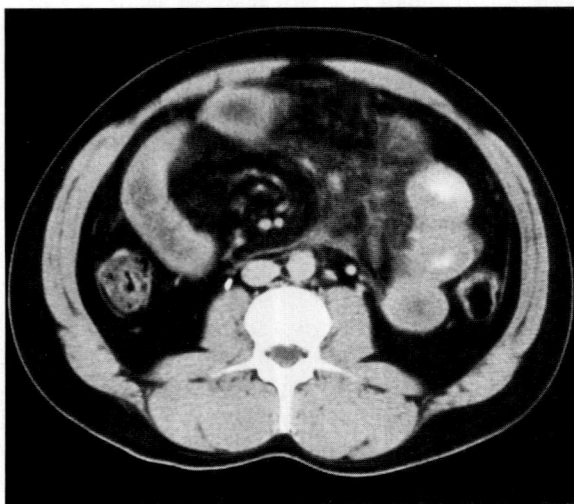

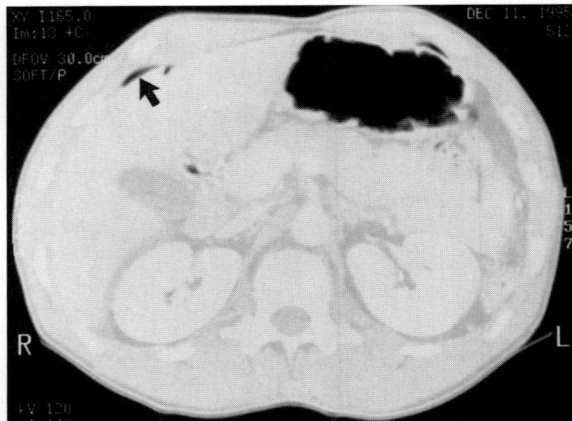

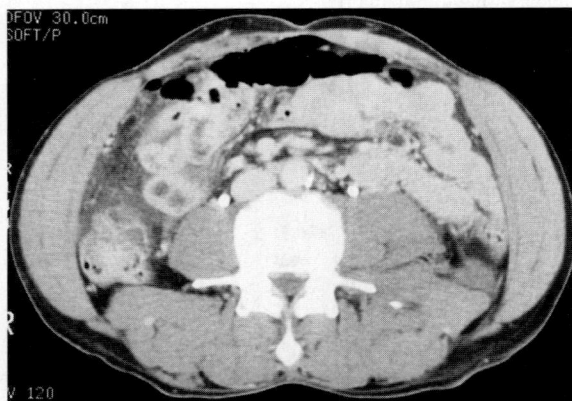

Fig. 15.15 a,b. Jejunal laceration. Intramural hematoma, mesenteric infiltration, and free intraperitoneal fluid (*arrow*) are present. Even though no extravasated contrast or free air was demonstrated, the jejunum was found to be lacerated at surgery

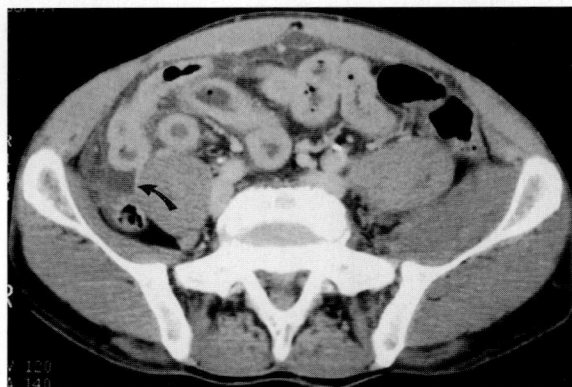

Fig. 15.16 a–c. Ileal laceration. **a** Wide window level imaging shows a small amount of free air (*arrow*). **b, c** Infiltrated mesenteric fat and triangular fluid collections (*curved arrow*) are in the mesentery adjacent to the ileal loops. Note mural thickening and enhancement due to peritonitis

Crohn's and ulcerative colitis, put these patients at increased risk for blunt intestinal rupture.

A modification of the standard CT protocol can be used to evaluate injury to the colon from blunt or penetrating trauma. Concern over missed injuries of the kidney or descending colon mandated surgical exploration in the past, but CT has proven valuable in evaluation of stab wounds of the back or flank. Contrast material (either air or iodinated aqueous solutions) can be introduced via a rectal tube and may be helpful in CT detection of colonic perforation. The depth of penetration of a knife (or shotgun pellets) and the relationship to kidney and colon are usually evident on CT. Confident CT evaluation of these patients frequently results in avoidance of surgery or, conversely, urgent surgery when critical lesions are identified.

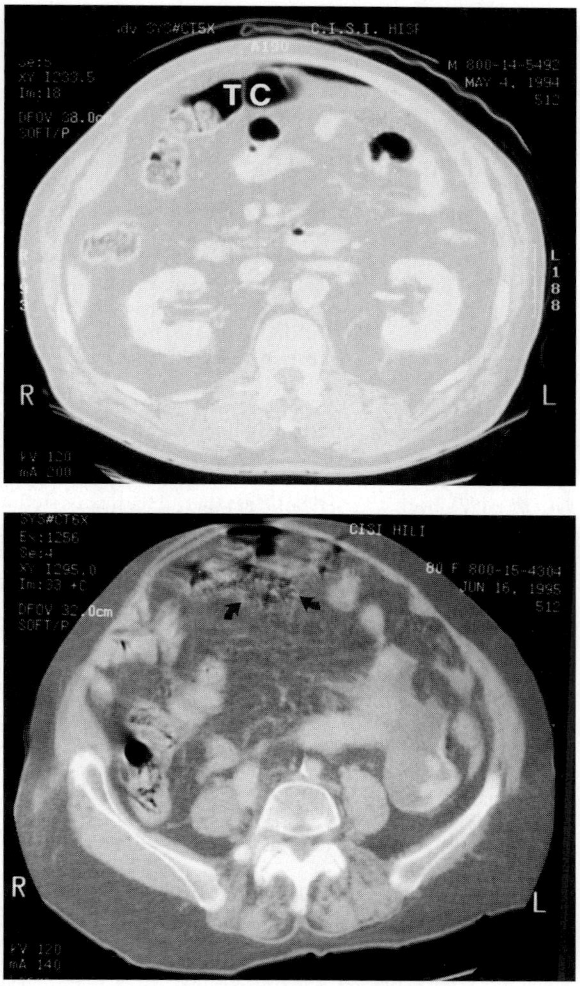

Fig. 15.17 a,b. Colon transection. Extraluminal gas is adjacent to the transverse colon (*TC*) along with disruption of the wall and fecal spillage (*arrows*). This patient also had transection of the jejunum (Fig. 15.7)

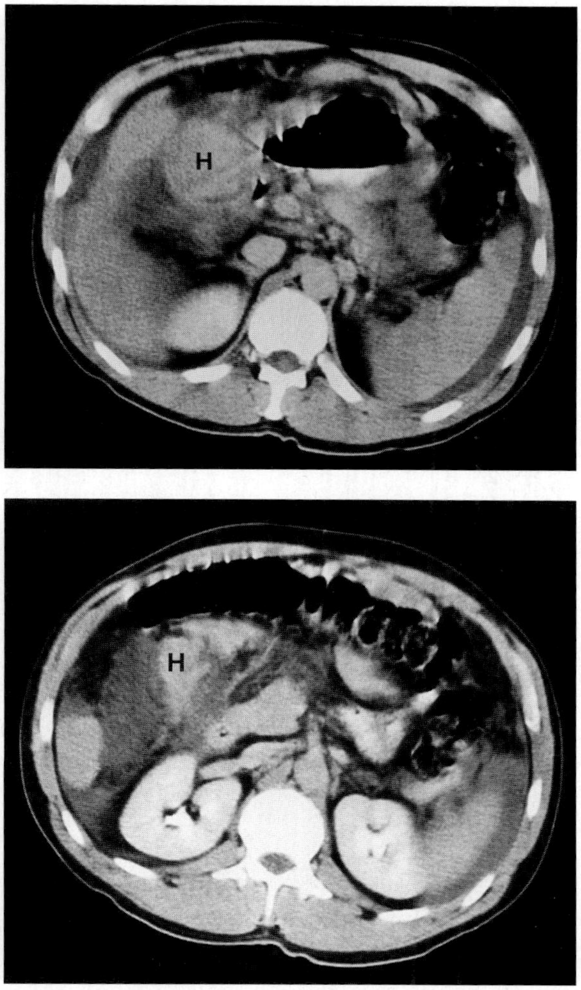

Fig. 15.18 a,b. Mesenteric hematoma. A focal high attenuation mass (*H*) is present in the mesentery along with lower density, more homogeneous blood in the peritoneal recesses. Torn mesenteric blood vessels were found at surgery but no bowel injury

15.3.3.5
Mesentery

Blunt trauma causes mesenteric hemorrhage 3 times more frequently than injury to the bowel itself. Many mesenteric injuries and minor and self-limiting but frequently lead to nontherpeutic laparotomy, especially on the basis of diagnostic peritoneal lavage. Disruption of larger mesenteric arteries or veins can result in major hemorrhage and bowel ischemia.

Signs of mesenteric injury include infiltration of the mesenteric fat, irregular or triangular fluid collections between mesenteric leaves or bowel segments, and a sentinel clot of high density within the mesentery (NGHIEM et al. 1993; ORWIG and FEDERLE 1989; RIZZO et al. 1989) (Fig. 15.18). Mesenteric bleeding usually spreads to dependent peritoneal recesses and along bowel loops. Mesenteric fluid collections are present in nearly all small intestinal and transverse colon injuries, in my experience. Once a mesenteric hematoma has been recognized on CT, a careful search should be made for signs of bowel or mesenteric vascular disruption. In some patients specific signs of bowel injury will not be found but surgery may still be needed to exclude significant bowel or vascular injury.

Table 15.1. CT signs of bowel or mesenteric trauma

Specific
Extraluminal gas
Extraluminal oral contrast medium
Intramural hematoma
Disruption of bowel wall
Extravasation of contrast medium from mesenteric vessels

Suggestive
Bowel wall thickening
Bowel wall enhancement
Free fluid without apparent source
Triangular mesenteric fluid collections
Sentinel clot in mesentery

15.3.3.6
Abdominal Wall

A rare but dramatic result of blunt trauma is acute disruption of the abdominal wall. Herniation of omental fat and bowel is noted on physical examination and on CT. Such injuries indicate massive trauma and surgical exploration is mandatory. Significant injuries to the bowel and mesentery are almost invariably present.

15.4
Summary

Blunt traumatic injuries to the bowel and mesentery are relatively uncommon but cause a disproportionate morbidity and mortality. Specific CT signs of bowel trauma include intramural hematoma, extravasated bowel contents, and free air. Indirect but important signs include the sentinel clot, triangular or irregular interloop fluid collections, and free intraperitoneal fluid without an apparent solid visceral injury (Table 15.1). CT findings can be subtle, particularly soon after the injury, and excellent CT technique is mandatory. CT findings become more evident with increasing delays after trauma, and there should be no hesitation to repeat a CT scan when warranted by continued clinical concern.

References

Asbun H, Irani H, Roe E, et al. (1990) Intraabdominal seatbelt injury. J Trauma 30:189–193

Brunsting L, Morton J (1987) Gastric rupture from blunt abdominal trauma. J Trauma 27:887–890

Buck G, Dalton M, Neely W (1986) Diagnostic laparotomy for abdominal trauma. Am Surg 52:41–43

Bulas DI, Taylor GA, Eichelberger MR (1989) The value of CT in detecting bowel perforation in children after blunt abdominal trauma. AJR 153:561–564

Burney R, Mueller G, Coon G, et al. (1983) Diagnosis of small bowel injury. Ann Emerg Med 12:71–74

Cook DE, Walsh JK, Vick CW, Brewer WH (1986) Upper abdominal trauma: pitfalls in CT diagnosis. Radiology 159:65–69

Courcy P, Soderstrom C, Brotman S (1984) Gastric rupture from blunt trauma: a plea for minimal diagnostics and early surgery. Am Surg 50:424–427

Cox E (1984) Blunt abdominal trauma: a 5-year analysis of 870 patients requiring celiotomy. Ann Surg 199:467–474

Donahue J, Federle M, Griffith B, et al. (1987) Computed tomography in the diagnosis of blunt intestinal and mesenteric injury. J Trauma 27:11–17

Fabian J, Mangiante E, White T, et al. (1986) A prospective study of 91 patients undergoing both computed tomography and peritoneal lavage following blunt abdominal trauma. J Trauma 26:602–608

Federle MP, Jeffrey RB Jr (1983) Hemoperitoneum studied by computed tomography. Radiology 148:187–192

Federle MP, Peitzman A, Krugh J (1995) Use of oral contrast material in abdominal trauma CT scans: is it dangerous? J Trauma 30:57–53

Fischer R, Beverlin B, Engran L, et al. (1978) DPL: 14 years and 2586 patients later. Am J Surg 136:701–704

Gur E, Michowitz M, Abu-Abeid S, et al. (1995) Traumatic rupture of the intestine in patients with inflammatory bowel disease. Am Surg 61:539–542

Hara H, Babyn PS, Bourgeois D (1992) Significance of bowel wall enhancement on CT following blunt abdominal trauma in childhood. J Comput Assist Tomogr 16:94–98

Hofer G, Cohen A (1989) CT signs of duodenal perforation secondary to blunt abdominal trauma. J Comput Assist Tomogr 13:430–432

Jeffrey RB Jr, Federle MP (1988) The collapsed inferior vena cava: CT evidence of hypovolemia. AJR 150:431–432

Jeffrey RB Jr, Cardoza JD, Olcott EW (1991) Detection of active intraabdominal arterial hemorrhage: value of dynamic contrast-enhanced CT. AJR 156:725–729

Kunin JK, Korobkin M, Ellis JH, et al. (1993) Duodenal injuries caused by blunt abdominal trauma: value of CT in differentiating perforation from hematoma. AJR 160:1221–1223

Kwauk S, Wallace K, Hyde P (1995) Gastrointestinal perforation or vascular injury? A diagnostic dilemma for computed tomography in blunt abdominal trauma (case report). Can Assoc Radiol J 46:57–59

Levine CD, Patel VJ, Wachsberg RH, et al. (1995) CT in patients with blunt abdominal trauma: clinical significance of intraperitoneal fluid detected on a scan with otherwise normal findings. AJR 164:1381–1385

Lucas C, Ledgerwood A (1975) Factors influencing outcome after blunt duodenal injury. J Trauma 15:839–846

Mee S, McAninch J, Federle M (1987) Computed tomography in bladder rupture: diagnostic limitations. J Urol 137:207–209

Mirvis SE, Shanmuganathan K (1994) Diffuse small bowel ischemia in hypotensive adults after blunt trauma (shock bowel): CT findings and clinical significance. AJR 163:1375–1379

Mirvis SE, Gens D, Shanmuganathan K (1992) Rupture of the bowel after blunt abdominal trauma: diagnosis with CT. AJR 159:1217–1221

Miyakawa K, Kaji T, Wakabayashi M, et al. (1992) CT of intestinal injuries following blunt trauma. Nippon Igaku Hoshasen Gakkai Zasshi 52:1653–1660

Nghiem HV, Jeffrey RB Jr, Mindelzun RE (1993) CT of blunt trauma to the bowel and mesentery. AJR 160:53–58

Orwig D, Federle M (1989) Localized clotted blood as evidence of visceral trauma on CT: the sentinel clot sign. AJR 153:747–749

Peitzman AB, Makoroun MS, Slasky BS, Ritter P (1986) Prospective study of CT in initial management of blunt trauma. J Trauma 26:585–591

Rizzo M, Federle M, Griffith B (1989) Bowel and mesenteric injury following blunt abdominal trauma: evaluation with CT. Radiology 173:143–148

Roman E, Silva Y, Lucas C (1971) Management of blunt duodenal injury. Surg Gynecol Obstet 132:7–14

Ryan J, Keyes F, Horner W, et al. (1986) Critical analysis of open peritoneal lavage in blunt abdominal trauma. Am J Surg 15:221–223

Scherk W III, Lonchyna V, Moylan J (1983) Preformation of the jejunum from blunt abdominal trauma. J Trauma 23:54–56

Shanmuganathan K, Mirvis S, Sover E (1993) Value of contrast-enhanced CT in detecting active hemorrhage in patients with blunt abdominal or pelvic trauma. AJR 161: 65–69

Strate R, Greico J (1983) Blunt injury to the colon and rectum. J Trauma 23:384–387

Taylor GA, Fallat ME, Eichelberger MR (1987) Hypovolemic shock in children: abdominal CT manifestations. Radiology 164:479–481

16 Perforations of the Alimentary Tract

G.G. Ghahremani

CONTENTS

16.1
Introduction

Even in the current era of modern medicine, perforations of the alimentary tract often present a formidable diagnostic and therapeutic challenge. The task of practicing radiologists is to promptly determine the occurrence of a perforation, its anatomic site and underlying cause, and the potential complications which may follow its conservative or surgical management.

The radiographic hallmark of alimentary tract perforation is extraluminal air, which, depending on its source, will collect in the mediastinum, peritoneal cavity, or retroperitoneal spaces. Unfortunately this important sign may not be visible on plain films in about 30% of cases when perforation is very small, self-sealed, or well contained by the adjacent structures (CHO and BAKER 1994). For example, the

two common entities of perforated appendicitis and diverticulitis are seldom associated with free air. On the other hand, the development of pneumoperitoneum might be due to various processes other than bowel perforation (MILLER et al. 1981). Therefore, the correct diagnosis will usually require opacification of the alimentary tract with radiopaque contrast material to demonstrate better the actual source of leakage at fluoroscopy or CT examination (GHAHREMANI 1993).

Until two decades ago the gastroduodenal ulcers were the major cause of perforation leading to spontaneous pneumoperitoneum. Since the introduction of potent antacid drugs, however, the incidence of this complication has been reduced to a remarkable extent. Nevertheless, perforations of the alimentary tract are being encountered with an increasing frequency and due to a broader spectrum of etiologic factors (Table 16.1). These account for approximately 50 000 cases of gastrointestinal perforations in the United States each year. Particularly significant are the iatrogenic injuries resulting from endoscopic instrumentation of the digestive tract in our aging population. Depending upon the patient's history and physical findings a tailored approach is required for the evaluation and management of suspected gastrointestinal perforations. Therefore, the purpose of this chapter is to provide an updated review of the clinical and radiologic features of perforations involving various segments of the alimentary tract.

16.2
Perforation of the Pharynx and Esophagus

16.2.1
Clinical Aspects

The hypopharynx and cervical esophagus are the most common sites of perforation caused by ingested foreign bodies, endoscopy, or intubation

G.G. GHAHREMANI, MD, Professor and Chairman, Department of Diagnostic Radiology, Evanston Hospital-McGaw Medical Center of Northwestern University, 2650 Ridge Avenue, Evanston, IL 60201, USA

Table 16.1. Etiology of alimentary tract perforations

1. Peptic and drug-induced gastroduodenal ulcers
2. Ischemic, inflammatory, or neoplastic lesions
3. Ingested foreign bodies and caustic agents
4. Blunt or penetrating abdominal trauma
5. Postoperative anastomotic leakage or dehiscence
6. Iatrogenic injuries during endoscopy or intubation
7. Technical mishaps during radiologic examination:
   a) Rectal perforation by enema tip or inflated balloon
   b) Rupture of an obstructed or overdistended colon
   c) Disruption of an ileostomy or colostomy
8. Miscellaneous (postemetic tears, perforated diverticula, etc.)

(GHAHREMANI 1989, 1994b). Less frequent sources are penetrating knife or gunshot wounds, blunt trauma sustained in whiplash injuries, and postoperative tears or leaks (FLYNN et al. 1989; JONES and GINSBERG 1992; KIM-DEOBALD and KOZAREK 1992).

Approximately 80% of accidentally swallowed sharp objects become entrapped in the pharyngoesophageal region. They can penetrate through the pyriform sinuses, valleculae, or the wall of cervical esophagus just below the cricopharyngeus muscle (GHAHREMANI 1989). These anatomic areas are also predisposed to iatrogenic instrumentation injuries. An autopsy study revealed pharyngoesophageal trauma in almost 60% of patients who had intubation or endoscopy during their final days of life (WOLFF and KESSLER 1973). It has been shown that a blindly inserted nasogastric tube or misdirected endotracheal tube may perforate the hypopharynx or cervical esophagus (GHAHREMANI et al. 1980). Fiberoptic endoscopes, with their bullet-shaped tip, can also crush the pharyngoesophageal mucosa against the cervical spine, particularly in elderly patients with osteoarthritic spurs and limited flexibility of their neck. Although modern endoscopes are flexible and inserted under direct vision, they induce pharyngoesophageal perforations in 0.1%–0.4% of the cases (EIMILLER 1992; MEYERS and GHAHREMANI 1975). This incidence is low but nevertheless significant because more than 0.5 million Americans undergo upper gastrointestinal endoscopy each year (GHAHREMANI 1994a; OVERHOLT 1984).

Patients with perforated hypopharynx or cervical esophagus usually experience pain and stiffness in the neck, increased oral secretion, odynophagia, sore throat or hoarseness, and respiratory distress. Localized or diffuse swelling of the neck with crepitation due to soft tissue emphysema develops in most cases.

Perforations of the thoracic esophagus may also complicate intubation or endoscopy (Fig. 16.1). Such iatrogenic injuries tend to occur particularly when the esophageal wall is friable due to preexisting inflammatory or neoplastic processes (FLYNN et al. 1989; GHAHREMANI 1993; KIM-DEOBALD and KOZAREK 1992). Since the esophagus has no serosal layer, the extraluminal leakage will promptly contaminate and incite a necrotizing inflammation in the mediastinum and pleural spaces. The clinical signs and symptoms typically include dysphagia or odynophagia, fever, tachycardia, cyanosis, hypotension, and respiratory distress. Most patients also experience severe chest pain in the retrosternal or interscapular regions, often aggravated by swallowing or breathing. These clinical findings can be further complicated by acute abdominal symptoms when the peritoneal cavity is also contaminated due to rupture of esophagogastric segment in Boerhaave syndrome or iatrogenic mishaps (BLADERGROEN et al. 1986; GHAHREMANI 1994b; HAN and TISHLER 1984).

16.2.2
Radiologic Diagnosis

The most useful initial radiograph when evaluating suspected pharyngoesophageal trauma due to an ingested foreign body or instrumentation is a lateral view of the neck (GHAHREMANI 1989, 1994b). It should be centered just below the angle of mandible to visualize the area between the skull base and thoracic inlet. The patient should preferably be in the upright or sitting position, with the neck extended while the shoulders are held low and posteriorly. In cases of foreign body ingestion, the patient should also be instructed to say "Eeee . . ." during film exposure. This phonation maneuver distends the pharyngolaryngeal region with air, thus enhancing the visibility of compartments where small sharp objects are often entrapped. The same technique can be used to obtain an anteroposterior view of the neck, though it is usually less informative than the lateral radiograph. Sometimes the sharp tip of a bone or needle pierces the pyriform sinus or pharyngoesophageal wall, while the rest of it projects into the air-containing lumen. In such cases the extraluminal leakage of air or contrast may not occur as long as the penetrating object blocks the transmural defect (Fig. 16.1a).

Following a large perforation of the pharynx or cervical esophagus, the radiographs will show exten-

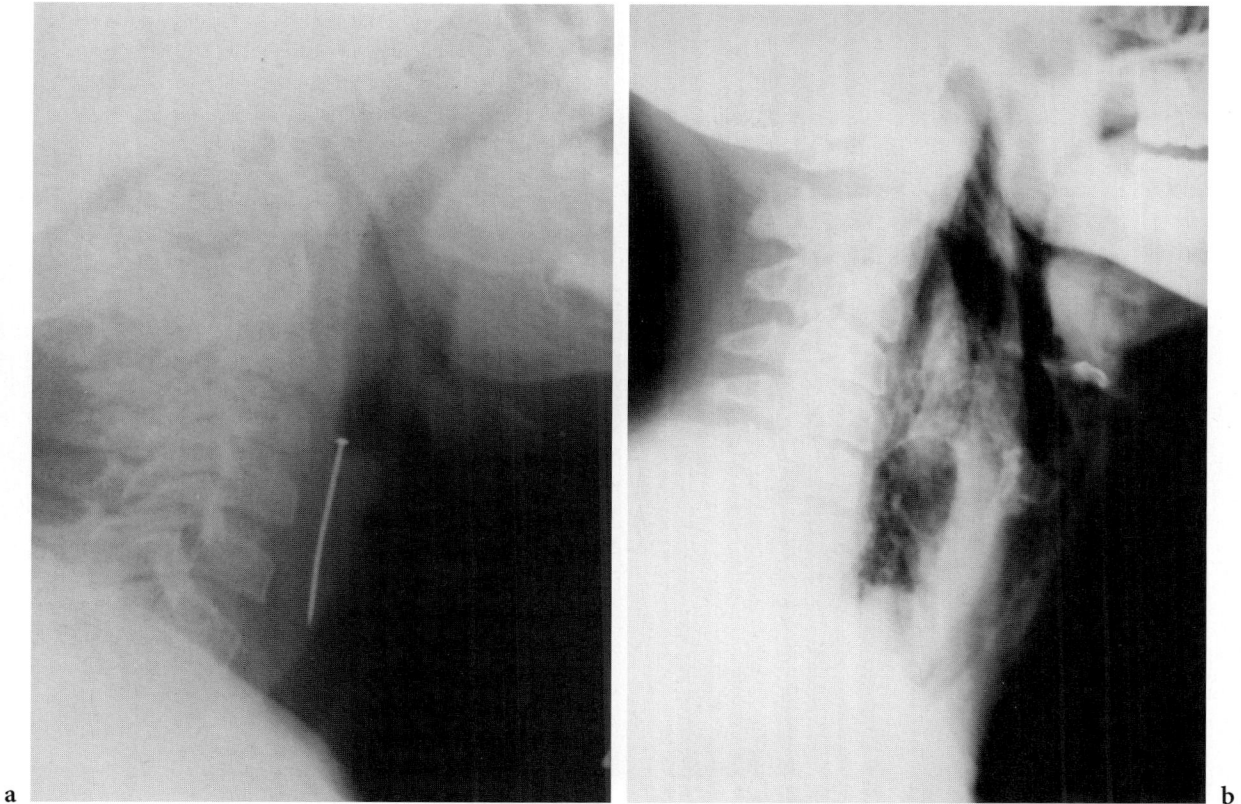

a   b

Fig. 16.1 a,b. Radiographic manifestations of pharyngoesophageal perforation in two patients. **a** Lateral view of the neck shows a swallowed pin piercing the left pyriform sinus and protruding into the prevertebral soft tissues. However, there is no extraluminal air leakage because the small perforation site is plugged by the foreign body. **b** Perforation of the hypopharynx by a misdirected endotracheal tube causing massive soft tissue emphysema of the neck

sive soft tissue emphysema of the neck and swelling of the retropharyngeal region due to edema, hematoma, or abscess (Fig. 16.1b). These findings are usually much more pronounced when the injury is induced by intubation or endoscopy because the misdirected instrument together with insufflated air during its insertion results in the development of a large extraluminal channel and massive emphysema of the neck (GHAHREMANI et al. 1980; MEYERS and GHAHREMANI 1975).

A false passage created by protruding tube or endoscope may persist and opacify during subsequent studies (Fig. 16.2). It could simulate and be mistaken for an esophageal duplication if the clinical history and previous radiographs are not available to the examining radiologist (GHAHREMANI 1981).

The exact site and extent of a pharyngoesophageal perforation is best delineated by extraluminal leakage of contrast media during consecutive swallows monitored by rapid sequence filming at fluoroscopy (Fig. 16.3). It is recommended that water-soluble io-dinated compounds such as diatrizoate meglumine (Gastrografin, Squibb, Princeton, N.J.) be used initially because of their relative safety and rapid absorption (BRICK et al. 1988; DODDS et al. 1982). If there is no obvious leakage or the findings are not clearly visible, however, the examination should be repeated promptly with barium. Experimental and clinical studies have shown that small perforations are much better demonstrated with barium due to its higher radiopacity and certain other physical characteristics (FOLEY et al. 1982).

Chest radiographs are the initial means for evaluating suspected perforations of the thoracic esophagus. The earliest sign is the presence of linear air collections in the mediastinum, fascial planes of the neck, and supraclavicular regions (HAN et al. 1985; O'CONNELL 1981). Further leakage of gas and fluid combined with inflammation and edema cause mediastinal widening, which is best appreciated in the paratracheal area. If the perforation extends to the adjacent pleura, an effusion with or without

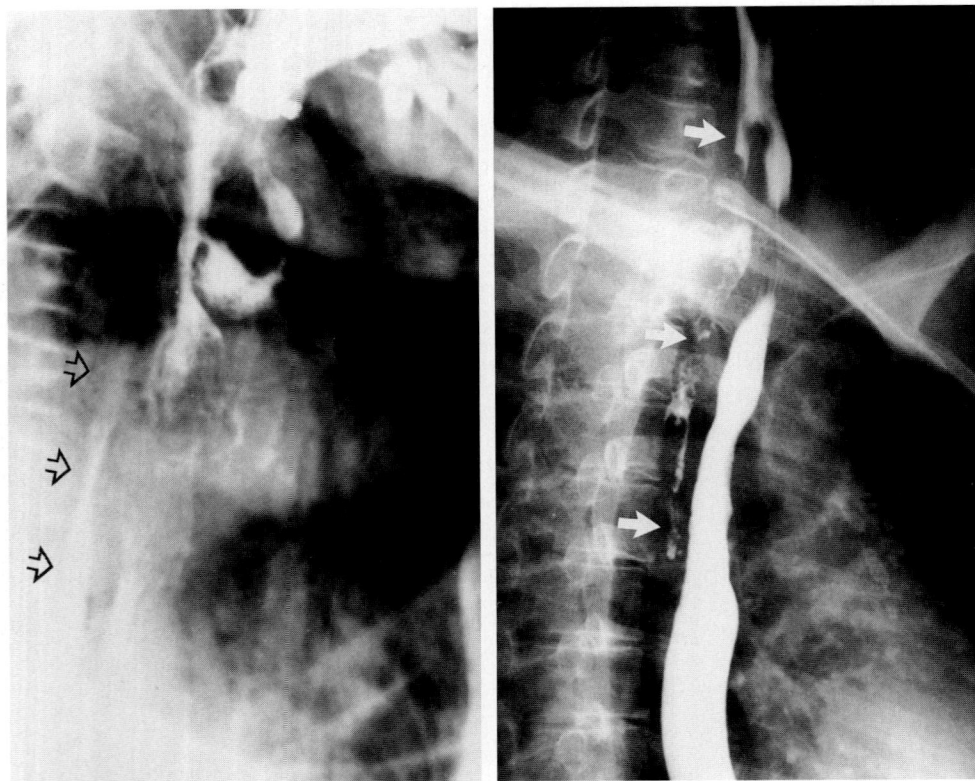

a

b

Fig. 16.2 a,b. Tube-induced perforation of the pharyngoesophageal region. **a** Spot film obtained during initial evaluation with water-soluble contrast material shows extraluminal leakage into the prevertebral false channel (*arrows*). It extends behind the cervical esophagus and is associated with extensive soft tissue emphysema of the neck. **b** Esophagogram 4 months after surgical drainage of the upper mediastinum shows the iatrogenic sinus track (*arrows*), simulating an esophageal duplication. (From GHAHREMANI 1994a)

hydropneumothorax will develop promptly. Even if the integrity of mediastinal pleura is not violated, however, a sympathetic effusion may appear within 48 h. It occurs on the left side in nearly 75% of cases, but can be on the right or bilateral in 5%–10% of the patients. Subsequent chest films may also reveal a left lower lobe consolidation or atelectasis (BLADERGROEN et al. 1986; HAN et al. 1985; KIM-DEOBALD and KOZAREK 1992).

It should be noted that chest radiographs will be normal when the perforation is intramural and thus contained within the esophageal wall. During an upper gastrointestinal endoscopy, for example, the rigid tip of fiberendoscope can lacerate the cervical esophagus and create a false channel as the instrument is advanced distally beneath the mucosa (FOLEY et al. 1982; GHAHREMANI 1994a). This type of intramural perforation is detectable only on a contrast esophagram. It will show the separation of true and false lumina by a thin mucosal stripe, similar to the angiographic appearance of an intimal flap in aortic dissection (Fig. 16.4).

The site of a transmural perforation can be demonstrated by esophagography in approximately 70%–80% of the patients, provided that multiple views of adequately distended esophagus are exposed during fluoroscopy (GHAHREMANI 1993). For this purpose the patient should be examined in a recumbent oblique position while swallowing the contrast material. In uncooperative or semiconscious patients the contrast agent can be injected through a nasogastric tube as it is being withdrawn into the esophagus. Sometimes the initial evaluation with Gastrografin does not show an obvious extravasation, but additional radiographs after administration of barium reveal the findings to better advantage (FOLEY et al. 1982; GHAHREMANI 1994b).

An extraluminal leakage may be minimal and not readily demonstrable if the perforation is very small, closed spontaneously due to focal edema and hematoma, or plugged by the offending object (Fig. 16.5). In the latter situation, the removal of such a foreign body during fluoroscopy would lead to leakage of air and contrast material.

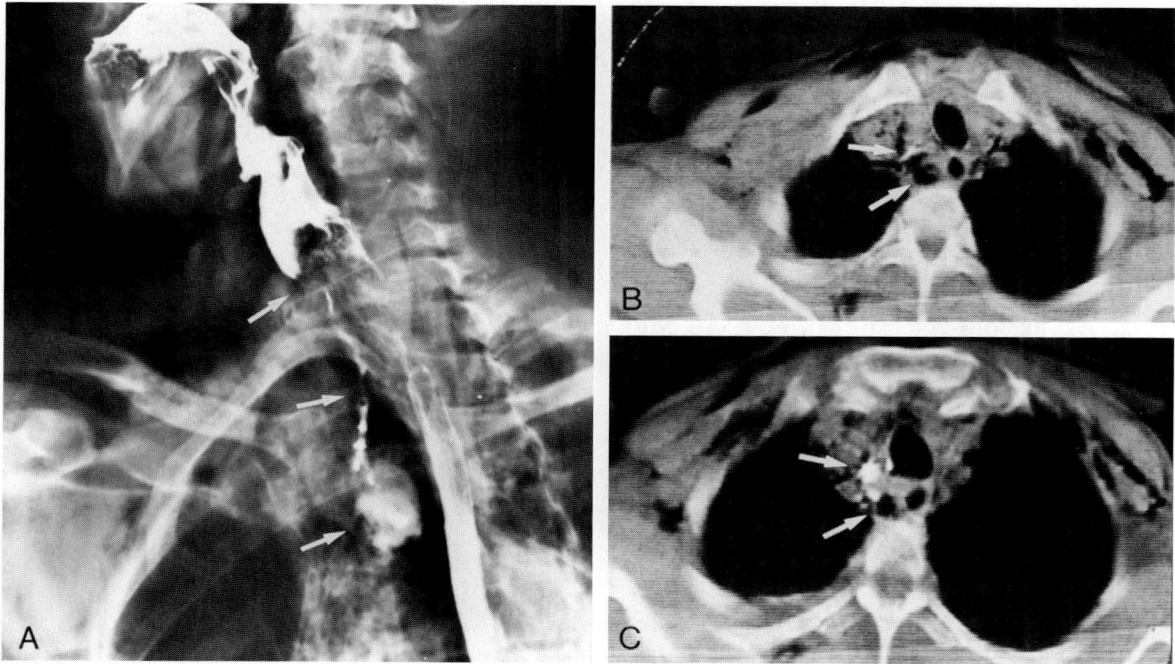

Fig. 16.3 a–c. Perforation of the hypopharynx during an attempted gastroscopy. **a** Evaluation with oral contrast material demonstrates the false passage from the apex of the pyriform sinus into the mediastinum (*arrows*). **b, c** CT sections of the chest show the extraluminal channel and contrast material (*arrows*), associated with pneumomediastinum, right pleural effusion, and massive soft tissue emphysema of the chest wall. (From GHAHREMANI 1994a)

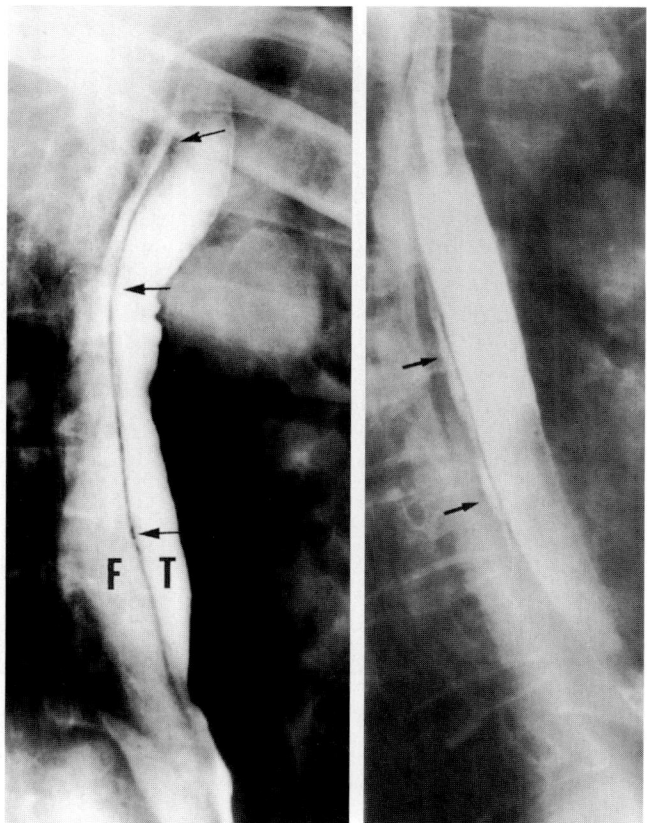

Fig. 16.4 a,b. Intramural dissection of the esophagus in two patients. **a** Longitudinal dissection resulting from submucosal passage of an endoscope after it had penetrated the wall of cervical esophagus. A thin mucosal flap (*arrows*) clearly separates the false channel (*F*) from true esophageal lumen (*T*), but there is no leakage of air or contrast into the mediastinum. **b** Submucosal collection of barium (*arrows*) following extraluminal passage of a guide wire used during dilatation of a distal esophageal stricture

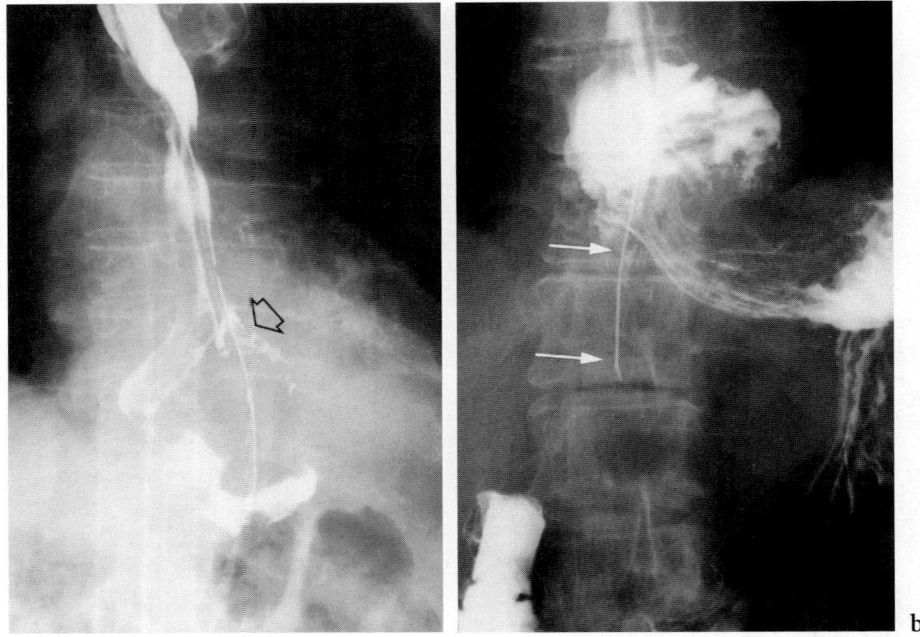

Fig. 16.5 a,b. Iatrogenic esophageal perforations. **a** Rupture of the distal esophagus by a nasogastric tube in an elderly man with reflux esophagitis (*arrow*). Note minimal extravasation around the extruded tube. **b** Perforation of the friable wall of a hiatus hernia in a woman, causing extraluminal protrusion of the nasogastric tube without any leakage of contrast material (*arrow*)

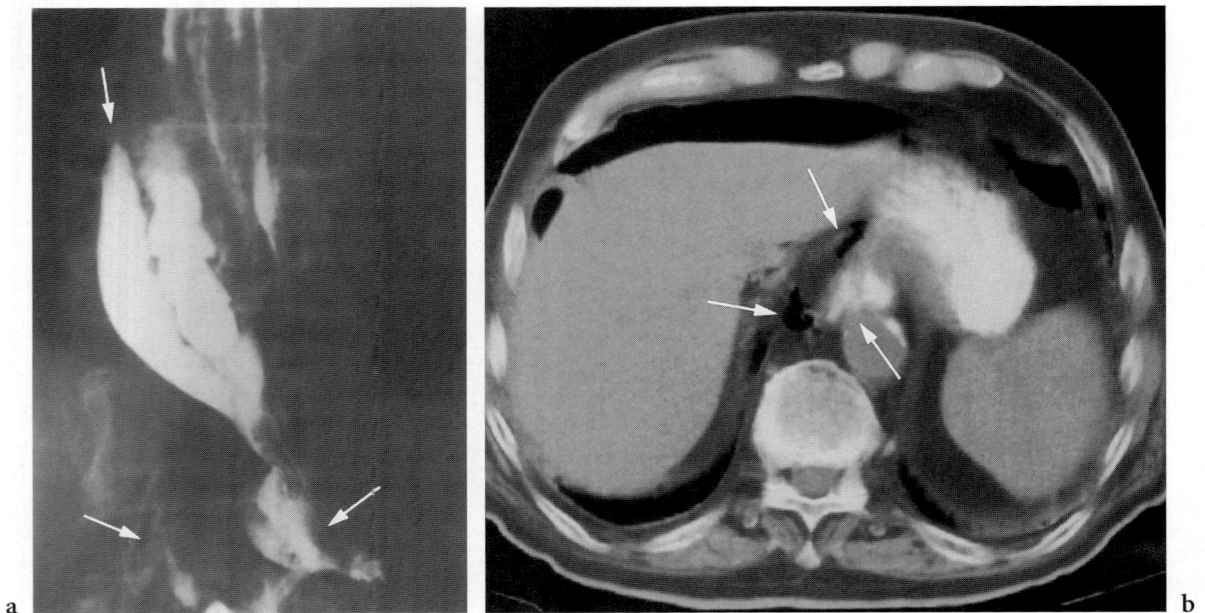

Fig. 16.6 a,b. Transmural rupture of the gastroesophageal segment during pneumatic dilatation for achalasia. **a** Esophagram reveals extravasation into the lower mediastinum and lesser sac (*arrows*). **b** CT section of the upper abdomen shows extraluminal air and contrast in the lesser sac (*arrows*), as well as a large pneumoperitoneum anterior to the liver

Rupture of the abdominal segment of the eso-phagus or the gastroesophageal junction occurs in Boerhaave syndrome and in 2%–4% of patients with achalasia undergoing pneumatic dilatation (GHAHREMANI 1981, 1994b). The radiographic ab-normalities in such cases typically involve both the chest and the abdomen; these are manifested by pneumomediastinum, pneumothorax or pleural ef-fusion, and extraluminal air collections in the upper abdomen (HAN and TISHLER 1984). Esophagogram reveals a markedly distorted lower esophagus with leakage of contrast material into the mediastinum, lesser sac, and upper retroperitoneal soft tissues (Fig. 16.6).

There have been a few reports concerning the use of CT in evaluating esophageal perforations (ALLEN et al. 1986; BAKER et al. 1990; WHITE et al. 1993). This technique allows the visualization of minute collec-tions of mediastinal air or contrast material due to small tears. It can also demonstrate some penetrat-ing foreign bodies that are faintly radiopaque and invisible on conventional radiographs (DOUGLAS and SISTROM 1991; GHAHREMANI 1993).

16.3
Gastroduodenal Perforations

16.3.1
Clinical Aspects

Gastroduodenal perforations associated with peptic ulcers or necrotic tumors were relatively common abdominal emergencies until a few decades ago, but these have become less frequent due to improved methods for earlier diagnosis and management. Concurrent with this medical progress, however, the incidence of gastroduodenal perforations resulting from iatrogenic and accidental injuries has increased (GHAHREMANI 1994a; WOLFMAN et al. 1992).

When performing fiberoptic gastroscopy there is approximately one perforation per thousand proce-dures (EIMILLER 1992; MEYERS and GHAHREMANI 1975). In most cases a transmural tear is caused just below the esophagogastric junction, where the poste-rior gastric wall is angulated anteriorly by the retro-peritoneal organs or due to its cascade shape. The head of a straightly advanced endoscope can pen-etrate this area and enter the lesser sac. The insuf-flated gas will then escape through the foramen of Winslow, causing a massive pneumoperitoneum.

Small transmural perforations induced by endoscopic lacerations or biopsy may seal spontane-ously and follow a benign course since the peritoneal contamination will be minimal if the stomach is empty at the time of iatrogenic trauma. Radiologic evaluation may not show any leakage of contrast material, thus prompting the designation "spon-taneous postgastroscopy pneumoperitoneum" (GHAHREMANI 1994a; MEYERS and GHAHREMANI 1975).

Endoscopic perforations of the anterior gastric wall or the duodenal bulb present a more serious problem. These may be caused by a deep endoscopic biopsy or penetration through a necrotic tumor, ulcer crater, or friable wall due to inflammatory or neoplastic processes. Such perforations are sel-dom sealed spontaneously and may lead to massive leakage complicated by peritonitis and abdominal abscesses.

Nasogastric tubes, balloon catheters, and bougies that are usually inserted without fluoroscopic guid-ance can perforate the gastric wall, particularly if it is already weakened by inflammatory or neoplastic processes (Fig. 16.7). Furthermore, the initially flex-ible NG-tubes tend to become rigid after a few days of exposure to the gastric secretions and they can perforate the intestinal walls during a subsequent manipulation or repositioning (GHAHREMANI et al. 1980).

Because of the intraperitoneal location of the stomach and duodenal bulb, perforations of them will lead to intraperitoneal leakage of gas and gas-troduodenal secretions. Both hydrochloric acid and digestive enzymes have irritant effects upon the peri-toneum, thereby causing severe abdominal pain and tenderness. About a third of cases, however, do not manifest with a pneumoperitoneum on abdominal radiographs (CHO and BAKER 1994; MADRAZO et al. 1984; RICE et al. 1982). The reasons may include an empty stomach at the time of perforation, prompt sealing of the defect by the greater omentum, or pen-etration into an adjacent solid organ like the pan-creas (JACOBS et al. 1991; JEFFREY et al. 1983).

The duodenal loop beyond the bulbar segment is retroperitoneal. Hence its perforations tend to be locally contained and rather insidious in clinical pre-sentation. Furthermore, these are usually the result of an injury rather than an intrinsic lesion. The prin-cipal causes of retroperitoneal perforations of the duodenum are blunt abdominal trauma due to seat belt or steering wheel injuries (HHYES et al. 1991; HOFER and COHEN 1989), endoscopic interventions during endoscopic retrograde cholangiopancreato-graphy and sphincterotomy (COTTON et al. 1991; KUHLMAN et al. 1989), and intubation for

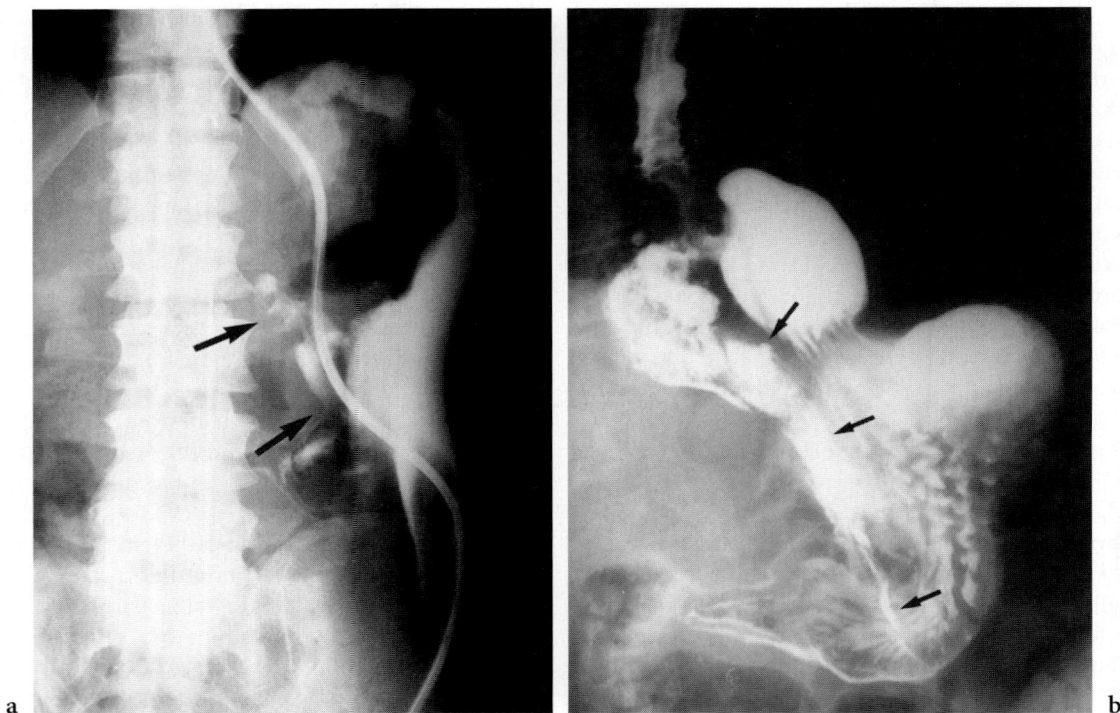

Fig. 16.7 a,b. Iatrogenic perforations of the stomach in two patients. **a** Rupture of gastrojejunal anastomosis by a nasogastric suction tube (*arrows*), which had been inserted without fluoroscopic control. This supine film reveals leakage of contrast material into the left paracolic gutter and subphrenic space. **b** Accidental passage of a dilatation bougie through the wall of an inflamed gastroesophageal stricture resulted in a large extraluminal collection along the herniated fundus and the lesser sac (*arrows*)

nasojejunal feeding or enteroclysis (Diner 1988; Ghahremani 1989; Siegle et al. 1976). Uncommon sources are perforating foreign bodies (Ghahremani 1989), duodenal diverticulitis (Gore et al. 1991; Pugash et al. 1990), postbulbar ulcers (Fultz et al. 1992), Crohn's disease, and necrotic tumors which originate in or secondarily involve the duodenal loop (Gore and Ghahremani 1986).

16.3.2
Radiologic Diagnosis

Large collections of intraperitoneal gas following gastroduodenal perforations are easily recognized on radiographs of the chest or abdomen (Fig. 16.8). With a small to moderate pneumoperitoneum, however, the diagnosis on supine films alone might be difficult. According to a recent report (Levine et al. 1991), in only 26 of 44 (59%) patients with pneumoperitoneum did the supine films demonstrate classic findings such as visualization of the bowel walls (Rigler's sign) or the falciform ligament.

Therefore, special imaging techniques must be employed for accurate diagnosis of perforations that are either contained or associated with minimal extraluminal air (Cho and Baker 1994; Fultz et al. 1992; Jeffrey et al. 1983).

An upright chest film can demonstrate as little as 1–2 ml of free air in the right subdiaphragmatic space, which is normally the uppermost region of the abdominal cavity and under a negative pressure (Miller et al. 1980). However, this radiographic sign may not be evident if the subphrenic space is obliterated by adhesions from previous inflammation or abdominal surgery (Fig. 16.8b). Small pockets of extraluminal air may also be entrapped beneath the viscera or mesenteric folds, and thereby not ascend to the subdiaphragmatic regions unless the patient is kept upright for 10–20 min. A more practical approach in evaluating critically ill patients is to obtain a left lateral decubitus film and carefully look for free air between the liver margin and right abdominal wall (Cho and Baker 1994; Rice et al. 1982).

A supine film of the abdomen is often the initial radiograph obtained in bedridden patients with gas-

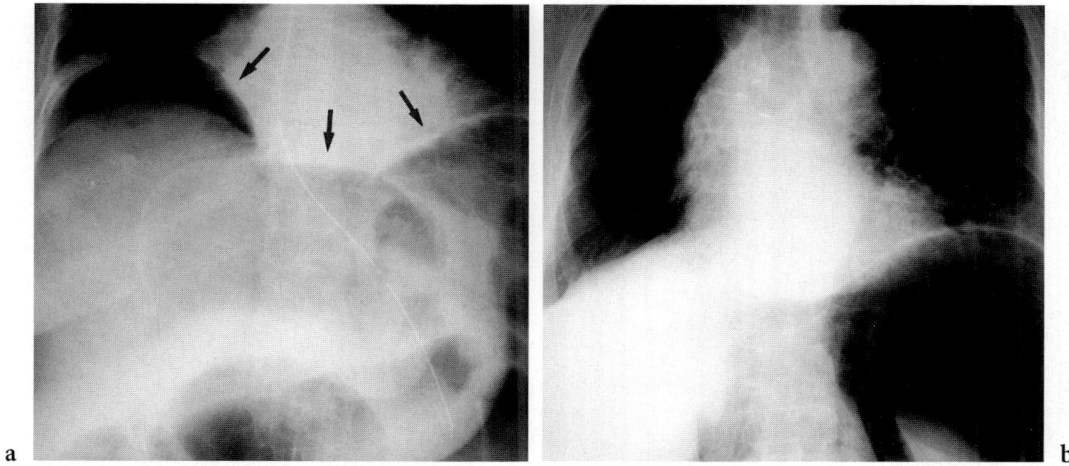

a

b

Fig. 16.8 a,b. Variable appearances of pneumoperitoneum in two patients with perforated stomach. **a** Radiograph of the abdomen following an endoscopic tear of the posterior gastric wall reveals large amounts of insufflated air within the lesser sac and subphrenic spaces (*arrows*) despite prompt insertion of a nasogastric suction tube. **b** In this patient with a perfo- rated antral ulcer there is free air only beneath the left hemidiaphragm because the right subphrenic space had been obliterated by adhesions following chest surgery. Note that the perforated stomach is collapsed and invisible in both in- stances. (From GHAHREMANI 1993)

trointestinal symptoms. Hence the radiologists must analyze it with utmost care in the search for the clas- sic signs of pneumoperitoneum. These include:

1. The *bas-relief or Rigler's sign*, which denotes clear visualization of the bowel wall as a 2- to 3-mm stripe outlined by radiolucent intraluminal and extraluminal gas. It is usually evident when at least 750 ml of free air is present.
2. The *triangle sign*, which represents the radio- lucent gas collection between two adjacent loops and the parietal peritoneum.
3. The *hyperlucent liver sign*, which is produced by accumulation of free air anterior to the liver.
4. The *hepatic edge sign*, caused by the interface of pneumoperitoneum with the inferior border of the liver.
5. The *falciform ligament sign*, which refers to the visualization of a 5- to 10-mm-thick band extend- ing obliquely from the umbilicus to the anterior surface of the liver.
6. The *ligamentum teres fissure sign*, which is due to air collection in the interlobar fissure.
7. The *urachus sign*, which appears as a thin and tubular midline structure between the urinary bladder and umbilical region.

Several other radiographic findings of extraluminal air collections in the peritoneal compartments such as the lesser sac or Morison's pouch have also been described (CHO and BAKER 1994). Nevertheless, the reported sensitivity of supine films in detecting pneumoperitoneum is only 50%–60% (LEVINE et al. 1991).

As noted earlier, about 30% of patients with perfo- rated ulcer do not exhibit pneumoperitoneum on abdominal radiographs (JACOBS et al. 1991; JEFFREY et al. 1983). In fact the presence of a penetrating ulcer may be first realized during fluoroscopic evaluation with barium sulfate, thus leading to massive intrap- eritoneal leakage and potential risk for subsequent development of adhesions (Fig. 16.9). An upper gas- trointestinal series utilizing water-soluble contrast material should be performed when there is a high index of clinical suspicion for gastroduodenal perfo- ration. Small perforations are sometimes difficult to visualize with water-soluble contrast medium as it diffuses rapidly into the peritoneal cavity and surrounding tissues. It is therefore recommended that questionable findings be reassessed promptly after administration of barium (FOLEY et al. 1982; GHAHREMANI 1993).

Another alternative approach is to perform a CT examination of the abdomen (CHO and BAKER 1994; HOFER and COHEN 1989; KANE et al. 1991), which can demonstrate minimal intraperitoneal leakage of gas or iodinated compounds (Fig. 16.10). Several studies have documented that abdominal CT is far more sensitive than plain film radiography for the detection of a small pneumoperitoneum and unsus- pected gastroduodenal perforations (JEFFREY et al.

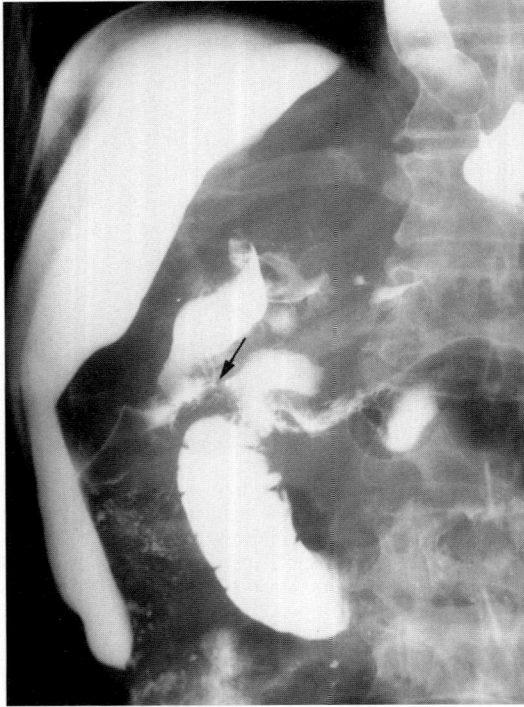

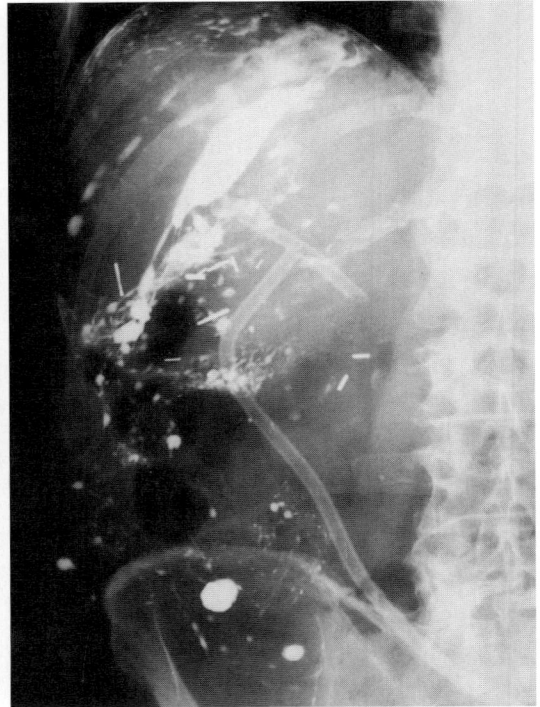

Fig. 16.9 a,b. Perforation of the duodenal bulb ulcer during upper gastrointestinal series. **a** Radiograph shows a deeply penetrating ulcer (*arrow*), causing massive leakage of barium into the right subphrenic and subhepatic spaces despite ab-sence of pneumoperitoneum. **b** Radiograph obtained 4 years later following cholecystectomy demonstrates residual barium in the peritoneal cavity, but it did not cause any complications

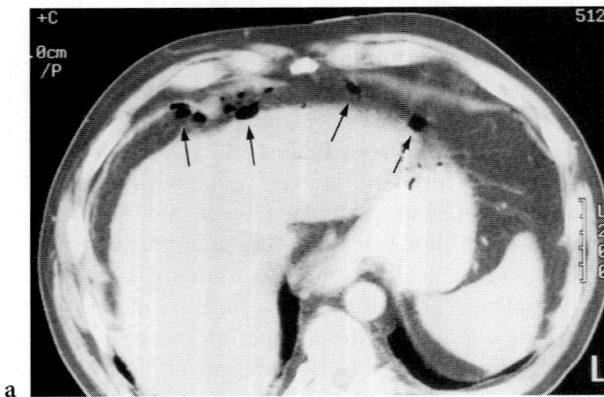

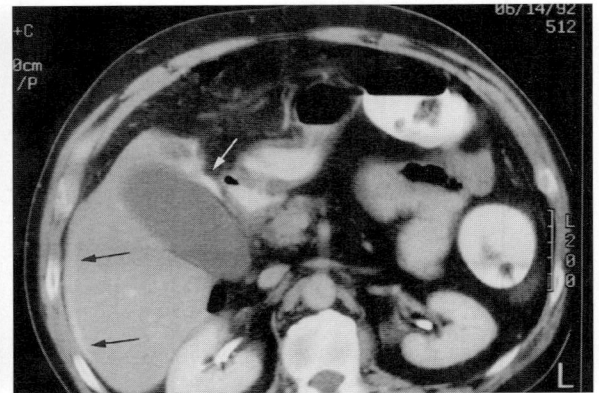

Fig. 16.10 a,b. CT diagnosis of a perforated duodenal ulcer. **a** CT of the upper abdomen demonstrates small pockets of free air entrapped beneath the omental fat (*arrows*). **b** Another section 8 cm caudad shows extravasation from the perforated duodenal bulb (*white arrow*), with minimal leakage into the gallbladder fossa and perihepatic region (*black arrows*). (From GHAHREMANI 1993)

1983; MADRAZO et al. 1984). According to a recent comparative study, upright chest films showed a small pneumoperitoneum in only 5 of 13 (38%) patients in whom free air was readily visible on CT scans (STAPAKIS and THICKMAN 1992). Tiny pockets of extraluminal gas trapped in the various peritoneal compartments and beneath the mesenteric leaves or greater omentum can be detected exclusively by CT, particularly on images with a lung window setting. Larger collections of free air are best seen in the upper abdomen and anterior to the liver due to su-pine position of the patient during CT examination.

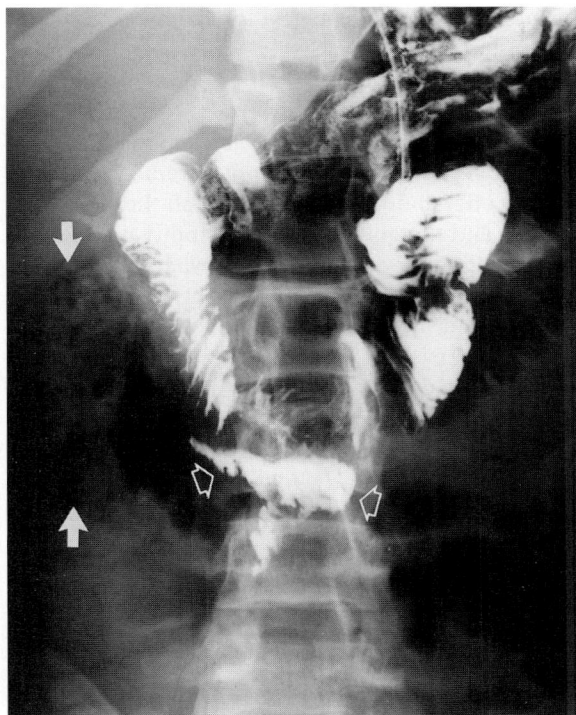

Fig. 16.11. Duodenal rupture due to blunt abdominal trauma. There is a localized retroperitoneal collection of contrast material (*open arrows*) adjacent to the ruptured third duodenal segment as it crosses the lumbar spine. Extraluminal gas is visible in the right anterior pararenal space (*solid arrows*), but not in the peritoneal cavity

There have been a few reports concerning the sonographic diagnosis of minimal pneumoperitoneum in patients undergoing evaluation for non-specific abdominal symptoms (LEE et al. 1990). In such cases, the free air often appeared as echogenic collections beneath the anterior abdominal wall in the right upper quadrant and produced characteristic posterior shadowing or reverberation artifact.

Due to the retroperitoneal position of the duodenal loop, its perforations are usually well contained and do not present as a pneumoperitoneum. On plain radiographs of the abdomen, however, pockets of extraluminal gas may be seen within the upper retroperitoneal soft tissues and in one or both anterior pararenal spaces. Fluoroscopic evaluation of the gastrointestinal tract with contrast material is crucial for establishing the correct diagnosis, particularly in patients with posttraumatic duodenal rupture (Fig. 16.11). The value of CT in demonstrating such perforations has also been well demonstrated (GLAZER et al. 1980; HAYES et al. 1991; HOFER and COHEN 1989; JACOBS et al. 1991; KUHLMAN et al. 1989).

16.4
Perforations of the Small Bowel

16.4.1
Clinical Aspects

Perforations of the small bowel are uncommon as compared with perforations of the rest of the alimentary tract. Nevertheless, they occur with a wide range of potential causes and clinical presentations.

Spontaneous intestinal perforation can develop in patients with ischemic or bacterial enteritis, Crohn's disease, jejunal or ileal diverticulitis, or ingested foreign bodies, or as the consequence of massive bowel dilatation due to obstructing tumors, adhesions, incarcerated hernias, volvulus, or intussusception.

Because the small bowel occupies most of the peritoneal cavity, it is prone to injury by penetrating stab wounds or gunshots. It can also rupture due to a forceful blunt trauma to the abdomen (BURNEY et al. 1983; PEVEC et al. 1991; WISNER and BLAISDELL 1992). Among the iatrogenic causes are perforations induced by nasojejunal feeding tubes, disrupted anastomoses, and inadvertent lacerations complicating laparoscopic surgery or other interventional procedures (GHAHREMANI 1981, 1994a; SIEGLE et al. 1976; WINEK et al. 1988).

Depending upon the size and nature of bowel perforation, variable amounts of air and intestinal secretions will spill into the peritoneal cavity. These can incite a peritoneal reaction causing abdominal pain, fever, chills, and sometimes a septic or hypovolemic shock. The clinical signs and symptoms may occasionally indicate a rather benign, insidious process, if the perforation is sealed promptly by the greater omentum or adjacent peritoneal folds (BURNEY et al. 1983; PEVEC et al. 1991).

16.4.2
Radiologic Diagnosis

The length and redundancy of small intestine, as well as its topographic relationships to other abdominal viscera, make it a difficult challenge to detect the presence and site of bowel perforation. Time lapse between the occurrence of perforation and subsequent radiologic studies can also affect the diagnostic accuracy since spontaneous closure of the defect and rapid resorption of free air are not uncommon. For these reasons, evidence for pneumoperitoneum may be seen in fewer than half the cases (BROWN et al. 1992; KANE et al. 1991).

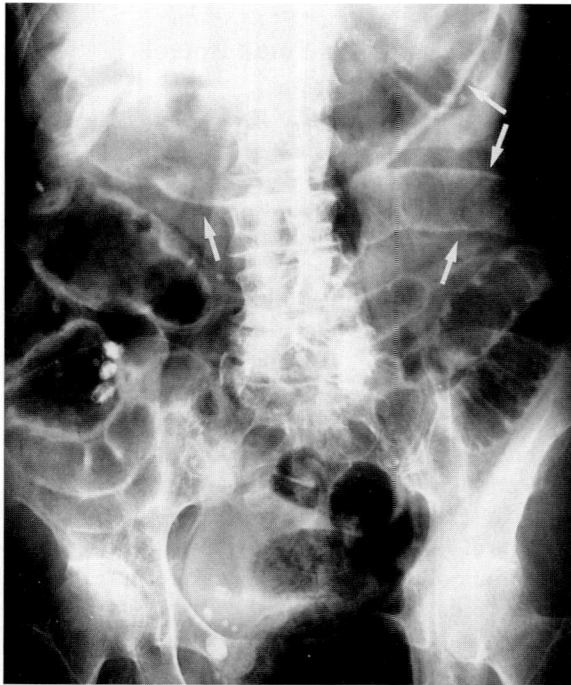

Fig. 16.12. Supine abdominal radiograph shows a large pneumoperitoneum, allowing clear visualization of the walls of the stomach and jejunum (*arrows*). These loops are well distended with gas, and therefore would not be the likely site of perforation. The actual cause of free air was ischemic colitis

If the small bowel perforation occurs while the bowel loops are distended with gas, a large pneumoperitoneum will be visible on abdominal radiographs. The perforated segment will appear collapsed as compared with the gas-filled proximal loops, which obviously would not remain distended if their walls had a defect. This can be a useful diagnostic clue for suggesting the approximate site of bowel perforation on plain radiographs (Fig. 16.12). Sometimes there is only minimal free air despite a massive leakage of intestinal secretions. Such an intraperitoneal fluid collection tends to pool in the more dependent pelvic fossae and paracolic gutters, and thereby become visible on a supine radiograph of the abdomen. Additional films in the upright or left lateral decubitus position may disclose a small pneumoperitoneum to support the diagnosis (CHO and BAKER 1994).

A postoperative perforation or anastomotic leakage can complicate reconstructive procedures such as gastrojejunostomy or ileocolostomy in up to 5% of cases (GHAHREMANI 1993). It is usually caused by ischemic necrosis and dehiscence of anastomosed margins within the first week of surgery. Plain films

of the abdomen can suggest the diagnosis by demonstrating a progressively enlarging pneumoperitoneum, associated with ileus, ascites, or abscesses (RICE et al. 1982).

In this context, it should be emphasized that pneumoperitoneum itself is an extremely common finding after abdominal surgery. Both the amount of free air and the duration of its visibility on abdominal radiography or CT are somewhat variable, depending on factors such as the patient's age, body habitus, and the type of operation (CHO and BAKER 1994; SELTZER 1984; WOLFMAN et al. 1992). In most cases a postsurgical pneumoperitoneum disappears in 3–5 days unless reaccumulated through abdominal drains or dehiscent incisions. However, persistent or progressively increasing free air in the abdomen beyond the first postoperative week would be highly indicative of anastomotic leakage or perforated viscus.

Small bowel examination with a contrast medium is the optimal technique for radiologic diagnosis of contained or free perforations. The selection of an iodinated compound versus barium should be based on the presence or absence of pneumoperitoneum at the time of evaluation (COHEN 1987). The extraluminal leakage of the contrast material and the source of such leakage can be demonstrated by careful fluoroscopy and serial radiographs, or by CT examination (Fig. 16.13). Small perforations are sometimes difficult to visualize with water-soluble agents such as Gastrografin, because it rapidly diffuses within the peritoneal cavity following extraluminal leakage. It is then resorbed and excreted promptly by the urinary tract. Accordingly, a positive urine test for iodine would indirectly confirm the suspected perforation (FOLEY et al. 1982).

16.5
Perforations of the Colon and Rectum

16.5.1
Clinical Aspects

Perforated appendicitis and diverticulitis of the colon are two common entities, but it is highly unusual for them to manifest with free intraperitoneal air. The gradual progression of these inflammatory processes will provide ample opportunity for the containment of perforation by surrounding soft tissues. Furthermore, the volvume of gas within the appendiceal lumen rarely exceeds 1–2 ml, and such a minute amount of free air released from a perforated

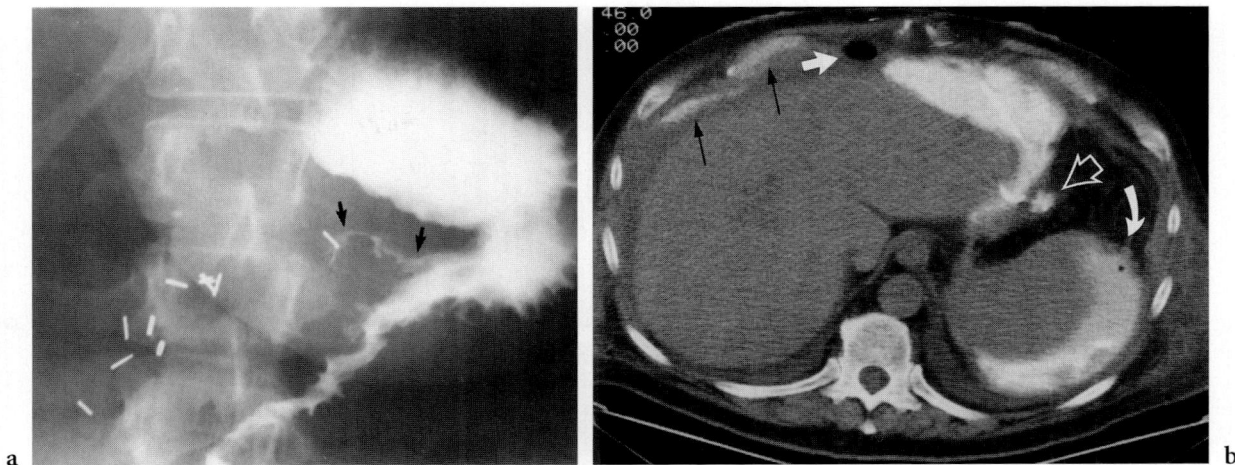

Fig. 16.13 a,b. Postsurgical pneumoperitoneum due to a leaking gastrojejunostomy. **a** Evaluation with Gastrografin shows minimal extravasation from the anastomosis (*arrows*). **b** CT reveals extraluminal contrast adjacent to the gastrojejunostomy (*open arrow*), in the left subphrenic space (*curved arrow*), and in the perihepatic region (*black arrows*). There is only a minimal amount of free air in the abdominal cavity (*white arrow*)

appendix is very difficult to detect on abdominal radiographs.

Spontaneous rupture of the large bowel can occur if its lumen is markedly dilated proximal to an obstructing lesion (e.g., tumor, volvulus, incarcerated hernia), or when the bowel wall is very friable (e.g., ischemic or ulcerative colitis, necrotic tumor). In such instances the perforation can result in massive peritoneal contamination and signs of an acute abdominal emergency.

Over the last few decades, the incidence of colorectal perforation due to abdominal trauma has increased (BROWN et al. 1992; HAYES et al. 1991; WISNER and BLAISDELL 1992). A recent study of 28 patients with colon injuries showed that seven of eight perforations from blunt trauma were in the left colon, whereas the majority of perforations from penetrating trauma involved the proximal half of the large bowel (BUGIS et al. 1992). In this context, it should be noted that the rectum and sigmoid are the predominant sites of iatrogenic injuries (GHAHREMANI 1994a).

Fiberoptic endoscopes are frequently utilized for evaluation and biopsy of colorectal lesions, as well as for polypectomy by means of an electrosurgical snare. These procedures cause perforation in 0.5%–3% of cases (EIMILLER 1992; KEVIN et al. 1992). In comparison, the average incidence of colorectal perforation during barium enema is 2–4 in every 10000 examinations (OTT and CHEN 1994; WILLIAMS and HARNED 1991). Transmural rectal tears may also be

induced during sexual assaults or insertion of foreign objects for erotic purposes (CRASS et al. 1981).

The clinical symptoms of traumatic colorectal perforations include rectal bleeding, fever, abdominal pain, and localized tenderness in the involved region. When the perforation occurs as the consequence of bowel obstruction and preexisting inflammatory or neoplastic lesions, however, its clinical features may be masked by those of the underlying disease.

16.5.2
Radiologic Diagnosis

Transmural perforation of the colon into the peritoneal cavity leads to the development of pneumoperitoneum, whereas a retroperitoneal leakage tends to be contained locally. A perforation complicating bowel obstruction or an endoscopic procedure is usually associated with a large amount of free air (WILLIAMS and HARNED 1991). In these instances, the intestinal gas or insufflated air promptly escapes into the peritoneal cavity and will be demonstrable on supine films as a hyperlucent abdomen with visualization of the falciform ligament, umbilical folds, and both sides of the bowel wall (CHO and BAKER 1994).

A transmural rectal tear below the peritoneal reflection leads to passage of gas into the perirectal fat and pelvic soft tissues. It will then extend bilaterally

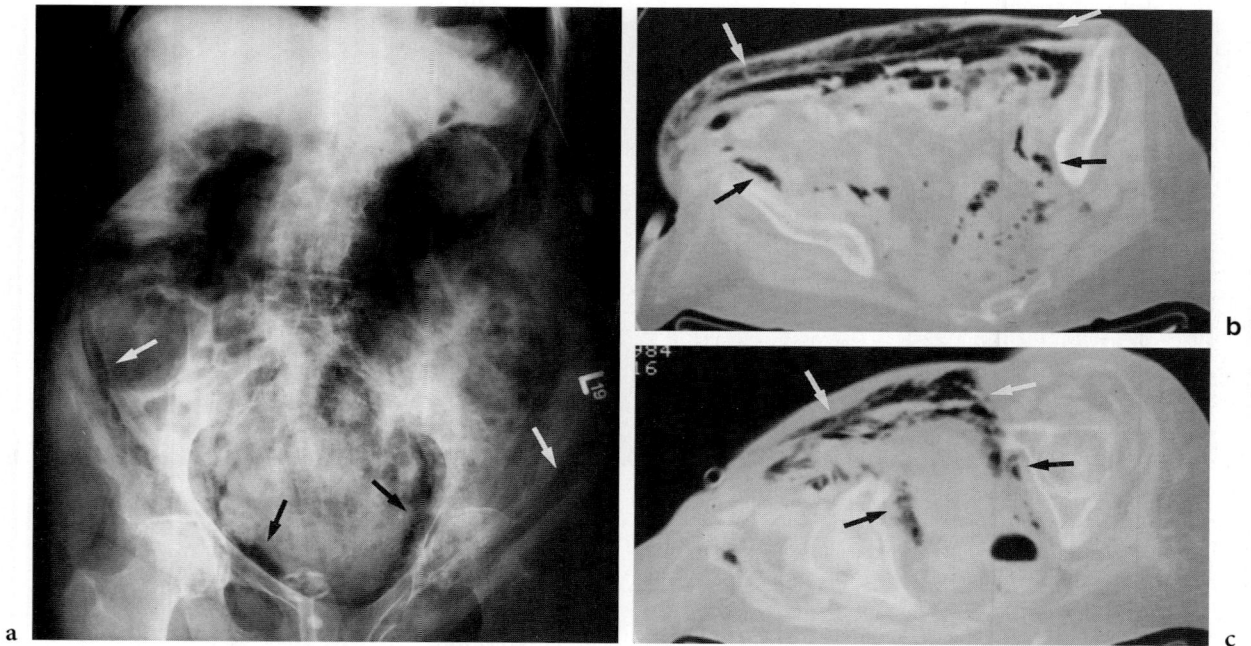

Fig. 16.14 a–c. Rectal perforation at colonoscopy. **a** Supine film of the abdomen demonstrates extraluminal air in the pelvis (*black arrows*) and abdominal walls (*white arrows*), but its retroperitoneal collection is ill-defined. **b, c** CT sections of the lower abdomen show dissection of perirectal gas along the pelvic walls (*black arrows*), causing subcutaneous emphysema of the anterior abdominal wall (*white arrows*). (From GHAHREMANI 1993).

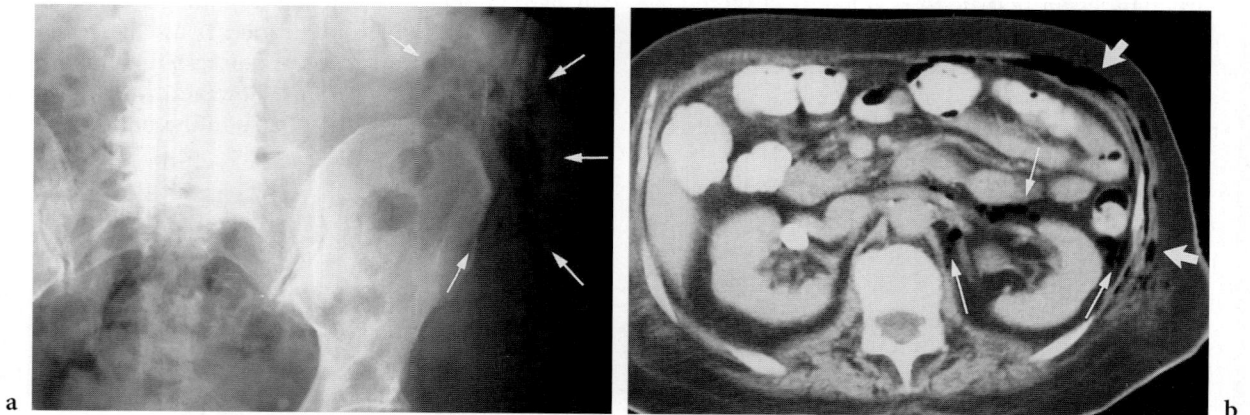

Fig. 16.15 a,b. Retroperitoneal perforation due to descending colon diverticulitis. **a** Plain film of the abdomen shows soft tissue emphysema in the left flank (*arrows*). **b** CT demonstrates extraluminal gas in the left pericolic and perirenal spaces (*small arrows*), with extension into the left abdominal wall (*large arrows*)

along the psoas muscles and posterior pararenal spaces into the flank stripes and abdominal wall. These findings may be confusing on plain radiographs of patients with massive emphysema of the anterior abdominal wall, but are easily appreciated on CT scans (Fig. 16.14).

Perforations involving the posterior aspect of ascending or descending colon are extraperitoneal.

Therefore, they tend to be contained and remain clinically silent for several hours or days prior to the correct diagnosis. These perforations may result from diverticulitis, endoscopic procedures, and blunt or penetrating injuries (BUGIS et al. 1992; GHAHREMANI 1994a; NELSON et al. 1982; NIVATVONGS 1988). The usual finding on abdominal radiograph is a localized extraluminal gas collection

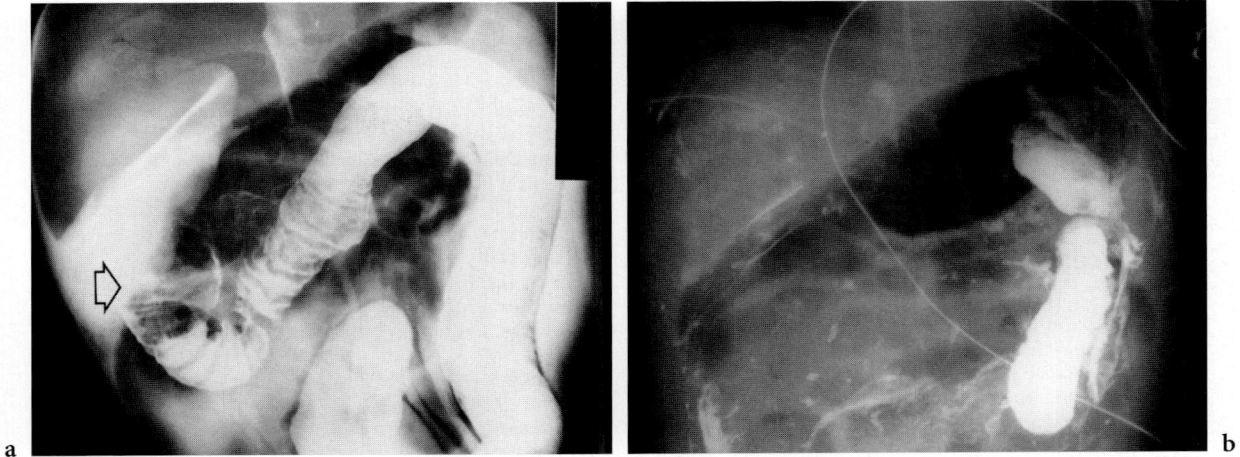

a b

Fig. 16.16 a,b. Perforation of the colon during barium enema. a Attempted hydrostatic reduction of an ileocolic intussusception (*arrow*) resulted in massive intraperitoneal leakage of barium. b Postoperative radiograph shows residual barium throughout the peritoneal cavity, but it did not induce any complications during the 10-year follow-up period

in the affected paracolic region or in the anterior pararenal space of the ipsilateral side. In the latter location, it presents as mottled radiolucencies between the medial border of psoas muscle and the spine, but usually does not extend to the contralateral side. On rare occasions, the extraluminal gas from perforated diverticulitis of the descending colon or sigmoid may dissect into the left flank and manifest as subcutaneous emphysema of the abdominal wall (Fig. 16.15). It can further extend into the buttocks and legs to incite a necrotizing fasciitis (JAGER et al. 1990; LIPSIT and LEWICKI 1979).

It is a common practice to examine the colon with water-soluble contrast material when a colorectal perforation is suspected on the basis of initial clinical and radiographic findings. Not infrequently, however, the existence of a free or contained perforation is first recognized during barium enema examination. As mentioned above, the procedure itself causes colorectal perforation in 2–4 of every 10 000 patients (OTT and CHEN 1994; WILLIAMS and HARNED 1991). The mechanism of injury is usually a transmural rectal tear by the inserted enema tip or an overinflated retention balloon. Other parts of the colon may rupture if the wall is already weak and friable due to inflammatory, ischemic, or neoplastic changes. Such an abnormal segment may perforate easily when the intraluminal pressure is increased during colon examination (Fig. 16.16). This also applies to focal areas of colonic wall damage caused by deep endoscopic biopsies or polypectomy. Following such procedures, therefore, it seems prudent to delay barium enema examination for at least 2–3 days

(GHAHREMANI 1994a; NELSON et al. 1982; WILLIAMS and HARNED 1991).

Depending on the location and extent of perforation, variable amounts of feces, gas, and contrast material may enter the abdominal cavity or extraperitoneal tissues. Prompt surgical repair of the perforated segment along with drainage of the contaminated area, diverting colostomy, and antibiotic therapy are the recommended approach (KEVIN et al. 1992; NELSON et al. 1982). However, small retroperitoneal leaks that are well contained can be managed conservatively, as in most instances of perforated diverticulitis.

Intraperitoneal barium leakage is generally considered a dreadful event because of the potential risk of barium-induced peritonitis, foreign body granulomas, and adhesions. This widely held and perpetuated concept is based on the clinical and experimental data published almost half a century ago. During the past two decades, however, there has been a remarkable improvement in the management of perforated viscus with barium leakage. Both the morbidity and the mortality of these complications have been reduced due to prompt diagnosis and surgical intervention, more effective antibiotics, and fluid replacement therapy. Practicing radiologists should be aware of the favorable prognosis following barium extravasation, since the majority of patients will not experience any long-term clinical symptoms such as barium-induced adhesive bowel obstruction (CORDONE et al. 1988; YAMAMURA et al. 1985).

Spontaneous passage of intestinal gas through the intact or ulcerated colorectal mucosa may occur if the lumen is overdistended. On rare instances the insufflated air during a double-contrast enema may dissect intramurally and extend into the mesocolon. Despite its striking radiographic appearance, however, this benign process will resolve uneventfully within a few days (OTT and CHEN 1994).

References

Allen KS, Siskind BN, Burrell MI (1986) Perforation of distal esophagus with lesser sac extension: CT demonstration. J Comput Assist Tomogr 10:612–614

Baker CL, LoCicero J, Hartz RS, et al. (1990) Computed tomography in patients with esophageal perforation. Chest 98:1078–1080

Bladergroen MR, Lowe JE, Postlethwait RW (1986) Diagnosis and management of esophageal perforation and rupture. Ann Thorac Surg 42:235–239

Brick SH, Caroline DF, Lev-Toaff AS, et al. (1988) Esophageal disruption: evaluation with iohexol esophagography. Radiology 169:141–143

Brown RA, Bass DH, Rode H, et al. (1992) Gastrointestinal tract perforation in children due to blunt abdominal trauma. Br J Surg 79:522–524

Bugis SP, Blair NP, Letwin ER (1992) Management of blunt and penetrating colon injuries. Am J Surg 163:547–550

Burney RE, Mueller GL, Coon WW, et al. (1983) Diagnosis of isolated small bowel injury following blunt abdominal trauma. Ann Emerg Med 12:71–74

Cho KC, Baker SR (1994) Extraluminal air: diagnosis and significance. Radiol Clin North Am 32:829–844

Cohen MD (1987) Choosing contrast media for the evaluation of the gastrointestinal tract of neonates and infants. Radiology 162:447–456

Cordone RP, Brandeis SZ, Richman H (1988) Rectal perforation during barium enema. Dis Colon Rectum 31:563–569

Cotton PB, Lehman G, Vennes J, et al. (1991) Endoscopic sphincterotomy complications and their management. Gastrointest Endosc 37:383–393

Crass RA, Tranbaugh RF, Kudsk KA, Trunkey DD (1981) Colorectal foreign bodies and perforation. Am J Surg 142:85–88

Diner WC (1988) Duodenal perforation during intubation for small bowel enema study. Radiology 168:39–41

Dodds WJ, Stewart ET, Vlymen WJ (1982) Appropriate contrast media for evaluation of esophageal disruption. Radiology 144:439–441

Douglas M, Sistrom CL (1991) Chicken bone lodged in the upper esophagus: CT findings. Gastrointest Radiol 16:11–12

Eimiller A (1992) Complications in endoscopy. Endoscopy 24:176–184

Flynn AE, Verrier ED, Way LW, et al. (1989) Esophageal perforation. Arch Surg 124:1211–1215

Foley MJ, Ghahremani GG, Rogers LF (1982) Reappraisal of contrast media used to detect upper gastrointestinal perforations. Comparison of ionic water-soluble media with barium sulfate. Radiology 144:231–237

Fultz PJ, Skucas J, Weiss SL (1992) CT in upper gastrointestinal tract perforations secondary to peptic ulcer disease. Gastrointest Radiol 17:5–8

Ghahremani GG (1981) Complications of gastrointestinal intubation. In: Meyers MA, Ghahremani GG (eds) Iatrogenic gastrointestinal complications. Springer, Berlin Heidelberg New York, pp 65–89

Ghahremani GG (1989) Ingested foreign bodies: radiological diagnosis and management. In: Thompson WM (ed) Common problems in gastrointestinal radiology. Year Book Medical Publishers, Chicago, pp 152–162

Ghahremani GG (1993) Radiologic evaluation of suspected gastrointestinal perforations. Radiol Clin North Am 31:1219–1234

Ghahremani GG (1994a) Iatrogenic gastrointestinal disorders. In: Gore RM, Levine MS, Laufer I (eds) Textbook of gastrointestinal radiology, vol II. Saunders, Philadelphia, pp 2583–2599

Ghahremani GG (1994b) Esophageal trauma. Semin Roentgenol 29:387–400

Ghahremani GG, Turner MA, Port RB (1980) Iatrogenic intubation injuries of the upper gastrointestinal tract in adults. Gastrointest Radiol 5:1–10

Glazer GM, Buy JN, Moss AA, et al. (1980) CT detection of duodenal perforation. AJR 137:333–336

Gore RM, Ghahremani GG (1986) Crohn's disease of the upper gastrointestinal tract. Crit Rev Diagn Imaging 25:305–331

Gore RM, Ghahremani GG, Kirsch MD, et al. (1991) Diverticulitis of the duodenum: clinical and radiological manifestations of seven cases. Am J Gastroenterol 86:981–985

Han SY, Tishler JM (1984) Perforation of the abdominal segment of the esophagus. AJR 143:751–754

Han SY, McElvein RB, Aldrete JS, Tishler JM (1985) Perforation of the esophagus: correlation of site and cause with plain film findings. AJR 145:537–540

Hayes CW, Conway WF, Walsh JW, et al. (1991) Seat belt injuries: radiologic findings and clinical correlation. Radiographics 11:23–26

Hofer GA, Cohen AJ (1989) CT signs of duodenal perforation secondary to blunt abdominal trauma. J Comput Assist Tomogr 13:430–432

Jacobs JM, Hill MC, Steinberg WM (1991) Peptic ulcer disease: CT evaluation. Radiology 178:745–748

Jager GJ, Rijssen HV, Lamers JH (1990) Subcutaneous emphysema of the lower extremity of abdominal origin. Gastrointest Radiol 15:253–258

Jeffrey RB, Federle MP, Wall S (1983) Value of computed tomography in detecting occult gastrointestinal perforation. J Comput Assist Tomogr 7:825–827

Jones WG, Ginsberg RJ (1992) Esophageal perforation: a continuing challenge. Ann Thorac Surg 53:534–543

Kane NM, Francis IR, Burney RE, et al. (1991) Traumatic pneumoperitoneum: implications of computed tomography diagnosis. Invest Radiol 26:574–578

Kevin H, Sinicrope F, Esker AH (1992) Management of perforation of the colon at colonoscopy. Am J Gastroenterol 87:161–167

Kim-Deobald J, Kozarek RA (1992) Esophageal perforation: an 8-year review of a multispecialty clinic's experience. Am J Gastroenterol 87:1112–1119

Kuhlman JE, Fishman EK, Milligan FD, Siegelman SS (1989) Complications of endoscopic retrograde sphincterotomy: computed tomographic evaluation. Gastrointest Radiol 14:127–132

Lee DH, Lim JH, Ko YT, Yoon Y (1990) Sonographic detection of pneumoperitoneum in patients with acute abdomen. AJR 154:107–109

Levine MS, Scheiner JD, Rubesin SE, et al. (1991) Diagnosis of pneumoperitoneum on supine abdominal radiographs. AJR 156:731–735

Lipsit ER, Lewicki AM (1979) Subcutaneous emphysema of the abdominal wall from diverticulitis with necrotizing fasciitis. Gastrointest Radiol 4:89–92

Madrazo BL, Halpert RD, Sandler MA, Pearlberg JL (1984) Computed tomographic findings in penetrating peptic ulcer. Radiology 153:751–754

Meyers MA, Ghahremani GG (1975) Complications of fiberoptic endoscopy. I. Esophagoscopy and gastroscopy. Radiology 115:293–300

Miller RE, Becker GJ, Slabaugh RA (1980) Detection of pneumoperitoneum: optimum body position and respiratory phase. AJR 135:487–490

Miller RE, Becker GJ, Slabaugh RD (1981) Nonsurgical pneumoperitoneum. Gastrointest Radiol 6:73–74

Nelson RL, Abcarian H, Prasad ML (1982) Iatrogenic perforation of the colon and rectum. Dis Colon Rectum 25:305–308

Nguyen BD, Beckman I (1992) Silent rectal perforation after endoscopic polypectomy: CT features. Gastrointest Radiol 17:271–273

Nivatvongs S (1988) Complications in colonoscopic polypectomy: lessons to learn from an experience with 1576 polyps. Am Surg 54:61–63

O'Connell DJ (1981) Perforation of the esophagus. In: Teplick JG, Haskin ME (eds) Surgical radiology, vol I. Saunders, Philadelphia, pp 368–378

Ott DJ, Chen YM (1994) Specific acute colonic disorders. Radiol Clin North Am 32:871–884

Overholt BF (1984) Gastrointestinal endoscopy in the 1980's: cost, challenge, and change. Gastrointest Endosc 30:325–328

Pevec WC, Peitzman AB, Udekwu AO, et al. (1991) Computed tomography in the evaluation of blunt abdominal trauma. Surg Gynecol Obstet 173:262–267

Pugash RA, O'Brien SE, Stevenson GW (1990) Perforating duodenal diverticulitis. Gastrointest Radiol 15:156–158

Rice RP, Thompson WM, Gedgaudas RK (1982) The diagnosis and significance of extraluminal gas in the abdomen. Radiol Clin North Am 20:819–837

Seltzer SE (1984) Abnormal intraabdominal gas collections visualized on computed tomography: a clinical and experimental study. Gastrointest Radiol 9:127–131

Siegle RL, Rabinowitz JG, Sarasohn C (1976) Intestinal perforation secondary to nasojejunal feeding tubes. AJR 126:1229–1232

Stapakis JC, Thickman D (1992) Diagnosis of pneumoperitoneum: abdominal CT vs. upright chest film. J Comput Assist Tomogr 16:713–716

White CS, Templeton PA, Attar S (1993) Esophageal perforation: CT findings. AJR 160:767–770

Williams SM, Harned RK (1991) Recognition and prevention of barium enema complications. Curr Probl Diagn Radiol 20:123–151

Winek TG, Mosely H, Grout H, et al. (1988) Pneumoperitoneum and its association with ruptured abdominal viscus. Arch Surg 123:709–712

Wisner DH, Blaisdell FW (1992) Visceral injuries. Arch Surg 127:687–693

Wolff AP, Kessler S (1973) Iatrogenic injury to the hypopharynx and cervical esophagus: an autopsy study. Ann Otolaryngol 82:778–783

Wolfman NT, Bechtold RE, Scharling ES, Meredith JW (1992) Blunt upper abdominal trauma: evaluation by CT. AJR 158:493–501

Yamamura M, Nishi M, Furubayshi H, et al. (1985) Barium peritonitis: report of a case and review of the literature. Dis Colon Rectum 28:347–352

Section 4: Surgery-Related Advances

17 Postoperative Findings

R.M. GORE and C. SMITH

CONTENTS

17.1
Introduction

Radiologic evaluation of patients who have undergone gastrointestinal (GI) tract surgery requires an understanding of the operative procedures and an appreciation of the normal postoperative appearance of the gut. The radiologist is frequently asked to define the postsurgical anatomy, to assess the efficacy of the procedure, to establish a postoperative baseline appearance, and to detect early and late postoperative complications. This chapter describes the more common operations performed on the GI tract, details the rationale for surgery, provides a basic approach to contrast examinations of postoperative patients, and illustrates normal appearances and common complications.

Surgery on the GI tract is performed for a number of reasons (Table 17.1) but most commonly to remove neoplastic and inflammatory tissue; to treat infection, perforation, bleeding, and obstruction; and to reconstruct portions of the gut to provide normal function. Postoperative contrast studies must be tailored to the nature of the surgery and the status of the patient.

17.2
Radiologic Technique

Before performing radiologic studies on a postoperative patient, it is vital to obtain as much information concerning the surgery as possible. Time spent pursuing this information is well invested. It is also important to obtain a plain film in the frontal and often lateral projections. The pattern of surgical clips, staples, and drains can provide valuable clues to postoperative anatomy and can detect residual contrast from prior studies that might be falsely interpreted as a new postoperative leak.

Patient positioning during the initial stages of a contrast study is important (GOLD and SEAMAN 1977) and staple patterns can help select the optimal starting position to best define the anatomy, particularly for patients who have had gastric surgery for weight control.

The selection of the contrast agent should be tailored to the clinical situation (JAMES et al. 1975). Water-soluble agents should be employed for pos-

R.M. GORE, MD, Professor and Vice Chairman, Department of Diagnostic Radiology, Evanston Hospital-McGaw Medical Center of Northwestern University, 2650 Ridge Avenue, Evanston, IL 60201, USA
C. SMITH, MD, Professor of Radiology, Section Director Gastrointestinal Radiology, Rush Presbyterian – St. Lukes' Medical Center, 1653 W. Congress Parkway, Chicago, IL 60612, USA

Table 17.1. Surgical procedures on the gastrointestinal tract

Patient problem	Surgery
Larynx and hypopharynx	
Neoplasm	Laryngectomy
	Partial
	Total
Esophagus	
Zenker's diverticulum	Cricopharyngeal myotomy with diverticulectomy or diverticulopexy
Achalasia	Pneumatic dilatation
	Esophagomyotomy
Neoplasm	Esophageal resection and reconstruction
	Gastric pull-up
	Colon interposition
	Jejunal interposition
Gastroesophageal reflux and esophagitis	Antireflux operations
refractory to medical therapy	Nissen fundoplication
	Belsey Mark IV
	Hill gastropexy
Paraesophageal hernia	Reduction and antireflux operation
Stomach	
Gastric ulcer refractory to medical therapy	Partial gastrectomy and reconstruction (Billroth I)
Hemorrhage	Optional vagotomy
Perforation	
Obstruction	
Neoplasm	Gastrectomy
	Partial with gastroenterostomy (Billroth II)
	Total gastrectomy with esophagojejunostomy
Dumping syndrome post-gastric surgery	Small bowel interposition
refractory to dietary manipulation	
Obesity	Gastric bypass
	Loop type anastomosis
	Roux-en-Y type anastomosis
	Vertical banded gastroplasty
Duodenum	
Duodenal ulcer	Vagotomy and antrectomy
	Highly selective vagotomy
	Truncal vagotomy and emptying procedures
Periduodenal neoplasm	Whipple procedure with or without gastric resection
	Biliary bypass and gastrojejunostomy
Small Bowel	
Localized bowel disease	Bowel resection with anastomosis
Colon	
Diffuse colon disease	Colectomy with ileostomy
	Continent ileostomy (Kock)
	End ileostomy
Neoplasm	Bowel resection and anstomosis
	With or without diverting colostomy
Diverticulitis	Bowel resection
	With or without diverting colostomy and second stage reconstruction
Ulcerative colitis	Proctocolectomy with ileal pouch and ileoanal anastomosis

sible anastomotic leaks. If no leak is encountered initially, barium should then be used because approximately 25% of anastomotic leaks are only demonstrated by barium contrast media (DODDS et al. 1982). Water-soluble contrast agents are also useful for evaluating patients with suspected obstructions, particularly in the postoperative esophagus, stomach, duodenum, and colon. Single-contrast barium studies are useful for detecting fistula and sinus tracts; evaluating the direction of flow and peristalsis; and examining patients who are unable to move easily. Although double-contrast barium studies provide superb mucosal detail, their use is limited in the immediate postoperative setting as patient mobility and cooperation are essential for these examinations.

The intravenous administration of glucagon is a useful adjunct in performing many studies because the hypotonia it induces can relieve spasm, maximize bowel distention to minimize postoperative artifacts, and slow down GI transit, affording more time to examine often complicated anatomy.

In patients who have an alimentary tract anastomosis, it is important to initially administer contrast material slowly and in small quantities. This is particularly true when the postoperative anatomy is unknown and following gastric surgery. If too much contrast is administered too quickly, the bowel will be "flooded," obscuring anatomic detail.

Retrograde contrast evaluation of patients with ileostomies and colostomies is often challenging. Commercially available devices and enema tips facilitate these studies. Alternatively, a Foley catheter introduced to its entire length may be used; the balloon should not be inflated while in the stoma, however. These tips and catheters should be held in place by having the patient exert manual pressure at the stomal site. When performing a double-contrast barium enema in these patients, less contrast material than normal is used because of difficulty in draining the barium (GOLDSTEIN and MILLER 1976). In patients who have had a right hemicolectomy, ready reflux of contrast through the enterocolic anastomosis should be anticipated.

Patients with temporary colostomies usually need evaluation of both limbs of the colon prior to their reanastomosis. Evaluation of the distal segment either per rectum or through the mucous fistula should be performed first, as demonstration of persistent severe disease in the distal segment may delay colostomy closure.

Whenever possible, contrast studies should be obtained before performing a new examination on a postoperative patient. Without old studies for comparison, perianastomotic surgical defects may be misdiagnosed as pathology and true abnormalities may be misinterpreted for postoperative bowel deformity.

17.3
Pharynx and Larynx

Surgery is performed on the larynx and pharynx primarily to palliate or cure neoplasms. Tumors that involve the epiglottis, arytenoids, and false vocal cords can be treated with hemilaryngectomy or supraglottic laryngectomy. These procedures preserve voice function, whereas total laryngectomy requires speech rehabilitation. In this later procedure, the airway and gastrointestinal tract are separated

with a permanent tracheostomy. The hyoid bone, the thyroid lamina, and muscles attached to the clavicles are dissected, and the larynx is separated from the pharynx and trachea and is then removed. The trachea is sectioned and exteriorized as a permanent tracheostomy.

After laryngectomy, the anterior wall of the pharynx is closed by a "key-shaped" closure. Vertical sutures along the axis of the upper esophagus cross with horizontal sutures that course from the lateral aspects of the base of the tongue and pharynx. These sutures meet in the midline and the anastomosis is reinforced by muscles of the inferior constrictor. This site should be examined closely as it is a common point of anastomotic breakdown (Fig. 17.1).

Postlaryngectomy patients must be studied with videotaping or rapid sequence camera. Examinations performed in the early postoperative period may show anastomotic leaks along the anterior pharyngeal wall (WIPPOLD and BALFE 1994). Later, muscular hypertrophy causing deformity of the contrast column may be found and may be difficult to differ-

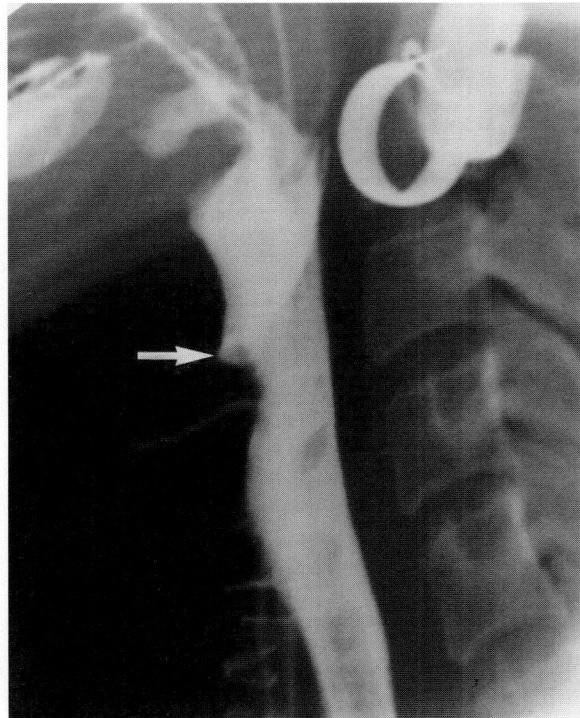

Fig. 17.1. Total laryngectomy: postoperative appearance. Lateral view of the cervical esophagus shows absence of the normal laryngeal structures. The *arrow* indicates the apex of the key-shaped closure, which is its weakest point and the most common site of anastomotic leak. (From SMITH et al. 1993)

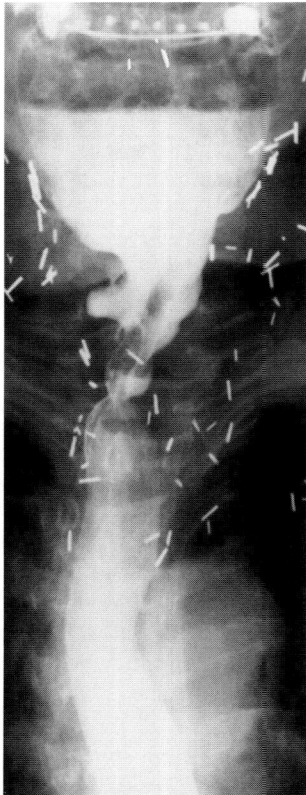

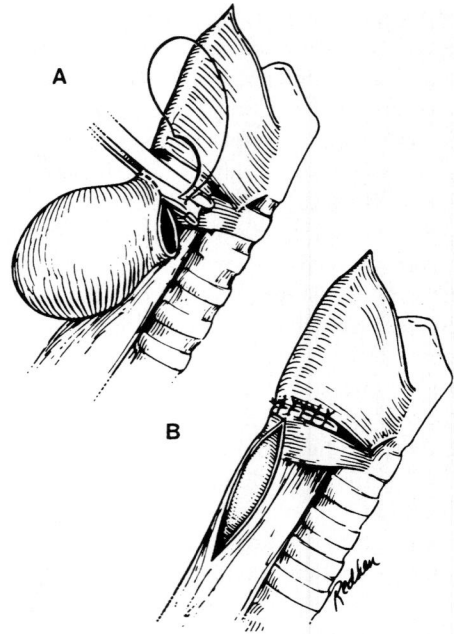

Fig. 17.3 a,b. Zenker's diverticulum surgery. a When large, these diverticula are best managed by excision. b A complementary division myotomy of the cricopharyngeus muscle reduces the chance of recurrence or postoperative dysphagia. (From MOODY and ROTH 1988)

Fig. 17.2. Total laryngectomy: chronic appearance. The contrast-filled neopharynx has a more undulating contour than seen in Fig. 17.1 in this patient 15 years post laryngectomy. Muscular hypertrophy, which causes this appearance, may be difficult to differentiate from a recurrent neoplasm in some patients. (From SMITH et al. 1993)

entiate from recurrent disease (Fig. 17.2) (BALFE et al. 1982).

17.4
Esophagus

Esophageal surgery is performed for a variety of reasons: resection of benign and malignant neoplasms, prevention and management of complications of gastroesophageal reflux, management of motility disorders, and treatment of esophageal diverticula or perforation (RUBESIN and ROSATO 1994).

17.4.1
Zenker's Diverticulum

Zenker's diverticulum is a mucosal and submucosal outpouching that arises at the junction of the

pharynx and esophagus in the posterior midline between the inferior constrictor of the pharynx and cricopharyngeus muscle. The etiology of this "false" diverticulum is controversial and a number of theories have been proposed: upper esophageal sphincter dysfunction, dis-coordination between pharyngeal contraction and upper esophageal sphincter relaxation, and gastroesophageal reflux (RUBESIN and YOUSEM 1994). Patients present with dysphagia, regurgitation of undigested food, halitosis, choking, and occasionally a neck mass. Treatment of this disorder is surgical and is indicated to alleviate dysphagia and prevent the sequelae of chronic aspiration. A cricopharyngeal myotomy with division of the fibers of the cricopharyngeus muscle is an absolutely essential feature of operative management (Fig. 17.3). If only a diverticulectomy is performed, both symptoms and the diverticulum will ultimately recur, as the underlying functional defect remains uncorrected (MOODY and ROTH 1988). Postoperative radiographic studies (Fig. 17.4) in these patients often demonstrate persistent posterior outpouchings (BALFE et al. 1982). They should not be interpreted as a recurrent diverticulum because the diverticulum has been resected.

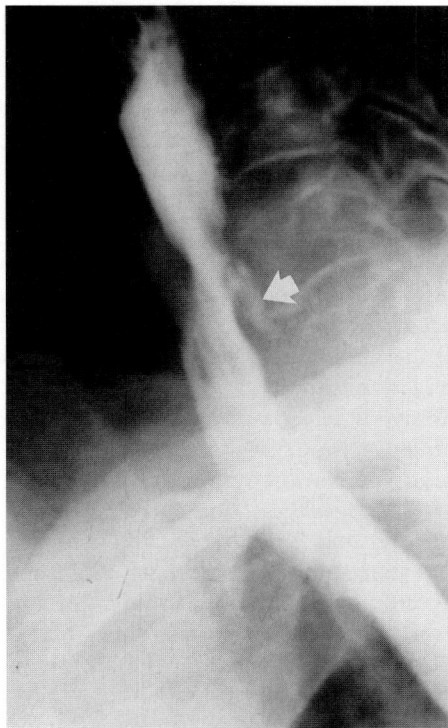

Fig. 17.4. Zenker's diverticulum: postoperative appearance. This patient underwent endoscopic cricopharyngeal myotomy and diverticulectomy. The small posterior outpouching (*arrow*) represents the widened esophagus at the site of the diverticulum

17.4.2
Achalasia

Achalasia is the most frequently encountered primary motor disorder of the esophagus and is characterized by aperistalsis of the esophageal body and dysfunction of the lower esophageal sphincter (LES), esophageal dilatation, and regurgitation.

Treatment of achalasia is directed at the LES, which in addition to having incomplete or no relaxation, is frequently hypertensive. Initial medical management includes the use of smooth muscle relaxants such as nitrates and calcium channel blocking agents in an attempt to decrease sphincteric resistance. These conservative measures usually do not significantly improve the patient's clinical status.

Pneumatic dilatation, open surgical myotomy, or a thoracoscopic or laparoscopic esophageal myotomy are the most effective treatment choices as they are directed at relieving the functional obstruction at the LES (RUBESIN et al. 1988; ZEGEL et al. 1979).

Pneumatic dilatation is the most reasonable initial therapy in patients with achalasia and consists in placement of a balloon catheter across the region of the LES and inflating it under fluoroscopic guidance. Contrast studies performed immediately following the procedure are helpful in detecting serious complications such as perforation.

An esophagomyotomy through the musculature that creates the LES is the mainstay of surgical treatment of achalasia. This operation can be performed through an open (Heller myotomy) or minimally invasive approach. Since simple esophagomyotomy may be complicated by reflux esophagitis and subsequent peptic strictures, some surgeons also reconstruct the hiatus and gastroesophageal junction with a Belsey Mark IV fundoplication to avoid postoperative gastroesophageal reflux. After a Heller myotomy, an outpouching resembling a diverticulum may develop at the lower end of the esophagus.

17.4.3
Carcinoma of the Esophagus

There are no simple, straightforward algorithms for treating patients with esophageal cancer. A number of treatment options are available, none of which are entirely satisfactory (O'REILLY and FORESTIERE 1996). Each treatment plan must be tailored to the individual patient based upon: (1) histologic features, grade, and stage of the tumor; (2) age and overall health of the patient; (3) social situation and access to care; (4) availability of specialized diagnostic, therapeutic, and support facilities; and (5) most importantly, the needs and desires of the patient (EISENBERG 1996).

17.4.3.1
Dilatation, Stenting, Photocoagulation

Since few patients are cured of their tumor, palliation for dysphagia is often the only therapeutic goal in patients with advanced esophageal cancer. Peroral dilatation can restore sufficient esophageal lumen patency in more than 90% of patients. When dilatation is not successful, a peroral polyvinyl prosthesis (Fig. 17.5), nitinol stent, Gianturo stent, or Wallstent may be inserted by pulsion technique through the stenosis, either radiologically or endoscopically (ACUNAS et al. 1996; NEVITT et al. 1996; COIA et al. 1994; WINKELBAUER et al. 1996). This has proven to be a safe and highly effective method for long-lasting

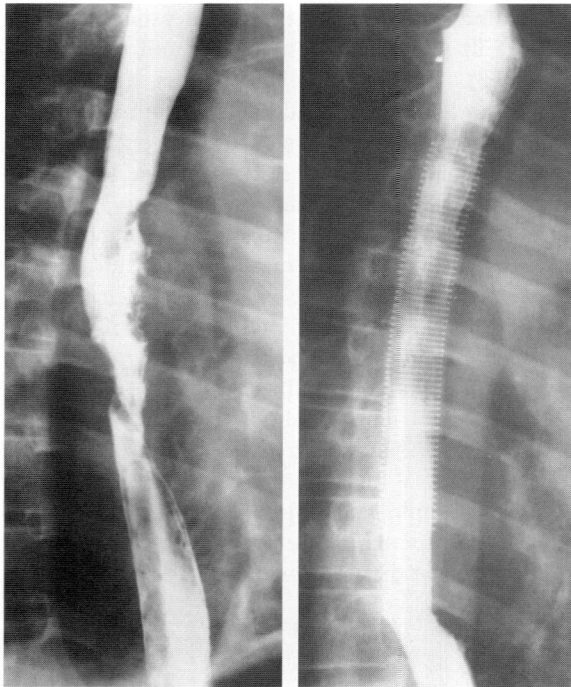

a,b

Fig. 17.5 a,b. Palliative stenting of esophageal carcinoma. **a** Esophagram demonstrates an ulcerating, constricting carcinoma in the mid-esophagus. This patient had severe dysphagia and disseminated metastases and did not respond to combined chemotherapy and radiation therapy. **b** Symptoms were alleviated by the peroral insertion of this polyvinyl stent

improvement of dysphagia (BOYCE 1993). In patients with esophagopulmonary or bronchial fistula, a perorally placed prosthesis blocks leakage and stops pulmonary soilage (BINKERT et al. 1996).

Transendoscopic ablation by laser photocoagulation of obstructing intraluminal tumors is a promising, safe technique for palliation of dysphagia (CARTER et al. 1993). Indeed, patients with unresectable esophageal cancer are best palliated either by peroral prosthesis or by combined therapy with laser ablation followed by external beam radiation (BARNETT 1996).

17.4.3.2
Surgery

Although advances in surgery have reduced postoperative mortality to half its former rate over the past decade, this has not led to increased survival, which remains at 25% at 1 year and 10% at 5 years after surgery. Only about 20% of lesions are resectable.

Survival rates increase dramatically if no lymph nodes are involved but this is rarely the case (FERGUSON and SKINNER 1996).

The choice of the surgical procedure is dependent on several factors: the preoperative condition of the patient, preoperative staging and findings at operation, and the surgeon's philosophy about en bloc resection versus palliative procedures.

An en bloc resection includes the entire tumor mass, a margin of normal esophagus and stomach to incorporate involved submucosal lymphatics, and all potential nodes. The surgical approach to an en bloc resection can be a right thoracotomy with laparotomy, a left thoracotomy with a thoracoabdominal incision, or separate abdominal and cervical incisions without thoracotomy.

With esophageal resection and a gastric pull-up, the approach may be either a combined transthoracic and transabdominal approach or a transhiatal esophagectomy without thoracotomy. The approach avoids the need for multiple gastrointestinal anastomoses. Although leakage from the anastomosis or oversewn gastric fundus may occur, the consequences are less devastating if the anastomosis has been performed in the neck since a leak in the cervical area can be managed more easily than one in the mediastinum.

With the transhiatal esophagectomy, the stomach is mobilized from an abdominal approach. Blunt dissection of the lower esophagus is accomplished through the diaphragmatic hiatus and the upper esophagus is mobilized through an incision in the left neck. Once the esophagus has been resected, the stomach is carefully positioned through the diaphragmatic hiatus into the posterior mediastinum (Fig. 17.6). As the fundus appears in the cervical neck incision, it is gently grasped and pulled into the wound. The cervico-esophagogastric anastomosis is performed on the anterior surface of the fundus ensuring that there is no tension. Pyloromyotomy accompanies the esophageal replacement procedure to ensure adequate gastric emptying (MATHISEN and WILKINS 1996). Because of its proximity, rich vascular supply, sufficient length to reach the anastomotic site, and need for only one anastomosis, the stomach is the preferred reconstructive organ (FOK and WONG 1988).

The concept of "blind" or transhiatal esophagectomy has been accepted over the past decade. The underlying principle is that carcinomas of the esophagus, especially of the middle third, are not usually curable by surgical means, so that palliation is the primary goal (AGHA and ORRINGER 1985).

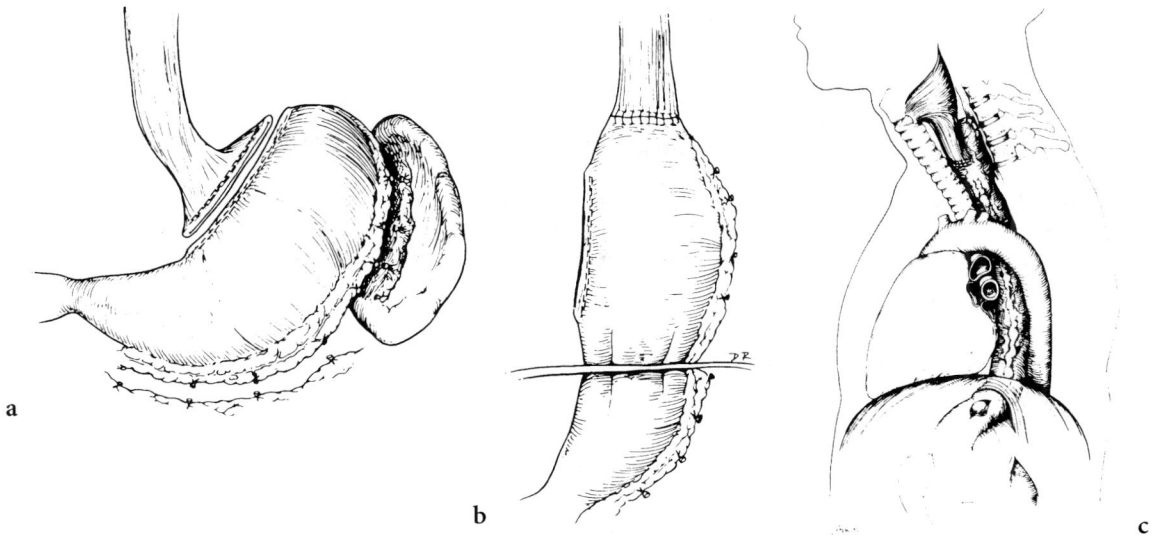

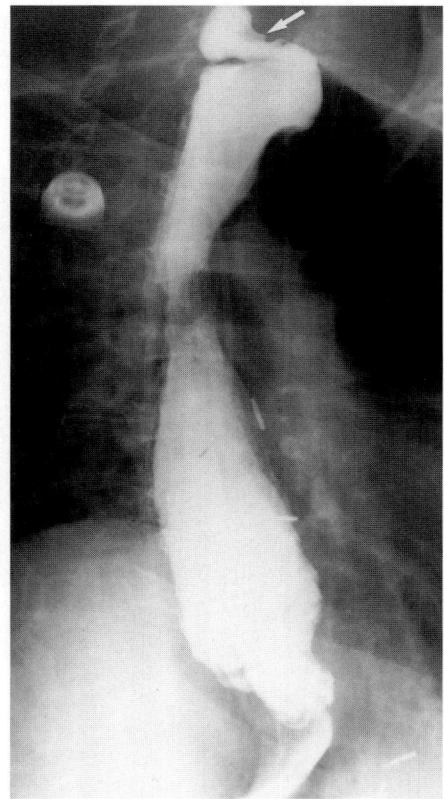

Fig. 17.6 a–d. Esophagectomy with esophagogastric anastomosis: gastric pull-up. a Initially there is resection along the greater curvature portion of the stomach. This allows the stomach to be fashioned into a tube and for removal of suspicious lymph nodes. b The stomach is pulled through the hiatus. The anastomosis can be end-to-end or the cardia can be oversewn with an end-to-side anastomosis. (From FERGUSON and SKINNER 1996). c The esophageal replacement is in the native esophageal bed. A pyloromyotomy is performed to facilitate gastric emptying. (From ORRINGER and SLOAN 1978). d Typical appearance of gastric pull-up as upper GI study: the anastomosis (arrow) is in the region of the cervical esophagus. (From SMITH et al. 1993)

If the tumor is small and has not invaded the full thickness of the esophageal wall, a case for direct visualization of the entire mediastinum and wide mediastinal dissection can be made. Transhiatal esophagectomy also does not permit accurate nodal staging and is not appropriate for tumors involving the tracheobronchial tree or major mediastinal vessels (ORRINGER and SLOAN 1978).

The radiographic appearance of esophageal replacement by a gastric pull-up is fairly standard. The cervical anastomosis may be an end-to-end type (Fig. 17.6) or it may be an end-to-side type where the proximal portion of the gastric fundus has been closed as a blind-ending pouch. The antrum and duodenum are generally subdiaphragmatic in location. The lesser curve of the stomach should be positioned to the right and may be identified by staple lines.

Replacement or bypass of the esophagus by a segment of colon (Fig. 17.7) can be performed for both malignant and benign diseases (CHRISTENSEN and SHAPIR 1986). As with esophagogastric anastomosis, it is safer to perform the bypass anastomosis in the neck, where an anastomotic leak is easier to recognize and manage. The distal anastomosis of the colon interposition is usually to the lesser curvature portion of the stomach.

Generally with colon interposition, an isoperistaltic segment of the descending colon with its intact vascular supply gives the best functional result. The esophageal replacement ideally should lie within the native esophageal bed. If there is significant residual tumor block in the posterior me-

diastinum, a substernal route can be used. Radiographically, the length of colon and its position varies. It is important to visualize both the proximal anastomosis and the cologastric anastomosis (CHRISTENSEN and SHAPIR 1986).

Other less common types of reconstruction of the esophagus include jejunal interposition and the formation of a reversed gastric tube from the greater curvature portion of the stomach.

17.4.4
Gastroesophageal Reflux

Operative treatment for gastroesophageal reflux is indicated when there is reflux esophagitis refractory to medical management, Barrett's esophagus, and respiratory complications such as asthma, aspiration, and laryngitis (BELSEY 1996). Pure anatomic repair of sliding hiatal hernias has been unsuccessful in correcting reflux disease. Surgery is now directed

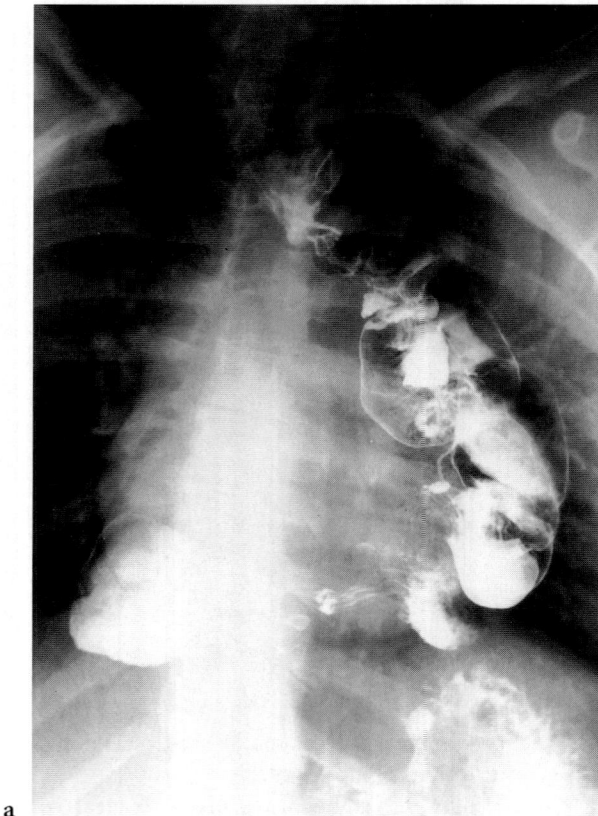

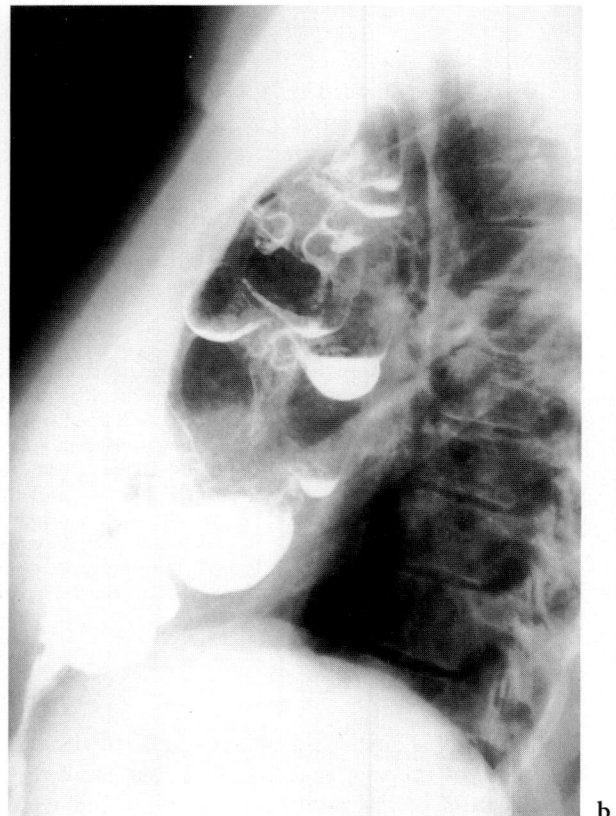

a
b

Fig. 17.7 a,b. Esophagectomy with colonic interposition. This patient's esophageal bed was obstructed by tumor and unresectable. The colon was interposed in a substernal loca-tion. This is the typical appearance of an interposition on an upper GI study: frontal (a) and lateral (b) views

toward correcting the physiologic abnormality by increasing the pressure that is transmitted to the LES (FEIGIN et al. 1974; HIEBERT 1996).

17.4.4.1
Nissen Fundoplication

The Nissen fundoplication has become the most common corrective procedure for gastroesophageal reflux (GOMPELS and HARRISON 1972). This is an antireflux operation in which the gastric fundus is wrapped completely around the gastroesophageal region (AGHA et al. 1985). The stomach is retracted inferiorly, the phrenicoesophageal ligament is stripped from the distal esophagus, 4–6 cm of the distal esophagus is freed, any hiatal hernia component is reduced, the diaphragmatic crura are approximated, and the anterior and posterior walls of the fundus are wrapped around the distal esophagus for 2–3 cm (Fig. 17.8a) (NAHRWOLD 1996). Sutures bind the fundus to itself, and incorporate the anterior muscular wall of the esophagus to the wrap to anchor it in place (POLK 1996). To insure that the wrap is not too tight, resulting in postoperative dysphagia or gas-bloat syndrome, appropriately sized dilators are placed in the esophagus as the wrap is constructed. The fundic wrap is preferably placed beneath the diaphragm, but may be left in the chest

and still function appropriately. This procedure produces a characteristic mass effect in the region of the gastric cardia on double-contrast barium studies (Fig. 17.8b,c) (GELFAND 1984; THOENI and MOSS 1979).

17.4.4.2
Noncircumferential Fundoplication

Other surgical variations can be performed where the wrap does not completely encircle the esophagus. These variations are generally performed when the patient is known to have a predisposing esophageal motility disorder that could be worsened by a total circumferential wrap. Noncircumferential fundoplication procedures include the Belsey Mark IV (BELSEY 1996), Hill (HILL 1996), and Toupet procedures. The radiographic appearance depends on the degree and orientation of the wrap.

Excessive gastroesophageal reflux should not be seen following a successful repair. Since the wrap is intentionally left loose to prevent esophageal obstruction, contrast material may insinuate around the wrap. Also, an apparent hiatal hernia will be seen on contrast studies if the wrap has been left in the chest or if the crura are not approximated. It is critical, as with other postoperative patients, to obtain consultation from the surgeon to determine the pro-

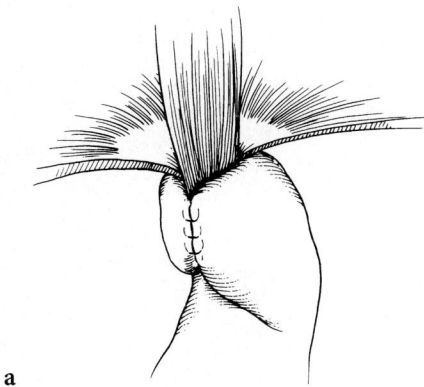

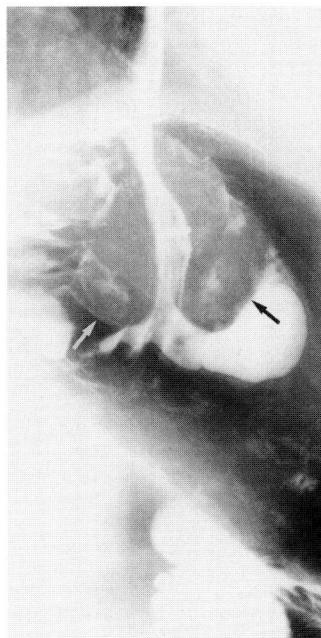

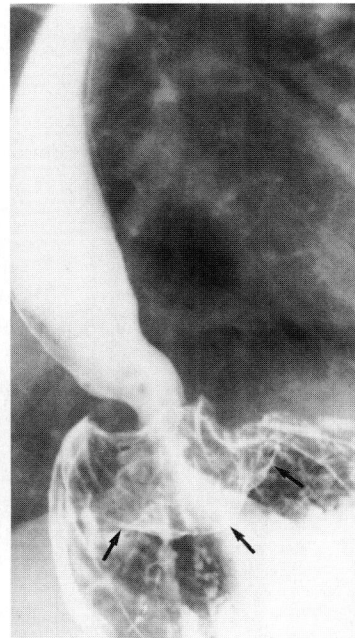

a

Fig. 17.8 a–c. Nissen fundoplication: normal appearance. a Schematic drawing shows that the anterior wrap is held by three structures. The wrap is placed in a subdiaphragmatic position and the crura are closed to maintain stability. On barium studies (b, c), the fundoplication causes a pseudotumor (*arrows*) in the region of the cardia that can simulate a tumor

b,c

cedure performed. Without this information, what appears to be a hiatal hernia may be erroneously interpreted as partial disruption of the wrap.

17.4.5
Postoperative Complications

Esophageal surgery is attended by one of the highest surgical morbidities and mortalities. Complications include: anastomotic leak; torsion or gangrene of the gastric, colonic, or jejunal "pull up"; subphrenic abscess; hemorrhage; wound infection and dehiscence; sepsis; anastomotic stricture; dumping syndrome; and reflux esophagitis. Complication rates are considerably higher for resection of the middle and proximal esophagus (Table 17.2). During the early postoperative period, the most common complications include stasis due to ileus or vagotomy, obstruction due to anastomotic edema, and perforation due to anastomotic breakdown (AHBARI et al. 1993). In the late postoperative period, the most common complications are gastroesophageal reflux, aspiration, anastomotic stricture, and recurrent tumor

(ORRINGER 1996). CT is an important adjunct in the evaluation of these patients. In the early postoperative period, CT is particularly useful for detecting abscesses that do not communicate with the gut and those that are missed by a fluoroscopic examination limited by the patient's clinical status. CT is also useful for demonstrating extraluminal recurrent tumor (HEIKEN et al. 1984).

Postoperative complications occur more commonly in the esophagus than other portions of the GI tract (RUBESIN and BEATTY 1994). Sutures and

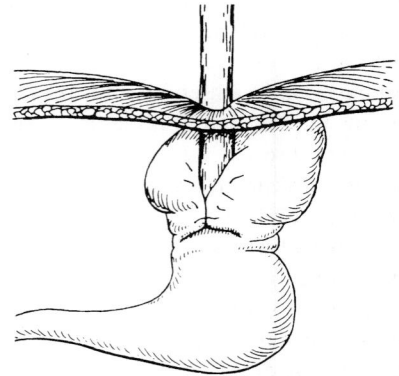

Table 17.2. Complications of esophageal surgery (modified from RUBESIN and BEATTY 1994)

Early complications
a) Common
   Gastroesophageal reflux
   Aspiration
   Anastomotic or staple-line leak
   Delayed bypass emptying
      Anastomotic edema
      Anastomotic narrowing
      Gastric/duodenal atony
      Obstruction at diaphragm
      Pyloric channel obstruction/spasm
b) Uncommon
   Pneumothorax
   Mediastinal hematoma
   Empyema
   Vocal cord paresis
   Chylothorax
   Ischemia of colonic or jejunal bypass
   Splenic injury

Late complications
a) Common
   Anastomotic stricture
   Aspiration
   Gastroesophageal reflux and its sequelae
   Recurrent carcinoma
b) Uncommon
   Delayed conduit emptying
   Tracheoesophageal fistula
   Anastomotic or staple-line leak

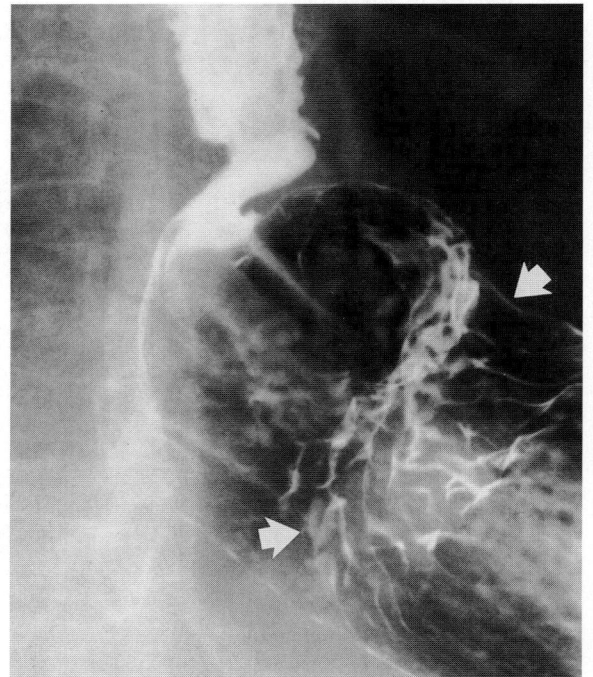

Fig. 17.9 a,b. Nissen fundoplication: disruption. **a** Disruption of one or all of the sutures will lead to distention of the stomach and the development of an abnormal pouch. **b** Upper GI study shows deformity (*arrows*) due to the disrupted fundoplication

staples hold less well in the esophagus because the esophagus lacks a serosa, the esophageal muscle is soft and stringy, and mucosa retracts from the cut esophageal margin because of great mobility between the squamous mucosa, the fatty submucosa, and muscularis propria (OWEN et al. 1983; RUBESIN and ROSATO 1994).

Following truncal vagotomy, the LES may fail to relax, giving a clinical and radiologic picture similar to achalasia. This is because the sensory and motor functions as well as the visceromotor neural control of esophageal function are interrupted. This complication, seen in approximately 1% of patients who undergo this treatment, usually resolves spontaneously but may occasionally require esophageal dilation (ORRINGER 1996).

Complications of antireflux procedures include esophageal or gastric obstruction and wrap dehiscence with recurrent reflux. Dysphagia may be due to transient edema in the first postoperative week. Persistent dysphagia occurs if the wrap or crural closure is too tight. The gas bloat syndrome, abdominal pain, and distension may also develop due to the inability to belch or vomit for relief.

Recurrent gastroesophageal reflux can occur with partial or complete disruption of the fundoplication (Fig. 17.9a). Radiographically, wrap dehiscence (Fig. 17.9b) appears as one or more contrast-filled projections from the fundus and the normal indentation from the gastric wrap is absent (HATFIELD and SHAPIR 1985).

Gastric obstruction results if the wrap "slips" from the distal esophagus and encircles a portion of the stomach.

17.5
Stomach

Operations are performed on the stomach for three major reasons: (1) for the treatment of peptic ulcer disease and its complications such as bleeding, perforation, and obstruction; (2) for resection of benign and malignant masses; and (3) for the management of obesity (NAHRWOLD 1996; SMITH et al. 1993).

17.5.1
Vagotomy and Pyloroplasty

Some type of vagotomy is critical in the operative management of duodenal ulcers. This procedure decreases acid secretion and parietal cell response to gastrin. Unfortunately, complete vagotomy induces gastric stasis and a pyloroplasty is required. This term is applied to any of several operations which widen the pyloric channel lumen to promote gastric emptying (Fig. 17.10a). The pylorus is incised longitudinally and reconstructed with vertical sutures (NAHRWOLD 1996). Radiologically, the normal contours of the pyloric channel are lost (Fig. 17.10b,c). This procedure is usually combined with a truncal vagotomy.

17.5.2
Billroth I Procedure

The Billroth I procedure is a hemigastrectomy or antrectomy which removes a significant bulk of the parietal cell mass as well as the gastrin-secreting antrum. If the duodenum is not inflamed or scarred, an end-to-end gastroduodenostomy (Fig. 17.11) is performed (SMITH et al. 1993). The goal in this surgery is to approximate the stomach and duodenum as closely as possible without compromising the gastric lumen. Gastric emptying and fluid dynamics are not dramatically altered by Billroth I surgery (NAHRWOLD 1996).

17.5.3
Billroth II Procedure

In the Billroth II procedure, subtotal gastrectomy is performed when anastomosis to the duodenum is not feasible. There is a gastroenterostomy linking the gastric pouch to the small bowel distal to the ligament of Treitz. There are several variations of this procedure which differ in the construction of the gastroenterostomy and in the way the jejunum is brought up to the anastomosis (NAHRWOLD 1996). A loop type gastrojejunostomy connects the jejunum to the stomach in one continuous segment. The configuration can be a right-to-left or antiperistaltic loop in which the afferent loop, or that part of the bowel bringing bile and bowel contents towards the stomach, is first anastomosed to the right or lesser curvature portion of the stomach and is then carried across to the left side (Fig. 17.12).

When creating a left-to-right or isoperistaltic loop, the anastomosis is situated so that the small bowel is brought first from the left side of the stomach and then to the right side so that the direction of peristalsis in the stomach and the attached jejunum are aligned (Fig. 17.13). Alternatively, a Roux-en-Y

Heineke-Mikulicz

Finney

a   Jaboulay

b   **c**

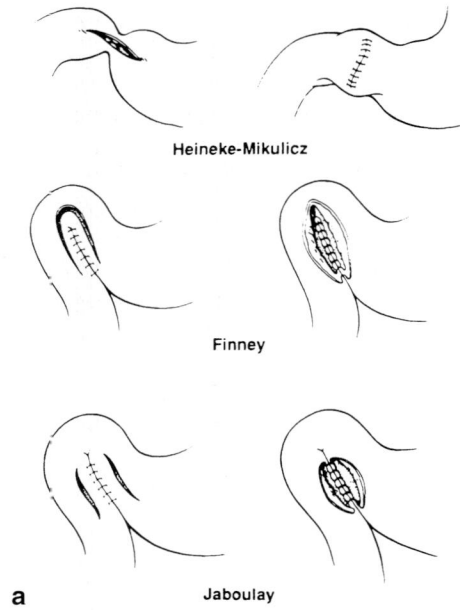

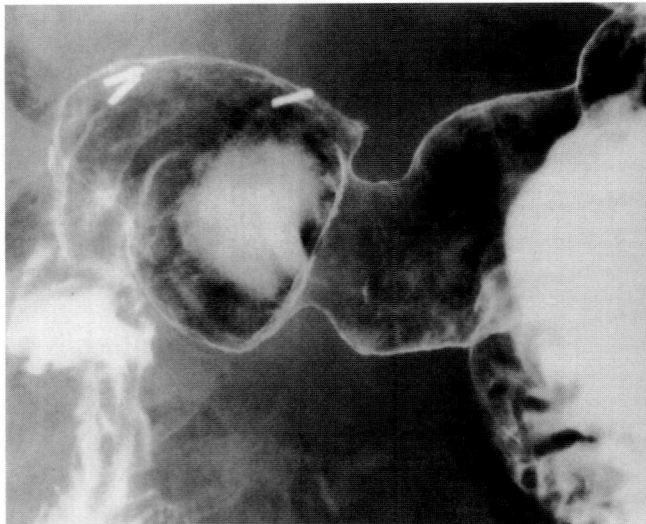

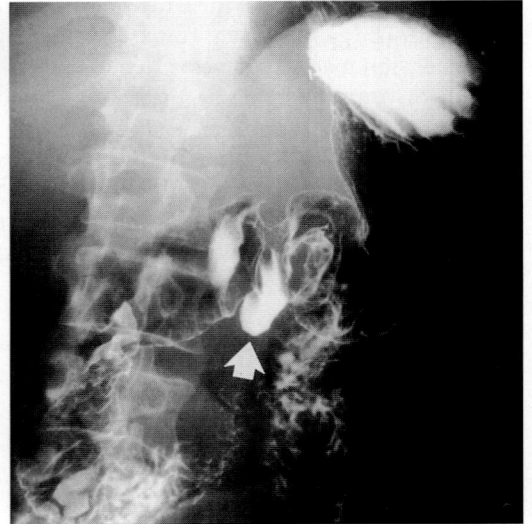

Fig. 17.10 a–c. Vagotomy and pyloroplasty. **a** Diagrams depicting the three major types of pyloroplasties. (From CHUNG 1992). The pyloroplasty may appear as a widened pylorus (**b**) or cause a pseudodiverticulum (*arrow*) (**c**) on barium studies

anastomosis can be performed. The jejunum is divided and the proximal end or side of the small bowel is attached to the stomach while the distal end is fashioned into an enteroenterostomy downstream (Fig. 17.14).

17.5.4
Surgery for Obesity

When medical and dietary therapy fail to control life- threatening obesity, surgically created gastric restrictive procedures can be effective (SMITH 1994b). Their purpose is to cause early satiety and decreased caloric intake by creating a small-capacity proximal stomach that leads to the distal stomach or small bowel by a very narrow channel or anastomosis (HOEHSTRA et al. 1993). The *gastric plication* (Figs. 17.15, 17.16) procedure consists in stapling a closure across the stomach just below the gastroesophageal junction, creating a small lumen between the small tubular pouch proximally and the remainder of the stomach distally (SMITH et al. 1994; SMITH and DEZIEL 1995). The channel must be reinforced

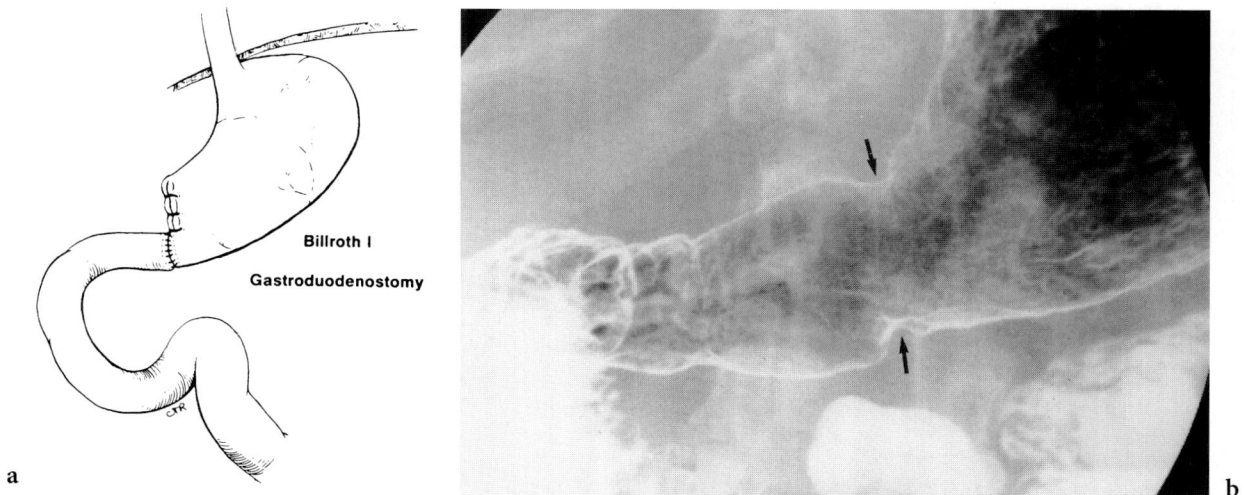

Fig. 17.11 a,b. Billroth I gastroduodenostomy. Several modifications have been devised but the basic operation ensures that the duodenal passage remains intact. **a** Diagram depicting the gastroduodenostomy. (From SMITH and DEZIEL 1995). **b** Upper GI series shows minimal indentation (*arrows*) at the widely patent anastomosis

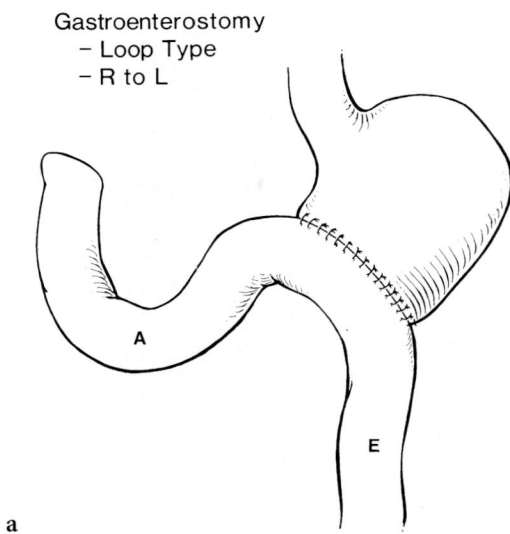

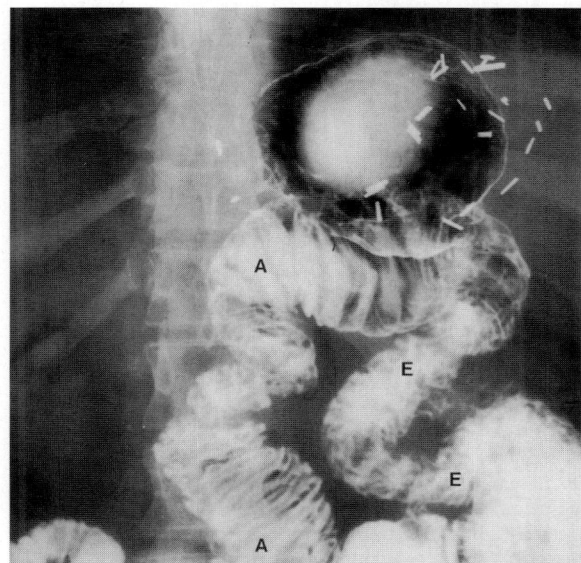

Fig. 17.12 a,b. Billroth II gastrojejunostomy: antiperistaltic configuration. **a** Diagram and **b** barium study show the loop-type, right-to-left configuration after gastric resection. The small bowel is first anastomosed to the right side of the stomach and is then carried to the left. The length of the afferent (*A*) loop varies; the efferent loop (*E*) carries contents away from the stomach. (From SMITH et al. 1993)

by an opaque band or nonopaque mesh. Stapling devices facilitate this otherwise laborious operation. This procedure has largely replaced the more complicated *gastric bypass* (Fig. 17.17), in which the small proximal gastric pouch is anastomosed to the jejunum via a loop or Roux-en-Y gastrojejunostomy (NAHRWOLD 1996, GELFAND 1984). With a Roux-en-Y type anastomosis, the jejunum is divided, the proximal end or side of the distal bowel is attached to the stomach, and the Roux-en-Y loop is anastomosed to the jejunum downstream. The stomach is separated from the food path but it is not transected. With a loop gastroenterostomy, the standard right-to-left anastomosis is performed (SMITH et al. 1985).

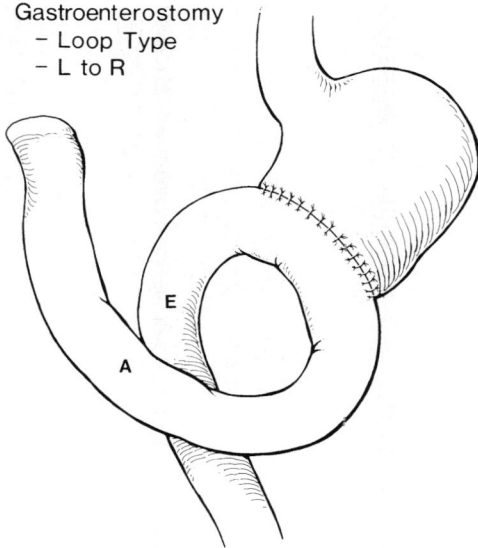

a

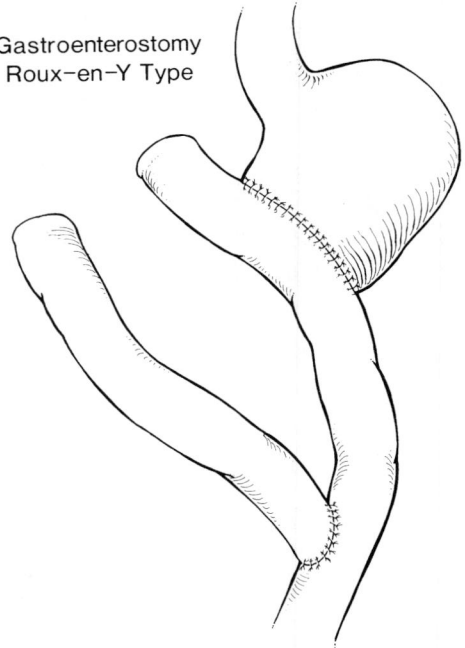

b

Fig. 17.13 a,b. Billroth II gastrojejunostomy: isoperistaltic configuration. a Diagram and b barium study showing loop-type, left-to-right configuration after gastric resection. In this modification, the afferent loop (A) swings to the left, and the anastomosis is carried from the greater curvature or left side of the stomach to the lesser curvature or right side. E, Efferent limb

17.5.5
Gastrectomy

A variety of procedures are used to treat gastric carcinomas (HANKS et al. 1995). In patients undergoing operation for potential cure, the location of the primary tumor dictates the choice of resection (ELLIS 1960; FUCHS and MAYER 1995). Tumors located

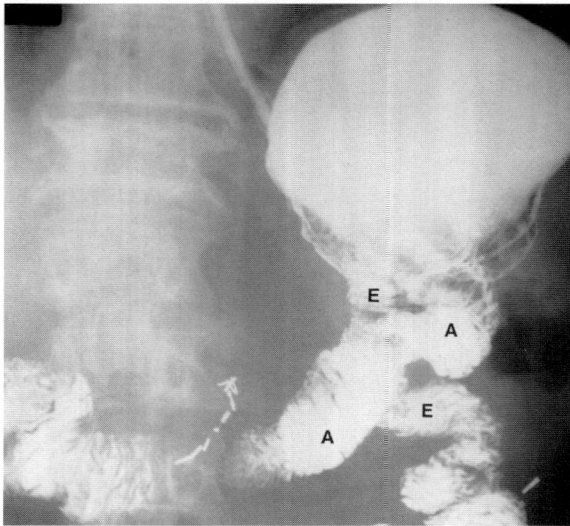

a

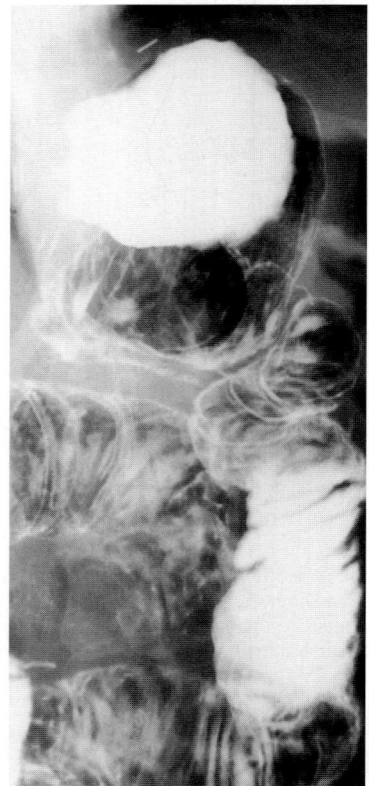

b

Fig. 17.14 a,b. Partial gastrectomy with Roux-en-Y gastrojejunostomy. a Diagram depicts the end-to-side gastrojejunostomy and enteroenterostomy. b Barium study shows that the Roux loop does not readily fill with contrast material and the distal enteroenterostomy may not be readily localized. Surgical clips are present at the gastroesophageal junctions from prior vagotomy. (From SMITH et al. 1993)

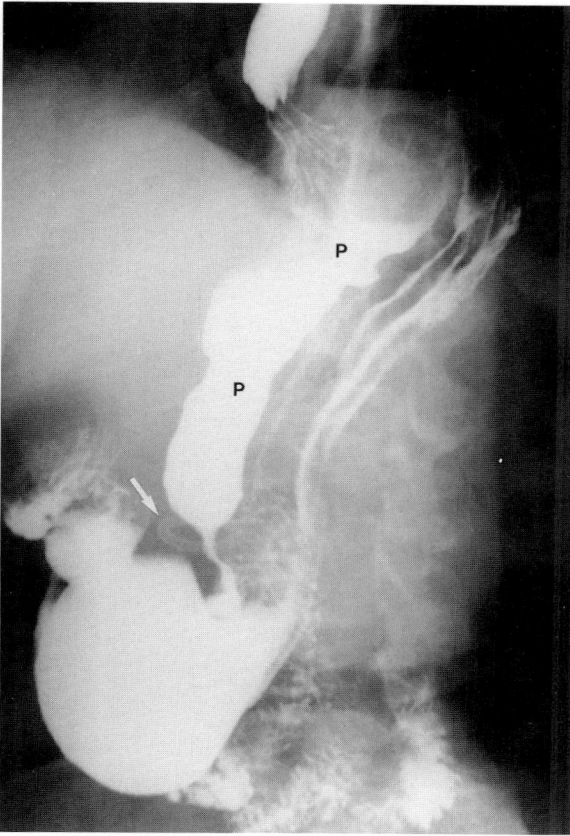

Fig. 17.15. Vertical banded gastroplasty. Stapling devices have facilitated this procedure. The lesser curvature proximal pouch (*P*) and channel are filled with barium. An opaque ring (*arrow*) reinforces the channel

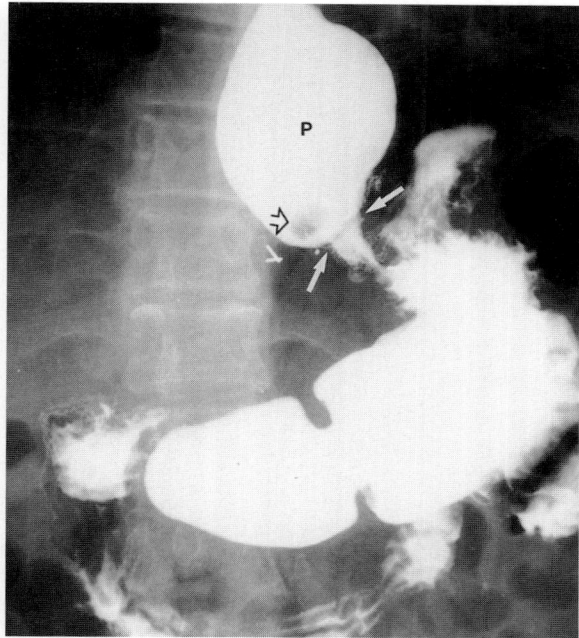

Fig. 17.16. Vertical banded gastroplasty with outlet obstruction. The proximal pouch (*P*) is distended by barium and retained food (*open arrow*). The channel lumen (*white arrows*) is only 2 mm. Postoperative deformity of the fundus is also seen. (From SMITH and DEZIEL 1995)

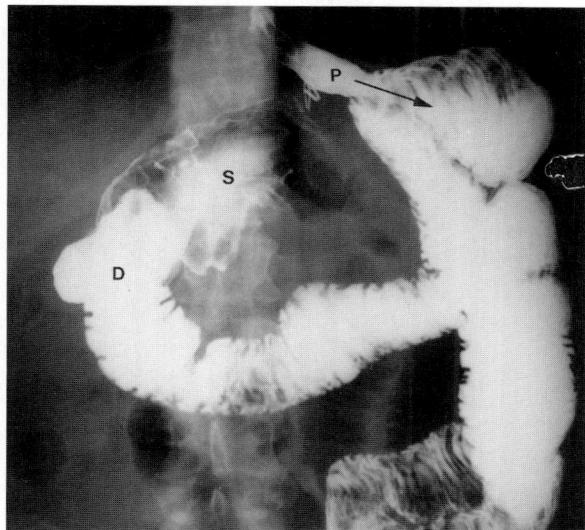

Fig. 17.17. Gastric bypass with loop gastrojejunostomy. The small proximal pouch (*P*) is anastomosed to the jejunum in a right-to-left loop type configuration (*arrow*). Contrast material has refluxed into the native duodenum (*D*) and distal stomach (*S*). (From SMITH et al. 1993)

within 5 cm of the gastroesophageal junction undergo proximal gastric resection, esophagogastric anastomosis, and pyloroplasty. With a loop type gastrojejunostomy, the stomach and jejunum are anastomosed in one contiguous segment (NAHRWOLD 1996). An alternative approach is total gastrectomy with or without splenectomy, but this approach is associated with greater postoperative morbidity due to complications of the reconstruction. For lesions located along the greater curvature, subtotal gastric resection for a distance of 5–6 cm around the lesion with omentectomy and splenectomy is performed, followed by creation of a gastroenterostomy or gastroduodenostomy (BURHENNE 1971). Antral cancers are removed by subtotal gastric resection with wide proximal margins. Some cancers require total gastrectomy and the distal esophagus is sutured to jejunum (Fig. 17.18) that has been brought up to the anastomosis as part of a Roux-en-Y (NAHRWOLD 1996).

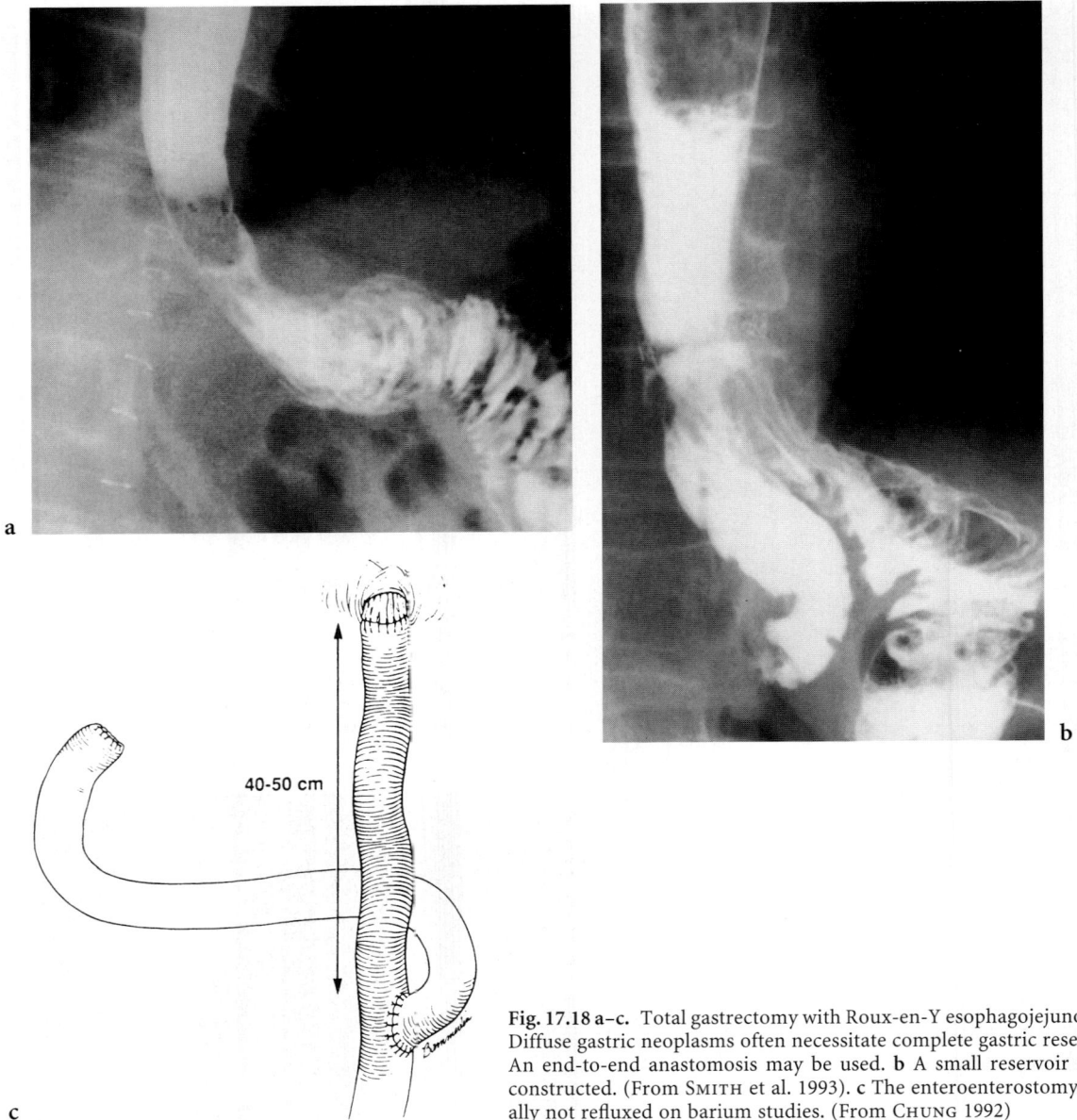

Fig. 17.18 a–c. Total gastrectomy with Roux-en-Y esophagojejunostomy. Diffuse gastric neoplasms often necessitate complete gastric resection. **a** An end-to-end anastomosis may be used. **b** A small reservoir may be constructed. (From SMITH et al. 1993). **c** The enteroenterostomy is usually not refluxed on barium studies. (From CHUNG 1992)

17.5.6
Complications of Gastric Surgery

Gastric surgery is fraught with considerable postoperative morbidity (Table 17.3) (SMITH et al. 1993). These complications can usually be diagnosed with conventional barium or water-soluble contrast studies but CT may be required to fully delineate their extent (SMITH 1994b).

17.5.6.1
Anastomotic Leaks

Breakdown of a suture line and surgical anastomosis can occur at any anastomosis between the stomach and small bowel and any enteroenteric anastomosis associated with gastric surgery, as well as at the oversewn proximal end of the duodenum following a Billroth II procedure (SMITH et al. 1994). These com-

Table 17.3. Complications that may follow gastric and duodenal surgery

Bowel dysmotility 　Postvagotomy hypotonia and stasis 　Dumping syndrome 　Generalized bowel ileus	Bowel obstruction 　Narrow anastomotic or channel diameter 　　Edema 　Marginal ulcer 　Stricture after ulcer healing 　　Prolapse and intussusception
Gastritis and gastric remnant ulcerations 　Technical factors 　　Indication for original operation 　　Type of operation 　　Experience of surgeon 　　Adequacy of surgery 　　Presence of unabsorbable sutures 　Presence of hypersecretory states 　　Incomplete vagotomy 　　Gastrinoma with Zollinger-Ellison syndrome 　　Antral G-cell hyperplasia 　　Retained antrum syndrome 　　Hyperparathyroidism 　Ulcerogenic substance use 　Alkaline reflux	Bezoar formation 　Afferent loop obstruction Metabolic effects 　Malabsorption 　　Steatorrhea with decreased vitamin D absorption 　　Shortened intestinal transit time 　　Inadequate mixture of pancreatic juices, bile salts, and food 　Iron deficiency anemia Inadequate diet 　Impaired resorption of dietary iron 　Chronic blood loss Vitamin B$_{12}$ anemia 　Decrease of gastric intrinsic factor 　Bacterial overgrowth
Neoplasm 　Recurrent tumor 　Gastric remnant cancer	Weight loss and malnutrition 　Insufficient caloric intake 　Incomplete digestion of food 　Inadvertent gastroileostomy 　Diarrhea
Anastomotic leak 　Bowel perforation 　Abscess 　Fistula	

plications are identified radiographically by contrast material exiting the gut lumen, filling an abscess cavity, fistula, or the peritoneal cavity. CT may be needed to fully define the abscess cavity and direct percutaneous drainage (HALPERT and GOODMAN 1993; GELFAND 1984).

17.5.6.2
Stomal Ulceration

Recurrent ulceration following Billroth I and II procedures for peptic ulcer disease commonly occurs on the duodenal or jejunal side of the anastomosis, respectively (SMITH 1994b). These marginal or postanastomotic ulcers develop in the following situations: inadequate gastric resection, retained antral remnant, gastrinoma, and excessively long afferent loop (SMITH and DEZIEL 1995). These ulcers are difficult to identify radiologically because the overlapping fold pattern and plication defects produced by surgery may obscure their detection (SMITH et al. 1993). When large, a frank ulcer crater may be identified (Fig. 17.19). Secondary signs include unusual stiffness at the anastomosis, an edematous appearing mass, or unusually thickened

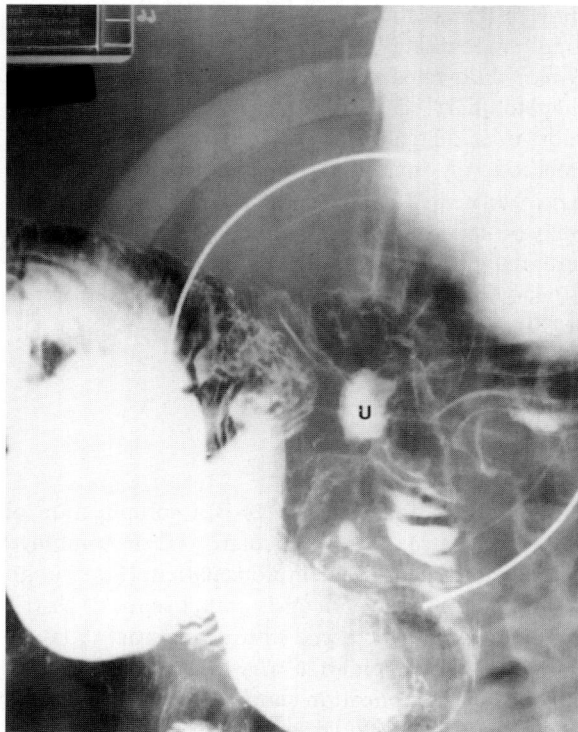

Fig. 17.19. Marginal ulcer. A large ulcer (*U*) is identified adjacent to the anastomosis of this gastrojejunostomy

folds (GELFAND 1984, HALPERT and GOODMAN 1993).

17.5.6.3
Jejunogastric Intussusception

Jejunogastric intussusception is a rare complication of Billroth II gastric surgery which can occur as an acute or chronic process (SMITH 1994b). Retrograde prolapse of the small bowel adjacent to the gastroenterostomy into the stomach can cause partial or complete obstruction and can occasionally cause vascular compromise. Radiologically, there is a large intraremnant filling defect (Fig. 17.20) often suggestive of intussusception in its configuration (GELFAND 1984; HALPERT and GOODMAN 1993).

17.5.6.4
Afferent Loop Syndrome

The afferent loop can become dilated in patients following Billroth II surgery for two reasons and cause considerable epigastric distress (SMITH et al. 1993). First, there may be partial obstruction of the afferent loop at the gastrojejunostomy leading to accumulation of pancreatic, biliary, and duodenal secretions and lumen dilatation (Fig. 17.21c). CT showing a dilated, fluid-filled afferent loop (Fig. 17.21b,c) and hepatobiliary scintigraphy revealing isotope retention in a dilated proximal segment are the main methods of establishing the diagnosis (GORE and GHAHREMANI 1994). Second, the gastrojejunostomy may be constructed so that food and fluid flow preferentially from the esophagus into the afferent loop (Fig. 17.21d), causing its dilatation (OP DEN ORTH 1992).

17.5.6.5
Bezoar

Bezoar formation (Fig. 17.22) is a complication of subtotal gastrectomy particularly when combined with vagotomy in an edentulous patient (EISENBERG 1996). Diminished peristalsis and absence of gastric acid allow poorly chewed fibrous material to be retained and form a matted mass (SALENA and HUNT 1993). This complication should be suspected radiologically whenever a large, discrete mass of food is encountered in a partially resected stomach in a fasting patient. Semisolid food will exit the stomach with

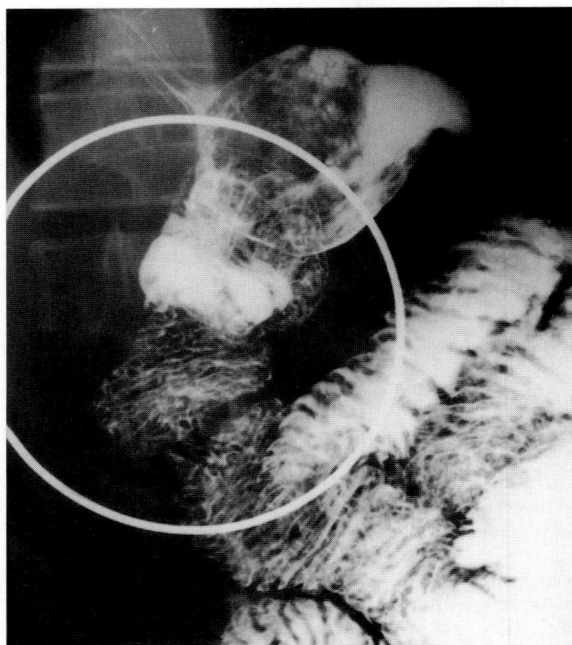

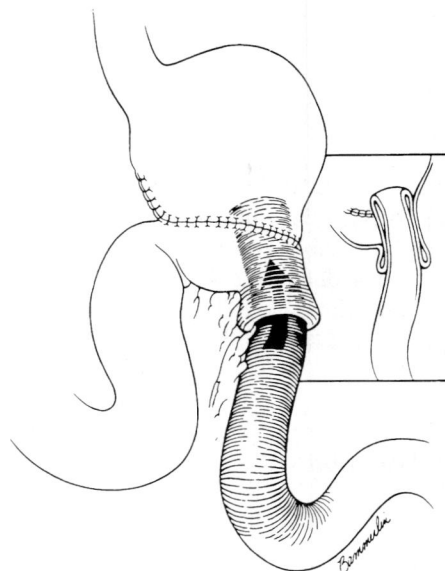

a

b

Fig. 17.20 a,b. Jejunogastric intussusception. Intussusception of the efferent limb is present on the GI study (**a**) and illustrated in the diagram (**b**). (From CHUNG 1992)

the barium flow while a bezoar remains in the stomach (GELFAND 1984; HALPERT and GOODMAN 1993).

17.5.6.6
Gastric Stump Carcinoma

Partial gastrectomy for benign disorders, particularly peptic ulcer disease, is associated with an in-

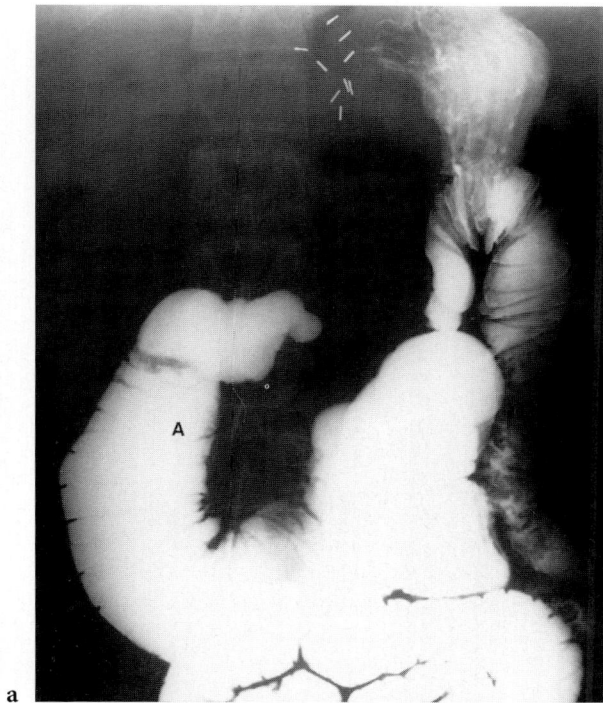

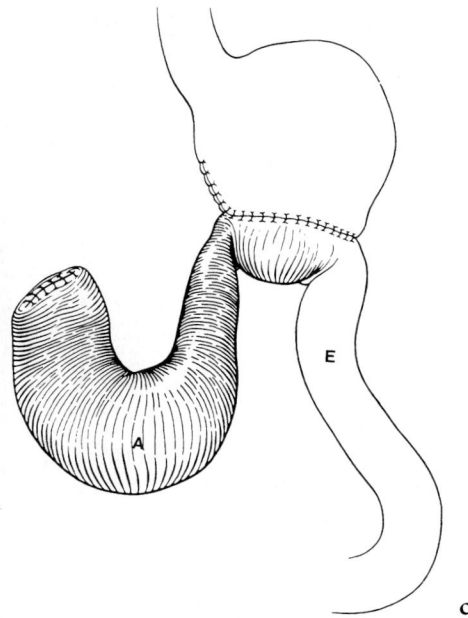

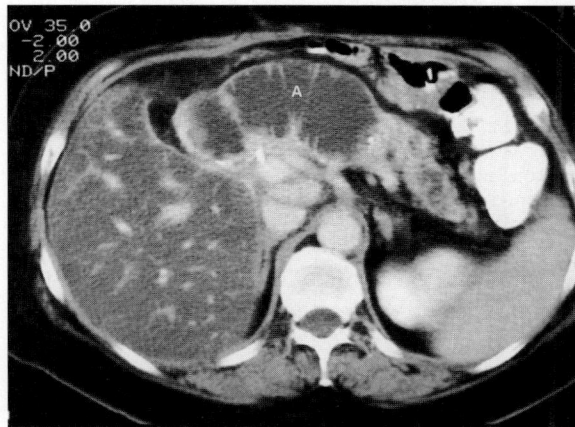

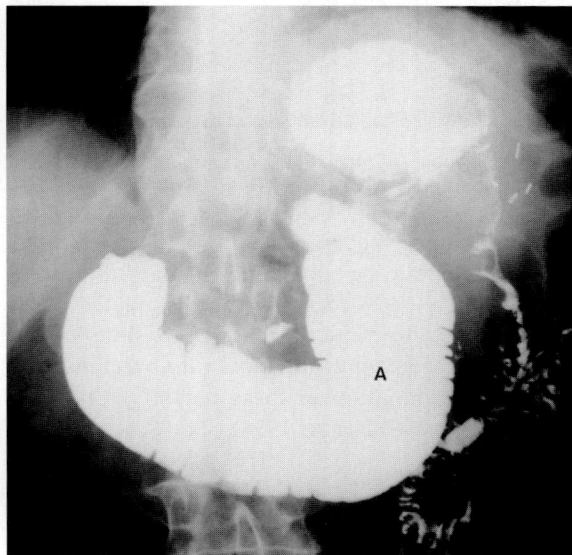

Fig. 17.21 a–d. Afferent loop syndrome. **a** Dilatation of a poorly emptying afferent loop (*A*) is demonstrated on a GI study. **b** CT scan performed on a different patient shows a dilated segment of jejunum (*A*) in the right upper quadrant. **c** Schematic depiction of afferent loop syndrome. (From Chung 1992). **d** Contrast material in this patient preferentially flows into the afferent (*A*) loop

creased risk of gastric stump cancer (Goodman et al. 1992). There is a 15- to 20-year latent period after which the relative risk increases three- to six-fold (Davis 1993). This delay probably reflects the time required for a gradual progression of normal mucosa to intestinal metaplasia to dysplasia and cancer (Fig. 17.23) as a result of prolonged achlorhydria and enterogastric reflux after enterostomy (Kondo et al. 1996). Truncal vagotomy, used to reduce gastric

acid, may potentiate this transition (Chandie Shaw and Op Den Orth 1994).

17.5.6.7
Recurrent Carcinoma

Patients who have had a partial gastrectomy for localized gastric cancer are at considerable risk for

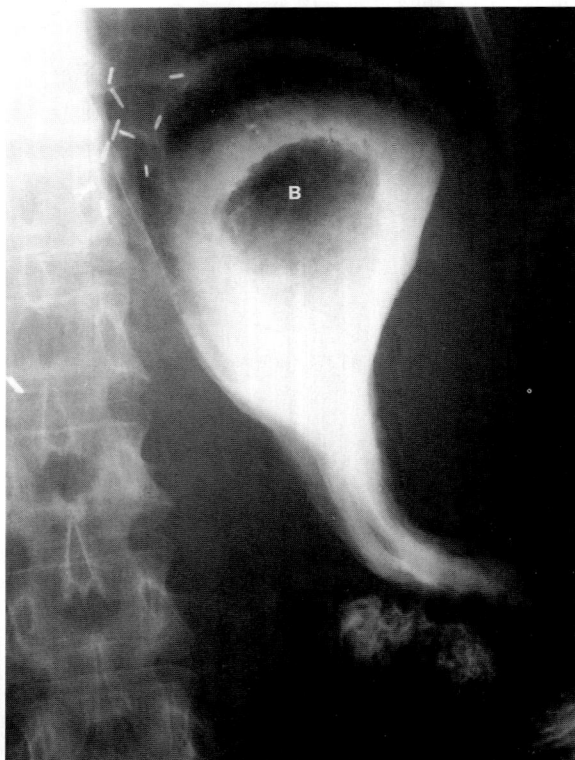

Fig. 17.22. Bezoar (*B*) formation is a common complication of Billroth II surgery

recurrent tumor. Recurrent tumor can appear infiltrating, polypoid, or ulcerating on barium studies (KODERA et al. 1996). Since surgically created plication defects can produce a mass effect simulating a malignancy, it is important to obtain a baseline postoperative examination in these patients (CHANDIE SHAW and OP DEN ORTH 1994).

17.5.6.8
Chronic Remnant Gastritis

One of the most common complications following gastric surgery is chronic gastritis (SMITH et al. 1993). Without an intervening pylorus, chronic reflux of bile and pancreatic secretions produces inflammatory change in the gastric remnant. This manifests radiologically (Fig. 17.24) as enlarged gastric rugal folds (SMITH et al. 1994).

17.6
Pancreas and Biliary Tract

Operations on the pancreas and biliary tract usually require anastomoses to the intestinal tract. This

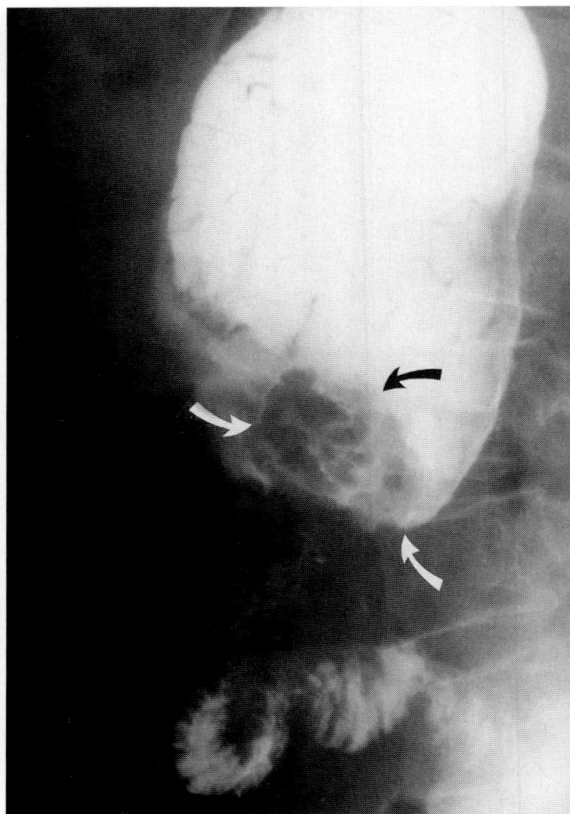

Fig. 17.23. Gastric carcinoma complicating Billroth II procedure. An irregular polypoid mass (*arrows*) is present at the gastrojejunostomy in this patient who had undergone surgery for benign peptic ulcer disease 18 years earlier

anatomy is often complex and requires careful planning before and during the radiologic study.

17.6.1
Whipple's Operation

Whipple's operation entails resection of the distal stomach, duodenum, and either part or all of the pancreas (Fig. 17.25). It is usually performed for removal of carcinoma of the pancreatic head or periampullary tumors (MICHELASSI et al. 1989). The GI tract must be reconstructed, which requires anastomosis of the jejunum to the pancreas, the biliary tree (usually the common bile duct), and the stomach. Vagotomy is usually performed as well to inhibit gastric acid secretion, thereby diminishing the potential for gastrojejunal ulceration. This reconstruction also requires that the inflow of alkaline bile and pancreatic juice be inserted proximal to the gastrojejunostomy to further protect against marginal ulceration (GORE and NAHRWOLD 1994).

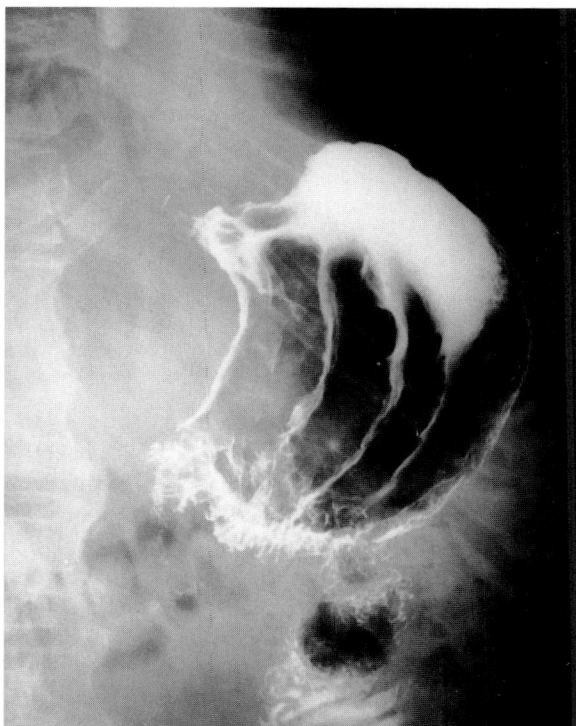

Fig. 17.24. Chronic remnant gastritis. There is diffuse thickening of the rugal folds in the gastric remnant in this patient who had undergone a Billroth II gastrectomy for intractable peptic ulcer disease

Fig. 17.25 a,b. Whipple's procedure. **a** In the classic procedure, there is resection of the distal stomach with an end-to-side, right-to-left gastrojejunostomy. There is an accompanying end-to-side choledochojejunostomy and a partial resection of the pancreas and pancreaticojejunostomy reconstruction. (From SMITH and DEZIEL 1995). **b** In the pylorus-sparing Whipple's procedure, the pylorus is spared to act as a sphincteric mechanism to prevent dumping symptoms. In the classic procedure the distal stomach and pylorus are resected. *A*, Afferent loop; *E*, efferent loop; *arrow*, gastrojejunostomy

On barium studies, a Billroth II gastrojejunostomy is identified, and there may be rapid filling of both jejunal afferent and efferent loops, which can obscure the anatomy. Early films with little distal small bowel opacification are the most diagnostic. If the afferent loop is sufficiently refluxed, the common bile duct may fill through the end-to-side anastomosis. Air in the biliary tree is often seen on plain films, CT scans, and ultrasound studies. On CT scans, the afferent loop can be positively identified in about half of cases when it is filled with oral contrast medium. When unopacified, these loops can be mistaken for an abscess or tumor recurrence. When the jejunum is brought up to the right upper quadrant via a retrocolic approach, it may be placed posterior to the superior mesenteric vessels and simulate the duodenum on CT studies. If unopacified, it can simulate lymphadenopathy. Serial postoperative CT scans should be obtained at 3- to 6-month intervals because pancreatic neoplasms usually quickly recur (GORE and NAHRWOLD 1994).

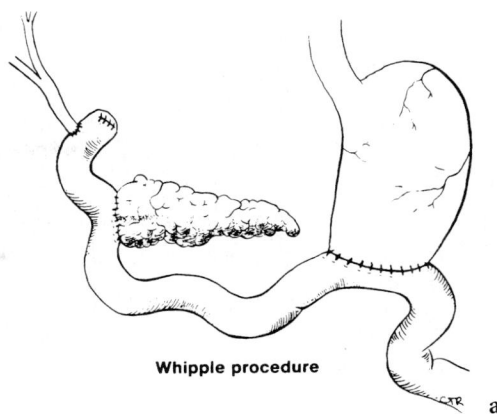

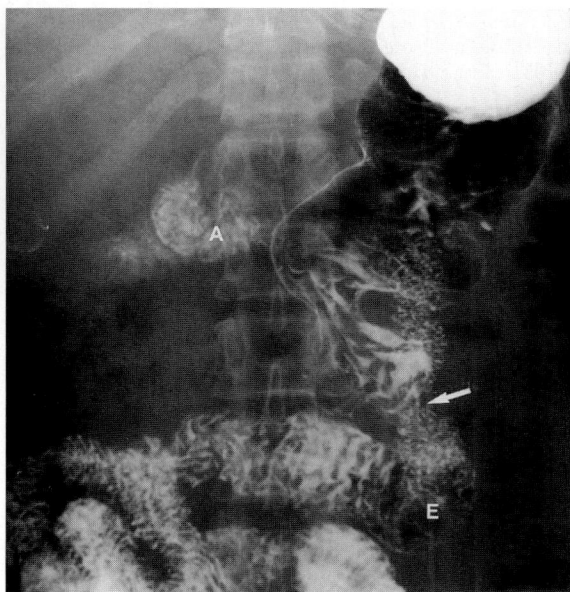

17.6.2
Bypass Procedures

Cholecystojejunostomy or choledochojejunostomy is performed to bypass unresectable pancreatic head neoplasms and severe distal common bile duct stone disease. Contrast medium and intestinal gas will reflux into the biliary system as a result (Fig. 17.26).

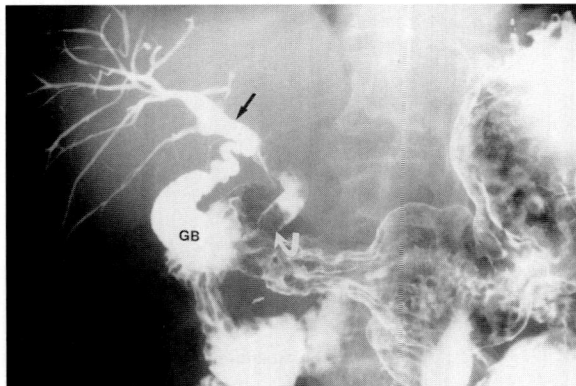

Fig. 17.26. Biliary bypass. This patient with a distal bile duct stone (*curved arrow*) has undergone a cholecysto-duodenostomy. Note the reflux of contrast into the gallbladder (*GB*) and biliary tree (*straight arrow*)

17.6.3
Sphincterotomy

Surgical or endoscopic sphincterotomy is one therapeutic approach to patients with sphincter of Oddi spasm and pancreas divisum. After this procedure, CT, ultrasound, and plain films may show intrabiliary and more rarely pancreatic ductal gas. On upper gastrointestinal studies, reflux of barium into the bile duct is common. Because the barium quickly empties into the duodenum, the reflux is generally not clinically significant.

17.6.4
Direct Pancreatic Ductal Drainage

In patients with chronic pancreatitis and ductal ectasia associated with multiple pancreatic duct strictures, a long longitudinal incision is made throughout the length of the duct until all the strictures are opened. The duct is then anastomosed to a Roux-en-Y loop of jejunum, which provides drainage at the obstructed regions. These patients usually do not show any abnormalities of the stomach, duodenum, or upper jejunum on gastrointestinal studies unless barium or air refluxes into the afferent loop. On rare occasions when barium does reflux, it is of no significance unless there is prolonged retention of contrast material by the afferent loop or fistula formation.

17.6.5
Pseudocyst Drainage

Cystogastrostomy or cystojejunostomy of pancreatic pseudocysts may be identified on upper GI series. On CT scans, these drained collections must be differentiated from abscess or undrained pseudocyst when there is no gas or contrast media in the cyst.

17.6.6
Choledochoduodenostomy

Choledochoduodenostomy is performed for a variety of reasons (GHAHREMANI 1994): multiple common bile duct calculi; papillary or ampullary stenosis; impacted distal stone in the absence of pancreatitis; intrahepatic calculi; perivaterian duodenal diverticula which cause recurrent cholangitis or pancreatitis; a massively dilated common bile duct without stones; tubular narrowing of the distal common bile duct segment (usually secondary to pancreatitis); and a low iatrogenic stricture. In order for this procedure to be successful, the common bile duct must be a minimum of 1.4 cm in diameter and the stoma size should be at least 2.5 cm. Choledochoduodenostomy should not be performed on a nondilated common bile duct, in patients with sclerosing cholangitis, in the decompression of the pancreatic duct for pancreatitis, or when there is significant duodenal inflammation or edema.

17.7
Small Bowel

Surgical interventions in the small intestine include enterotomy for removal of polyps or foreign bodies; enteroplasty to resolve a stricture; enterectomy for the resection of obstructed, traumatized, neoplastic, or necrotic segments; plication to prevent small intestinal obstruction; and the creation of ostomies or mucous fistulas for feeding or drainage purposes (LAPPAS and MAGLINTE 1994; GREAGER et al. 1995). The small intestine is also used for the construction of reservoirs following gastrectomy and proctocolectomy and for reconstitution of biliary or pancreatic flow into the gastrointestinal tract (LIU and WALKER 1996). Surgical bypass of the small intestine has also been performed in an attempt to control morbid obesity or lower serum cholesterol.

Most postoperative radiologic studies of the small bowel are performed to define the anatomy (Fig.

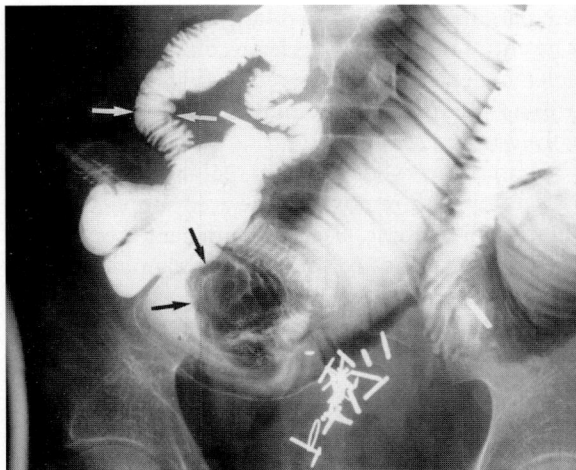

Fig. 17.27. Ileostomy study: tumor recurrence. This retrograde ileostomy study was performed on a patient with familial adenomatous polyposis who had undergone a total proctocolectomy for polyps and small bowel resection for adenocarcinoma. Tumor has recurred at the anastomotic site (*black arrows*). The small bowel proximally is dilated and obstructed; the distal ileum (*white arrows*) is normal in caliber

17.27) or to investigate complications (Fig. 17.28). It may be difficult to localize the entero-enterostomy with a traditional small bowel follow-through study, and an enteroclysis examination may be needed.

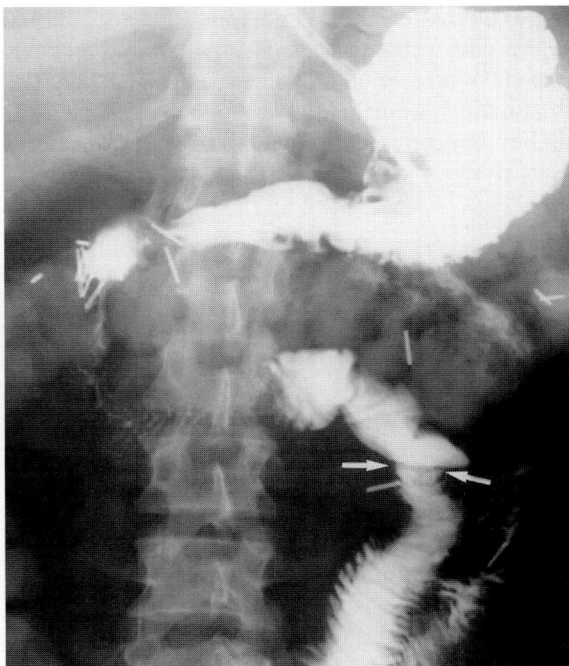

Fig. 17.28. Enteroenterostomy. This film from a small bowel follow-through shows that the patient has had a small bowel resection and anastomosis between the jejunum near the ligament of Treitz and the distal jejunum. There is some perianastomotic deformity (*arrows*) but the lumen is widely patent. (From SMITH et al. 1993)

17.8
Colon

Colon surgery is performed for a variety of reasons (CONDON 1996): resection of malignant and benign masses; diverticular disease with bleeding, diverticulitis, or stricture; obstruction due to cancer, diverticulitis, volvulus, or hernia; angiodysplasia with hemorrhage; ischemia and gangrene; perforation; and inflammatory bowel disease. Radiologists are frequently asked to evaluate the colon to exclude complications such as anastomotic dehiscence, fistula, stricture, and abscess formation. The postoperative colon is also evaluated for the following indications: assessment of anastomotic healing, resolution of inflammatory disease prior to colostomy closure, and detection of tumor recurrence following resection for tumor.

In most situations, surgeons will perform a primary anastomosis after colon resection for benign and malignant disorders. A colostomy may be needed, however, when there is extensive infection, inflammation, and ischemia, or in emergency situations when the colon is unprepared. End colostomies

are performed without an associated anastomosis; diverting colostomies are often designed to protect a distal anastomosis. A "double-barrel" colostomy entails complete division of the colon and exteriorizing both ends. This prevents spill-over of bowel contents from the proximal to the distal loop. The anterior wall of the colon is slit and exteriorized with a loop colostomy; the posterior wall of the colon is intact (DENT et al. 1987).

When an end colostomy is created with a distal anastomosis, the distal remnant of colon and rectum may be handled in one of two ways. With the Hartmann's procedure, the tumor or diseased segment of sigmoid is resected, a colostomy is created, and the distal rectal stump is closed, leaving the distal rectum and anus intact. The resulting pouch becomes a blind segment of colon from the anus to the sealed stump. Alternatively, if the distal segment of rectosigmoid is of adequate length, it can be exteriorized to the abdominal wall as a mucous fistula.

In the early postoperative period, anastomotic leak is the major indication for a contrast enema. Water-soluble contrast should be employed, because barium leakage into the peritoneal cavity may lead to granuloma formation and adhesions and will interfere with subsequent studies since it is not absorbed. Water-soluble contrast material, on the other hand, is absorbed so that follow-up studies will not be compromised by residual contrast from a previous study.

17.8.1
Colon Cancer

The primary treatment of colorectal cancer is surgical resection. The goal of surgery is a wide resection of the involved segment of colon together with removal of regional lymphatic drainage (SIGURDSON 1995). The resection should include a segment of colon at least 5 cm on either side of the tumor although wider margins may be required because of obligatory ligation of the arterial blood supply (LOGGIE 1996).

Cancers of the right colon require removal of the right colon, the proximal two-thirds of the transverse colon, and a short segment of terminal ileum and appendix combined with resection of attached mesenteric blood vessels and regional lymph channels and nodes (Fig. 17.29). This wide resection is essential because of the numerous lymphatic channels from the colon that join the ileocolic and middle colic vessels. This rich lymphatic network is a reflection of the absorptive function of the right colon.

Cancers of the transverse colon often have the worst prognosis because the lymphatics drain into the paraduodenal and peripancreatic lymph nodes. The entire right and transverse colon along with the splenic flexure must be resected if lymph nodes around the origin of the middle colic artery are involved (Fig. 17.30).

With cancers of the left colon, a left hemicolectomy with removal of the area supplied by the inferior mesenteric artery is sufficient. Lesser segmental resections are adequate for sigmoid cancers (Fig. 17.31).

The surgical approach to patients with rectal cancer depends upon the location of the tumor and its size. Lesions located in the rectosigmoid and upper rectum can be treated with a low anterior resection through an abdominal incision followed by primary anastomosis. If a distal margin of at least 2 cm of normal bowel can be resected below the lesion, even low rectal carcinomas can have a sphincter-saving resection. This is facilitated by new end-to-end stapling devices. Indeed, low anterior resection is now the rule for cancers within the distal 6 cm of rectum provided they are not too large or fixed. Increasingly sphincter-saving operations with or without preoperative radiation are performed for cancers 3–4 cm from the anal verge (VERNAVA and GOLDBERG 1996). Unlike tumors of the colon, large rectal tumors may not allow an adequate resection margin and mandate an abdominoperineal resection (BLOCK and HURST 1996).

An abdominoperineal resection is indicated if an adequate distal margin cannot be obtained, if the tumor is large and bulky deep within the pelvis, if there is extensive local spread of rectal cancer, or if

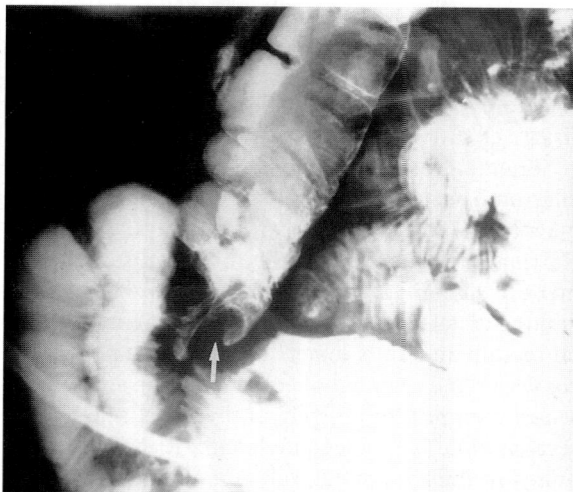

Fig. 17.29. Right hemicolectomy with end-to-side anastomosis. On this barium enema, the anastomotic site is patent and there is free reflux of contrast material into the small bowel. There is, however, recurrent tumor (*arrow*) at the anastomosis

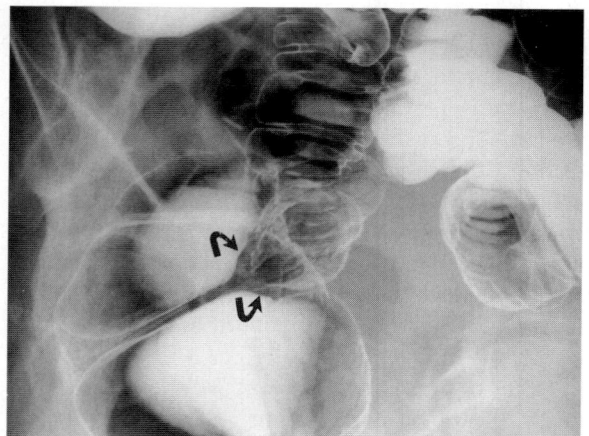

Fig. 17.30. Subtotal colectomy with anastomosis between the small bowel and rectum. Double-contrast barium enema demonstrates a widely patent anastomosis (*arrows*) approximately 9 cm proximal to the anus. (From SMITH et al. 1993)

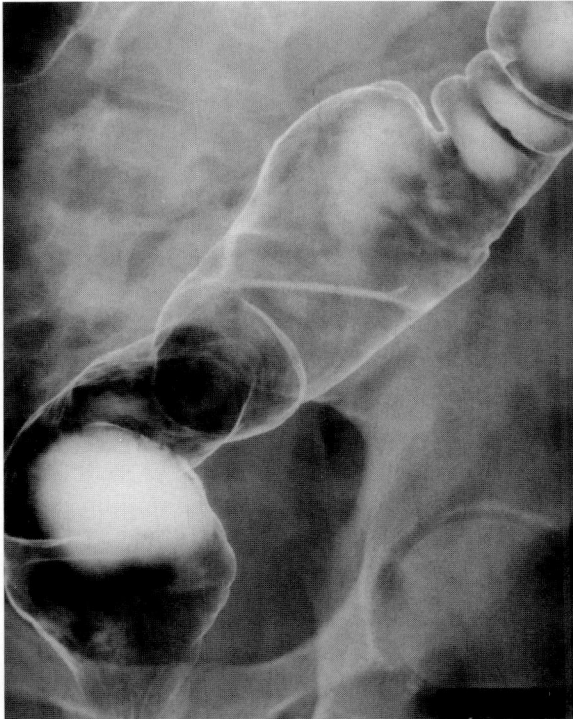

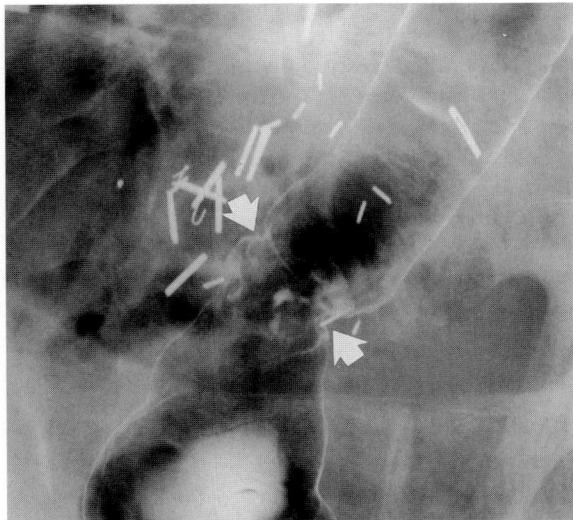

Fig. 17.31 a,b. Sigmoidectomy: normal appearance versus recurrent tumor. **a** Double-contrast barium enema demonstrates a widely patent end-to-end anastomosis. The caliber varies between the descending colon and sigmoid. **b** Mucosal nodularity (*arrows*) is present at this anastomosis, suggesting recurrent tumor that was confirmed at colonoscopy. (From SMITH et al. 1993)

there is a poorly differentiated morphology. In this procedure, the distal sigmoid, rectosigmoid, rectum, and anus are removed via a combined abdominal and perineal approach, and a permanent sigmoid

colostomy is established. Postoperatively, these patients typically have varying degrees of urinary retention, and impotence is characteristically present in males; wound infections are quite common.

In patients with advanced disease at the time of presentation, surgical removal is still indicated to prevent obstruction or bleeding. If the patient has multiple medical problems making surgery too risky, endoluminal stents and tumor fulguration may help palliate the patient's symptoms.

Patients who present with obstruction or perforation have a much worse prognosis, particularly when systemic symptoms are present. Overall mortality is 25%. Surgery is usually done in stages; a subtotal colectomy is recommended for obstructed left-sided lesions to avoid a temporary colostomy (BOKEY et al. 1995).

Recurrent tumor will develop in 40% of patients who undergo curative surgery. The goals of postoperative surveillance are the detection of recurrent cancer at a stage when it is still curable and the detection and prevention of metachronous carcinoma (NWILOH 1991).

Recurrent colorectal cancer may present as a local, regional, or distant tumor. The most common site of recurrent disease is distant, with liver or lung metastases or both. Localized recurrent tumor (Figs. 17.27, 17.31b) which is amenable to surgical resection is rare. The incidence of anastomotic recurrence is quite low (0.7%) after right hemicolectomy and ileocolic anastomosis. Local anastomotic recurrence is more common in colocolic and colorectal anastomoses and quite high in rectal resection. Thus, surveillance barium studies after right hemicolectomy are primarily performed for the detection of metachronous polyps and cancers. For rectal cancers, periodic barium studies can detect recurrent tumor at the suture line which often represents ingrowth of tumor cells from the outer surface of the rectum into the mucosal surface. Exophytic growth cannot be assessed by colonoscopy or barium studies. These techniques also cannot evaluate patients following abdominoperineal resection. For this, computed tomography and/or magnetic resonance imaging is necessary.

17.8.2
Diverticulitis

When medical therapy with or without percutaneous abscess drainage performed under imaging guidance is ineffective in treating diverticulitis, sigmoid resection and primary anastomosis are performed. When a primary anastomosis is contraindicated, sigmoid resection is followed by an end colostomy and formation of either a Hartmann's pouch (Fig. 17.32) or a mucous fistula as previously described. The colostomy is taken down and intestinal continuity is re-established after the inflammation has resolved (BALTHAZAR 1994).

17.8.3
Ulcerative Colitis

Although proctocolectomy is always curative for ulcerative colitis, this procedure carries an operative risk, and not all patients are willing to accept an ileostomy. Consequently, colectomy is not indicated for patients who are easily managed medically. There are several major indications for surgery in ulcerative colitis: (a) massive, unremitting colonic hemorrhage; (b) toxic megacolon with impending or frank perforation; (c) fulminant colitis despite intensive steroid therapy; (d) obstruction from a stricture; and

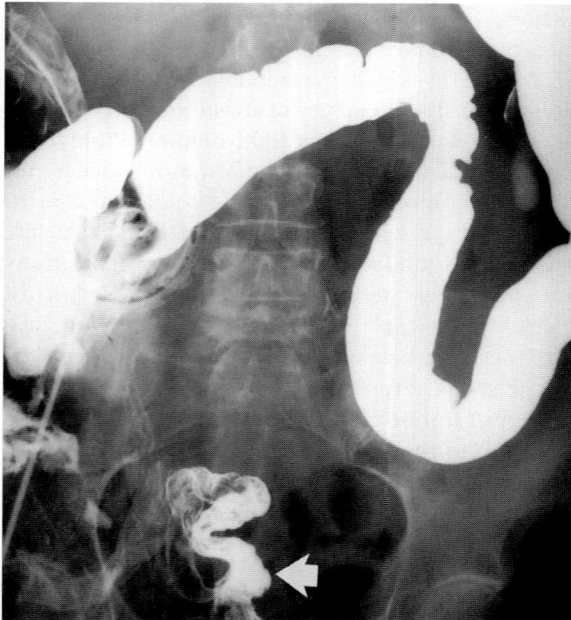

Fig. 17.32. Diverting colostomy and Hartmann's pouch. This patient underwent an emergency procedure for diverticular disease. A primary anastomosis could not be performed, so a protective double-barrel colostomy was made. Contrast was injected into both stomas of the colostomy, filling the ascending colon as well as portions of the descending colon. There is also contrast in the rectosigmoid (*arrow*) that was introduced prior to the colostomy study to examine the distal pouch. (From SMITH et al. 1993)

(e) suspicion or demonstration of colon cancer (GORE and LAUFER 1994). Less immediate and definite indications for colectomy are: (a) intractable, chronic disease that becomes a physical and social burden to the patient; (b) failure of children to mature at an acceptable rate; and (c) high-grade dysplasia in a patient with pancolitis. Fulminant acute disease accounts for approximately 13%–25% of colectomies in patients with ulcerative colitis. Many of the extraintestinal complications of ulcerative colitis, such as uveitis and pyoderma gangrenosum, will also be eliminated by colectomy. The course of hepatobiliary disease and ankylosing spondylitis, however, is usually not altered by surgery.

In the past two decades, tremendous advances have been made in the surgical approach to ulcerative colitis that offer the patient and surgeon a variety of options.

17.8.3.1
Proctocolectomy with Brooke Ileostomy

This is the standard procedure in which a proctocolectomy is performed, followed by passing the end of the ileum through an opening in the mid aspect of the right rectus muscle at a point beneath the umbilicus that allows convenient placement of the forepiece of an ileostomy bag. This procedure is curative and requires one operation, but the patient must constantly wear an external ileostomy appliance that needs to be emptied 4–8 times per day. Perineal wound problems, stoma revision, and small bowel obstruction occur in approximately 10%–25% of patients. While this is the fastest and safest operation, it dramatically alters body image in many patients, particularly younger ones (SCHOLZ 1994).

17.8.3.2
Proctocolectomy with Continent Ileostomy (Kock's Pouch)

In this procedure, a continent ileostomy is made by creating a pouch out of terminal ileum to hold the intestinal contents, an ileal conduit that leads from the pouch to the stoma, and an intervening intestinal valve (Fig. 17.33). Patients empty the pouch by passing a tube through the valve via the stoma. The ileostomy is continent, so an external appliance is not needed. The nipple valve is created by intussuscepting the terminal ileum in a retrograde manner into the pouch for 3–4 cm. Anatomic complications

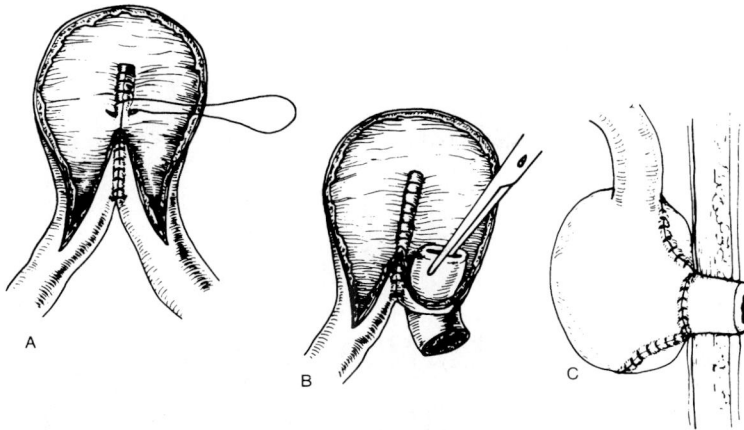

Fig. 17.33 a–c. Kock's pouch construction. **a** A 30-cm segment of ileum is sewn together, leaving a 10-cm afferent limb; the loop is opened. **b** A one-way value is created by intussuscepting the afferent limb back into the pouch. **c** The pouch is folded together and sewn closed. The pouch is brought through the abdominal wall and left flush with the skin surface. (From SMITH 1989)

requiring reoperation develop in 40%–50% of these patients.

17.8.3.3
Total Colectomy with Ileorectal Anastomosis

This procedure is no longer popular because of a fairly high complication rate and an unpredictable functional result.

17.8.3.4
Total Proctocolectomy, Rectal Mucosal Stripping, and Ileal Pouch Formation

This procedure involves an abdominal colectomy and a mucosal proctectomy. A "J," "S," or "W" pouch is fashioned out of ileum (Fig. 17.34). This reservoir is then anastomosed to the anus. The endorectal ileal pouch-anal anastomosis is given 9 weeks to heal by diverting the gut through a conventional ileostomy (KREMERS et al. 1985).

The advantages of this procedure are that no stoma is required and fecal continence is usually maintained, albeit with four to eight bowel movements per day. This is a technically demanding procedure that requires two operations. Complications include postoperative abscess, pouch fistulas, stenosis, small bowel obstruction, and pouchitis. Some 15% of patients require reoperation, and some ultimately require a conventional ileostomy (MANN 1992).

Pouchitis is an inflammatory process that can cause tenesmus, bloody diarrhea, and constitutional symptoms similar to those of ulcerative colitis.

17.8.4
Crohn's Disease

There is a high rate of recurrence (30%–53%) of Crohn's disease after resection of diseased bowel. It is possible that Crohn's disease affects, at least at a microscopic level, the entire gut from the outset, so the disease cannot be cured by surgery. Therefore, operative therapy should be reserved for certain complications of the disease or for unequivocal failure to respond to optimal medical therapy. These guidelines are particularly applicable to two groups of patients: (a) those who have previously undergone small bowel resection and present with recurrent disease of an obstructive nature and (b) those who have diffuse disease and multiple small bowel strictures. Removal of all the diseased areas in these patients may lead to the short bowel syndrome (SIMPKINS and GORE 1994).

The major indications for surgery in Crohn's disease are obstruction, perforation, hemorrhage, and carcinoma. Abscesses and fistulas should first be treated by the interventional radiologist because this may save the patient from having surgery.

Strictureplasty is effective in treating short stenosis Crohn's lesions of the small bowel that cause obstruction. Short fibrous strictures in patients who have not had an acute inflammatory flare-up of the

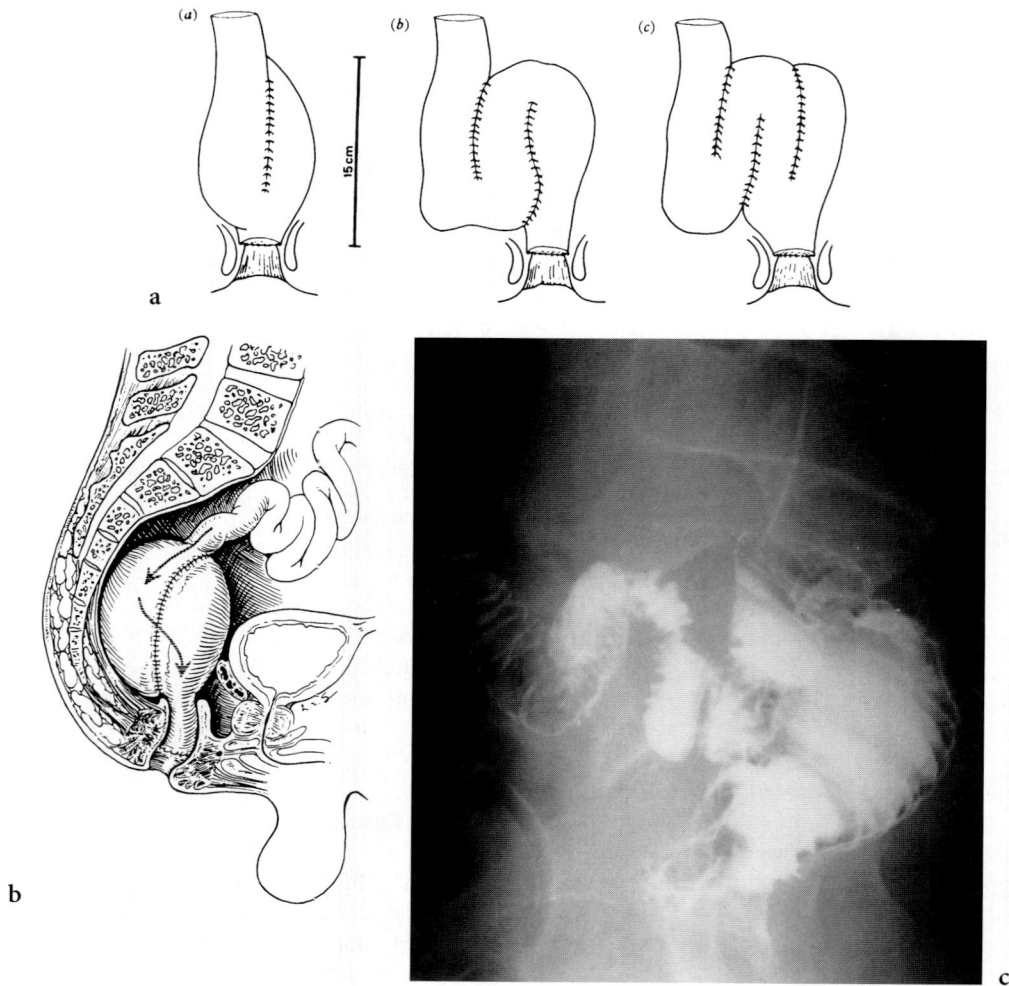

Fig. 17.34 a–c. Ileo-anal anastomosis. a A substitute rectum is made from joined folds of ileum to form an expanded "pouch" of small intestine. Three ways of forming a pouch are illustrated: (a) a simple revered "J"; (b) an "S" pouch; (c) a "W" pouch. (From MANN 1992). b The pouch is then placed through the denuded rectal stump to the pectinate line, where it is anastomosed to anoderm. (From SCHROCK (1991). c The integrity of the small bowel pouch is confirmed with a retrograde contrast study. The small bowel proximal to the pouch has also been refluxed

disease segment are most amenable to strictureplasty. The recurrence rate after strictureplasty is similar to that after primary resection for small intestinal Crohn's disease (SCHROCK 1991).

Radiologically guided balloon dilatation has proven useful in treating colonic strictures due to Crohn's disease, but is not suitable for Crohn's strictures located in the small bowel.

References

Acunas B, Rozanes I, Akpinar S, et al. (1996) Palliation of malignant esophageal strictures with self-expanding nitinol stents: drawbacks and complications. Radiology 199:648–652

Agha FP, Orringer MB (1985) Gastric interposition following transhiatal esophagectomy: radiographic evaluation. Gastrointest Radiol 10:17–24

Agha FP, Trenkner SW, Orringer MB, et al. (1985) The combined Collis gastroplasty-Nissen fundoplication: surgical procedure and radiographic evaluation. AJR 145:729–734

Anbari M, Levine MS, Cohen R, et al. (1993) Delayed leaks and fistulas after esophagogastrectomy: radiologic evaluation. AJR 160:1212–1220

Balfe DM, Koehler RE, Setzen M, et al. (1982) Barium examination of the esophagus after total laryngectomy. Radiology 143:501–506

Balthazar EJ (1994) Diverticular disease. In: Gore RM, Levine MS, Laufer I (eds) Textbook of gastrointestinal radiology. Saunders, Philadelphia, pp 1072–1097

Barnett JL (1996) Esophageal carcinoma: palliation with intubation and laser. In: Zuidema GA (ed) Shackelford's surgery of the alimentary tract, 4th edn. Saunders, Philadelphia, pp 358–368

Belsey R (1996) The Belsey Mark IV antireflux procedure. In: Zuidema GD (ed) Shackelford's surgery of the alimentary tract, 4th edn. Saunders, Philadelphia, pp 204–213

Binkert CA, Jost R, Steiner A, et al. (1996) Benign and malignant stenoses of the stomach and duodenum: treatment with self-expanding metallic endoprostheses. Radiology 199:335–338

Block GE, Hurst RD (1996) Abdominoperineal resection. In: Zuidema GD (ed) Shackelford's surgery of the alimentary tract, 4th edn. Saunders, Philadelphia, pp 245–252

Bokey EL, Chapuis PH, Fung C, et al. (1995) Postoperative morbidity and mortality following resection of the colon and rectum for cancer. Dis Colon Rectum 38:480–487

Boyce HW (1993) Stents for palliation of dysphagia due to esophageal cancer. N Engl J Med 329:1345–1346

Burhenne HJ (1971) Postoperative defects of the stomach. Semin Roentgenol 6:182–192

Carter R, Smith JS, Anderson JR (1993) Laser recanalization versus endoscopic intubation in the palliation of malignant dysphagia: a randomized prospective study. Br J Surg 79:1167–1170

Chandie Shaw P, Op den Orth JO (1994) Postoperative stomach and duodenum. Radiol Clin North Am 32:1275–1291

Christensen LR, Shapir J (1986) Radiology of colonic interposition and its associated complications. Gastrointest Radiol 11:233–240

Chung RS (1992) Peptic ulcer surgery and its complications. In: Achkar E, Farmer RG, Fleshler B (eds) Clinical gastroenterology. Lea and Febiger, Philadelphia, pp 261–273

Coia LR, Ahmad N, Rosenthal SA (1994) Expansile stents in esophageal cancer. N Engl J Med 330:790–791

Condon RE (1996) Resection of the colon. In: Zuidema GD (ed) Shackelford's surgery of the alimentary tract, 4th edn. Saunders, Philadelphia, pp 207–224

Davis GR (1993) Neoplasms of the stomach. In: Sleisenger MH, Fordtran JS (eds) Gastrointestinal disease, 5th edn. Saunders, Philadelphia, pp 763–848

Dent TL, Kukora JS, Nejman JH (1987) The colon, rectum, and anus. In: Hardy JD (ed) Hardy's textbook of surgery, 2nd edn. Lippincott, Philadelphia, pp 582–636

Disario JA, Burt RW, Vargas H, et al. (1994) Small bowel cancer: epidemiological and clinical characteristics from a population-based registry. Am J Gastroenterol 89:699–701

Dodds WJ, Stewart ET, Vlymen WJ (1982) Appropriate contrast media for evaluation of esophageal disruption. Radiology 144:439–441

Eisenberg BL (1996) Surgical palliation of upper gastrointestinal cancer. Curr Probl Cancer 19:338–347

Ellis FH Jr (1960) Treatment of carcinoma of the esophagus and cardia. Mayo Clin Proc 35:363–650

Feigin DS, James AE, Stitik FR, et al. (1974) The radiological appearance of hiatal hernia repairs. Radiology 110:71–77

Ferguson MK, Skinner DB (1996) Carcinoma of the esophagus and cardia. In: Zuidema GA (ed) Shackelford's surgery of the alimentary tract, 4th edn. Saunders, Philadelphia, pp 305–332

Fok M, Wong J (1988) Esophagogastrectomy for carcinoma of the abdominal esophagus and gastric cardia. In: Nyhus LLM, Baker RJ (eds) Masters of surgery. Little, Brown & Co, Boston, pp 731–740

Fuchs CS, Mayer RJ (1995) Gastric carcinoma. N Engl J Med 333:32–41

Gelfand D (1984) Gastrointestinal radiology. Churchill Livingstone, New York, pp 195–220

Ghahremani GG (1994) Postsurgical and traumatic lesions of the biliary tract. In: Gore RM, Levine MS, Laufer I (eds) Textbook of gastrointestinal radiology. Saunders, Philadelphia, pp 1762–1778

Gold RP, Seaman WB (1977) The primary double-contrast examination of the postoperative stomach. Radiology 124:295–305

Goldstein HM, Miller RH (1976) Air contrast colon examination in patients with colostomies. AJR 127:607–610

Gompels BM, Harrison GK (1972) Barium studies following the Nissen-Rossetti operation for oesophageal stricture due to reflux. Br J Radiol 45:137–141

Goodman PC, Levine MS, Gohil MN (1992) Gastric carcinoma after gastrojejunostomy for benign disease: radiographic findings. Gastrointest Radiol 17:211–213

Gore RM, Ghahremani GG (1994) CT evaluation of the stomach: current status. The Radiologist 1:345–355

Gore RM, Laufer I (1994) Ulcerative and granulomatous colitis: idiopathic inflammatory bowel disease. In: Gore RM, Levine MS, Laufer I (eds) Textbook of gastrointestinal radiology. Saunders, Philadelphia, pp 1098–1141

Gore RM, Nahrwold DL (1994) Pancreatic trauma and surgery. In: Gore RM, Levine MS, Laufer I (eds) Textbook of gastrointestinal radiology. Saunders, Philadelphia, pp 2193–2202

Greager JA, Eckhauser ML, Pennington LR, et al. (1995) Neoplasms of the small intestine. In: Zuidema GA (ed) Shackelford's surgery of the alimentary tract, 4th edn. Saunders, Philadelphia, pp 1393–1401

Halpert RD, Goodman P (1993) Gastrointestinal radiology: the requisites. Mosby, St. Louis, pp 33–82

Hanks JB, Jones RS, Minasi JS (1995) Tumors of the stomach and duodenum. In: Zuidema GA (ed) Shackelford's surgery of the alimentary tract, 4th edn. Saunders, Philadelphia, pp 88–96

Hatfield M, Shapir J (1985) The radiologic manifestations of failed antireflux operations. AJR 144:1209–1214

Heiken JP, Balfe DM, Roper CL (1984) CT evaluation after esophagogastrectomy. AJR 143:555–560

Hiebert CA (1996) Overview: hiatal hernia, gastroesophageal reflux, and their complications. In: Zuidema GD (ed) Shackelford's surgery of the alimentary tract, 4th edn. Saunders, Philadelphia, pp 179–191

Hill L (1996) The Hill procedure. In: Zuidema GD (ed) Shackelford's surgery of the alimentary tract, 4th edn. Saunders, Philadelphia, pp 192–203

Hoehstra SM, Lucas CE, Ledgerwood AM (1993) A comparison of gastric bypass and gastric wrap for morbid obesity. Surg Gynecol Obstet 176:262–266

James AE, Montali RJ, Chaffee V, et al. (1975) Barium or gastrografin: which contrast media for diagnosis of esophageal tears? Gastroenterology 698:1103–1113

Kodera Y, Yamamura Y, Torii A, et al. (1996) Gastric remnant carcinoma after partial gastrectomy for benign and malignant gastric lesions. J Am Coll Surg 182:1–6

Kondo K, Yokoyama Y, Yokoyama I, et al. (1996) Early gastric cancer after gastro-jejunostomy: clinical and pathologic aspects. Am J Gastroenterol 90:2213–2216

Kremers PW, Scholz FJ, Schoetz DJ Jr, et al. (1985) Radiology of the ileoanal reservoir. AJR 145:559–567

Lanza FL (1995) Benign and malignant tumors of the stomach other than carcinoma. In: Haubrich WS, Schaffner F (eds) Bockus gastroenterology, 5th edn. Saunders, Philadelphia, pp 841–858

Lappas JC, Maglinte DDT (1994) Postoperative small intestine. In: Gore RM, Levine MS, Laufer I (eds) Textbook of gastrointestinal radiology. Saunders, Philadelphia, pp 984–996

Liu KJM, Walker FW (1996) Surgical procedures of the small intestine. In: Zuidema GD (ed) Shackelford's surgery of the alimentary tract, 4th edn. Saunders, Philadelphia, pp 267–288

Loggie BW (1996) Surgical concepts in the treatment of colorectal cancer. Semin Roentgenol 31:111–117

Lynch PM (1995) Polyposis syndromes. In: Haubrich WS, Schaffner F (eds) Bockus gastroenterology, 5th edn. Saunders, Philadelphia, pp 1731–1743

Mann CV (1992) The small and large intestines. In: Mann CV, Russell RCG (eds) Bailey & Love's short practice of surgery, 21st edn. Chapman & Hally London, pp 1125–1167

Mathisen DJ, Wilkins EW (1996) Techniques of esophageal reconstruction. In: Zuidema GA (ed) Shackelford's surgery of the alimentary tract, 4th edn. Saunders, Philadelphia, pp 389–413

Michelassi F, Errol F, Dawson PJ, et al. (1989) Experience with 647 and consecutive tumors of the duodenum ampulla, head of pancreas and distal CBD. Ann Surg 210:544–554

Moody FG, Roth JA (1988) The esophagus and diaphragmatic hernias. In: Hardy JD (ed) Hardy's textbook of surgery, 2nd edn. Lippincott, Philadelphia, pp 485–513

Moon M, Schulte W, Haasler G, et al. (1992) Transhiatal and transthoracic esophagectomy for adenocarcinoma of the esophagus. Am J Surg 127:951–955

Nahrwold DL (1996) Gastric resection and reconstruction. In: Zuidema GD (ed) Shackelford's surgery of the alimentary tract, 4th edn. Saunders, Philadelphia, pp 152–165

Nakajima T, Ota K, Ishikara S, et al. (1993) Extended radical gastrectomy for advanced gastric cancer. Surg Clin North Am 32:467–481

Nevitt AW, Kozarek RA, Kidd R (1996) Expandable esophageal prostheses: recognition, insertion techniques, and positioning. AJR 167:1009–1013

Nwiloh J, Dardik H, Dardik M, et al. (1991) Changing patterns in morbidity and mortality of colorectal surgery. Am J Surg 162:83–85

Op den Orth JO (1992) The postoperative stomach. In: Laufer I, Levine MS (eds) Double contrast gastrointestinal radiology. Saunders, Philadelphia, pp 287–320

O'Reilly S, Forastiere AA (1996) Multimodality therapy for esophageal carcinoma. In: Zuidema GA (ed) Shackelford's surgery of the alimentary tract, 4th edn. Saunders, Philadelphia, pp 349–357

Orringer MB (1996) Complications of esophageal surgery. In: Zuidema GD (ed) Shackelford's surgery of the alimentary tract, 4th edn. Saunders, Philadelphia, pp 446–476

Orringer MB, Sloan H (1978) Esophagectomy without thoracotomy. J Thorac Cardiovasc Surg 76:643–654

Owen JW, Balfe DM, Koehler RE, et al. (1983) Radiologic evaluation of complications after esophagogastrectomy. AJR 140:1163–1169

Polk HC (1996) The Nissen fundoplication: operative technique and clinical experience. In Zuidema GD (ed) Shackelford's surgery of the alimentary tract, 4th edn. Saunders, Philadelphia, pp 214–221

Rubesin SE, Beatty SM (1994) The postoperative esophagus. Semin Roentgenol 29:401–410

Rubesin SE, Rosato EF (1994) Postoperative esophagus. In: Gore RM, Levine MS, Laufer I (eds) Textbook of gastrointestinal radiology. Saunders, Philadelphia, pp 542–556

Rubesin SE, Yousem DM (1994) Structural abnormalities of the pharynx. In: Gore RM, Levine MS, Laufer I (eds) Textbook of gastrointestinal radiology. Saunders, Philadelphia, pp 244–276

Rubesin SE, Kennedy M, Levine MS, et al. (1988) Distal esophageal ballooning following Heller myotomy. Radiology 167:345–347

Salena BJ, Hunt RH (1993) Bezoars. In: Sleisinger MH, Fordtran JS (eds) Gastrointestinal disease, 5th edn. Saunders, Philadelphia, pp 758–762

Scholz FJ (1994) Postoperative colon. In: Gore RM, Levine MS, Laufer I (eds) Textbook of gastrointestinal radiology. Saunders, Philadelphia, pp 1342–1351

Schrock TM (1991) Large intestine. In: Way LW (ed) Current surgical diagnosis and treatment, 9th edn. Appleton & Lange, Norwalk, Conn, pp 663–680

Sigurdson ER (1995) Surgical palliation of colorectal cancer. Curr Prog Surg 19:348–359

Simpkins KC, Gore RM (1994) Crohn's disease. In: Gore RM, Levine MS, Laufer I (eds) Textbook of gastrointestinal radiology. Saunders, Philadelphia, pp 2660–2681

Smith C (1994a) Radiology of the stomach after gastric surgery for obesity. In: Freeny PC, Stevenson JW (eds) Margolis and Burhenne's alimentary tract radiology. Mosby, St. Louis, pp 455–467

Smith C (1994b) Postoperative stomach and duodenum. In: Gore RM, Levine MS, Laufer I (eds) Textbook of gastrointestinal radiology. Saunders, Philadelphia, pp 742–758

Smith C, Deziel DJ (1995) Radiology of the postoperative stomach. In: Taveras JM, Ferrucci JT (eds) Radiology: diagnosis – imaging – intervention. Lippincott, Philadelphia, pp 1–16

Smith C, Gardiner R, Kubicka RA, et al. (1984) Gastric restrictive surgery for obesity: early radiologic evaluation. Radiology 153:321–327

Smith C, Gardiner R, Kubicka RA, et al. (1985) Radiology of gastric restrictive surgery. Radiographics 5:193–216

Smith C, Deziel DJ, Kubicka RA (1993) Appearances of the postoperative alimentary tract. Radiol Clin North Am 31:1235–1254

Smith C, Deziel DJ, Kubicka RA (1994) Evaluation of the postoperative stomach and duodenum. Radiographics 14:67–86

Smith LE (1989) Surgical therapy in ulcerative colitis. Gastroenterol Clin North Am 18:99–110

Thoeni RF, Moss AA (1979) The radiographic appearance of complications following Nissen fundoplication. Radiology 131:17–21

Vernava AM, Goldberg SM (1996) Low anterior resection. In: Zuidema GD (ed) Shackelford's surgery of the alimentary tract, 4th edn. Saunders, Philadelphia, pp 225–244

Walsh TN, Noonan N, Hollywood D, et al. (1996) A comparison of multimodality therapy and surgery for esophageal adenocarcinoma. N Engl J Med 335:462–467

Winkelbauer FW, Schöfl R, Niederle B, et al. (1996) Palliative treatment of obstructing esophageal cancer with Nitinol stents: value, safety, and long-term results. AJR 166:79–84

Wippold FJ, Balfe DM (1994) Imaging the postoperative neck. In: Gore RM, Levine MS, Laufer I (eds) Textbook of gastrointestinal radiology. Saunders, Philadelphia, pp 277–291

Zegel HG, Kressel HY, Levin NS, et al. (1979) Delayed perforation after pneumatic dilatation for the treatment of achalasia. Gastrointest Radiol 4:219–221

18 Advances in Interventional Radiology of the Alimentary Tract

D.H.W Grönemeyer, A. Melzer, T. Vogl, J. Plassmann, and R. Seibel, A. Schmidt

D.H.W. Grönemeyer, MD, Professor and Chairman, Department of Radiology and Microtherapy, University of Witten/Herdecke, D-58448 Witten, Germany
A. Melzer, MD, Department of Radiology and Microtherapy, University of Witten/Herdecke, D-58448 Witten, Germany
J. Plassmann, MD, Department of Radiology and Microtherapy, University of Witten/Herdecke, D-58448 Witten, Germany
R. Seibel, MD, Department of Radiology and Microtherapy, University of Witten/Herdecke, D-58448 Witten, Germany
A. Schmidt, MD, Department of Radiology and Microtherapy, University of Witten/Herdecke, D-58448 Witten, Germany
T. Vogl, MD, Professor, Virchow Klinikum, Medizinische Fakultät der Humboldt-Universität zu Berlin, Augustenburger Platz 1, D-13353 Berlin, Germany

18.1 Introduction

Percutaneous interventional procedures in the abdomen and pelvis are usually performed for biopsies, but also may be done for sympathectomy, for drainage, and, increasingly, for cancer therapy.

As long ago as 1967, Nordenstrom reported the first series of percutaneous fluoroscopically guided lymph node biopsies. Since then, different approaches, e.g., transperitoneal, translumbar, and transvascular, using different image modalities have been described (Göthlin 1976; Grönemeyer and Seibel 1990a; Haaga et al. 1977, 1983; Jaques et al. 1989; MacErlean et al. 1980; Macintosh et al. 1979; Pagani 1983; Ruttimann 1968; Seibel et al. 1990b).

Fine-needle biopsies are most often performed for cytologic and histologic diagnosis in the abdomen, retroperitoneum, pelvis, lymph nodes, bones, and joints. In general, the results with percutaneous aspiration techniques are very good: success rates of more than 80% have been reported for the achievement of cytologic diagnosis (Macintosh et al. 1979; Pereiras et al. 1978; Seibel et al. 1990b).

Ultrasound (US)- and computed tomography (CT)-guided biopsies are established diagnostic techniques; however, US-guided methods have increasingly been replaced by CT guidance (Grönemeyer and Seibel 1990a; Haaga and Alfidi 1976). Magnetic resonance imaging (MRI) techniques for clinical treatments are new (Dumoulin et al. 1993; Grönemeyer et al. 1990c,e; Herman et al. 1996; Lufkin et al. 1987; Mueller et al. 1986; Silverman et al. 1995). They have the potential to replace conventional techniques, but currently must be used carefully in so-called low-risk Areas, where no vital structures are vulnerable (Grönemeyer et al. 1995b). Today the routine use of tomographic scanners permits biopsies of tumor masses and drainage of fluid collections like cysts or abscesses, as well as percutaneous tumor therapy with ethanol ablation (Grönemeyer and Seibel

1989, 1990c; LIVRAGHI et al. 1986; SEKI et al. 1989; SHEU et al. 1987; SILVERMAN 1996; UNGER 1994), radiofrequency (RF) (ANZAI et al. 1995), or lasers (JOLESZ et al. 1988; VOGL et al. 1995) and also interventional pain therapy (GRÖNEMEYER and SEIBEL 1990b). When real-time diagnosis of histologic or cytologic pathology is available, the tumor treatment may be performed directly after the biopsy through the same guidance cannula. This shortens the therapy time and is emotionally helpful for the patient. In the field of pain therapy, especially if the tumor mass is infiltrating bony structures, percutaneous sympathectomy with ethanol will reduce this kind of pain at once in more than 75% of patients.

The detailed and accurate measurement of the size and/or volume of pathologic structures, and their distance from the skin, vessels, neural structures, and surrounding organs, is only possible by CT or MRI. The density and resolution of abnormal masses are also often better defined by these techniques. The major advantages of MRI and CT over US guidance are:

1. Less training is needed to orient the image.
2. The system itself is not moved; consequently exact reproduction of the scan level is possible.
3. When using US guidance for biopsy, more time is needed to place the transducer over the area of pathology, especially when repeated examinations are necessary.

On the other hand, the trained examiner with US has a method at his disposal which can interactively demonstrate the structures two-dimensionally. This interactive advantage over CT alone is lost when using fluoroscopy or keyhole techniques in MRI or US or fluoroscopy guidance in conjunction with CT or MRI (GRÖNEMEYER et al. 1995b).

18.2
Equipment

18.2.1
Scanner Technology

The key feature of all access techniques is the hybrid combination of imaging systems: CT, MRI, ultrasound, x-ray, and endoscopy. One of the new access techniques is a combined interventional procedure: for this technique, an x-ray C-arm is placed directly at the CT or the ultrafast electron beam tomography (EBT) scanner. By combining use of a

mobile fluoroscope with or without digital subtraction angiography and CT/EBT, the structures to be punctured can be visualized three-dimensionally with excellent morphologic differentiation in real time.

Another possibility is to use an open MRI scanner for guidance technology. With the addition of CT, EBT, and MRI, all interstitial and bone structures can be defined with high accuracy. Therefore, the treatment and the approach to the region of therapy can be planned and controlled precisely. The thickness and extension of muscles, fat, lymph nodes, and tendons are also visible, as are risk areas such as nerves, vessels, or the dural sac. Complications can be detected at an early stage and therapeutic effects documented interactively.

18.2.2
Hybrid Scanner: CT Scanner
and Fluoroscopy Unit

For minimal access treatments CT scanners with gantry openings for the patient of more than 60 cm are required. Our treatments are performed in a spiral CT scanner with a 70-cm gantry (Somatom Plus S and Plus 4; Siemens, Erlangen, Germany). The distance between the patient couch and the gantry must be between 0.5 and 1.0 m, so that a fluoroscopy unit can be installed close to the gantry with optimal space for the therapist in all directions. The table has to be moved to defined positions in- and outside the gantry, depending upon the operative field. Monitors, laser systems, endoscopy, and US units are placed close to the gantry.

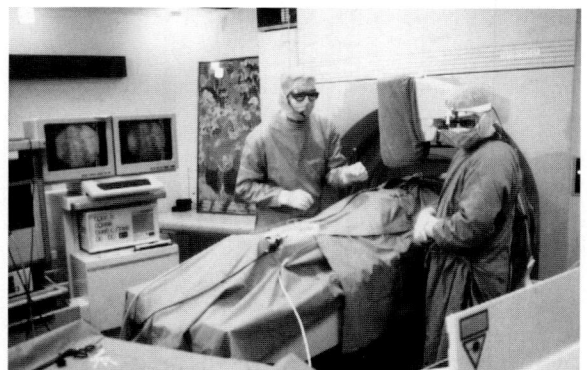

Fig. 18.1. Hybrid EBT unit (Imatron, Siemens). The fluoroscopy unit is installed near to the gantry, and the electronic equipment is located around it

18.2.3
Hybrid scanner: Electron Beam Tomograph and Fluoroscopy Unit

The recent revolution in advanced digital imaging technologies widens the field for interventional scanners. Ultrafast EBT has been developed for noninvasive calcification screening (BOYD et al. 1979) in coronary arteries (produced by Imatron Inc. Los Angeles, Calif., USA; marketed by Siemens). One important requirement for minimal access procedures is that the gantry opening is 90 cm in diameter: this is important for minimally invasive guidance procedures with long instruments like endoscopes or forceps. We initially reported this technique in 1989 (JASCHKE et al. 1989), and today we are combining a C-arm for the fluoroscopy unit with EBT (Fig. 18.1) to achieve a three-dimensional (3D) view of the operative field. During scanning mode, an electron beam is focused to a 1- to 2-mm focal spot that is deflected across a series of four semicircular tungsten targets around the patient. Each target can produce a beam of x-radiation. Frame rates of up to 34 images per second (conventional CT: 1 per second) are possible (simultaneous multilevel scan acquisition in 50 ms). Two detector rings are installed above the patient so that a pair of EBT images can be obtained each time any one of the tungsten rings is "swept" by the electron beam. Thus up to eight levels can be scanned at the same time without moving the patient table. Scans can be acquired at two, four, six, or eight levels during a single acquisition. Instruments can be followed through several planes at the same time.

In the future, ultrafast scanning and fast 3D reconstruction will also be helpful for virtual endoscopy examination of the alimentary tract. Such ultrafast imaging does not lose any structural information in respect of moving organs and can be performed within a matter of seconds.

18.2.4
Open MRI Systems

The advantages of MRI guidance using an open system for interventional procedures are twofold: the avoidance of x-ray, multiplanar imaging and the possibility of operating with fast MRI-fluoroscopic modes inside the magnet. The ultra-low-field MRI scanner, developed by KAUFMAN et al. in 1987, was the first open MR system. This MRI unit (ACCESS, Toshiba MRI, Inc., San Francisco, Calif., USA) uti-

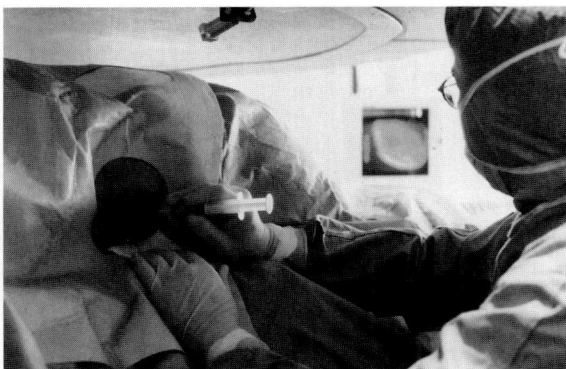

Fig. 18.2. Microinvasive therapy inside a magnet (0.064T, Toshiba)

lizes a permanent magnet with a field strength of 0.064 T. The vertical field magnets of this scanner permit circumferential open access at the four lateral sides, as with the 0.3- and 0.6-T units from Fonar Inc. Since 1993 other open MRI unit configurations with different field strengths (U-shaped, 0.2 T: Siemens, Picker; mid field, 0.5 T: GE Medical Systems; 0.3 T: Hitachi, Fonar) have been developed (Fig. 18.2).

In the past, the diagnostic potential of open MRI was underestimated. The efficiency and the possibilities of open magnets and low-field MRI are currently undergoing extensive research. Compared with the narrow, tube-like MRI scanners, the open systems are generally more comfortable. As a result, patients tend to be more cooperative and amenable to diagnosis and percutaneous procedures. Additionally "claustrophobic" and frightened patients can be examined more easily. (Table 18.1)

18.2.5
Electronic Equipment, Software, and Instruments

Shielding the electronic equipment for MRI allows the use of lasers, endoscopic systems, monitors, light boxes, etc. close to the magnets. Because the images of flat LED monitors are not sensitive to magnetic distortion, they can be used for screening MRI scans and for endoscopy, US, or other imaging. In order to avoid projectile effects and artifacts in MRI, mechanical instruments and endoscopes have to be developed using special nonferromagnetic materials like titanium, platinum, stainless steel, special plastics, or superelastic nitinol (MELZER et al. 1996). With CT or EBT every instrument which is used in conventional minimally invasive therapy can be

Table 18.1. MRI units for interventional procedures (increasing field strength) (from GRÖNEMEYER et al. 1996a)

Producer	Field strength (T)	Magnet type	Design	Interventional capabilities
Toshiba ACCESS	0.064	Permanent	Open four-sided (360°) restricted vertical access	Open system with horizontal access fluoroscopy, general interventions
Inner Vision	0.14	Permanent	Open three-sided restricted vertical access	Dedicated system for head and extremities
Siemens OPEN	0.2	Resistive iron core	C form open three-sided restricted vertical access	Open system, suitable for intervention, fast imaging possible
GE Profile	0.2	Permanent	Open two-sided restricted vertical access	Open system, suitable for intervention, fast imaging possible
PICKER Outlook	0.23	Resistive iron core	Open three-sided restricted vertical access	Intervention, fast imaging possible
Hitachi AIRIS	0.3	Permanent	270° access, restricted vertical access	Open system, suitable for intervention, fast imaging possible
Fonar	0.3	Hybrid permanent	Open four-sided limited vertical access	Open system, suitable for interventions
Magnalab	0.3	Permanent	C form open three-sided	Dedicated system for extremities
GE MRT	0.5	High temperature superconducting	"Double donut" full vertical limited horizontal access	Developed especially for intervention, fast imaging possible
Picker ASSET	0.5	Superconducting	Tube two-sided access	Only restricted, suitable as tube system
Philips NT	0.5–1.5	Superconducting	Tube two-sided access	Only restricted suitable as tube system, integrated LCD monitor
Fonar	0.6	Hybrid permanent	Open four-sided horizontal	Open system, suitable for interventions

guided without changing materials and without major problems.

A new laser positioning device (Micromed Inc., Bochum, Germany) can transfer the given entry point and puncture angle automatically to the skin. The laser light is projected directly onto the hub end of the instruments and is so positioned that the cross-hairs of the laser beam are projected onto the target surfaces of the endoscopes, forceps, cannulas, etc. Speech control enables movement of the patient couch in all directions. These technologies have been developed by our group.

18.3
2D Versus 3D Imaging for Interventional Procedures

Today, all cross-sectional imaging modalities such as US, CT, MRI, positron emission tomography, single-photon emission tomography, and EBT allow 3D re-constructions in the postprocessing mode. Real-time processing is not yet possible. The advantage of 3D over 2D imaging is the rapid recognition of anatomic regions that it allows, especially for nonspecialist doctors. Transparent surfacing and several processing modalities enable the doctor to look onto organ structures such as surfaces, vessels, and nerves. Also, increasingly 3D reconstructions of inner surfaces of intestinal organs for virtual endoscopy are under development.

Nevertheless, in comparison to cross-sectional 2D slices the regional and density resolution is poor. For access and guidance techniques, the therapist needs high resolution for tip tracking and if possible also ultrafast or real-time imaging. Tissue changes such as regional edema, bleeding, or lesions caused by energetic treatments (laser, RF, cryotherapy, etc.) in between operating manipulations can only be controlled by high-resolution imaging. For this reason, 3D or virtual guidance must be combined interactively with actual and not with prescanned slices.

Three-dimensional imaging is also an important tool for postprocessing documentation of therapeutic effects such as drug distribution (e.g., percutaneous ethanol instillation for cancer therapy or sympathectomy), laser-induced tissue changes, or implantations. 3D models are very helpful for operative planning as well as for education and training, especially if animal studies can be avoided (GRÖNEMEYER et al. 1995b).

18.4
Minimal Access Technique for CT, EBT, and MRI Guidance

The patient is positioned in accordance with the best possible access to the lesion. Due to the minimal trauma from the microinstruments and the use of local anesthesia, premedication is not required in most cases. The procedure is performed as follows: First a CT, EBT, or MRI scan of the region of interest is performed. An i.v. injection of contrast medium is required for CT/EBT in those regions (e.g., the mediastinum) where vascular structures are not visible in soft tissues (for MRI, contrast media are only used for differentiation of tumor and scar tissue). Then, the entry point, the puncture angle, and the distance to the therapeutic region are electronically determined and visualized at the monitor. After disinfection, local anesthesia is performed with 1% mepivacaine using a special guidance coaxial set (EZEM, US; Cook, Denmark; Micromed, Germany); the direction and postion of the cannulae are then checked with CT, EBT, or MRI.

All instruments such as lasers, endoscopes, and forceps, are introduced through the guidance cannula. The distance from the skin level to the structure which has to be reached can always be determined through the centimeter scale on the instrument's shaft. Injury to high-risk structures such as lung, nerves, or vessels in the path of the instruments is avoided by injecting local anesthetic and saline solution while they are advanced, which helps to push these structures away from the tip of the cannula [so-called hydraulic assisted cannula insertion: HACI (GRÖNEMEYER et al. 1995b; MELZER et al. 1996)]. Percutaneous procedures using an open-field MRI system can be approached in a similar manner as with either fluoroscopically or sonographically guided techniques. After imaging the patient can be treated inside the gantry or removed from the center of the magnet for the performance of major interventional procedures requiring greater access. For biopsies special reduced artifact instruments are available from Somatex and Daum (both Germany) and EZEM (USA). Therapeutic sets for cancer therapy are also available from Somatex. When using CT or MRI, diluted contrast medium (e.g., gadolinium) has to be injected prior to intratumoral drug instillation in order to document the drug distribution. With CT or EBT, the patient couch has to be moved out of the gantry several times for the treatments.

18.5
Therapy Phases

There are four major therapy phases for each procedure, and each phase requires different imaging modalities (GRÖNEMEYER et al. 1996a):

Phase 1: Localization: slice definition and electronic measurement (high resolution)
Phase 2: Guidance: introduction of instruments (fast imaging, low resolution)
Phase 3: Treatment: control of therapeutic effects (high resolution, 3D imaging)
Phase 4: Documentation: of treatment (high resolution, several planes, 3D imaging)

18.6
Biopsy Guidance

There are different forms of guidance technique, based on different concepts. Normally physicians are used to performing biopsies with frameless devices in US and CT. With all MRI systems this technique can be adopted (Fig. 18.3) in nearly the same way as with CT scanners (SCHMIDT et al. 1996; SILVERMAN 1996; SILVERMAN et al. 1995). Another approach, long employed in neurosurgery, is the use of stereotactic frames for guidance procedures in predefined virtual image environments. Furthermore, interactive guidance systems which are connected with the instruments via robotic arms (e.g., "viewing wand," ISG, Toronto, Canada) or directly with the instruments (e.g., Radionics, Mass., USA) are in use (GRÖNEMEYER et al. 1996a). These units are stand-alone systems and helpful in all MRI units by installation of a separate workstation. The guidance procedure is only possible with prescanned images in a virtual volume. The best interactive approach is

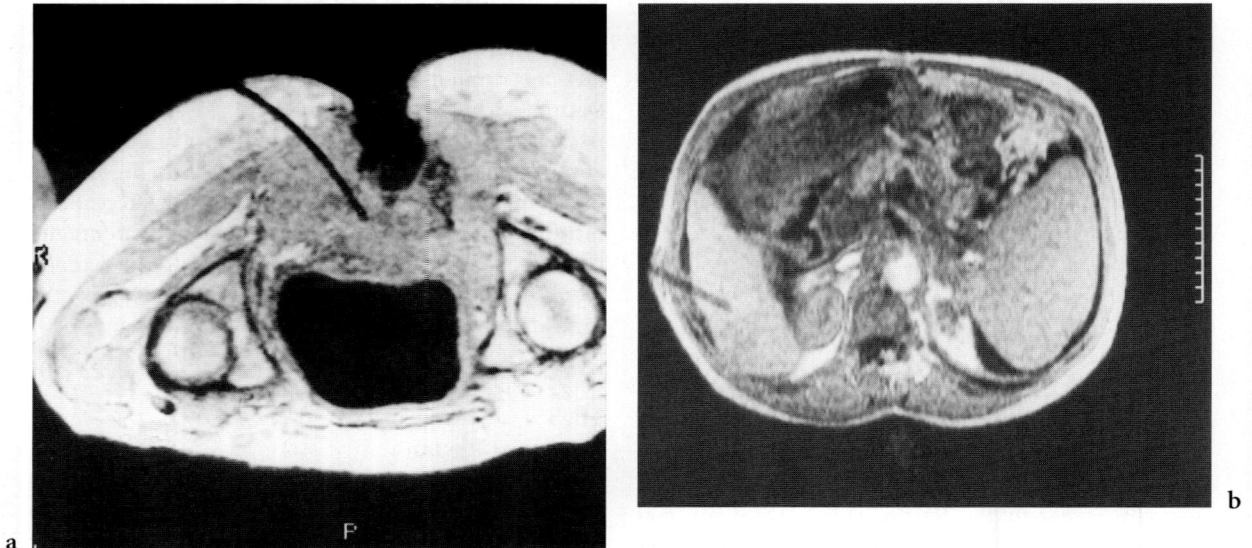

Fig. 18.3. a MRI-guided biopsy of a carcinoma of the colon below open surgery (0.064T, Toshiba). **b** Liver biopsy (0.2 T, Siemens)

achieved with the dedicated open MRI system of GE. Here the image plane is automatically referenced to a hand-held or a fixed probe over the region of therapy. The position of the probe is constantly identified and the radiologist can define up to three orthogonal image planes that are related to the axis of the probe interactively (SILVERMAN et al. 1995). The organ with the highest risk for biopsies is the liver, because enormous bleeding can appear.

18.6.1
Contraindications

Contraindications to biopsy are the use of anticoagulant therapy and the presence of blood clotting disorders. Prior to each biopsy the clotting status and platelet count must be determined. For safety reasons the prothrombin value should not be below 50%–60%. No other general contraindications are known.

18.6.2
Complications

Complications are rare if CT-guided techniques are used in high-risk areas and MRI-guided techniques are carefully employed in low-risk areas with artifact-free instruments by physicians with long experience. No complication has occurred since

1988 in our clinic, when we commenced clinical interventional procedures in CT, EBT, and open MRI (GRÖNEMEYER et al. 1996a). Today we are using two Toshiba ACCESS units and one Siemens OPEN unit as well as a Somatom Plus S and Plus 4 and two EBT scanners for interventional tomography.

18.6.3
Guidance Technique in MRI

In MRI a large belt coil (Siemens, Toshiba, Fonar) or flexible coil (GE) is fixed around or on the patient prior to the biopsy, with the target volume in the center of the coil. Using T1-weighted 2D-FLASH sequences in "breath-hold," the intervention is planned in a comparable way to a CT intervention. The distance from an anatomic landmark within the image plane that can be palpated accurately is determined on the screen. From the palpated structure the entry point is marked on the skin. Subsequent to disinfection and sterile covering, an MRI-compatible cannula is introduced and advanced under a "fluoroscopic" FISP- or FLASH-2D sequence. An image rate of 1 per second can be achieved in Toshiba ACCESS or 1 per 2 s in Siemens OPEN. Verifying the needle position with a 2D-FLASH sequence in breath-hold, the biopsy is performed (SCHMIDT et al. 1996).

Before biopsy the patient is positioned in a comfortable way, so that the probe can be introduced in the easiest puncture direction, avoiding vital structures. Following introduction of the guidance cannula, local anesthetic is injected into the skin and areas where the patient is feeling pain. The procedure takes about 35 min on average.

18.7
Liver Biopsies

18.7.1
Indications

The radiologic differential diagnosis of focal liver lesions is subject to considerable uncertainty. This uncertainty is the cause for the increasing interest in CT- and, increasingly, MRI-guided procedures. The CT-guided technique is safer than US- and MRI-guided biopsy (GRÖNEMEYER et al. 1995b, 1996a), especially in small and/or deep-seated lesions. Furthermore, the ability to avoid high-risk biopsy routes and to collect material from the non-necrotic tumor margins is also best with CT. A general advantage of the CT-guided biopsy is the better control of the needle tip and the improved documentation of the needle position. CT-guided liver biopsy is indicated for any focal lesions where a suspicion of malignancy cannot be excluded and where obtaining the diagnosis can be followed by therapy.

18.7.2
Contraindications

A significant coagulopathy is a contraindication to this technique. Earlier reports estimated a high risk from hemangioma puncture, but more recent articles have shown a much lower risk of hemorrhage (KRAMANN 1989). Prior to the puncture of any cystic lesion, echinococcosis must be excluded serologically.

18.7.3
Technique

The route of access to a liver lesion is determined by the topography. Normally, the shortest route is preferred; however, in cases where a hemangioma is included in the differential diagnosis, a longer intraparenchymatous puncture tract should be selected. This longer tract can self-tamponade after a hemorrhagic puncture (HAAGA et al. 1983). The longer puncture tract is especially helpful for lesions located close to the liver surface. In cases of subphrenic masses, transpleural access is technically easier than puncture-directed medial and superior access, which avoids the pleural space. If a pleurocentesis cannot be circumvented with a maximum inspiration, then it is recommended that the puncture be performed at maximum expiration or with the patient in the lateral position, because under these conditions the pleural recesses will contain little or no lung tissue (HAAGA et al. 1983).

We normally use an 18-G set for fine-needle aspiration (FNA). PAGANI (1983) reported a sensitivity of 84% with the utilization of 14-G and 18-G needles. High success rates of biopsies with large-diameter cannulas in comparison to needles with a small lumen have also been reported by other authors (FEUERBACH 1988; LÜNING et al. 1989). Additionally, the specificity of a cutting biopsy is higher than that of an FNA biopsy, because histochemical examinations can also be conducted. LÜNING et al. (1989) pointed out that a large number of aspirates per biopsy are needed; therefore, he recommended that biopsy material be obtained at least four different times.

The possibility of incorrect cytologic diagnosis is well known. Apart from the quality of the material and its preparation, difficulties can arise from the differentiation of pseudoatypical changes caused by inflammation from genuine atypical cells, which is always difficult and sometimes impossible. The value of a cutting biopsy is often greater than that of an FNA, especially in cases of benign processes. CT-guided fine-needle punctures with needles smaller than 20 G should preferably be performed only in the neighborhood of high-risk structures, such as the vicinity of the porta of the liver or within the subphrenic region. Otherwise, it is recommended that a 20-G needle (DTMB 20-15 SIN, Cook, Denmark) be used, because even with this small caliber, a cutting biopsy is still possible. Another advantage of the 20-G needle is that it can be inserted in a fan-like fashion into different tumor areas, as with the puncture for aspiration biopsy.

Magnetic resonance imaging is helpful in lesions more than 1.5 cm in diameter, because the tip of the instrument is otherwise not exactly detectable; on the other hand no MR fluoroscopy mode exists for nearly real-time guidance and multiplanar imaging. Real-time pathologic analysis helps to shorten the therapy time for the patient. If guidance cannulas are used for biopsy, the tumor could be treated through the same cannulas with laser, drugs, etc.

18.8
Cancer Therapy

In patients with cancer or metastatic disease, infiltration into abdominal tissues like the liver or pancreas can be painful, and especially bone infiltration gives rise to one of the most intense forms of pain known to man (BONICA 1953). Effective tumor therapy therefore has to achieve three important goals: fast pain relief, effective reduction of tumor growth, and stabilization of bone or of the vertebral body to prevent paralysis. Now, new effective and less traumatic treatment approaches involving tomographic guidance are available for these patients.

Normally, nearly all treatment modalities which have been used in the past under CT or US guidance would be possible using MRI. Currently, however, only a small number of instruments and items of electronic equipment for artifact-free MRI guidance are available on the market. The easiest method of percutaneous cancer therapy is the local application of a high concentration of ethanol (PEI: percutaneous ethanol instillation) or chemotherapeutic agents (PDI: percutaneous drug instillation) (GRÖNEMEYER and SEIBEL 1993; LIVRAGHI et al. 1991). The disadvantage of this technique is that precise control of the spread of fluid within tissue is not possible; nevertheless, ethanol instillation is helpful for fast pain relief and for calcification and stabilization of infiltrated bony structures (GRÖNEMEYER and SEIBEL 1990c).

Other possibilities are intratumoral hyperthermia or vaporization, e.g., in liver, neck, or brain, using Nd:YAG laser applications (GEWIESE et al. 1994; HIGUCHI et al. 1992; KAHN et al. 1994; VOGL et al. 1996), RF ablations (ANZAI et al. 1995; ORGAN 1976), cryotherapy (GILBERT et al. 1985), hyperenergetic ultrasound (CLINE et al. 1994; YANG et al. 1993), or brachytherapeutic treatments. Imaging of temperature changes in tissues is only possible with MRI, and the therapist can control exactly the depth of the temperature infiltration. New imaging modalities employing the open MRI system using temperature-sensitive sequences and interactive image subtraction have been developed and are helpful for control of the predefined treatment area.

Percutaneous sympathectomy at all levels of the spine is also helpful as a first step in pain therapy using CT or ultrafast EBT with or without endoscopy and RF ablation or 96% ethanol instillation (GRÖNEMEYER and SEIBEL 1993; SEIBEL and GRÖNEMEYER 1990c).

18.8.1
Psychological Diagnosis

Besides radiologic and interventional examinations prior to therapy, psychological diagnosis is very important for the therapeutic approach to cancer patients. The diagnosis of "cancer" incites six types of fear in the patient (SCHARA 1986):

1. Fear of death
2. Fear of bodily deterioriation
3. Fear of inadequate therapy
4. Fear of intractable pain
5. Fear of being helpless
6. Fear of being socially isolated

Therefore, an essential aspect of tumor therapy is to initiate individual strategies for overcoming these fears and clear diagnostic and therapeutic approaches. Additionally, the pain level can be reduced when the physician devotes more time to the tumor patient (GRÖNEMEYER and SEIBEL 1990c).

A detailed history and interdisciplinary examinations are necessary prior to any treatment, especially if new symptoms appear in addition to those of the primary diagnosis. A questionnaire is helpful for analyzing the stage of tumor illness as well as the quality and quantity of pain. To characterize the quality, localization, and intensity of tumor pain can be very difficult due to the complexity of the pain, the psychological situation, and the perception of pain in these tumor patients. Furthermore, it is not possible to predict whether a tumor will cause pain or what form of pain is due to which tumor. Bone pain and retroperitoneal pain are almost always very intense, and nerve infiltrations and compressions and abdominal obstructions can also result in severe pain. However, tissue tumors and parenchymal tumors often do not produce pain.

Against this background, every doctor dealing with oncologic patients has to have a comprehensive knowledge of the different pain patterns of malignant diseases, the diagnostic procedures, and the treatment strategies.

18.8.2
Imaging Guidance and Tumor Pain Therapy

Among the various procedures in the field of interventional tumor therapy, PEI and laser therapy are the most commonly used. PEI was first used for small liver tumors in conjunction with US guidance (LIVRAGHI et al. 1986; SCHILD et al. 1989).

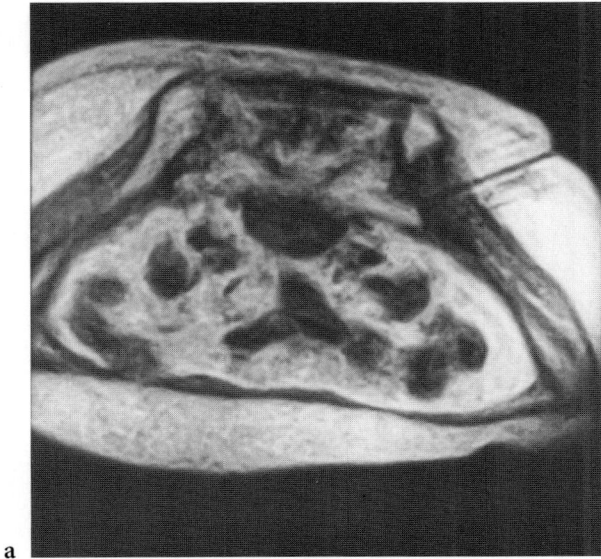

a

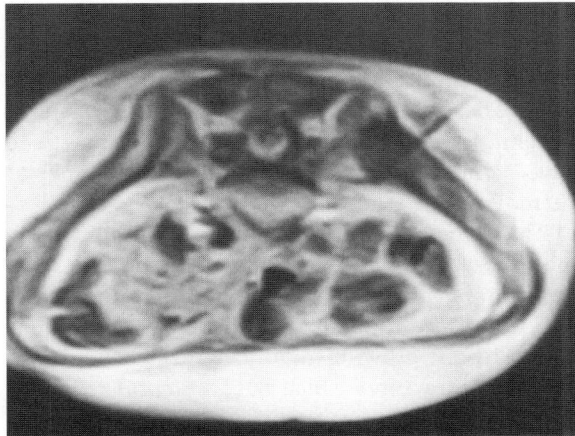

b

Fig. 18.4 a,b. Percutaneous ethanol instillation under MRI guidance (0.064 T, Toshiba) for the treatment of a bony metastasis in the os ilium in a patient with breast carcinoma. a Before and b After contrast medium and ethanol instillation

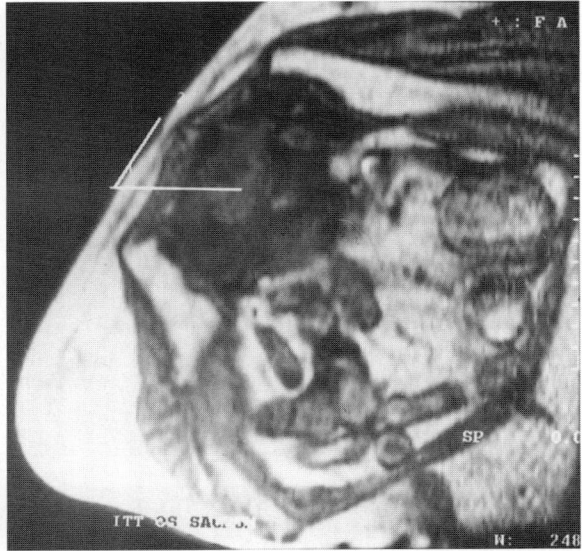

a

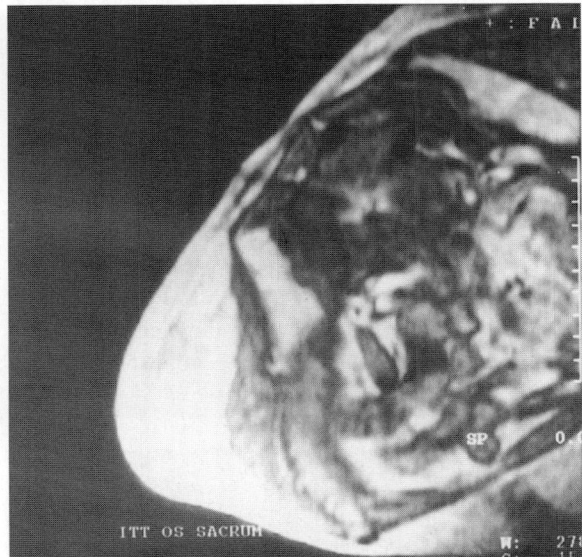

b

Fig. 18.5 a,b. MRI guidance for PEI into a bony metastasis in the os sacrum (0.2 T, Siemens). Microinvasive therapy inside a magnet a a Before and b After contrast medium and ethanol instillation

Today, hybrid combinations of different imaging systems with CT and, increasingly, MRI (Figs. 18.4, 18.5) are used for interventional microtherapy. Both techniques are far superior to fluoroscopy and US (Figs. 18.6, 18.7): they provide not only precise, detailed, and reproducible images of the anatomy, but also high resolution and high-contrast information on the pathology. Even less well trained physicians can become familiar with cross-sectional CT/MRI images in a much shorter time than is required for the moving real-time images of US. Tomographic images allow accurate reproducibility of specific slices at any time for the purpose of cancer therapy and drug instillation in high-risk areas. Tumor pain therapy has been successfully performed in our institution since 1988. Especially in tumor patients who continue to have intractable pain in spite of pain-relieving therapy (oral opiates, antiphlogistics, peridural anesthesia, local radiation therapy), percutaneous neurolysis of the sympathetic system at multiple levels can be very successful.

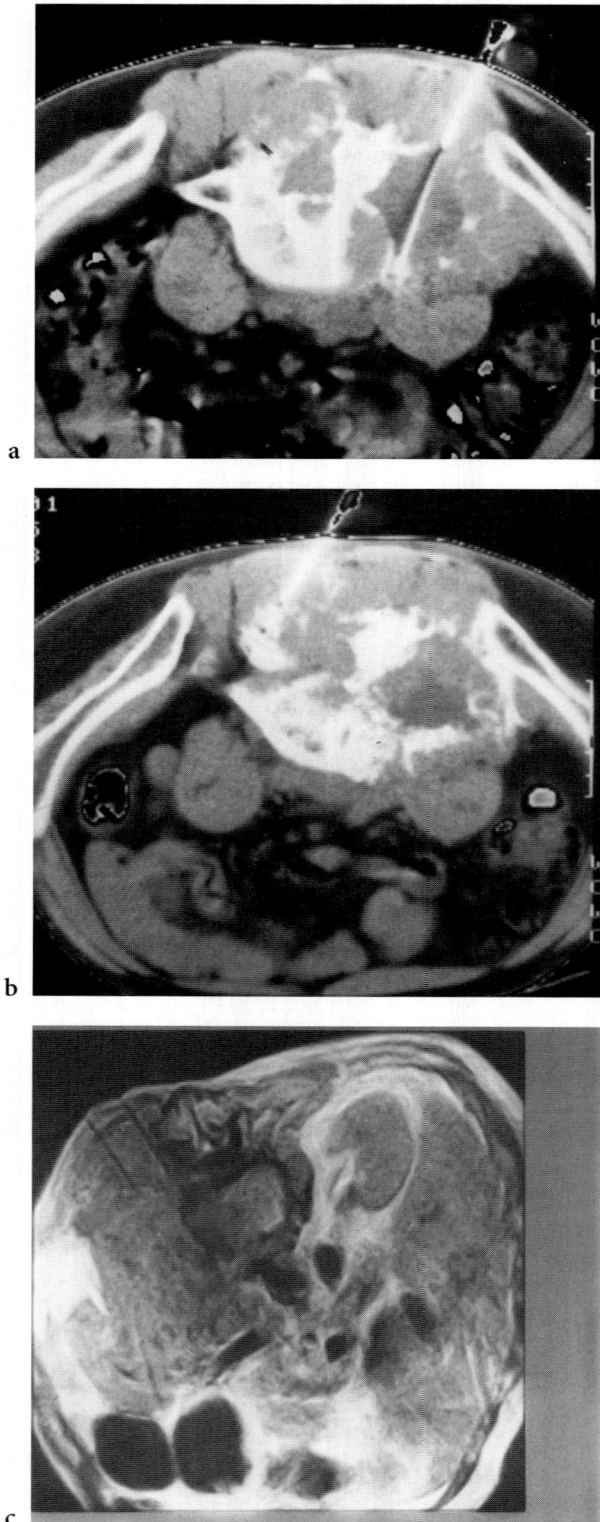

Fig. 18.6 a–c. Percutaneous treatment (PEI) of metastasis from a renal cell carcinoma to the lumbar spine/os ilium area. a CT before treatment; b 3 months later, calcification and stabilisation between the lumbar spine and os ilium is seen; c MRI guidance (0.064 T, Toshiba)

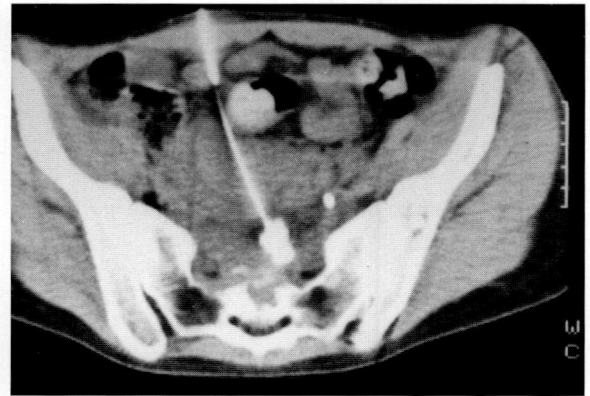

Fig. 18.7. Percutaneous transabdominal treatment of metastatic carcinoma of the colon, under CT guidance

18.8.2.1
Reqirements and Indications for Drug Instillation

We regard drug instillation under imaging guidance to be appropriate in patients who have tumor progression after surgery, radiation therapy, and/or systemic chemotherapy, and in patients who have contraindications to radiation therapy or chemotherapy.

The principal indication for CT/MRI-guided tumor therapy is cancer of stage M1. Such lesions can be treated for a relatively long period. Further indications are tumor pain and neurologic deficits caused by fast-growing tumors. Bone metastases and pathologic fractures which have immobilized a patient are very sensitive to this kind of therapy.

18.8.2.2
Technique of Intratumoral Drug Instillation

After prescanning the tumor region, the entry point of the treatment is defined. Either a transabdominal or a dorsal approach can be used. After local anesthesia of the skin through a guidance cannula, the therapy needle is inserted very carefully into the tumor area. This procedure has to be carried out stepwise by interactive CT/MRI scanning and injection of saline solution for hydraulic tissue deviation (HACI) as well as for anesthetic reasons. For intratumoral therapy, double the amount of local anesthetic agent in relation to ethanol or to a chemotherapeutic drug like mitoxantrone (an anthracycline which is locally well tolerated, and is only used close to vital structures) is necessary. In order to avoid pain due to drug instillation, a short-acting local anesthetic agent (1% mepivacaine) is combined with a long-acting agent (0.5% Carbostesin) in a ratio of 1:1 and is injected into the tumor before the drug instillation. In addition, diluted contrast medium is instilled into the tumor before the treatment. This is important for safety reasons, i.e., documentation that the needle tip is located outside vessels, as well as for visualization of the drug distribution.

The injection with a 15- to 20-cm 22-G cannula is performed with 1.5–5 cc 50%–96% ethanol or with a local-acting cytostatic drug of low toxicity, such as mitoxantrone in a volume of 2–20 ml (2–10 mg). We currently use low-dose ethanol, diluted by 50% when the injection is close to vital structures. Depending on the size of the tumor, treatment sessions are necessary every 3–14 days. On each occasion, the drug instillation is performed at another location within the tumor (GRÖNEMEYER and SEIBEL 1989).

18.8.2.3
Complications

In general the most likely complications when performing punctures using a fine needle are infection and hemorrhage. If a motor nerve is punctured, neurolysis is possible. If the spinal canal is hit, arachnoiditis, neurolysis, shock, and even death may occur. Treatment of the pancreas entails the possibility of pancreatitis. Vascular complications (false aneurysms) have to be considered if arteries are lacerated. Thus far we have not seen any of these complications in the patients we have treated.

18.8.2.4
Discussion

Treatment with alcohol can produce severe pain if the doses of local anesthetic and drugs are not precisely calculated according to the individual clinical situation of the patient (GRÖNEMEYER and SEIBEL 1990c, 1993). Sometimes a burning sensation and muscular aches lasting for several days occur following treatment with ethanol, and can be controlled by antiphlogistic drug therapy. The syndrome of neurolysis after accidental injection of ethanol into a motor nerve can only be treated with opiates. The toxic effects of ethanol in human tissues are well known, i.e., local dehydration with denaturation of proteins and necrosis (GRÖNEMEYER and SEIBEL 1990b) and denervations [e.g., lumbar sympathicolysis (SEIBEL et al. 1990)]. Complications after intravascular ethanol injection are also described.

In 1982, COX et al. and RABE et al. described colon/renal infarctions and abscesses, LAMMER et al. reported skin necrosis in 1985, and the same group observed an anterior spinal syndrome when ethanol was injected intravascularly.

In our department we have never experienced complications after injecting ethanol [we perform about 1000 facet joint denervations, PEIs for local cancer therapy, and sympathicolyses per year (GRÖNEMEYER et al. 1996a)]. Nevertheless, given the reported complications, only diluted ethanol (50%) in small volumes (<2 ml) should be delivered in the vicinity of vital structures (intestine, skin, spinal canal). Injection of contrast medium before the injection of alcohol is absolutely necessary in order to demonstrate the distribution of the volume. Following each action (change of the angulation of the needle, injection of fluid) a new CT scan of the region of interest has to be performed to ensure that the needle is still safely positioned. The distribution of the contrast medium has to be followed in a craniocaudal fashion with a slice thickness of 8 mm. Three-dimensional reconstruction images would be ideal, and a three-dimensional volume would also facilitate the calculation of the ethanol fractions to be injected. We recommend pretreatment calculation of the entire tumor volume (similar to the planning prior to radiation therapy) and the amount of the ethanol fractions. The tumor has to be divided into several sections and the amount and concentration of the ethanol to be instilled can then be calculated. At a distance of 1 cm from the spinal canal the ethanol should be diluted by 50%; alternatively, if the needle tip will lie very close to the spinal canal, mitoxantrone should be used because it has no toxic effect on vital structures such as nerves. It is known that at a concentration of 50% or less, ethanol only damages the sympathetic nerve fibers, i.e., it does not affect motor nerve fibers.

The excellent success of ethanol instillation for pain therapy is probably due to the fact that it eliminates small sensitive neural branches. The effect of further dilution of ethanol remains to be elucidated, as does that of combinations of ethanol and local cytotoxic agents. It is still unclear whether the amount of injected drugs should be varied in accordance with the size and histology of the tumor. The successful intratumoral treatment with ethanol of small hepatic, abdominal, and tracheobronchial tumors has been described by various authors (BURGENER and STEINMETZ 1987; FUJISAWA et al. 1986; SEKI et al. 1989; SIRONI et al. 1991; VARGAS et al. 1991). Indeed, a 100% survival rate has been reported following treatment of single small hepatocarcinomas with a diameter of less than 20 mm (LIVRAGHI et al. 1986). While use of high doses of ethanol (8–50 cc) for intratumoral therapy is common (UNGER 1994) , we prefer the low-dose ethanol application technique in order to avoid the above-mentioned complications.

The possibilities and prospects of direct intratumoral application of cytotoxic agents have to be further evaluated. We have already successfully started to treat soft tissue metastases in the lower abdomen and metastatic disease to the spinal cord with mitoxantrone. In contrast to radiation treatment, PEI into bone metastases causes an immediate drastic relief of pain and the stabilizing effect on the area of tumor destruction seems to start earlier. Further controlled studies should evaluate whether intratumoral therapy could also be used before radiation therapy or hyperthermia.

Single or repeated neurolysis of the sympathetic nervous system should be immediately added to the therapeutic armamentarium of every physician dealing with patients suffering from metastatic disease.

18.8.3
Laser-Induced Thermotherapy

Laser-induced thermotherapy (LITT) is a new minimally invasive technique for local tumor therapy. Well-defined coagulative necrosis can be achieved by low-power lasers with delivery of light energy through thin optical fibers. The tumor will be destroyed by direct heating without damage to the surrounding structures. Pilot clinical studies have shown a palliative effect of this treatment in patients with hepatic tumors. Only with MRI is real-time monitoring of the extent of thermal damage possible (VOGL 1994; VOGL et al. 1995).

18.8.3.1
Laser System

A neodymium:YAG laser with a wavelength of 1064 nm and a special diffusing laser applicator, which is mounted on a 400-μm silica fiber, are used (Dornier, Zeiss, Germany). The applicator diffuses its light homogeneously and emits laser light to an effective distance of 12–15 mm.

The application kit (Somatex, Germany) consists of a puncturing needle (20 cm, 4 Ch), a cannula (15 cm, 10 Ch), and a protective catheter with a closed end (43 cm, 7 Ch) for prevention of contact between tissue and applicator and to enable complete removal of the applicator even in cases of damage. The catheter is stable to a temperature of 400°C and is transparent to x-rays; the light is transmitted to the MRI scanning area with a 10-m-long fiber optic cable.

18.8.3.2
Technique

The procedure commences with CT documentation of the tumor. Thereafter, 20 ml of 1% lidocaine is infiltrated, and the 7-French catheter and then a thermostable plastic catheter are introduced. A special software program is used to calculate parameters like energy and application time. The patient is then moved to the MRI unit. Here the laser fiber is inserted into the guidance catheter and the treatment can start under the control of a turbo-FLASH sequence (TR 300–400 ms) for MR thermometry, which is sensitive for thermal-induced changes in signal and morphology. The turbo-FLASH sequence has to start precontrast and with a short delay (6 s) postcontrast over a total duration of 180 s. Posttherapeutic imaging is performed 1 week, 4 weeks, 3 months, and 6 months later.

There is a reproducible loss of signal intensity corresponding to increasing tissue temperature. The maximum diameter of signal loss in a treated area with 5 W and an application time of 12 minutes is 25 mm. With the turbo-FLASH sequence a nearly linear, inverse correlation between signal intensity and temperature is possible, but the FLASH-2D sequence provides higher spatial resolution and clearer delineation of topographic structures (Fig. 18.8).

18.8.3.3
Discussion

After lung and breast cancer, colorectal cancer is the third leading cause of death in Western countries. At the time of death, metastases are found in the liver in approximately two-thirds of patients with colorectal cancer. Only 20% of patients with liver metastases are suitable for radical operations, and liver surgery carries a mortality of about 5%.

New therapeutic alternatives like LITT or PEI are helpful in terms of improving treatment safety. Both LITT and PEI are very effective, but LITT needs a CT

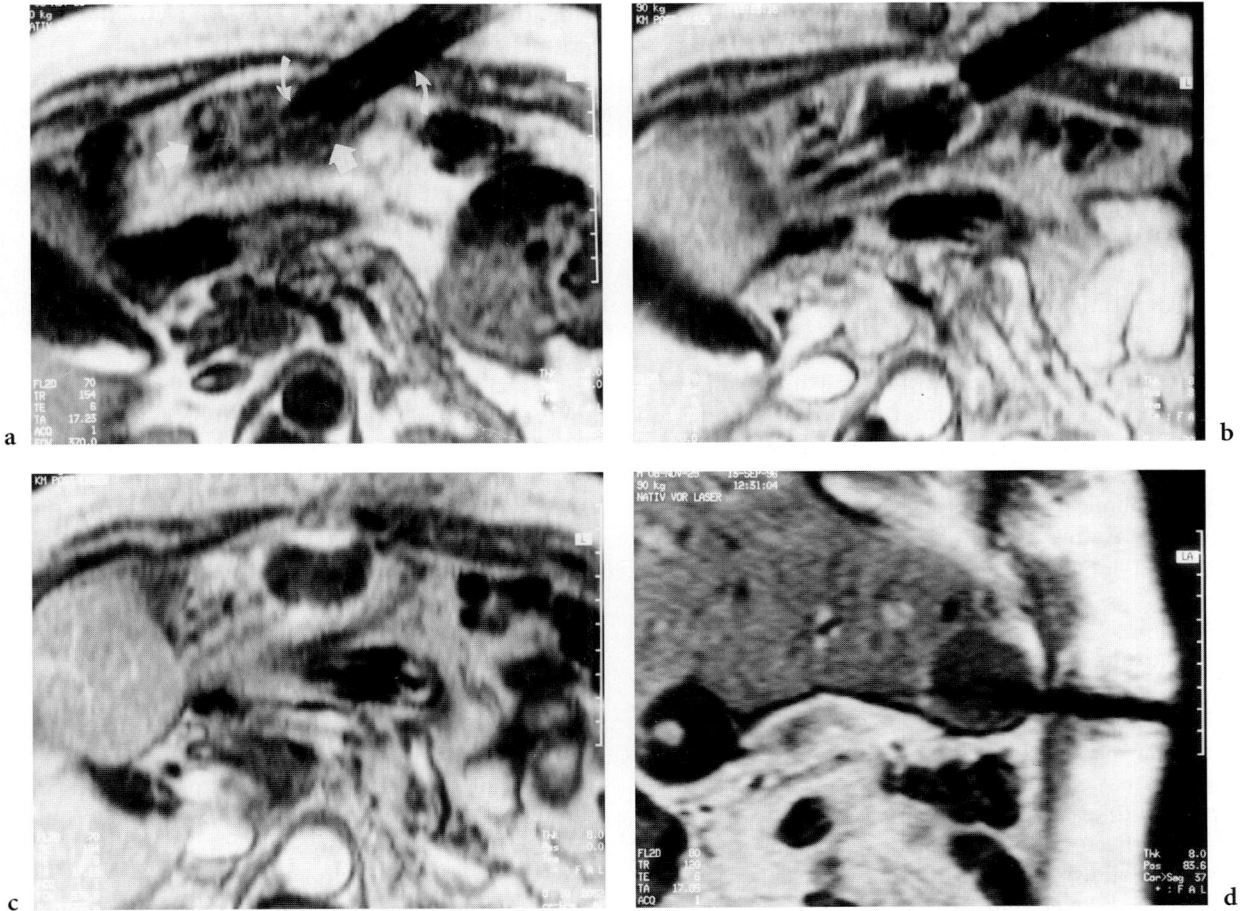

Fig. 18.8 a–e. MR-guided LITT of a liver metastasis of colorectal carcinoma in segment 2 of the liver. **a** Gradient-echo sequence, FLASH-2D, TR/TE = 154/6. Note the metastasis with low signal intensity (*straight arrows*) in segment 2. The interventionally placed laser catheters are identified by low signal intensity due to superparamagnetic markers (*curved arrows*). **b** Gradient-echo sequence, TR/TE = 154/6, Gadolinium-enhanced. Note the strong signal intensity with rim enhancement after LITT, and the low signal intensity of the central necrosis. **c** MR control, 2 days post LITT. As a result of the interventional MR-guided LITT, a huge area of central necrosis with some peripheral enhancement due to reactive changes is identified. **d** Sagittal orientation with a low signal intensity metastasis. The position of the laser applicator is shown. **e** Sagittal orientation. Note the high signal intensity of the surrounding rim after LITT and the central necrosis

scanner for exact needle placement and an MRI unit for thermometry. On the other hand, the diameter of the necrosis can be defined and planned very precisely. PEI is possible with US and, more precisely, with CT; also, guidance with MRI is increasingly being used. Thus in PEI can be performed every therapeutic center, but the drug distribution in tissue is diffuse and there is no method for exact planning. A painkiller effect is possible with PEI, especially in cases where metastases are infiltrating bones. Surrounding tissues can be damaged (fistula, aneurysm, etc.). With both LITT and PEI the best results are documented in lesions less than 2 cm in diameter.

There are three factors that favor the clinical success of MRI-guided LITT (VOGL et al. 1996):

1. Optimal localization of the applicator in the center of the tumor
2. Optimal "on-line monitoring" of the temperature
3. Exact documentation of local tumor dose application

LITT and PEI have to be integrated into interdisciplinary oncologic strategies and will increasingly be able to replace surgical interventions. Combination with other cancer treatments such as radiation therapy, systemic or locoregional chemotherapy, and embolization techniques is desirable. Controlled studies are required.

18.8.4
Percutaneous Neurolysis for Pain Therapy

The first use of surgery on the sympathetic nervous system was by ALEXANDER, who in 1889 unsuccessfully attempted to cure epileptics by the removal of the superior sympathetic trunk ganglions. After this sympathectomy was used for a number of indications. Following an attempt to treat spastic paralysis, ROYLE discovered in 1924 that after sympathectomy vasoconstriction was eliminated. Later, sympathectomy was used for the treatment of angina pectoris, bronchial asthma, hemoptysis, lung embolysis, hypertension, esophageal pain, and aortic pain (STILLER 1960).

We recommend that prior to tomographic cancer therapy in patients with tumor pain, chemical neurolysis of sympathetic nerves is performed at the segmental level of the upper pole of the tumor. Currently this can be achieved only with CT. The tip of a 22-G needle is advanced under CT guidance into the surrounding area of the plexus or ganglion. Here, injection of 1% Scandicain and 0.5% Carbostesin (ratio, 1:1) at nearly the same volume as ethanol is performed, followed by an injection of contrast medium (Iopamidol: Ultravist 150, Schering). The amount and the concentration of ethanol, which is injected carefully after the contrast medium, as well as the specific procedure, vary for different regions (celiac plexus: 50 cc of 50% ethanol; thoracic spine: 1.5 cc of 96% ethanol; lumbar spine: 4 cc of 96% ethanol; sacral plexus: 2 cc of 96% ethanol). If the treatment is insufficient, a second or third

sympathectomy at different segments below the first treatment is often helpful.

For thoracic sympathectomy the needle tip is advanced at a safe distance to the foramen intervertebrale. The space between the vertebral body and pleura is widened from about 1 mm to 4–5 mm by the injection of saline solution and local anesthetic agents. With this technique injury to the lung and pleura is avoided. The interventional needle must be advanced under contact with the vertebral body (SEIBEL et al. 1990a). Before lumbar sympathectomy, a scan with intravenous contrast medium at the level L2–4 is important for documentation of the ureters, which have to be at a safe distance (about 2 cm) from the ethanol instillation area. The major potential disadvantages of this technique are fistulas and ethanol-induced fibrotic obstruction of the ureters. Increasingly, combined techniques with CT-guided endoscopic RF ablation are possible (Figs. 18.9, 18.10).

18.8.4.1
Neurolysis of the Celiac Plexus

The value of neurolysis of the celiac plexus for pain therapy has long been recognized. Such blockades have been performed intraoperatively, percutaneously with or without fluoroscopic control, under sonographic guidance, and, finally, under CT guidance. Today, the CT-guided procedure is the technique of choice for celiac plexus blocks owing to its accuracy (SCHILD et al. 1989).

18.8.4.1.1
INDICATIONS
Neurolysis of the celiac plexus is indicated for the treatment of chronic pain which can no longer be alleviated by other means. The major causes of this type of intractable pain are diseases of the epigastric organs. However, successful plexus neurolyses have also been performed for pain caused by diseases of other abdominal organs and of retroperitoneal structures.

The most common diseases warranting this form of palliative therapy are pancreatic carcinoma and chronic pancreatitis, though it is also used for a wide variety of other diseases (i.e., liver metastases, lymphomas, Crohn's disease, and carcinomas of the bile ducts and gallbladder, kidney, stomach, colon, rectum, uterus, and ovaries) (BRIDENBAUGH et al. 1964; BUY et al. 1982; FILSHIE et al. 1983; GORBITZ and LEAVENS 1971; HAAGA et al. 1984;

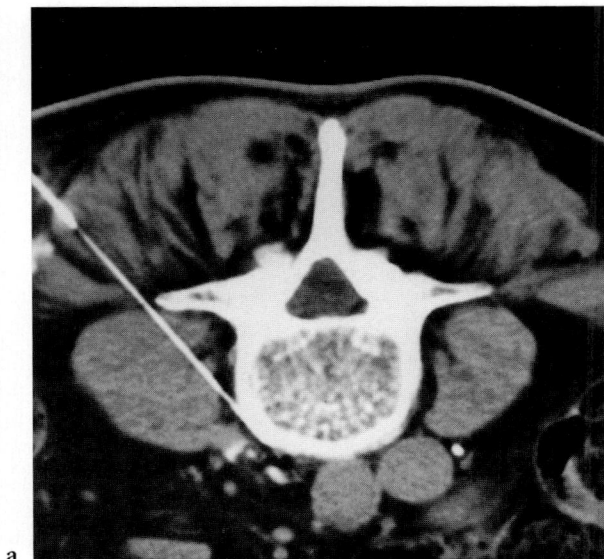

a

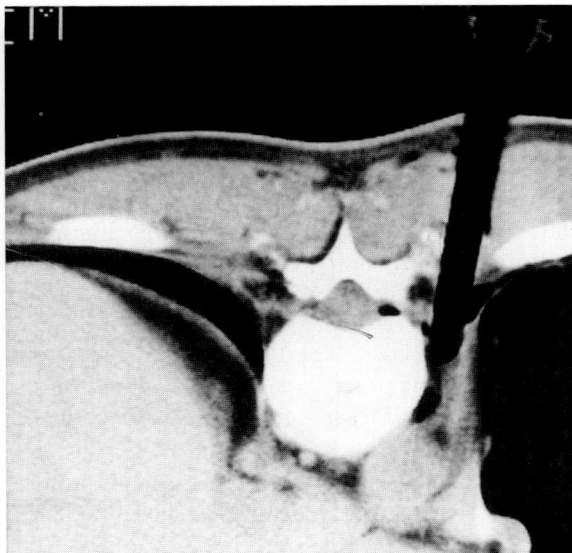

a

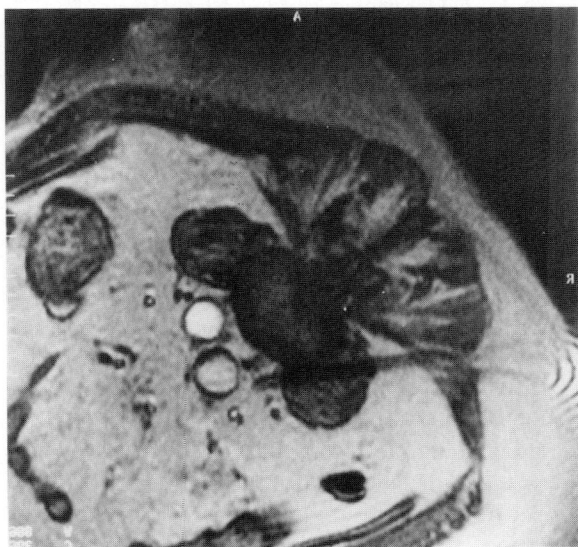

b

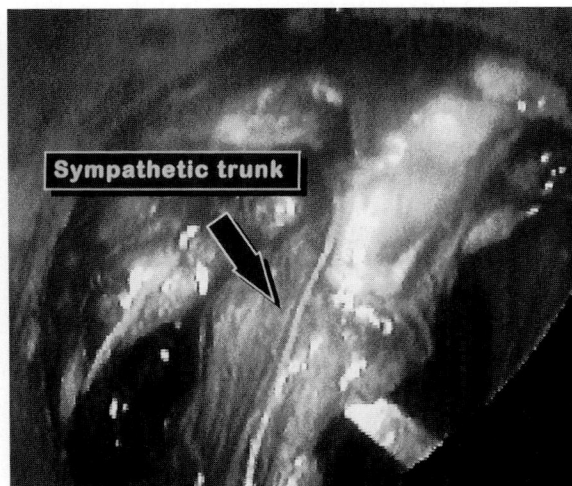

b

Fig. 18.9. Percutaneous lumbar sympathectomy under **a** CT and **b** MRI guidance (0.2 T, Siemens)

Fig. 18.10 a,b. Combined CT and endoscopy-guided sympathectomy at the T11/12 level. **a** CT-guided dilatation of the paravertebral space between the lung and vertebra for the trocar (12 mm). **b** Endoscopic view before RF sympathectomy

Hanowell et al. 1980; Moore et al. 1981; Muehle et al. 1987).

18.8.4.1.2
REQUIREMENTS

The requirements for CT-guided celiac plexus neurolysis are:

1. Normal blood clotting tests
2. Effective test block with a local anesthetic (during the same session)

18.8.4.1.3
TECHNIQUE

First, for the purpose of planning, CT scans from the lower end of the T12 vertebral body to the middle of the L2 vertebral body are requested. The decision regarding the appropriate side for the puncture, or whether to puncture both sides, depends on the potential complications which could occur given the existing anatomy, e.g., puncture of the liver, aorta, vena cava, or kidney. After CT identification of the celiac artery trunk, an entry point is defined on the skin. From this point a puncture of the area anterior to the aorta immediately above the celiac artery trunk can be performed. Normally neurolysis is performed at the level of the L1 vertebral body. A fine needle with a maximum diameter of 0.7 mm is used. Many access routes are possible because of the low risk of injury with this fine needle. Furthermore, neurolyses have been performed transabdominally from an anterior, transhepatic, or translumbar approach, the last-mentioned also involving a transaortic puncture (Fig. 18.11).

The following procedure is normally independent of the approach (i.e., anterior, transhepatic, or translumbar). After local anesthesia of the skin through a guidance cannula, the treatment needle is introduced and local anesthetic is injected as the needle is advanced. When the needle tip is just anterior to the aorta, immediately above or – less desirable but in most cases also acceptable – immediately below the celiac artery trunk, an aspiration is performed. After a negative aspiration (if aspiration is positive the needle position must be corrected), 1–2 ml diluted contrast medium (Ultravist 300, Schering; Solutrast 300, Byk-Gulden; diluted 1:5–7 with physiologic saline solution) is injected.

If the CT scan demonstrates that the injected contrast medium is distributed anterior to the aorta and on both sides, then a test blockade is performed with 5–10 ml 2% lidocaine. If there are no complications and the patient experiences alleviation of pain, a permanent blockade is performed. Many physicians use pure, high-proof alcohol for the neurolysis. However, 96% alcohol can cause severe pain and also can carry an increased risk of complications. For neurolysis of the celiac plexus we therefore prefer an injection of 20–50 ml of the following:

- Six to seven parts absolute ethanol (caution: alcohol must be suitable for parenteral application!)
- Three to four parts of a long-acting local anesthetic, e.g., 0.5% bupivacaine (Carbostesin).
- Approximately 1 part contrast medium (compatible with the mixture) for which we use iopamidol (Ultravist 300, Schering, Germany; Solutrast 300, Byk-Gulden, Germany).

Due to the local anesthetic, the injection is almost painless. The addition of the contrast medium allows observation of the distribution of the solution. A CT scan is used to monitor the injection after the first half of the injection and at the end of the injection.

Alternatively we often use a 1:1 mixture of 96% ethanol with bupivacaine 1% without the addition of

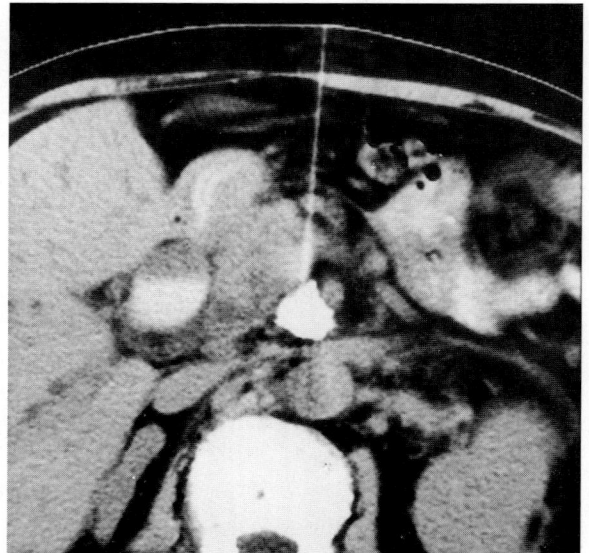

Fig. 18.11. PEI for neurolysis of the celiac plexus

contrast medium. The distribution of this mixture can also be documented with CT due to the negative contrast of the solution.

If the CT scan shows that the neurolytic solution is not distributed equilaterally about the celiac artery trunk region or the aorta, then in the same session, a second puncture can be performed. However, the positioning of the second needle tip can be difficult due to the contrast medium already injected. The total amount of the injected solution should not exceed 60–70 ml. An alternative approach, which we believe to be more logical, is to wait for the clinical results of the original injection and only then to reach a decision about a second injection. Because of the possibility of hypotension or other cardiovascular problems after the neurolysis the patient remains in hospital for 24 h (Buy et al. 1982; Filshie et al. 1983; Haaga et al. 1984; Ischia et al. 1983; Moore et al. 1981; Muehle et al. 1987).

18.8.4.1.4
SIDE-EFFECTS

Pain during and after the injection caused by irritation of abdominal structures frequently appears only after the use of a pure alcohol solution. Such pain can be avoided to a great extent by the addition of a local anesthetic to the neurolytic solution.

A significant drop in blood pressure has been described in the literature in up to 20% of the cases;

however, this has rarely been observed by us with the use of the above procedure. An improvement in the impaired bowel function is often observed after neurolysis, often to the delight of the patients.

18.8.4.1.5
COMPLICATIONS

Complications such as infection or bleeding, and in the case of a pancreatic puncture the possibility of pancreatitis, are associated with any kind of fine-needle puncture. However, we have not observed any of these complications using the transabdominal procedure from an anterior approach. Complications of CT-guided plexus blockade from a posterior approach, as reported in the literature, are:

1. Temporary hematuria from a kidney puncture
2. Spinal canal puncture without consequences
3. Disk puncture without consequences

In the literature, there are reports of the following major complications after fluoroscopically guided plexus blockades:

1. Paraplegia (spinal ischemia can be caused by an intramural injection or injection at/into a lumbar artery supplying the spinal cord)
2. Partial leg paralysis through the influence of the neurolytic solution on the lumbar plexus

There are also reports of sexual dysfunction and urination disorders. However, the fear that a plexus blockade could mask the symptoms of an acute abdomen has not been verified (BRIDENBAUGH et al. 1964; BUY et al. 1982; HAAGA et al. 1984; HEGEDUES 1979; ISCHIA et al. 1983; MOORE et al. 1981; MUEHLE et al. 1987).

18.8.4.2
Presacral Neurolysis

CT-guided neurolysis of the presacral and precoccygeal sympathetic trunk is another important method for local pain therapy. In patients with tumoral infiltration of the pelvis (mostly from colorectal or gynecologic carcinomas), we were able to achieve very good results with neurolysis of the presacral and precoccygeal sympathetic trunk (SEIBEL and GRÖNEMEYER 1990c).

18.8.4.2.1
INDICATIONS

Indications are pelvic or leg pain caused by tumoral infiltration of the pelvis.

18.8.4.2.2
TECHNIQUE

In contrast to lumbar sympathetic trunk and celiac plexus neurolysis, presacral and precoccygeal neurolysis normally requires multiple treatments. Generally, we perform four separate treatments bilaterally at two levels. At each treatment we inject between 2 and 4 ml alcohol into the plexus. The puncture most often is performed from a lateral approach, but can sometimes also be made from an anterior approach. The needle tip is positioned just presacrally or precoccygeally. However, in the presacral puncture, anterior access is sometimes required. In precoccygeal neurolysis, a puncture from lateral or posterolateral is the most convenient approach. As in each neurolysis procedure, documentation of the potential alcohol distribution has to be performed prior to the injection of alcohol. Therefore, dilute contrast medium is injected after the placement of the needle tip. Additionally, after 2–3 weeks, the procedure is repeated (Fig. 18.12).

18.9
Drainage of Fluid Accumulations

Diagnosis of abscesses and fluid accumulations was made predominately by operative measures until the development of US, CT, and MRI. These imaging modalities (especially CT and MRI) are today considered the diagnostic tools of choice for documentation and description of the topography, expansion, and internal structure of fluid collections as well as for interventional therapy.

The first step in the development of nonsurgical catheter placement was CT- and US-guided fine-needle punctures for diagnostic serologic and/or bacteriologic studies. The image quality of CT is superior to that of US, especially for drainage placement. The access route and positioning of the catheter within the fluid collection can be determined prior to the procedure by means of CT. The selection of a catheter depends on the amount, contents, and structure of the fluid accumulation.

For interventional therapy planning in respect of thoracic or abdominal abscesses or fluid accumulations, it may be necessary to use a bolus CT technique at the planned puncture level to show larger vessels, so that they can be avoided during puncture. As a matter of principle, the shortest access route should be selected. However, in particular cases, it may be necessary to select a longer access route, often transhepatic, to avoid injuries of abdominal

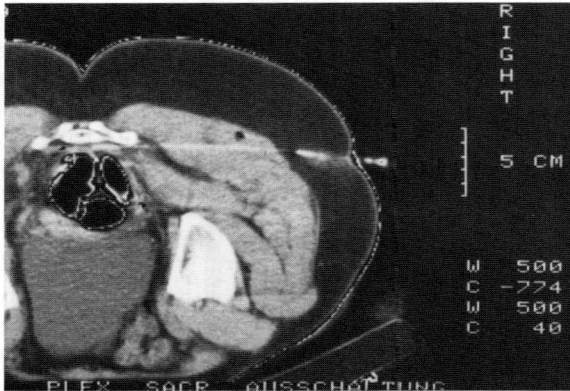

Fig. 18.12. PEI for neurolysis of the presacral plexus

structures (i.e., intestine, stomach, kidneys, and large vessels). Also, the expected duration of drainage has to be taken into consideration when determining the access route. A subphrenic or subhepatic abscess can heal in 1–2 weeks with systemic medication and drainage, whereas a pancreatic pseudocyst can take more than 3 months to heal completely.

The majority of these drainage cases are patients who have had one or more operations, so most are willing to tolerate a drainage catheter for an extended period. It is crucial that the tip of the catheter rests in the lowest area to be drained. In patients with infected drainage material, periodic flushes with antibiotics are performed. The appropriate antibiotics are determined by an antibiogram. These antibiotic flushes are first performed at short intervals, and then at longer intervals later in the treatment. For non-necrotic fluid accumulations, a simple drainage bag without suction can be used. After a short period in hospital, patients can return home under the care of the family doctor for continued treatment. Plain films, with contrast medium if needed, and CT are often useful for follow-up in patients with long-term drainage.

18.9.1
Instruments

Catheters suitable for drainage should have the following properties:

1. Sliding capability, relatively sturdy, and made of x-ray dense material
2. A row of holes with a large lumen along the inner curve of a pigtail or curved catheter; a terminal

lumen with an additional mushroom configuration is also possible
3. At least one large interior lumen and, if needed, a second thinner lumen in tandem position for flushing
4. A Luer-Lok nozzle for connection with the drainage bag
5. Availability in 6–24 French

18.9.2
Technique

First, the puncture depth and angle are determined on the CT monitor. Then, after local anesthesia, under CT guidance a relatively thin Teflon-coated cannula is inserted into the area to be drained. After removal of the mandrin and aspiration of a few milliliters of fluid for serology, bacteriology, and possibly cytology, a guide wire is inserted without removal of large amounts of fluid. Combined CT and fluoroscopy is necessary for the remainder of the procedure. After dilation of the tract to the desired lumen under CT and fluoroscopic control, the final catheter can be inserted using the Seldinger technique. Small amounts of a diluted contrast medium are injected in the abscesses or fluid collections to help visualize their extent (Fig. 18.13). After final positioning, the drainage catheter is fixed to the skin and covered with a sterile dressing (SEIBEL et al. 1989; WEIGAND 1990).

18.10
CT or MRI for Guidance Techniques?

Although CT is our current gold standard for instrument guidance, MRI will gain in importance due to the newly developed "open" systems. In contrast to CT, MRI does not produce x-rays. This is important not only for the therapist, but also for the patient. In addition, imaging in three planes can be achieved almost in real time. Also, without contrast medium, arteries and veins can be documented, as can changes in tissue contrast after heating with laser or cooling with cryotherapy or the application of hyperenergetic ultrasound for tissue ablation. The use of this patient-friendly open device is advantageous not only in corpulent persons but also in children and persons who suffer from claustrophobia. The advantage becomes apparent when parents, relatives, or medical staff can accompany anxious patients.

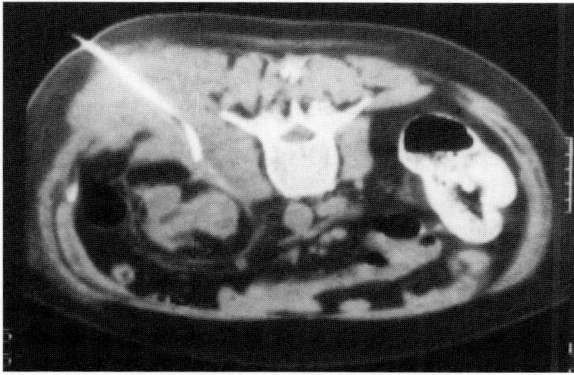

Fig. 18.13. Fluid collection of abdominal mass. Combined CT and x-ray fluoroscopic guidance. Precise tip tracking of the catheter is possible with CT

In open MRI systems, operations can be carried out quite comfortably inside the gantry without the patient being moved, and with nearly real-time guidance using fast keyhole sequences (GRÖNEMEYER et al. 1995b, 1996a).

If there are vital structures such as nerves and vessels in the target region (high-risk area), we regard CT as the gold standard for guidance (GRÖNEMEYER et al. 1996b). With CT the precision of tip guidance is $1\,mm^3$, the edges of the instruments are sharply displayed, and the tip can be defined to within $\pm 0.2\,mm$. In many cases correct and safe access can be achieved by CT/EBT for interstitial therapy such as drug injection or placement of prostheses and implants. Another area of application for CT/EBT is osteosynthesis, i.e., to assist drilling and fixation at the correct angle. Hybrid tomographic systems may prove useful for balloon dilatation as well as for laser treatments or stent implantation. With this kind of technique, by means of tip tracking the catheter can be placed very precisely inside the vessel, in the optimal position in relation to the arterial or venous wall. As already pointed out, EBT has the largest gantry (90 cm) and the fastest acquisition time, but current computer processing is too slow.

The best access for treatments is provided by the open MRI systems with nearly real-time guidance using special fast keyhole sequences. This technique is faster than CT, but offers lower quality imaging. For high-quality scans, the total scan time is much longer than with CT. For high-resolution documentation, a T1- and T2-weighted sequences have to be acquired after MR-fluoroscopy mode for guidance procedure in almost one more plane. Special materials are required for the instruments because conven-

tional instruments cause artifacts in the displayed scans. Some special nonferromagnetic cannulas are now available for interventional MRI. However, a major drawback is that the resolution of the tip and longitudinal edges of the instruments is only $\pm 3.5\,mm$ (GRÖNEMEYER et al. 1995b). Open MRI is useful in low-risk areas. Organs which are affected by breathing should be imaged during breath-holding. It should be noted that it is possible to start with CT for the guidance procedure and then to change to MRI for visualization of treatment effects such as laser ablation. Another advantage of MRI in comparison to CT/EBT is the possibility of temperature mapping (CLINE et al. 1994) and of measuring metabolic changes with imaging or spectroscopy mode in high-field (1.5 T) systems. With all tomographic systems preoperative planning is possible, as is 3D reconstruction before and after the treatment.

We believe that in about 10 years these tomography systems (CT, EBT, and MRI) will be available in many operating theaters as a hybrid combination of endoscopy systems and US or x-ray units. The conventional x-ray devices that provide only a shadowy image of the body structures will disappear. At the same time, the cost of high-tech systems will be comparable to that of classical x-ray units due to the widespread installation of tomographs.

In the future, dedicated CT/EBT (GRÖNEMEYER et al. 1995b, 1996a) or MRI systems should be available for all diagnostic or microinvasive procedures. The different procedures are complementary to and not competitive with each other.

18.11
Conclusion and Future Outlook

In the near future more interventional procedures will be performed in the abdomen and pelvis. Especially for the treatments of tumors, RF, cryotherapy, and laser techniques are of great potential, if the necessary equipment is available. The introduction of endoscopic minimally invasive therapeutic procedures and minimized open surgery in open MRI systems in the abdomen and retroperitoneum will be one of the next steps in the development of new surgical treatments. If endocoils and/or MRI-compatible endoscopic systems are developed, combined MRI and endoscopy will become a routine technique, especially for obstetrics and in the gallbladder, urinary tract, and colon. First experiences with such a technique have already been reported from London (DESOUZA 1994) and by our group (GRÖNEMEYER et al. 1995a; MELZER et al. 1996). Today, MRI-guided sympathectomies are being performed in experimental studies because tip tracking is of importance near to vital structures such as the aortic branches, ureter, and spinal canal, where complications are easily possible. CT guidance is now standard technology in minimally invasive and microinvasive abdominal interventions (GRÖNEMEYER et al. 1996b).

References

Alexander W (1889) The treatment of epilepsy. Nat Libr Cat 1955–1959

Anzai Y, Desalles AAF, Black KL, et al. (1993) Interventional MR imaging. RadioGraphics 13:897–904

Anzai Y, et al. (1995) Preliminary experience with a technique for MR-guided thermal ablation of brain tumors. AJNR 16:39–48

Bonica JJ (1953) The management of cancer pain. In: Zimmermann M, Irings P, Wagner R (eds) Pain in cancer patients. Springer, Berlin Heidelberg New York Tokyo (Recent results in cancer research 83:13–27)

Boyd D, Gold R, Quinn J, Sparks R, Stanley R, Hermannsfeldt W (1979) A proposed dynamic cardiac 3-D densitometer for easy detection and evaluation of heart disease. IEEE Trans Nucl Sci NS 26:2724

Bridenbaugh LD, et al. (1964) Management of upper abdominal cancer pain. J Am Med Assoc 190:877

Burgener FA, Steinmetz SD (1987) Treatment of experimental adenocarcinomas by percutaneous intratumoral injection of absolute ethanol. Invest Radiol 22:472–477

Buy JN, et al. (1982) CT-guided celiac plexus and splanchnic nerve neurolysis. J Comput Assist Tomogr 6:315

Cline H, et al. (1994) MR temperature mapping of focused ultrasound surgery. Magn Reson Med 31:628–636

Cox GG, Lee KR, Price HJ, Gunter K, Noble MJ, Mebust WK (1982) Colonic infarction following ethanol embolization of renal carcinoma. Radiology 145:343–345

DeSouza N (1994) MR-guided application in the body. In: Black K, Lufkin R (eds) Interventional MRI. Marina del Ray, 13–14 August 1994, 162–163

Dumoulin CL, et al. (1993) Real-time position monitoring of invasive devices using magnetic resonance. Magn Reson Med 29:411–415

Feuerbach S (1988) Perkutane Biopsie. In: Clausen C, Felix R (eds) Quo vadis CT? Springer, Berlin Heidelberg New York, p 284

Filshie J, et al. (1983) Unilateral computerised tomography guided celiac plexus block: a technique for pain relief. Anesthesia 38:498

Fujisawa T, Hongo H, Yamaguchi Y, et al. (1986) Intratumoral ethanol injection for malignant tracheobronchial lesions: a new bronchofiberscopic procedure. Encoscopy 18:188–189.

Gewiese B, et al. (1994) Magnetic resonance imaging-controlled laser – induced interstitial thermotherapy. Invest Radiol 29:345–351

Gilbert J, et al. (1985) Real time ultrasonic monitoring of hepatic cryosurgery. Cryobiology 22:319–330

Gorbitz C, Leavens ME (1971) Alcohol block of the celiac plexus for control of upper abdominal pain caused by cancer and pancreatitis. J Neurosurg 34:575

Göthlin JH (1976) Post-lymphographic percutaneous fine needle biopsy of lymph nodes, guided by fluoroscopy. Radiology 120:205

Grönemeyer DHW, Seibel RMM (1989). Neue Formen der Interventionellen Tumortherapie in der Radiologie. In: Grönemeyer DHW, Seibel RMM (eds) Interventionelle Computertomographie. Ueberreuter Wissenschaft Berlin, pp 201–224

Grönemeyer DHW, Seibel RMM (1990a) Atlas of CT guided biopsies. In: Seibel RMM, Grönemeyer DHW (eds) Interventional computed tomography. Blackwell, Oxford, pp 3–6

Grönemeyer DHW, Seibel RMM (1990b) CT-guided cervical blockades and methods of cancer therapy for lesions of the cervicobrachial plexus. In: Seibel RMM, Grönemeyer DHW (eds) Interventional computed tomography. Blackwell, Oxford, pp 161–179

Grönemeyer DHW, Seibel RMM (1990c) New forms of interventional tumor therapy in radiology. In: Seibel RMM, Grönemeyer DHW (eds) Interventional computed tomography. Blackwell, Oxford, pp 137–138

Grönemeyer DHW, Seibel RMM (1993) Microinvasive CT-guided cancer therapy of soft tissue and bone metastases. WMW 12:313–321

Grönemeyer DHW, Seibel RMM (1995c) Interventional CT and MRI, a challenge for safety and cost reduction in health care system. Health Care Technology Policy II, SPIE 2499:132–148

Grönemeyer DHW, Seibel RMM, Busch M, et al. (1990d) Interventional magnetic resonance imaging. In: Seibel RMM, Gronemeyer DHW. Interventional computed tomography. Blackwell, Oxford, pp 289–305

Grönemeyer DHW, Seibel RMM, Kaufman L, et al. (1990e) Interventional procedures in low field magnetic resonance imaging. Diagnostic Imaging International 11/12:32–36.

Grönemeyer DHW, Seibel RMM, Melzer A, Schmidt A, Deli M, Friebe MH, Busch M (1995a) Future of advanced guidance techniques by interventional CT and MRI. Minimally Invasive Therapy and Allied Technologies 2:251–259

Grönemeyer DHW, Seibel RMM, Melzer A, Schmidt A (1995b) Image guided access technique. Endosc Surg Allied Technol 1:69–75

Grönemeyer DHW, Seibel RMM, Erbel R, et al. (1996a) Equipment configuration and procedures-preferences for interventional microtherapy. J Dig Imag 9:81–96

Grönemeyer DHW, et al. (1996b) Image-guided access enhances microtherapy. Diagn Imag 11:2–5

Haaga JR, et al. (1983) Clinical comparison of small- and large-caliber cutting needles for biopsy. Radiology 146:665

Haaga JR, Alfidi RJ, Havrilla TR, et al. (1977) CT detection and aspiration of abdominal abscess. Am J Roentgenol 128:465

Haaga JR, et al. (1984) Improved technique for CT-guided celiac ganglia block. Amer J Roentgenol. 142:1201

Haaga JR, Alfidi RJ (1976) Precise biopsy localization by computed tomography. Radiology 118:603

Hanowell S, et al. (1980) Celiac plexus block: diagnostic and therapeutic applications in abdominal pain. South Med J 33:1330

Hegedues V (1979) Relief of pancreatic pain by radiography-guided block. Am J Roentgenol 133:1101

Herman SD, et al. (1986) Incidental prostatic carcinoma detected by MRI and diagnosed by MRI/CT-guided biopsy. Am J Roentgenol. 146:351–352

Higuchi N, et al. (1992) Magnetic resonance imaging of the acute effects of interstitial neodymium:YAG laser irradiation on tissues. Invest Radiol 27:814–821

Ischia S, et al. (1983) A new approach to the neurolytic block of the celiac plexus: the transaortic technique. Pain 16:333

Jaques PF, Staab E, Richey W, et al. (1978) CT-assisted pelvic and abdominal aspiration biopsy in gynecological malignancy. Radiology 128:651

Jaschke W, Grönemeyer DHW, Seibel RMM, Boyd DP (1989) Perspektiven für CT-gesteuerte Punktionstechniken durch Ultra-Fast-Cine-CT. In: Grönemeyer DHW, Seibel RMM (eds) Interventionelle Computertomographie. Ueberreuter Wissenschaft, Berlin, pp 291–295

Jolesz FA, Bleier AR, Jakob P, et al. (1988) MR imaging of laser tissue interactions. Radiology 168:249–253

Kahn T, et al. (1994) MRI-guided laser induced interstitial thermotherapy of cerebral neoplasms. J Comput Assist Tomogr 18:519–532

Kaufman L, Crooks L, Mitsuaki A, Hoenninger J, Watts J, Winkler M (1987) Admin Radiol 6:32–38

Klose KC, Gunther RW (1988) CT-gesteuerte Punktionen. In: Gunther RW, Thelen M (eds) Interventionelle Radiologie. Thieme Stuttgart, p 459

Kramann B (1989) CT-gesteuerte Leber Biopsie. In: Grönemeyer DHW, Seibel RMM (eds) Interventionelle Computertomographie. Ueberreutes Wissenschaft, Berlin, pp 291–295

Lackner M, et al. (1989) CT-gesteuerte Punktionen. In: Friedmann G, Steinbrich W (eds) Angioplastie, Embolisation, Punktion, Drainagen. Interventionelle Methoden in der Radiologie. Springer, Konstanz, p 147

Lammer J, Justich F, Schreyer H, Pettek R (1985) Complications of renal tumor embolization. Cardiovasc Intervent Radiol 8:31–35

Livraghi T, Festi D, Monti F, et al. (1986) US-guided percutaneous alcohol injection of small hepatic and abdominal tumors. Radiology 161:309–310

Livraghi T, Vettore C, Lazzaroni S (1991) Liver metastases: results of percutaneous ethanol injection in 14 patients. Radiology 179:709–712

Lufkin R, et al. (1987) New needle for MR-guided aspiration cytology of the head and the neck. Am J Roentgenol 149:380–382

Lüning M, et al. (1989) CT-gestützte Feinnadelbiopsien bei Leberraumforderungen. Ein Vergleich der Ergebnisse einer Arbeitsgruppe von zwei Zeiträumen. Rontgenpraxis 42:1974

MacErlean DP, et al. (1980) Pancreatic pseudocyst. Management by ultrasonically guided aspiration. Gastrointest Radiol 5:255

Macintosh PK, Thomson KR, Barbaric ZL (1979) Percutaneous transperitoneal lymph-node biopsy as a means of improving lymphographic diagnosis. Radiology 131:647

Martino CT, et al. (1984) CT-guided liver biopsies: eight years' experience. Radiology 152:755

Matsumoto R, et al. (1992) Monitoring of laser and freezing-induced ablation in the liver with T1–weighted imaging. J Magn Res Imag 2:555–562

Melzer A, et al. (1996) Prerequisites for magnetic resonance image guided interventions and endoscopic surgery. Minimally Invasive Therapy and Allied Technologies 5:255–262

Moore DC, et al. (1981) Celiac plexus block: a roentgenographic anatomic study of technique and spread of solution in patients and corpses. Anaesth Analg 60:369

Muehle C, et al. (1987) Radiographically guided alcohol block of the celiac ganglia. Semin Intervent Radiol 4:195

Mueller PR, et al. (1986) MR-guided aspiration biopsy: needle design and clinical trials. Radiology 161:605–609

Nordenstrom B (1967) Paraxiphoid approach to the mediastinum for mediastinography and mediastinal needle biopsy: a preliminary report. Invest Radiol 2:141

Organ L (1976) Electrophysiologic principles of radio-frequency lesion making. Appl Neurophysiol 39:69–76

Pagani J (1983) Biopsy of focal hepatic lesions. Comparison of 18 and 22 gauge needles. Radiology 147:673

Pereiras PV, Meiers W, Kunhardt B, et al. (1978) Fluoroscopically guided thin needle aspiration biopsy of the abdomen and retroperitoneum. Am J Roentgenol 131:197

Rabe FE, Yun HY, Richmond BD, Klatte EC (1982) Renal tumor infarction with absolute ethanol. Am J Roentgenol 139:1139–1144

Royle ND (1924) A new treatment of spastic paralysis by sympathetic ramisection. Experimental basis and clinical results. Surg Gynecol Obstet 39:701–720

Rüttimann A (1968) Iliac lymph node aspiration biopsy through paravascular approach: preliminary report. Radiology 90:150

Schara J (1986) Tumorschmerz. Schmerz-Pain-Douleur 2:41–42

Schild HH, et al. (1989) Perkutane Neurolyse des Plexus Coeliacus. In: Grönemeyer DHW, Seibel RMM. Interventionelle Computertomographie. Ueberreuter Wissenschaft, Berlin, pp 291–295

Schmidt A, et al. (1996) Tomographic guided biopsy and cell aspiration' of neoplasms. Minimally Invasive Therapy and Allied Technologies 3:249–254

Seibel RMM, Grönemeyer DHW, Werner WR, Starck E, Arlart IP (1989) Die thorakale und abdominelle perkutane CT-gesteuerte Abszessdrainage. In: Grönemeyer DHW, Seibel RMM. Interventionelle Computertomographie. Ueberreuter Wissenschaft, Berlin, pp 241–272

Seibel RMM, Grönemeyer DHW, Balzer K, Carstensen G, Sehnert C (1990a) The CT-guided lumbar sympathetic trunk neurolysis for the treatment of the occlusive arterial disease. In: Seibel RMM, Grönemeyer DHW (eds) Interventional computed tomography. Oxford, Blackwell, pp 211–225

Seibel RMM, Grönemeyer DHW, Weigand H (1990b) Thorax – Biopsy: Lunge – Pleura – Mediastinum. In: Seibel RMM, Gronemeyer DHW (eds) Interventional computed tomography. Blackwell, Oxford, pp 15–26

Seibel RMM, Grönemeyer DHW (1990c) CT-guided neurolysis of the presacral and precoccygeal sympathetic trunk. In: Seibel RMM, Grönemeyer DHW (eds) Interventional computed tomography. Blackwell, Oxford, pp 193–199

Seki T, Nonaka T, Kubota Y, Mizuno T, Samashima Y (1989) Ultrasonically guided percutaneous ethanol injection therapy for hepatocellular carcinoma. Am J Gastroenterol 84:1400–1407

Sheu JC, Huang GT, Chen DS, et al. (1987) Small hepatocellular carcinoma: intratumor ethanol treatment using new needle and guidance systems. Radiology 163:43–44

Silverman S (1996) Percutaneous abdominal biopsy: recent advances and future directions. Semin Interv Radiol, 13:3–15

Silverman S, et al. (1995) Interactive MR-guided biopsy in an open-configuration MR imaging system. Radiology 197:175–181

Sironi S, et al. (1991) Small hepatocellular carcinoma treated with percutaneous ethanol injection: MR imaging findings. Radiology 180:333–336

Stiller H (1960) Indikation und Erfolg der Sympathikuschirurgie. Fortschr Med 78:425–428

Unger E (1994) MR-guided alcohol ablation of the body. In Black K, Lufkin R (eds) Interventional MRI. Marina del Rey: 13–14 August 1994, pp 154–158

Vargas H, et al. (1991) Ethanol injection of hepatic tumors. J Invest Surg 4:291–298

Vogl T (1994) MR-guided laser induced thermotherapy (LITT) of liver metastasis and experimental and clinical results. In: Black K, Lufkin R (eds) Interventional MRI. Marina del Ray, 13–14 August 1994, pp 150–152

Vogl TJ, et al. (1995) Malignant liver tumors treated with MR imaging-guided laser induced thermotherapy: technique and prospective results. Radiology 196:257–265

Vogl TJ, et al. (1996) MR imaging-guided laser-induced thermotherapy. Minimally Invasive Therapy and Allied Technologies 5:243–248

Weigand H (1990) Drainage technique in interventional radiology. In: Seibel RMM, Grönemeyer DHW (eds) Interventional computed tomography. Blackwell, Oxford, pp 279–283

Yang R, et al. (1993) Liver cancer ablation with extracorporal high – intensity focused ultrasound. Eur Urol 23 (Suppl): 17–22

Subject Index

List of Contributors

Masao Ando, MD
Department of Gastroenterology
JR Sendai Hospital
1-3-1 Itsutsubashi Aoba-ku
Sendai 980
Japan

Susan M. Ascher, MD
Associate Professor of Radiology
Director, Body MRI
Department of Radiology
Georgetown University Medical Center
3800 Reservoir Road NW
Washington DC 20007-2197
USA

Yasumasa Baba, MD
Division of Internal Medicine
Cancer Institute Hospital
1-37-1 Kami-Ikebukuro Toshima-ku
Tokyo 170
Japan

Albert L. Baert, MD
Professor, Department of Radiology
University Hospital K.U.Leuven
Herestraat 49
3000 Leuven
Belgium

Clive I. Bartram, FRCP, FRCR
Intestinal Imaging 4V
St. Mark's Hospital
Northwick Park
Harrow HA1 3UJ
UK

Akimichi Chonan, MD
Department of Gastroenterology
JR Sendai Hospital
1-3-1 Itsutsubashi Aoba-ku
Sendai 980
Japan

Kulwinder S. Dua, MD
Assistant Professor of Medicine
Medical College of Wisconsin
Division of Gastroenterology & Hepatology
Director, GI Diagnostic Laboratory, VAMC
Froedtert Memorial Lutheran Hospital
9200 West Wisconsin Avenue
Milwaukee, WI 53226-3596
USA

Caryn S. Easterling, MS/CCC
Clinical Supervisor, Speech Pathology
Curative Rehabilitation Services
Froedtert Memorial Lutheran Hospital
9200 West Wisconsin Avenue
Milwaukee, WI 53226-3596
USA

Michael P. Federle, MD
Department of Radiology
University of Pittsburgh Medical Center
DeSota at O'Hara Street
Pittsburgh, PA 15213
USA

Gary G. Ghahremani, MD
Professor and Chairman
Department of Diagnostic Radiology
Evanston Hospital – McGaw Medical Center of
Northwestern University
2650 Ridge Avenue
Evanston, IL 60201
USA

Richard M. Gore, MD
Professor and Vice Chairman
Department of Diagnostic Radiology
Evanston Hospital – McGaw Medical Center of Northwestern
University
2650 Ridge Avenue
Evanston, IL 60201
USA

Dietrich H.W. Grönemeyer, MD
Professor and Chairman
Department of Radiology and Microtherapy
University of Witten/Herdecke
58448 Witten
Germany

Shunkichi Kai, MD
Division of Internal Medicine
Cancer Institute Hospital
1-37-1 Kami-Ikebukuro Toshima-ku
Tokyo 170
Japan

Sachio Kaku, MD
Division of Internal Medicine
Cancer Institute Hospital
1-37-1 Kami-Ikebukuro Toshima-ku
Tokyo 170
Japan

K. KOIZUMI, MD
Division of Internal Medicine
Cancer Institute Hospital
1-37-1 Kami-Ikebukuro Toshima-ku
Tokyo 170
Japan

JOHN C. LAPPAS, MD
Professor of Radiology
Indiana University School of Medicine
Wishard Memorial Hospital
1001 West Tenth Street
Indianapolis, IN 46202
USA

DEAN D.T. MAGLINTE, MD, FACR
Clinical Professor of Radiology
Indiana University School of Medicine
Methodist Hospital of Indiana
1701 North Senate Boulevard
Indianapolis, IN 46206
USA

ALEXANDER R. MARGULIS, MD
Professor of Radiology
University Advancement and Planning
University of California, San Francisco
3333 California Street
Laurel Heights, Suite 16
San Francisco, CA 94143-0292
USA

MASAKAZU MARUYAMA, MD
Division of Internal Medicine
Cancer Institute Hospital
1-37-1 Kami-Ikebukuro Toshima-ku
Tokyo 170
Japan

ANDREAS MELZER, MD
Department of Radiology and Microtherapy
University of Witten/Herdecke
58448 Witten
Germany

MORTON A. MEYERS, MD, FACR, FACG
Professsor of Radiology and Medicine
Department of Radiology
School of Medicine
Health Sciences Center
SUNY at Stony Brook
Stony Brook, NY 11794-8460
USA

F.H. MILLER, MD
Assistant Professor and Chief of Gastrointestinal Radiology
Nortwestern Memorial Hospital
Nortwestern University Medical School
710 N. Fairbanks
Ct, Chicago, IL 60611
USA

ROBERT E. MINDELZUN, MD, FACR
Associate Professor of Radiology
Department of Radiology
School of Medicine
Stanford University
300 Pasteur Drive, Room H 1307
Stanford, CA 94305-5105
USA

FUKUJI MOCHIZUKU, MD
Department of Gastroenterology
JR Sendai Hospital
1-3-1 Itsutsubashi Aoba-ku
Sendai 980
Japan

D.J. NOLAN, MD
Consultant Radiologist
John Radcliffe Hospital
Oxford, OX 3 9DU
UK

STEVEN H. OMINSKY, MD
Department of Radiology
University of California, San Francisco
505 Parnassus Avenue, Box 0628, A344a
San Francisco, CA 94143-0628
USA

JÜRGEN PLASSMANN, MD
Department of Radiology and Microtherapy
University Witten/Herdecke
58448 Witten
Germany

TATSUYA SAKAI, MD
Division of Internal Medicine
Cancer Institute Hospital
1-37-1 Kami-Ikebukuro Toshima-ku
Tokyo 170
Japan

ARMIN SCHMIDT, MD
Department of Radiology and Microtherapy
University of Witten/Herdecke
58448 Witten
Germany

RAINER SEIBEL, MD
Department of Radiology and Microtherapy
University of Witten/Herdecke
58448 Witten
Germany

CLAIRE SMITH, MD
Professor of Radiology
Section Director Gastrointestinal Radiology
Rush Presbyterian, St. Luke's Medical Center
1653 W. Congress Parkway
Chicago, IL 60612
USA

EDWARD T. STEWART, MD, FACR
Professor of Radiology
Medical College of Wisconsin
Chief, GI Radiology
Froedtert Memorial Lutheran Hospital
9200 West Wisconsin Avenue
Milwaukee, WI 53226-3596
USA

NORISHIGE TAKEMOTO, MD
Division of Internal Medicine
Cancer Institute Hospital
1-37-1 Kami-Ikebukuro Toshima-ku
Tokyo 170
JAPAN

Z.C. TRAILL, MD
Department of Radiology
John Radcliffe Hospital
Oxford, OX 3 9DU
UK

DIRK VANBECKEVOORT, MD
Department of Radiology
University Hospital K.U. Leuven
Herestraat 49
3000 Leuven
Belgium

LIEVEN VAN HOE, MD
Department of Radiology
University Hospital K.U. Leuven
Herestraat 49
3000 Leuven
Belgium

THOMAS VOGL, MD
Professor
Virchow Klinikum
Medizinische Fakultät der Humboldt-Universität zu Berlin
Augustenburger Platz 1
13353 Berlin
Germany

SUSAN D. WALL, MD
Professor, Department of Radiology
University of California, San Francisco
Chief, Angiography and Interventional Radiology
Assistant Chief of Radiology
Veterans Affair Medical Center
4150 Clement Street
San Francisco, CA 94121
USA

JUDY YEE, MD
Assistant Professor of Radiology
University of California, San Francisco
Chief, Computed Tomography
and Gastrointestinal Radiology
Department of Radiology
Veterans Affair Medical Center
4150 Clement Street
San Francisco, CA 94121
USA

MEDICAL RADIOLOGY
Diagnostic Imaging and Radiation Oncology

Titles in the series already published

MEDICAL RADIOLOGY
Diagnostic Imaging and Radiation Oncology

Titles in the series already published